Fifth Edition

MEDICAL TERMINOLOGY
with HUMAN ANATOMY

Jane Rice, RN, CMA-C

Former Medical Assisting Program Director
Coosa Valley Technical College
Rome, Georgia

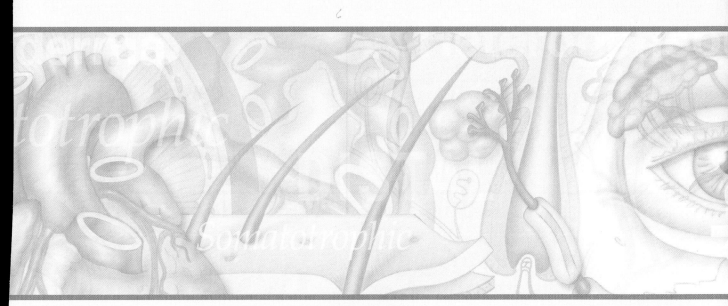

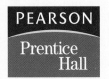

PEARSON

Prentice
Hall

Upper Saddle River, New Jersey 07458

Library of Congress Cataloging-in-Publication Data

Rice, Jane.
    Medical terminology with human anatomy / Jane Rice.—5th ed.
        p. ; cm.
        Includes index.
        ISBN 0-13-048706-6
  1. Medicine—Terminology 2. Human anatomy—Terminology.
    [DNLM: 1. Medicine—Terminology—English 2. Human anatomy—Terminology—English. W 15 R496m 2005] I. Title
        R123.R523 2005
        610'.1'4—dc22

                                        2004002207

Notice: Care has been taken to confirm the accuracy of the information presented in this book. The authors, editors, and the publisher, however, cannot accept any responsibility for errors or omissions or for the consequences for application of the information in this book and make no warranty, express or implied, with respect to its contents.

The authors and the publisher have exerted every effort to ensure that drug selections and dosages set forth in this text are in accord with current recommendations and practice at time of publication. However, in view of ongoing research, changes in government regulations, and the constant flow of information relating to drug therapy and drug reactions, the reader is urged to check the package inserts of all drugs for any change in indications of dosage and for added warnings and precautions. This is particularly important when the recommended agent is a new and/or infrequently employed drug.

Publisher: Julie Levin Alexander
Assistant to Publisher: Regina Bruno
Senior Acquisitions Editor: Mark Cohen
Associate Editor: Melissa Kerian
Editorial Assistant: Jaquay Felix
Media Editor: John J. Jordan
Development Editor: Elena Mauceri
Director of Production and Manufacturing: Bruce Johnson
Managing Production Editor: Patrick Walsh
Production Liaison: Danielle Newhouse
Production Editor: Jessica Balch, Pine Tree Composition
Manufacturing Manager: Ilene Sanford
Manufacturing Buyer: Pat Brown

Design Director: Cheryl Asherman
Design Coordinator: Christopher Weigand
Interior Designer: Donna Wickes
Cover Designer: Joseph DePinho
Electronic Art Creation: Barb Cousins, Hutchinson Studio
Director of Marketing: Karen Allman
Channel Marketing Manager: Rachele Strober
Manager of Media Production: Amy Peltier
New Media Project Manager: Stephen Hartner
New Media Production: Horus Development
Composition: Pine Tree Composition, Inc.
Printer/Binder: R.R. Donnelley & Sons
Cover Printer: Phoenix Color Corp.

Pearson Prentice Hall™ is a trademark of Pearson Education, Inc.
Pearson® is a registered trademark of Pearson plc.
Prentice Hall® is a registered trademark of Pearson Education, Inc.

Pearson Education Ltd., *London*
Pearson Education Australia Pty. Limited, *Sydney*
Pearson Education Singapore, Pte. Ltd.
Pearson Education North Asia Ltd., *Hong Kong*
Pearson Education Canada, Ltd., *Toronto*
Pearson Educación de Mexico, S.A. de C.V.
Pearson Education—Japan, *Tokyo*
Pearson Education Malaysia, Pte. Ltd.
Pearson Education, Upper Saddle River, New Jersey

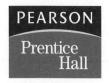

10 9 8 7 6 5 4 3 2
ISBN 0-13-048706-6

In special memory of my parents, Warren Galileo and Elizabeth Styles Justice.

CONTENTS IN BRIEF

DETAILED CONTENTS

CHAPTER 4   THE SKELETAL SYSTEM   89

CHAPTER 5   THE MUSCULAR SYSTEM   127

CHAPTER 9   THE RESPIRATORY SYSTEM   289

CHAPTER 10   THE URINARY SYSTEM   321

CHAPTER 14 · SPECIAL SENSES: THE EYE · 463

CHAPTER 15 · THE FEMALE REPRODUCTIVE SYSTEM · 493

PREFACE

The fifth edition of *Medical Terminology with Human Anatomy* continues its tradition of excellence with a new and refreshed approach to covering all aspects of medical terminology.

Over the years, this book has helped thousands gain a firm grasp of the challenging, yet exciting, new language of medicine. This revised edition embraces the philosophy that has made the book so successful, and incorporates fresh new features that will be sure to engage readers of all learning styles.

There are two driving goals of this text:

1. To teach students how to build medical terms by using word parts, and
2. To teach the basics of anatomy and physiology.

NEW TO THIS EDITION

- *Medical Terminology with Human Anatomy*'s unique **word building** approach has been further strengthened, and **pathology** has been highlighted in new and exciting ways: The terminology and vocabulary sections that were present in the 4th edition have been updated and rearranged into one feature entitled **Building Your Medical Vocabulary**, so that students can learn about terms that are built from word parts concurrently with vocabulary words. This more logical approach groups each important term by relevance in a single study list. The list is alphabetical, which is important because words with common prefixes follow each other, thereby creating a repetition that aids learning. Words listed in black are shown with their component word parts, while words in pink represent vocabulary terms that are not build from word parts. Pronunciations are provided for all terms.

- This section is followed by **Pathology Spotlights** and **Pathology Checkpoints**—new features that embody our initiative to fortify the pathology content in this edition. Pathology Spotlights highlight 4–6 conditions related to the chapter content, with artwork and links to media as well as the CD-ROM. Pathology Checkpoints provide the student with a concise list of the pathology terms they have encountered in the chapter. Students may check off those terms that they understand, and go back and review any that are not clear.

- Nearly 75 **new** illustrations and photos have been added to highlight important areas of the text.

- The Spanish component of the text has been removed and will now be included, along with French and German, as part of a **Terminology Translator** feature on the **free** CD-ROM (found at the back of the text). This Terminology Translator provides an innovative tool to translate medical words into Spanish, French, and German.

- A **free** CD-ROM is included with every text, and provides a wide variety of interactive activities such as labeling, word building, spelling, multiple-choice, true/false, fill-in-the-blank, and a variety of quiz games. An audio pronunciation glossary is included, along with a custom flashcard generator on the CD-ROM, that allows students to select glossary terms and print out flashcards for any or all terms for study. Finally, pathology concepts come alive with the presentation of one feature video per chapter that correlates to selected content in the Pathology Spotlight sections of the text.

MEDICAL WORD BUILDING TECHNIQUE—A TIME-PROVEN APPROACH

The fifth edition of *Medical Terminology with Human Anatomy* is still organized by body systems and specialty areas, with the component parts of medical words presented as they relate to each system of the body and specialty area. Prefixes and suffixes are repeated throughout the text, while word roots and combining forms are presented according to the system or specialty area to which they relate. Once the material in Chapters 1 and 2 has been mastered, the student should know approximately 87 prefixes, 68 roots/combining forms, and 77 suffixes. To build a medical vocabulary, all the student has to do is recall the word parts that they have learned and link them with the new component parts presented in each chapter. This word-building technique, while not complicated, is different from other terminology texts that have students learn prefixes, roots, combining forms and suffixes as separate entities generally not related to the terminology of a body system. It is much easier to learn component parts directly associated with a body system or specialty area and this is the key to the time-proven approach of *Medical Terminology with Human Anatomy*.

KEY FEATURES

- **Chapter Outlines and Objectives**   These appear at the beginning of each chapter. The outlines identify the organizational content of the chapter. The objectives state the learning concepts that should be obtained by the learner.

- **A Full Color Art Presentation**   Art provides visual references of diseases, disorders, and/or conditions. Color photographs are strategically placed throughout the text.

- **Full Color Illustrations**   Beautiful anatomy and physiology illustrations give the student access to essential diagrams of the human body. This is a perfect complement to the discussion of the anatomy and physiology overview in Chapters 2–16.

- **Anatomy and Physiology Overview** (Chapters 2–16)   Comprehensive coverage of the structure and function of the body with full-color art and tables.

- **Life Span Considerations**   Presents interesting facts about the human body as it relates to the child and the older adult.

- **Building Your Medical Vocabulary—NEW!**   This section provides the foundation for learning medical terminology. By connecting various word parts in an organized sequence, thousands of words can be built and learned. In this text the word list is alphabetized so one can see the variety of meanings created when common prefixes and suffixes are repeatedly applied to certain word roots and/or combining forms. Words shown in **pink** are additional words related to the content of the chapter that are not built from word parts. These words are included to enhance the student's vocabulary. Each medical word has a pronunciation guide directly under it.

- **Terminology Translator—NEW!** This feature, found on the **free** CD-ROM, provides an innovative tool to translate medical words into Spanish, French, and German. In our multicultural society, it is becoming more and more important that students be able to communicate in a variety of languages.

- **Pathology Spotlights—NEW!** This feature provides an in-depth focus on diseases and conditions related to the topic of the chapter. Presented are current findings in medicine along with interesting facts about the various medical conditions that are spotlighted.

- **Pathology Checkpoint—NEW!** This feature provides a concise list of pathology-related terms that the student has seen in the chapter. The student should review this checklist to make sure they are familiar with the meaning of each term before moving on to the next section.

- **Drug Highlights** Presents essential drug information that relates to the subject of the chapter.

- **Diagnostic and Laboratory Tests** Provides a snapshot of current tests and procedures that are used in the physical assessment and diagnosis of certain conditions/diseases.

- **Abbreviations** Selected abbreviations with their meanings are included in each chapter. These abbreviations are in current use and directly associated with the subject of the chapter.

- **Study and Review** Provides the student with the opportunity to write in or identify correct answers for questions that relate to each section of the chapter.

- **Case Studies** Highlight a disease, disorder, and/or condition that relates to the subject of the chapter. A synopsis of a patient's visit to a physician is presented with present history, signs and symptoms, diagnosis, treatment, and prevention. Case study questions follow the synopsis, and answers are provided at the back of the text.

COMPREHENSIVE TEACHING–LEARNING PACKAGE

To enhance the teaching and learning process, an attractive media-focused supplements package for both students and faculty has been developed for *Medical Terminology with Human Anatomy*. The various components of the package is also described on the inside front cover of this text. The full complement of supplemental teaching materials is available to all qualified instructors from your Prentice Hall sales representative.

Student CD-ROM

The Student CD-ROM is packaged **free** with every copy of the textbook. It includes:

- Custom flashcard generator
- Audio glossary with pronunciations of the key terms presented in the text
- Terminology Translator

- Pathology Spotlights videos, with additional content and weblinks related to diseases and conditions

- Medical terminology exercises, games, and activities that quiz students on spelling, word-building concepts, anatomy, and more.

Instructor's Resource Manual

This manual contains a wealth of material to help faculty plan and manage the medical terminology course. It includes lecture suggestions and outlines, learning objectives, a complete test bank, and more for each chapter. Through MediaLink boxes, the IRM also guides faculty on how to assign and use the text-specific Companion Website, www.prenhall.com/rice, and the CD-ROM that accompany the textbook.

Instructor's Resource CD-ROM

Packaged with the Instructor's Resource Manual, the Instructor's Resource CD-ROM provides many resources in an electronic format. First, the CD-ROM includes the complete test bank that allows instructors to generate customized exams and quizzes. Second, it includes a comprehensive turn-key lecture package in PowerPoint format. The lectures contain discussion points along with embedded color images from the textbook as well as bonus animations and videos to help infuse an extra spark into the classroom experience. Instructors may use this presentation system as it is provided, or they may opt to customize it for their specific needs.

Companion Website and Syllabus Manager®

Students and faculty will both benefit from the free Companion Website at www.prenhall.com/rice. This website serves as a text-specific, interactive online workbook to *Medical Terminology with Human Anatomy*. The Companion Website includes:

- A variety of quizzes in multiple-choice, true/false, labeling, fill-in-the-blank, and essay formats. Instant feedback and rationales are provided.

- An audio glossary in which key terms, as well as their component word parts, are pronounced.

- Instructors adopting this textbook for their courses have **free** access to an online Syllabus Manager with a whole host of features that facilitate the students' use of this Companion Website and allow faculty to post their syllabi online for their students. For more information or a demonstration of Syllabus Manager®, please contact your Prentice Hall sales representative or visit www.prenhall.com/demo, click on Companion Websites, and select Syllabus Manager Tour.

Finally, those instructors wishing to facilitate on-line courses will be able to access our premium on-line course management option, which is available in WebCT, Blackboard, or CourseCompass formats. For more information or a demonstration of our on-line course systems, please contact your Prentice Hall sales representative or visit www.prenhall.com/demo.

ACKNOWLEDGMENTS

It does not seem possible, but *Medical Terminology with Human Anatomy*, my "dream" text, is 18 years old. During these 18 years many people have stood by my side, guided me, and helped me in so many ways. A special thank you to all the Medical Assisting, Radiologic Technology, Respiratory Therapy, Nursing, and Business and Office Technology students that I have had the privilege to teach.

To Elena Mauceri, because of your hard work, your diligent persistence, and your knowledgeable foresight, the fifth edition is the best of the best. Words cannot express my gratitude, but a very special thank you goes to you, Julie Levin Alexander, Mark Cohen, and Melissa Kerian for believing in my book.

There are many other special people who help me in all that I do and I extend to each of you my warmest appreciation and gratitude:

Patrick Walsh   Mary Ellen Ruitenberg
Cheryl Asherman   John Jordan
Christopher Weigand   Nicole Benson
Danielle Newhouse   Amy Peltier
Jessica Balch   Barbara Cousins

I would like to express my appreciation to the following people for their valuable contributions to the supplements:

CD-ROM

Pamela A. Eugene, B.A.S., L.R.T. (R)
Delgado Community College
New Orleans, Louisiana

Patricia McLane, RHIA, MA
Henry Ford Community College
Dearborn, Michigan

Mindy A. Goldberg, PA-C, MPH
Pellissippi State Technical Community
   College
Knoxville, Tennessee

Instructor's Resource Manual

Pamela A. Eugene, B.A.S., L.R.T. (R)
Delgado Community College
New Orleans, Louisiana

I would also like to express my appreciation to the following reviewers for their valuable input:

Judy Anderson, MEd
Coastal Carolina Community College
Jacksonville, North Carolina

Ann Barton, CMT
Riverside, California

Cheryl Bernhardt, MS
John A. Logan College
Carterville, Illinois

Jamie L. Flower, MS, RN
University of Arkansas—Fort Smith
Fort Smith, Arkansas

Rebecca L. Gibson, MSTE, CMA, ASPT
The University of Akron
Akron, Ohio

Laura C. Gilliam, BS, MS
Western Piedmont Community College
Morganton, North Carolina

Marta Lopez, LM, CPM
Miami-Dade Community College
Miami, Florida

Ford Matipa, MD
The New York School for Medical
and Dental Assistants
Forest Hills, New York

Mildred Norris, BS, RHIT, CCS, CPC
Hillsborough Community College
Tampa, Florida

Martha L. Rew, MS, RD, LD
Texas Woman's University
Denton, Texas

Marie Rogers, RNC, MSN, MA
Kalamazoo Valley Community College
Kalamazoo, Michigan

Jonathan Allen Thorsen, BS, RRT
Long Beach City College
Long Beach, California

Linda G. Toomer, MSN, RN
J. Sargeant Reynolds Community
College
Richmond, Virginia

Renee Twibell, DNS, RN
Ball State University
Muncie, Indiana

Portions of the Pathology Spotlights sections are from Discovery Communications (www.discovery.com) and Adam, Inc. We thank them for their contributions.

ABOUT THE AUTHOR

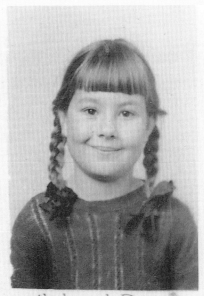

School Days
1946-47

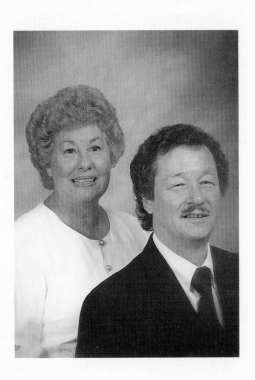

I would like for you to close your eyes and go back in time with me. To a time before most of you were born. The year is 1947 and I am a little girl with brown hair that is braided into pigtails. I am very shy and afraid—for, you see, I am in the second grade and I cannot read. Not one little word. The teacher discovered this and made me sit on a tall metal stool in front of the classroom with a dunce cap on my head. Still to this day, I get very nervous when I have to get up in front of a crowd of people.

My mother taught me to read because back then, there were no special classes for children with learning disabilities. I did not learn "phonetics," but memorized everything. I still have trouble pronouncing words, but I can tell you all you want to know about a medical word.

After the death of two brothers, my father, and the impending death of my mother, I prayed for something else to do, something that would help take away the pain and the hurt. In 1982 my prayers were answered with a most precious gift: *Medical Terminology with Human Anatomy*, which was first published in September of 1985.

I owe so much to God and my best friend and husband, Charles Larry Rice. Larry helps me in all that I do. We have a lovely adopted daughter, Melissa, who came into our lives 34 years ago when she was 3 weeks old. She has blessed us with a son-in-law, Doug, and five precious grandchildren: Zachary, Benjamin, Jacob, Mary Katherine, and Elizabeth Ann.

Although I am now retired, I had a wonderful teaching career. Because of my childhood experiences I became a caring and devoted teacher. As Medical Assisting Program Director at Coosa Valley Technical Institute, I developed the original curriculum for the medical assisting program and taught my favorite subject, medical terminology, for 29 years. I am grateful to my many wonderful students who taught me so much and touched my life with their unique qualities.

Jane Rice, RN, CMA-C

Build student SUCCESS with these time-proven tools!

Start with a strong foundation of anatomy and physiology . . .

BODY SYSTEMS ORGANIZATION

The chapter organization clearly places medical terms in context with their related body system.

BRIEF CONTENTS

THE CARDIOVASCULAR SYSTEM 7

Anatomy and Physiology Overview

Through the cardiovascular system, blood is circulated to all part the action of the heart. This process provides the body's cells nutritive elements and removes waste materials and carbon dio a muscular pump, is the central organ of the system, which also include and **capillaries.** The various organs and components of the cardiovas described in this chapter, along with some of their functions.

ANATOMY AND PHYSIOLOGY

Found at the beginning of each chapter, this section provides a comprehensive yet concise overview of the body system to which the terminology relates.

FULL COLOR ARTWORK

Our high-quality art provides a visual reference drawn with a consistent style throughout the book–fostering a comfortable experience for visual learners. **Nearly 75 new photos and illustrations** have been added to this edition!

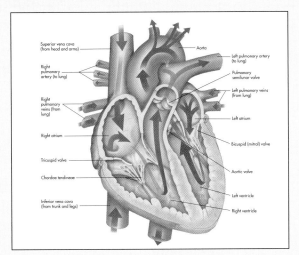

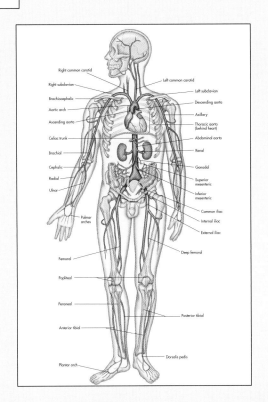

. . . and a unique word building approach

BUILDING YOUR MEDICAL VOCABULARY

This section provides the foundation for learning medical terminology. Medical words can be made up of four different types of word parts:

MEDICAL WORD	WORD PARTS (WHEN APPLICABLE)			DEFINITION
	Part	Type	Meaning	
coronary heart disease (CHD)				Coronary heart disease (CHD), also referred to as coronary artery disease (CAD), refers to the narrowing of the coronary arteries sufficient to prevent adequate blood supply to the myocardium. ✱ See Pathology Spotlight: Coronary Heart Disease.
cyanosis (sī-ă n-ō′ sĭs)	cyan -osis	R S	dark blue condition of	A dark blue condition of the skin and mucus membranes caused by oxygen deficiency
diastole (dī-ăs′ tō-lē)	diast -ole	R S	to expand small	The relaxation phase of the heart cycle during which the heart muscle relaxes and the heart chambers fill with blood
dysrhythmia (dĭs-rĭth′ mē-ă)	dys rhythm -ia	P R S	difficult rhythm condition	An abnormal, difficult, or bad rhythm. ✱ See Pathology Spotlight: Dysrythmias.
echocardiography (ĕk″ ō-kăr″ dē-ŏg′ rah-fē)	ech/o cardi/o -graphy	CF CF S	echo heart recording	A noninvasive ultrasound method for evaluating the heart for valvular or structural defects and coronary artery disease
electrocardiograph (ē-lĕk″ trō-kăr′ dĭ-ō-grăf)	electr/o cardi/o -graph	CF CF S	electricity heart to write, record	A device used for recording the electrical impulses of the heart muscle
electrocardio- phonograph (ē-lĕk″ trō-kăr″ dĭ-ō-fō′ nō-grăf)	electr/o cardi/o phon/o -graph	CF CF CF S	electricity heart sound to write, record	A device used to record heart sounds
embolism (ĕm′ bō-lĭzm)	embol -ism	R S	a throwing in condition of	A condition in which a blood clot obstructs a blood vessel; *a moving blood clot*
endarterectomy (ĕn″ dăr-tĕr-ĕk′ tō-mē)	end arter -ectomy	P R S	within artery excision	Surgical excision of the inner portion of an artery
endocarditis (ĕn″ dō-kăr-dī′ tĭs)	endo card -itis	P R S	within heart inflammation	Inflammation of the endocardium. See Figure 7–16.
endocardium (ĕn″ dō-kăr′ dē-ŭm)	endo card/i -um	P CF S	within heart tissue	The inner lining of the heart

BUILDING YOUR MEDICAL VOCABULARY

This feature is at the core of the book's approach. Students can learn about terms that are built from word parts **concurrently** with vocabulary words. This logical approach groups each important term by relevance in a single study list.

Highlights of this feature are:

- Medical word and pronunciation are included in the left column.

- Components word parts in the center colum each clearly identify a prefix (P), root (R), combining form (CF), or suffix (S).

- The list is alphabetical, which places similar words together, thereby creating repetition that aids learning.

- Words shown in pink represent vocabulary words that are not built from word parts.

- Words related to diseases and conditions are integrated into this section. Those that are covered in the Pathology Spotlights section are highlighted with an asterisk icon ✱

- A CD icon indicates a corresponding media element such as an animation or video.

Add focused pathology coverage . . .

Two new features embody our initiative to fortify the pathology content in this edition. With these features, readers can focus their learning on the most common diseases and disorders related to the body system.

PATHOLOGY SPOTLIGHTS

These features highlight 4-6 common conditions related to the chapter content, with illustrations and photos.

PATHOLOGY SPOTLIGHTS

Coronary Heart Disease (CHD)

Coronary heart disease (CHD) is the most common form of heart disease. It is also referred to as coronary artery disease (CAD) and refers to the narrowing of the coronary arteries that supply blood to the heart. It is a progressive disease that increases the risk of myocardial infarction (heart attack) and sudden death.

CHD usually results from the buildup of fatty material and plaque (**atherosclerosis**). See Figures 7–27, 7–28, and 7–29. As the coronary arteries narrow, the flow of blood to the heart can slow or stop. Blockage can occur in one or many coronary arteries.

Small blockages may not always affect the heart's performance. The person may not have symptoms until the heart needs more oxygen-rich blood than the arteries can supply. This commonly occurs during exercise or other activity. The pain that results is called stable angina.

If a blockage is large, angina pain can occur with little or no activity. This is known as unstable angina. In this case, the flow of blood to the heart is so limited that the person can-

✔ PATHOLOGY CHECKPOINT

Following is a concise list of the pathology-related terms that you've seen in the chapter. Review this checklist to make sure that you are familiar with the meaning of each term before moving on to the next section.

Conditions and Symptoms

- ❏ aneurysm
- ❏ anginal
- ❏ angiocarditis
- ❏ angioma
- ❏ angiostenosis
- ❏ aortomalacia
- ❏ arrhythmia
- ❏ arteriosclerosis
- ❏ arteritis
- ❏ atheroma
- ❏ atherosclerosis
- ❏ bradycardia
- ❏ bruit
- ❏ cardiomegaly
- ❏ cardiomyopathy
- ❏ cardiopathy
- ❏ carditis
- ❏ claudication
- ❏ constriction
- ❏ coronary heart disease (CHD)
- ❏ cyanosis
- ❏ dysrhythmia
- ❏ embolism
- ❏ endocarditis
- ❏ heart failure (HF)
- ❏ hemangiectasis
- ❏ hemangioma
- ❏ hypertension
- ❏ hypotension
- ❏ infarction
- ❏ ischemia
- ❏ mitral stenosis
- ❏ murmur
- ❏ myocardial infarction (MI)
- ❏ myocarditis
- ❏ occlusion
- ❏ palpitation
- ❏ pericarditis
- ❏ phlebitis
- ❏ Raynaud's phenomenon
- ❏ rheumatic heart disease
- ❏ shock
- ❏ spider veins
- ❏ tachycardia
- ❏ telangiectasis
- ❏ thrombophlebitis
- ❏ thrombosis
- ❏ vasoconstrictive
- ❏ vasospasm

Diagnosis and Treatment

- ❏ anastomosis
- ❏ angiocardiography
- ❏ artificial pacemaker
- ❏ auscultation
- ❏ cardiocentesis
- ❏ cardiometer
- ❏ cardiotonic
- ❏ catheterization
- ❏ coronary bypass
- ❏ echocardiography
- ❏ electrocardiograph
- ❏ electrocardiophonograph
- ❏ endarterectomy
- ❏ extracorporeal circulation
- ❏ heart-lung transplant
- ❏ heart transplant
- ❏ oximetry
- ❏ percutaneous transluminal coronary angioplasty
- ❏ phlebotomy
- ❏ sphygmomanometer
- ❏ stethoscope
- ❏ vasodilator
- ❏ venipuncture

PATHOLOGY CHECKPOINTS

Provide a concise list of the pathology terms covered in the chapter. Readers can "check off" those terms that they understand, and go back and review any that are not clear. Consistent headings are provided to separate Conditions/Symptoms from Diagnosis/Treatment.

. . . and practical applications

LIFESPAN
CONSIDERATIONS

■ THE CHILD

The development of the fetal heart is usually completed during the first 2 months of intrauterine life. It is
completely formed and functioning by 10 weeks. At 16
weeks fetal heart tones can be heard with a **fetoscope**.
Oxygenated blood is trasported by the umbilical

mal aging heart is able to pr
output. But in some older ad
harder to pump blood beca
arteries (arteriosclerosis) and
in the arterial walls (ather
gradually become stiff and lo
aorta and arteries supplying

LIFESPAN CONSIDERATIONS

Presents interesting facts about the human
body as it relates to the child and the older
adult. Learning about these populations
and their special needs prepares readers to
work in a variety of settings.

DRUG HIGHLIGHTS

Presents essential drug information that relates to the subject of
the chapter.

DRUG HIGHLIGHTS

Drugs that are generally used for cardiovascular diseases and disorders i
tions, antiarrhythmic agents, vasopressors, vasodilators, antihypertensi
demic, antiplatelet drugs, and thrombolgtic agents.

Digitalis Drugs   Strengthen the heart muscle, increase the force and velocity of
contraction, slow the heart rate, and decrease conduction velo

DIAGNOSTIC & LAB TESTS

TEST	DESCRIPTION
angiogram (ăn′ jē-ō-grăm)	A test used to determine the size and shape of arteries and veins of organs and tissu A radiopaque substance is injected into the blood vessel, and x-rays are taken.
angiography (ăn′′ jē-ŏg′ ră-fē)	The x-ray recording of a blood vessel after the injection of a radiopaque substance Used to determine the condition of the blood vessels, organ, or tissue being studie

DIAGNOSTIC AND LAB TESTS

Provides a snapshot of current tests
and procedures that are used in the
physical assessment and diagnosis of
certain diseases and conditions

ABBREVIATIONS

Selected abbreviations with their meanings
are included in each chapter. These abbreviations are in current use and are directly
associated with the subject of the chapter.

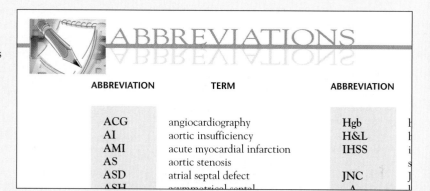

ABBREVIATIONS

ABBREVIATION	TERM	ABBREVIATION	
ACG	angiocardiography	Hgb	
AI	aortic insufficiency	H&L	
AMI	acute myocardial infarction	IHSS	
AS	aortic stenosis		
ASD	atrial septal defect	JNC	
ASH	asymmetrical septal		

And reinforce learning with integrated media . . .

MedMedia

Included at the beginning of each chapter, this feature prompts readers to use the various media components on the accompanying CD-ROM and Companion Website. MedMedia serves as a gateway to deeper understanding.

MedMedia
www.prenhall.com/rice

Additional interactive resources and activities for this chapter can be found on the Companion Website. For Terminology Translator, animations, video, audio glossary, and review, access the accompanying CD-ROM in this book.

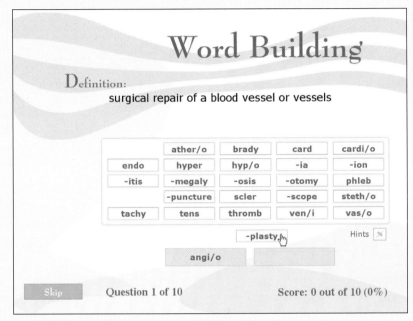

CD-ROM

A **free** CD-ROM is included with every text, and provides a wide variety of interactive games, animations, videos, an audio glossary, as well as exercises such as labeling, word building, spelling, and more. A custom flashcard generator is also available on the CD-ROM–allowing students to select glossary terms and printout flashcards for any or all terms for study.

TERMINOLOGY TRANSLATOR

This unique NEW feature, found on the FREE CD-ROM, provides an innovative tool to translate medical words into **Spanish, French,** and **German**. In our multicultural society, it is becoming more and more important that students be able to communicate in a variety of languages.

ON-LINE LEARNING

This text breaks new ground by offering on-line options in both a **free-access** Companion Website as well as **premium-level** distance learning courses. The Companion Website (www.prenhall.com/rice) serves as a text-specific, interactive online workbook and includes a variety of quizzes, links, and an audio glossary. Instructors adopting this textbook for their courses have **free** access to an online Syllabus Manager with a host of features that facilitate the students' use of this Companion Website and allow faculty to post their syllabi online for their students. Finally, those instructors wishing to facilitate on-line courses will be able to access our premium on-line course management option, which is available in **WebCT, Blackboard** or **CourseCompass** formats. For more information or a demonstration of our on-line course please visit www.prenhall.com/demo.

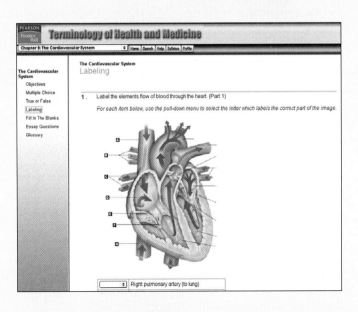

. . . and tools for student success

STUDY AND REVIEW

This section provides the student with the opportunity to review and reinforce their knowledge with activities that relate to each section of the chapter. Students can check their answers in the back of the book.

A variety of activities can be found in this section, including:

- Anatomy and physiology fill-in questions
- Word part definition fill-in exercises
- Identifying Medical Terms
- Spelling exercises
- Matching exercises
- Abbreviation exercises

STUDY AND REVIEW

Anatomy and Physiology

Write your answers to the following questions. Do not refer to the text.

1. The cardiovascular system includes:

   a. _____   b. _____

   c. _____   d. _____

2. Name the three layers of the heart.

   a. _____   b. _____

   c. _____

PREFIXES

Give the definitions of the following prefixes:

1. a- _____

3. brady- _____

5. end- _____

Identifying Medical Terms

In the spaces provided, write the medical terms for the following meanings:

1. _____ A tumor of a blood vessel

2. _____ The germ cell from which blood vessels develop

3. _____ Surgical repair of a blood vessel or vessels

Spelling

In the spaces provided, write the correct spelling of these misspelled terms:

1. astomosis _____   2. athrosclerosis _____

3. atriventrcular _____   4. endcarditis _____

5. extracoporal _____

Matching

Select the appropriate lettered meaning for each word listed below.

_____ 1. cholesterol

_____ 2. claudication

_____ 3. dysrhythmia

a. The two separate heart sounds that can be h with the use of a stethocope

b. Quivering of muscle fiber

c. Fat and protein molecules that are bound together

Abbreviations

Place the correct word, phrase, or abbreviation in the space provided.

1. acute myocardial infarction _____

2. atrioventricular _____

3. BP _____

CASE STUDIES

This feature highlights a disease, disorder, and/or condition that relates to the subject of the chapter. A patient scenario includes present history, signs and symptoms, diagnosis, treatment, and prevention. Case Study questions follow the synopsis, and answers are provided in the back of the text.

CASE STUDY — ANGINA PECTORIS

Read the following case study and then answer the questions that follow.

A 45-year-old male was seen by a cardiologist; the following is a synopsis of his visit.

Present History: The patient states that during a workout session he felt tightness in his chest, became short of breath, and felt very apprehensive. He states that this uncomfortable sensation went away after he stopped exercising.

Signs and Symptoms: Tightness in his chest, dyspnea, apprehension.

Diagnosis: Angina pectoris. Diagnosis was determined by a complete physical examination, an electrocardiogram, and blood enzyme studies.

Treatment: Nitroglycerin sublingual tablets 0.4 mg as needed for chest pain. The patient is instructed to seek medical attention without delay if the pain is not relieved by three tablets, taken one every 5 minutes over a 15-minute period.

Prevention: Teach the patient to avoid situations that precipitate angina attacks. Proper rest and diet, stress management, lifestyle changes, avoidance of alcohol and tobacco are recommended.

CASE STUDY QUESTIONS

1. Signs and symptoms of angina pectoris include tightness in the chest, _____ (shortness of breath), and apprehension.

2. The diagnosis of angina pectoris was determined by a complete physical examination, an _____ _____, and blood enzyme studies.

3. The medication regimen prescribed included _____ 0.4 mg as needed for chest pain.

4. If the patient follows the recommended medication regimen and it does not relieve the pain, he should _____.

FUNDAMENTAL WORD STRUCTURE

1

OBJECTIVES

On completion of this chapter, you will be able to:

- Describe the fundamental elements that are used to build medical words.
- List three guidelines that will assist you with the identification and spelling of medical words.
- Analyze, build, spell, and pronounce medical words.
- Describe selected medical and surgical specialties, giving the scope of practice and the physician's title.
- Identify and define selected abbreviations.
- Successfully complete the study and review section.

MedMedia
www.prenhall.com/rice

Additional interactive resources and activities for this chapter can be found on the Companion Website. For Terminology Translator, animations, videos, audio glossary, and review, access the accompanying CD-ROM in this book.

Understanding Fundamental Word Structure

Medical terminology is the study of terms that are used in the art and science of medicine. It is a specialized language with its origin arising from the Greek influence on medicine. Hippocrates was a Greek physician who lived from 460 to 377 BC and whose vital role in medicine is still recognized today. He is called "The Father of Medicine" and is credited with establishing early ethical standards for physicians. Because of advances in scientific computerized technology, many new terms are coined daily; however, most of these terms are composed of word parts that have their origins in ancient Greek or Latin. Because of this foreign origin, it is necessary to learn the English translation of terms when learning the fundamentals of word structure.

FUNDAMENTALS OF WORD STRUCTURE

The fundamental elements in medical terminology are the component parts used to build medical words. The terms for component parts used in this text are P = **prefix**, R = **root**, CF = **combining form**, and S = **suffix**. Each of these component parts is described in detail below.

Prefix

The term **prefix** means to fix before or to fix to the beginning of a word. A prefix may be a syllable or a group of syllables united with or placed at the beginning of a word to alter or modify the meaning of the word or to create a new word.

For example: the word **abnormal** means pertaining to away from the normal. Note its component parts below:

ab	P or prefix meaning	away from
norm	R or root meaning	rule
-al	S or suffix meaning	pertaining to

Word Root

A **root** is a word or word element from which other words are formed. It is the foundation of the word. The root conveys the central meaning of the word and forms the base to which prefixes and suffixes are attached for word modification.

For example: the word **autonomy** means condition of being self-governed. Note its component parts below:

auto	P or prefix meaning	self
nom	R or root meaning	law
-y	S or suffix meaning	condition

Combining Form

A **combining form** is a word root to which a vowel has been added to join the root to a second root or to a suffix. The vowel "o" is used more often than any other to make combining forms. Combining forms may be found at the beginning of a word or within the word.

For example: the word **chemotherapy** means treatment of disease by using chemical agents. Note the relation of its component parts:

chem/o	CF or combining form meaning	chemical
-therapy	S or suffix meaning	treatment

Suffix

The term **suffix** means to fasten on, beneath, or under. A suffix may be a syllable or group of syllables united with or placed at the end of a word to alter or modify the meaning of the word or to create a new word.

For example: the word **centigrade** means having 100 steps or degrees and the word *centimeter* means one-hundredth of a meter:

centi	P or prefix meaning	a hundred
-grade	S or suffix meaning	a step
centi	P or prefix meaning	a hundred
-meter	S or suffix meaning	measure

In many medical terminology textbooks, all the prefixes and suffixes used throughout the text are grouped into one or two beginning chapters. Under this arrangement, you are forced to refer repeatedly to these chapters to identify or define these word elements. In this book, however, prefixes and suffixes, along with their definitions, are integrated into each chapter throughout the text and provide a ready reference. Naturally, many of these same prefixes and suffixes will be used in each chapter. This repetition serves to reinforce the learning of the terms and their definitions and makes this text an improved learning tool.

Word roots and combining forms, together with their definitions, are included in each chapter according to the cell, tissue, organ, system, or element they describe. This arrangement makes it possible for you to form associations between medical terms and the various body systems. To reinforce this relation, this text provides you with a general anatomy and physiology overview for each of the body systems that it includes.

PRINCIPLES OF COMPONENT PARTS

As you learn definitions for prefixes, roots, combining forms, and suffixes, you will discover that some component parts have the same meanings as others. This occurs most often with words that relate to the organs of the body and the diseases that affect them. The existence of more than one component part for a particular meaning can be traced to differences in the Greek or Latin words from which they originated. Most of the terms for the body's organs originated from Latin words, whereas terms describing diseases that affect these organs have their origins in Greek.

For example:

- **Uterus**—a Latin word for one of the organs of the female reproductive system
- **Hyster**—a Greek R (root) for womb
- **Hysterectomy**—surgical excision of the womb from hyster R (root) meaning womb + -ectomy S (suffix) meaning surgical excision
- **Metr/i**—a Greek CF (combining form) for uterus
- **Myometrium**—muscular tissue of the uterus from my/o CF meaning muscle + metr/i CF meaning uterus + -um S meaning tissue

Many prefixes and suffixes have more than a single definition. When learning medical terminology, you must learn to use the definition that best describes the term. The following are commonly used prefixes that have more than a single definition:

PREFIXES WITH MORE THAN ONE MEANING

Prefix	Meanings	Prefix	Meanings
a-, an-	no, not, without, lack of, apart	extra-	outside, beyond
ad-	toward, near, to	hyper-	above, beyond, excessive
bi-	two, double	hypo-	below, under, deficient
de-	down, away from		
di-	two, double	in-	in, into, not
dia-	through, between	mega-	large, great
dif-, dis-	apart, free from, separate	meta-	beyond, over, between, change
dys-	bad, difficult, painful	para-	beside, alongside, abnormal
ec-, ecto-	out, outside, outer	poly-	many, much, excessive
		post-	after, behind
end-, endo-	within, inner	pre-	before, in front of
ep-, epi-	upon, over, above	pro-	before, in front of
eu-	good, normal	super-	above, beyond
ex-, exo-	out, away from	supra-	above, beyond

The following prefixes and their meanings have been selected to aid you in building a medical vocabulary:

PREFIXES THAT PERTAIN TO POSITION OR PLACEMENT

Prefix	Meanings	Prefix	Meanings
ab-	away from	hyper-	above, excessive
ad-	toward	hypo-	below, deficient
ana-	up	infra-	below
ante-	before	inter-	between
cata-	down	intra-	within
circum-, peri-	around	meso-	middle
endo-	within	para-	beside, alongside
epi-	upon, above	retro-	backward
ex-	out, away from	sub-	below, under
extra-	outside, beyond	supra-	above, beyond

PREFIXES THAT PERTAIN TO NUMBERS AND AMOUNTS

Prefix	Meanings	Prefix	Meanings
ambi-	both	poly-	many
bi-	two, double	primi-	first
centi-	a hundred	quadri-	four
deca-	ten	quint-	five
dipl-	double	semi-, hemi-	half
di(s)-	two, apart	tetra-	four
milli-	one-thousandth	tri-	three
multi-	many, much	uni-	one
nulli-	none		

PREFIXES THAT ARE DESCRIPTIVE AND ARE USED IN GENERAL

Prefix	Meanings	Prefix	Meanings
a, an-	without, lack of	hetero-	different
anti-, contra-	against	homeo-	similar, same
auto-	self	hydro-	water
brachy-	short	mega-	large, great
brady-	slow	micro-	small
cac-, mal-	bad	oligo-	scanty, little
dia-	through	pan-	all
dys-	bad, difficult	pseudo-	false
eu-	good, normal	sym-, syn-	together

The following are commonly used suffixes that have more than a single definition:

SUFFIXES WITH MORE THAN ONE DEFINITION

Suffix	Meanings	Suffix	Meanings
-ate	use, action	-plasm	a thing formed, plasma
-blast	immature cell, germ cell		
-ectasis	dilatation, dilation, distention	-plegia	stroke, paralysis
-gen	formation, produce	-ptosis	prolapse, drooping
-genesis	formation, produce	-rrhea	flow, discharge
-genic	formation, produce	-scopy	to view, examine
-gram	weight, mark, record	-spasm	tension, spasm
-ic	pertaining to, chemical	-stasis	control, stopping
-ive	nature of, quality of	-staxia	dripping, trickling
-lymph	serum, clear fluid	-trophy	nourishment, development
-lysis	destruction, to separate		
-megaly	enlargement, large	-y	process, condition, pertaining to
-penia	lack of, deficiency		

The following suffixes and their meanings have been selected to aid you in building a medical vocabulary:

SUFFIXES THAT PERTAIN TO PATHOLOGIC CONDITIONS

Suffix	Meanings	Suffix	Meanings
-algia, -dynia	pain	-pathy	disease
-cele	hernia, tumor, swelling	-penia	deficiency
-emesis	vomiting	-phobia	fear
-itis	inflammation	-plegia	paralysis, stroke
-lith	stone	-ptosis	drooping
-lysis	destruction, separation	-ptysis	spitting
-malacia	softening	-rrhage	bursting forth
-megaly	enlargement, large	-rrhagia	bursting forth
-oid	resemble	-rrhea	flow, discharge
-oma	tumor	-rrhexis	rupture
-osis	condition of		

SUFFIXES USED IN DIAGNOSTIC AND SURGICAL PROCEDURES

Suffix	Meanings	Suffix	Meanings
-centesis	surgical puncture	-pexy	surgical fixation
-desis	binding	-plasty	surgical repair
-ectomy	excision	-rrhaphy	suture
-gram	a weight, mark, record	-scope	instrument
-graph	to write, record	-scopy	to view
-graphy	recording	-stasis	control, stopping
-meter	instrument to measure, measure	-stomy	new opening
		-tome	instrument to cut
-opsy	to view	-tomy	incision

SUFFIXES THAT ARE USED IN GENERAL

Suffix	Meanings	Suffix	Meanings
-blast	immature cell, germ cell	-phraxis	to obstruct
-cyte	cell	-physis	growth
-ist	one who specializes, agent	-pnea	breathing
-logy	study of	-poiesis	formation
-phagia	to eat	-therapy	treatment
-plasia	formation, produce	-trophy	nourishment, development
-phasia	to speak		
-philia	attraction	-uria	urine

IDENTIFYING MEDICAL WORDS

When identifying medical words you will learn to distinguish between and select the appropriate component parts for the meaning of the word. It is most important that you learn the words as they are listed, for the slightest change in the arrangement of a medical word's component parts can change its meaning.

For example: the word **microscope** means an instrument used to view small objects. Compare the following:

micro + -scope   Proper placement of component parts (P + S) although the definitions translate micro = small and scope = instrument.

-scope + micro   Improper placement of component parts (S + P). Although incorrect, this arrangement of word parts seems to correspond to the term's definition.

SPELLING

Medical words of Greek origin are often difficult to spell because many of them begin with a silent letter or have a silent letter within the word. The following are examples of words that begin with silent letters:

Silent Beginning	Pronounced	Medical Term	Pronunciation Guide
cn	n	**c**nemial	(nē′mĭ-al)
gn	n	**g**nathic	(năth′ĭk)
kn	n	**k**nuckle	(nŭk′ĕl)
mn	n	**m**nemic	(nē′mĭk)
pn	n	**p**neumonia	(nū′-mō′nĭ-ă)
ps	s	**p**sychiatrist	(sī-kī′ă-trĭst)
pt	t	**p**tosis	(tō′sĭs)

The following are examples of medical terms that contain silent letters within the word:

Silent Letter	Medical Term	Pronunciation Guide
g	phle**gm**	(flĕm)
p	ble**ph**aro**pt**osis	(blĕf″ă-rō-tō′ sis)

Correct spelling is extremely important in medical terminology, as the addition or omission of a single letter may change the meaning of a word to something entirely different. The following examples illustrate this point:

Term/Letter Change	Meaning of Term	Term/Letter Change	Meaning of Term
abduct	To lead **away** from the middle	arte**ritis**	Inflammation of an **artery**
adduct	To lead **toward** the middle	arth**ritis**	Inflammation of a **joint**

Listed below are some of the prefixes and suffixes that often contribute to spelling errors:

PREFIXES AND SUFFIXES THAT ARE FREQUENTLY MISSPELLED

Prefix	Meaning	Suffix	Meaning
ante-	before	-poiesis	formation
anti-	against	-ptosis	prolapse, drooping
		-ptysis	spitting
ecto-	outside		
endo-	within	-rrhagia	bursting forth
		-rrhage	bursting forth
hyper-	above, beyond, excessive		
hypo-	below, under, deficient	-rrhaphy	suture
		-rrhea	flow
		-rrhexis	rupture
inter-	between	-scope	instrument
intra-	within	-scopy	to view
para-	beside, alongside, abnormal	-tome	instrument to cut
peri-	around	-tomy	incision
per-	through	-tripsy	crushing
pre-	before	-trophy	nourishment, development
pro-	before		
super-	above, beyond		
supra-	above, beyond		

The following guidelines are provided to help with the identification and spelling of medical words:

1. If the suffix begins with a vowel, drop the combining vowel from the combining form and add the suffix.

   For example: hemato + -oma becomes hematoma when we drop the "o" from hemato.

2. If the suffix begins with a consonant, keep the combining vowel and add the suffix to the combining form.

   For example, kilo + -gram becomes kilogram and we keep the "o" on the combining form kilo.

3. Keep the combining vowel between two or more roots in a term.

   For example: electro + cardio + -gram becomes electrocardiogram and we keep the combining vowels.

FORMING PLURAL ENDINGS

To change the following singular endings to plural endings, substitute the plural endings as illustrated:

Singular Ending	Plural Ending	Singular Ending	Plural Ending
a as in burs**a**	to **ae** as in burs**ae**	**ix** as in append**ix**	to **ices** as in append**ices**
ax as in thor**ax**	to **aces** as in thor**aces** or **es** as in thor**ax**es	**nx** as in phala**nx**	to **ges** as in phala**nges**
		on as in spermatozo**on**	to **a** as in spermatozo**a**
en as in foram**en**	to **ina** as in foram**ina**	**um** as in ov**um**	to **a** as in ov**a**
is as in cris**is**	to **es** as in cris**es**	**us** as in nucle**us**	to **i** as in nucle**i**
is as in ir**is**	to **ides** as in ir**ides**	**y** as in arter**y**	to **i** and add **es** as in arter**ies**
is as in femor**is**	to **a** as in femor**a**		

PRONUNCIATION

Pronunciation of medical words may seem difficult; however, it is very important to pronounce medical words with the same or very similar sounds to convey their correct meanings. As in spelling, one mispronounced syllable can change the meaning of a medical word. This text uses a phonetically spelled pronunciation guide adapted from *Taber's Cyclopedic Medical Dictionary*, and you should practice speaking each term aloud when working with the various lists of medical terms or vocabulary words. Accent marks are used to indicate stress on certain syllables. A single accent mark (′) is called a primary accent and is used with the syllable that has the strongest stress. A double accent (″) is called a secondary accent and is given to syllables that are stressed less than primary syllables.

Diacritics are marks placed over or under vowels to indicate the long or short sound of the vowel. In this text, the macron (‾) shows the long sound of the vowel, the breve (˘) shows the short sound of the vowel, and the schwa (ə) indicates the uncolored, central vowel sound of most unstressed syllables [for example: antiseptic (an″ ti-sep′ tik) or diathermy (di′ ə-thĕr″ mē)].

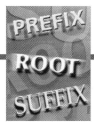

BUILDING YOUR MEDICAL VOCABULARY

This section provides the foundation for learning medical terminology. Medical words can be made up of four different types of word parts:

- Prefixes (P)
- Roots (R)
- Combining forms (CF)
- Suffixes (S)

By connecting various word parts in an organized sequence, thousands of words can be built and learned. In this text the word list is alphabetized so one can see the variety of meanings created when common prefixes and suffixes are repeatedly applied to certain word roots and/or combining forms. Words shown in pink are additional words related to the content of this chapter that are not built from word parts. These words are included to enhance your vocabulary.

MEDICAL WORD	WORD PARTS (WHEN APPLICABLE)			DEFINITION
	Part	Type	Meaning	
abate (ă-bāt′)				To lessen, decrease, or cease
abnormal (ăb-nōr′ măl)	ab norm -al	P R S	away from rule pertaining to	Pertaining to away from the normal or rule
abscess (ăb′ sĕs)				A localized collection of pus, which may occur in any part of the body
acute (ă-cūt′)				Sudden, sharp, severe; a disease that has a sudden onset, severe symptoms, and a short course
adhesion (ăd′ hē-zhŭn)	adhes -ion	R S	stuck to process	The process of being stuck together
afferent (ăf′ ĕr ĕnt)				Carrying impulses toward a center
ambulatory (ăm′ bŭ-lăh-tŏr″ ē)				The condition of being able to walk, not confined to bed
antidote (ăn′ tĭ-dōt)				A substance given to counteract poisons and their effects
antipyretic (ăn″ tĭ-pī-rĕt′ĭk)	anti pyret -ic	P R S	against fever pertaining to	Pertaining to an agent that works against fever

MEDICAL WORD	WORD PARTS (WHEN APPLICABLE)			DEFINITION
	Part	Type	Meaning	
antiseptic (ăn″ tĭ-sĕp′ tĭk)	anti sept -ic	P R S	against putrefaction pertaining to	Pertaining to an agent that works against sepsis; *putrefaction*
antitussive (ăn″ tĭ-tŭs′ ĭv)	anti tuss -ive	P R S	against cough nature of, quality of	Pertaining to an agent that works against coughing
apathy (ăp′ ă-thē)				A condition in which one lacks feelings and emotions and is indifferent
asepsis (ā-sĕp′ sĭs)	a -sepsis	P S	without decay	Without decay; *sterile,* free from all living microorganisms
autoclave (ŏ′ tō-klāv)	auto -clave	P S	self a key	An apparatus used to sterilize articles by steam under pressure
autonomy (ăw-tŏ′ nōm-ē) (ŏ-tŏ′ nōmē)	auto nom -y	P R S	self law condition	The condition of being self-governed; to function independently
axillary (ăks′ ĭ-lār-ē)	axill -ary	R S	armpit pertaining to	Pertaining to the armpit
biopsy (bĭ′ ŏp-sē)	bi(o) -opsy	R S	life to view	Surgical removal of a small piece of tissue for microscopic examination; used to determine a diagnosis of cancer or other disease processes in the body
cachexia (kă-kĕks′ ĭ-ă)	cac -hexia	P S	bad condition	A condition of ill health, malnutrition, and wasting
centigrade (sĕn′ tĭ-grād)	centi -grade	P S	a hundred a step	Having 100 steps or degrees, like the Celsius temperature scale; boiling point = 100°C and freezing point = 0°C
centimeter (sĕn′ tĭ-mē-tĕr)	centi -meter	P S	a hundred measure	Unit of measurement in the metric system; one hundredth of a meter
centrifuge (sĕn′ trĭ-fūj)	centr/i -fuge	CF S	center to flee	A device used in a laboratory to separate solids from liquids
chemotherapy (kē″ mō-thĕr′ ă-pē)	chem/o -therapy	CF S	chemical treatment	Treatment using chemical agents
chronic (krŏn ik)				Pertaining to time; a disease that continues over a long time, showing little change in symptoms or course

MEDICAL WORD	WORD PARTS (WHEN APPLICABLE)			DEFINITION
	Part	Type	Meaning	
diagnosis (dī″ ăg-nō′ sĭs)	dia -gnosis	P S	through knowledge	Determination of the cause and nature of a disease
diaphoresis (dī″ ă-fō-rē′ sĭs)	dia -phoresis	P S	through to carry	To carry through sweat glands; *profuse sweating*
disease (dĭ-zēz′)				Lack of ease; an abnormal condition of the body that presents a series of symptoms that sets it apart from normal or other abnormal body states
disinfectant (dĭs″ ĭn-fĕk′ tănt)	dis infect -ant	P R S	apart infection forming	A chemical substance that destroys bacteria
efferent (ĕf′ ĕr ĕnt)				Carrying impulses away from a center
empathy (ĕm′ pă-thē)				A state of projecting one's own personality into the personality of another to understand the feelings, emotions, and behavior of the person
epidemic (ĕp″ i-dĕm′ ik)	epi dem -ic	P R S	upon people pertaining to	Pertaining to among the people; the rapid, widespread occurrence of an infectious disease
etiology (ē″ tē-ŏl′ ō-jē)	eti/o -logy	CF S	cause study of	The study of the cause(s) of disease
excision (ĕk-si′ zhŭn)	ex cis -ion	P R S	out to cut process	The process of cutting out, surgical removal
febrile (fē′ brĭl)				Pertaining to fever
gram (grăm)				A unit of weight in the metric system; a cubic centimeter or a milliliter of water is equal to the weight of a gram
heterogeneous (hĕt″ ĕr-ō-jē′ nĭ-ŭs)	hetero gene -ous	P R S	different formation, produce pertaining to	Pertaining to a different formation
illness (ĭl′ nĭs)				A state of being sick

MEDICAL WORD	WORD PARTS (WHEN APPLICABLE)			DEFINITION
	Part	Type	Meaning	
incision (ĭn-sĭzh′ ŭn)	in cis -ion	P R S	in, into to cut process	The process of cutting into
kilogram (kĭl′ ō-grăm)	kil/o -gram	CF S	a thousand a weight	Unit of weight in the metric system; *1000 g*
liter (lē′ tĕr)				A unit of volume in the metric system; equal to 33.8 fl oz or 1.0567 qt
macroscopic (măk″ rō-skŏp ĭk)	macr/o scop -ic	CF R S	large to examine pertaining to	Pertaining to objects large enough to be examined by the naked eye
malaise (mă-lāz′)				A bad feeling; a condition of discomfort, uneasiness; often felt by a patient with a chronic disease
malformation (măl″ fōr-mā′ shŭn)	mal format -ion	P R S	bad a shaping process	The process of being badly shaped, deformed
malignant (mă-lĭg′ nănt)	malign -ant	R S	bad kind forming	A bad wandering; pertaining to the spreading process of cancer from one area of the body to another area
maximal (măks′ ĭ-măl)	maxim -al	R S	greatest pertaining to	Pertaining to the greatest possible quantity, number, or degree
microgram (mī′ krō-grăm)	micro -gram	P S	small a weight	A unit of weight in the metric system; *0.001 mg*
microorganism (mī″ krō-ōr′ găn-ĭzm)	micro organ -ism	P R S	small organ condition	Small living organisms that are not visible to the naked eye
microscope (mī′ krō-skōp)	micro -scope	P S	small instrument	An instrument used to view small objects
milligram (mĭl′ ĭ-grăm)	milli -gram	P S	one-thousandth a weight	A unit of weight in the metric system; *0.001 g*
milliliter (mĭl′ ĭ-lē″ tĕr)	milli -liter	P S	one-thousandth liter	A unit of volume in the metric system; *0.001 L*
minimal (mĭn″ ĭ-măl)	minim -al	R S	least pertaining to	Pertaining to the least possible quantity, number, or degree
multiform (mŭl′ tĭ-form)	multi -form	P S	many, much shape	Occurring in or having many shapes

MEDICAL WORD	WORD PARTS (WHEN APPLICABLE)			DEFINITION
	Part	**Type**	**Meaning**	
necrosis (nĕ-krō′ sis)	necr -osis	R S	death condition of	A condition of death of tissue
neopathy (nē-ŏp′ ă-thē)	neo -pathy	P S	new disease	A new disease
oncology (ŏng-kŏl′ ō-jē)	onc/o -logy	CF S	tumor study of	The study of tumors
pallor (păl′ or)				Paleness, a lack of color
palmar (păl′ mar)	palm -ar	R S	palm pertaining to	Pertaining to the palm of the hand
paracentesis (păr″ ă-sĕn-tē′ sĭs)	para -centesis	P S	beside surgical puncture	Surgical puncture of a body cavity for fluid removal
prognosis (prŏg-nō′ sĭs)	pro -gnosis	P S	before knowledge	A condition of foreknowledge; the prediction of the course of a disease and the recovery rate
prophylactic (prō-fi-lăk′ tĭk)	prophylact -ic	R S	guarding pertaining to	Pertaining to preventing or protecting against disease
pyrogenic (pī″ rō-jĕn′ ĭk)	pyr/o -genic	CF S	heat, fire formation, produce	Pertaining to the production of heat; *a fever*
radiology (rā″ dē-ŏl′ ō-jē)	radi/o -logy	CF S	ray study of	The study of radioactive substances
rapport (ră-pōr′)				A relationship of understanding between two individuals, especially between the patient and the physician
syndrome (sĭn′ drōm)	syn -drome	P S	together, with a course	A combination of signs and symptoms occurring together that characterize a specific disease
thermometer (thĕr-mŏm′ ĕ-tĕr)	therm/o -meter	CF S	hot, heat instrument to measure	An instrument used to measure degree of heat. See Figure 1–1.
topography (tō-pŏg′ răh-fē)	top/o -graphy	CF S	place recording	A recording of a special place of the body
triage (trē-ahzh′)	tri -age	P S	three related to	The sorting and classifying of injuries to determine priority of need and treatment

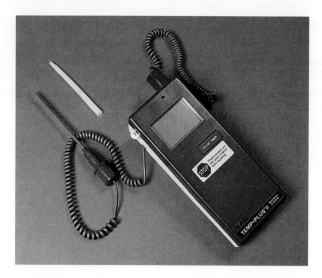

FIGURE 1–1

Electronic thermometer.

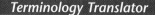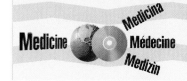
MEDICAL AND SURGICAL SPECIALTIES

Today, the practice of medicine involves many areas of specialization. The American Board of Medical Specialties (ABMS) was founded in 1933. This board established standards for and monitoring of specialty practice areas. A physician who has met standards beyond those of admission to licensure and has passed an examination in a specialty area becomes board certified. There are various medical professional organizations that establish their own standards and administer their own board certification examinations. Individuals successfully completing all requirements are called Fellows, such as Fellow of the American College of Surgeons (FACS) or Fellow of the American College of Physicians (FACP). Board certification may be required by a hospital for admission to the medical staff or for determination of a staff member's rank. See Table 1–1 for selected medical and surgical specialties and Table 1–2 for types of surgical specialties with description of practice.

TABLE 1–1 SELECTED MEDICAL AND SURGICAL SPECIALTIES

Specialty and Scope of Practice/Physician/Word Parts

Allergy and Immunology: The branch of medicine concerned with diseases of an allergic nature. The physician is an **allergist** or **immunologist** (*immun/o—immune; log—study of; -ist—one who specializes*).

Anesthesiology: The branch of medicine concerned with appropriate anesthesia for partial or complete loss of sensation. The physician is an **anesthesiologist** (*an—without; esthesi/o—feeling; log—study of; -ist—one who specializes*).

Cardiology: The branch of medicine concerned with diseases of the heart, arteries, veins, and capillaries. The physician is a **cardiologist** (*cardi/o—heart; log—study of; -ist—one who specializes*).

Dermatology: The branch of medicine concerned with diseases of the skin. The physician is a **dermatologist** (*dermat/o—skin; log—study of; -ist—one who specializes*).

Endocrinology: The branch of medicine concerned with diseases of the endocrine system. The physician is an **endocrinologist** (*endo—within; crin/o—to secrete; log—study of; -ist—one who specializes*).

Epidemiology: The branch of medicine concerned with epidemic diseases. The physician is an **epidemiologist** (*epi—upon; demi/o—people; log—study of; -ist—one who specializes*).

Family Practice: The branch of medicine concerned with the care of members of the family regardless of age and/or sex. The physician is a **Family Practitioner.**

Gastroenterology: The branch of medicine concerned with diseases of the stomach and intestines. The physician is a **gastroenterologist** (*gastr/o—stomach; enter/o—intestine; log—study of; -ist—one who specializes*).

Geriatrics: The branch of medicine concerned with aspects of aging. The physician is a **gerontologist** (*geront/o—old age; log—study of; -ist—one who specializes*).

Gynecology: The branch of medicine that studies diseases of the female reproductive system. The physician is a **gynecologist** (*gynec/o—female; log—study of; -ist—one who specializes*).

Hematology: The branch of medicine that studies diseases of the blood and blood-forming tissues. The physician is a **hematologist** (*hemat/o—blood; log—study of; -ist—one who specializes*).

Infectious Disease: The branch of medicine concerned with diseases caused by the growth of pathogenic microorganisms within the body.

Internal Medicine: The branch of medicine concerned with diseases of internal origin, those not usually treated surgically. The physician is an **internist** (*intern—within; -ist—one who specializes*).

Nephrology: The branch of medicine concerned with diseases of the kidney and urinary system. The physician is a **nephrologist** (*nephr/o—kidney; log—study of; -ist—one who specializes*).

Neurology: The branch of medicine concerned with diseases of the nervous system. The physician is a **neurologist** (*neur/o—nerve; log—study of; -ist—one who specializes*).

Obstetrics: The branch of medicine concerned with treating the female during pregnancy, childbirth, and the postpartum. The physician is an **obstetrician.** The Latin word element *obstetrix* means midwife.

Oncology: The branch of medicine that studies tumors. The physician is an **oncologist** (*onc/o—tumor; log—study of; -ist—one who specializes*).

Ophthalmology: The branch of medicine concerned with diseases of the eye. The physician is an **ophthalmologist** (*ophthalm/o—eye; log—study of; -ist—one who specializes*).

Orthopedic Surgery (*Orthopaedic*): The branch of medicine concerned with diseases and disorders involving locomotor structures of the body. The physician is an **orthopedist** (*orthopaedist*) (*orth/o—straight; ped—child; -ist—one who specializes*).

Otorhinolaryngology: The branch of medicine concerned with diseases of the ear, nose, and larynx. The physician is an **otorhinolaryngologist** (*ot/o—ear; rhin/o—nose; laryng/o—larynx; log—study of; -ist—one who specializes*).

TABLE 1–1 SELECTED MEDICAL AND SURGICAL SPECIALTIES (CONTINUED)

Specialty and Scope of Practice/Physician/Word Parts

Pathology: The branch of medicine that studies structural and functional changes in tissues and organs caused by disease. The physician is a **pathologist** (*path/o—disease; log—study of; -ist—one who specializes*).

Pediatrics: The branch of medicine concerned with diseases of children. The physician is a **pediatrician** (*ped—child; iatr—treatment; -ician—physician*).

Physical Medicine and Rehabilitation: The branch of medicine concerned with the treatment of disease by physical agents. The physician is a **physiatrist** (*phys—nature; iatr—treatment; -ist—one who specializes*).

Psychiatry: The branch of medicine concerned with diseases of the mind. The physician is a **psychiatrist** (*psych/o—mind; iatr—treatment; -ist—one who specializes*).

Pulmonary Disease: The branch of medicine concerned with diseases of the lungs. The physician is a **pulmonologist** (*pulmon/o—lung; log—study of; -ist—one who specializes*).

Radiology: The branch of medicine that studies radioactive substances and their relationship to prevention, diagnosis, and treatment of disease. The physician is a **radiologist** (*radi/o—ray; log—study of; -ist—one who specializes*).

Rheumatology: The branch of medicine concerned with rheumatic diseases. The physician is a **rheumatologist** (*rheumat/o—rheumatism; log—study of; -ist—one who specializes*).

Urology: The branch of medicine concerned with diseases of the urinary system. The physician is a **urologist** (*ur/o—urine; log—study of; -ist—one who specializes*).

TABLE 1–2 TYPES OF SURGICAL SPECIALTIES
WITH DESCRIPTION OF PRACTICE

Surgical Specialty	*Description of Practice*
Surgery is defined as the branch of medicine dealing with manual and operative procedures for correction of deformities and defects, repair of injuries, and diagnosis and cure of certain diseases.	
Cardiovascular	Surgical repair and correction of cardiovascular dysfunctions
Colon and Rectum	Surgical repair and correction of colon and rectal dysfunctions
Cosmetic, Reconstructive, Plastic	Surgical repair, reconstruction, revision, or change the texture, configuration, or relationship of contiguous structures of any part of the human body
General	Surgical repair and correction of various body parts and/or organs
Maxillofacial	Surgical treatment of diseases, injuries, and defects of the human mouth and dental structures
Neurologic	Surgical repair and correction of neurologic dysfunctions
Orthopedic (Orthopaedic)	Surgical prevention and repair of musculoskeletal dysfunctions
Thoracic	Surgical repair and correction of organs within the rib cage
Trauma	Surgical repair and correction of traumatic injuries
Vascular	Surgical repair and correction of vascular (vessels) dysfunctions

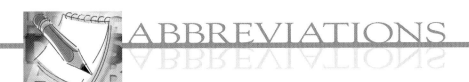

ABBREVIATIONS

ABBREVIATION	MEANING	ABBREVIATION	MEANING
AB	abnormal	FACP	Fellow of the American College of Physicians
ABMS	American Board of Medical Specialties	FACS	Fellow of the American College of Surgeons
ac	acute	FP	family practice
ax	axillary	g	gram
Bx	biopsy	GYN	gynecology
C	centigrade, Celsius	kg	kilogram
cm	centimeter	L	liter
CT	computerized tomography	mcg	microgram
CVD	cardiovascular disease	mg	milligram
D/C	discontinue	mL, ml	milliliter
derm	dermatology	OB	obstetrics
Dx	diagnosis	Peds	pediatrics
DRGs	diagnosis related groups	Psy	psychiatry, psychology
ENT	otorhinolaryngology		

STUDY AND REVIEW

Word Parts

1. In the spaces provided, write the definition of these prefixes, roots, combining forms, and suffixes. Do not refer to the listings of medical words. Leave blank those words you cannot define.

2. After completing as many as you can, refer back to the medical word listings to check your work. For each word missed or left blank, write the word and its definition several times on the margins of these pages or on a separate sheet of paper.

3. To maximize the learning process, it is to your advantage to do the following exercises as directed. To refer to the word building section before completing these exercises invalidates the learning process.

PREFIXES

Give the definitions of the following prefixes:

1. a- _____

2. ab- _____

3. anti- _____

4. auto- _____

5. cac- _____

6. centi- _____

7. dia- _____

8. hetero- _____

9. mal- _____

10. micro- _____

11. milli- _____

12. multi- _____

13. neo- _____

14. para- _____

15. pro- _____

16. syn- _____

17. tri- _____

18. dis- _____

19. epi- _____

20. ex- _____

21. in- _____

ROOTS AND COMBINING FORMS

Give the definitions of the following roots and combining forms:

1. adhes _____

2. axill _____

3. centr/i _____

4. chem/o _____

5. format _____

6. gene _____

7. kil/o _____

8. macr/o _____

9. necr _____

10. nom _____

11. norm _____

12. onc/o _____

13. organ _____

14. pyret _____

15. pyr/o _____

16. radi/o _____

17. scop _____

18. sept _____

19. therm/o _____

20. top/o _____

21. tuss _____

22. infect _____

23. dem _____

24. eti/o _____

25. cis _____

26. malign _____

27. maxim _____

28. minim _____

29. palm _____

30. prophylact _____

SUFFIXES

Give the definitions of the following suffixes:

1. -age _____

2. -al _____

3. -ary _____

4. -centesis _____

5. -clave _____

6. -drome _____

7. -form _____

8. -fuge _____

9. -genic _____

10. -gnosis _____

11. -grade _____

12. -gram _____

13. -graphy _____

14. -hexia _____

15. -ic _____

16. -ion _____

17. -ism _____

18. -ive _____

19. -liter _____

20. -logy _____

21. -meter _____

22. -osis _____

23. -ous _____

24. -pathy _____

25. -phoresis _____

26. -scope _____

27. -sepsis _____

28. -therapy _____

29. -ar _____

30. -y _____

Identifying Medical Terms

In the spaces provided, write the medical terms for the following meanings:

1. _____ Process of being stuck together

2. _____ Without decay

3. _____ Pertaining to the armpit

4. _____ Treatment using chemical agents

5. _____ Pertaining to a different formation

6. _____ Process of being badly shaped, deformed

7. _____ An instrument used to view small objects

8. _____ Occurring in or having many shapes

9. _____ A new disease

10. _____ The study of tumors

Spelling

In the spaces provided, write the correct spelling of these misspelled terms:

1. antseptic _____

2. autnomy _____

3. centmeter _____

4. diphoresis _____

5. miligram _____

6. necosis _____

7. parcentesis _____

8. radilogy _____

Matching

Select the appropriate lettered meaning for each word listed below.

_____ 1. abate

_____ 2. antipyretic

_____ 3. cachexia

_____ 4. diagnosis

_____ 5. disease

_____ 6. etiology

_____ 7. illness

_____ 8. prognosis

_____ 9. prophylactic

_____ 10. triage

a. Lack of ease
b. A state of being sick
c. Pertaining to protecting against disease
d. Pertaining to an agent that works against fever
e. The sorting and classifying of injuries to determine priority of need and treatment
f. To lessen, decrease, or cease
g. Determination of the cause and nature of a disease
h. A new disease
i. The prediction of the course of a disease and the recovery rate
j. A condition of ill health, malnutrition, and wasting
k. The study of the cause(s) of disease

Abbreviations

Place the correct word, phrase, or abbreviation in the space provided.

1. AB _____

2. ax _____

3. biopsy _____

4. CVD _____

5. DRGs _____

6. otorhinolaryngology _____

7. family practice _____

8. gram _____

9. GYN _____

10. Peds _____

**MedMedia
Wrap-Up**
www.prenhall.com/rice

Additional interactive resources and activities for this chapter can be found on the Companion Website. For animations, videos, audio glossary, and review, access the accompanying CD-ROM in this book.

Audio Glossary
Medical Terminology Exercises & Activities
Terminology Translator
Animations
Videos

Objectives
Medical Terminology Exercises & Activities
Audio Glossary
Drug Updates
Medical Terminology in the News

THE ORGANIZATION OF THE BODY

2

OBJECTIVES

On completion of this chapter, you will be able to:

- Define terms that describe the body and its structural units.
- List the systems of the body and give the organs in each system.
- Define terms that are used to describe direction, planes, and cavities of the body.
- Understand word analysis as it relates to Head-to-Toe Assessment.
- Analyze, build, spell, and pronounce medical words.
- Review Drug Highlights presented in this chapter.
- Identify and define selected abbreviations.
- Successfully complete the study and review section.

MedMedia
www.prenhall.com/rice

Additional interactive resources and activities for this chapter can be found on the Companion Website. For Terminology Translator, animations, videos, audio glossary, and review, access the accompanying CD-ROM in this book.

Anatomy and Physiology Overview

This chapter introduces you to terms describing the body and its structural units. To aid you, these terms have been grouped into two major sections: the first offers an overview of the units that make up the human body, and the second covers terms used to describe anatomical positions and locations. The human body is made up of atoms, molecules, organelles, cells, tissues, organs, and systems. See Figure 2–1. All of these parts normally function together in a unified and complex process. During **homeostasis** these processes allow the body to perform at its maximum potential.

THE HUMAN BODY: LEVELS OF ORGANIZATION

Atoms

An **atom** is the smallest chemical unit of matter. It consists of a nucleus that contains protons and neutrons and is surrounded by electrons. The **nucleus** is at the center of the atom and a **proton** is a positively charged particle, while a **neutron** is without an electrical charge. The **electron** is a negatively charged particle that revolves about the nucleus of an atom.

Chemical elements are made up of atoms. In chemistry, an **element** is a substance that cannot be separated into substances different from itself by ordinary chemical means. It is the basic component of which all matter is composed. There are at least 105 different chemical elements that have been identified.

Elements found in the human body include aluminum, carbon, calcium, chlorine, cobalt, copper, fluorine, hydrogen, iodine, iron, manganese, magnesium, nitrogen, oxygen, phosphorus, potassium, sodium, sulfur, and zinc. See Table 2–1.

TABLE 2–1 ELEMENTS FOUND IN THE HUMAN BODY

Symbol	Element	Atomic Weight
Al	aluminum	13
C	carbon	6
Ca	calcium	20
Cl	chlorine	17
Co	cobalt	27
Cu	copper	29
F	fluorine	9
H	hydrogen	1
I	iodine	53
Fe	iron	26
Mn	manganese	25
Mg	magnesium	12
N	nitrogen	7
O	oxygen	8
P	phosphorus	15
K	potassium	19
Na	sodium	11
S	sulfur	16
Zn	zinc	30

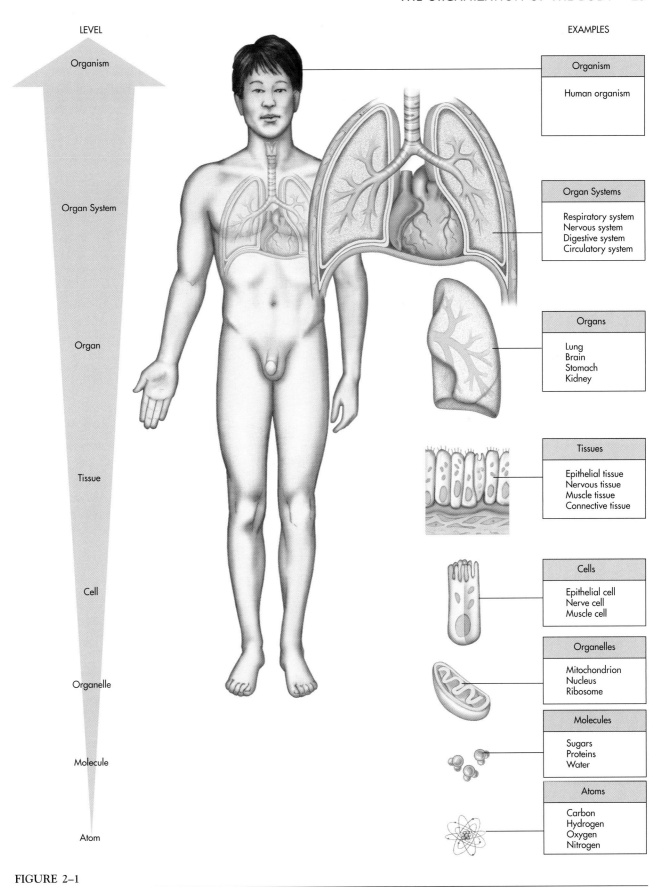

LEVEL

Organism

Organ System

Organ

Tissue

Cell

Organelle

Molecule

Atom

EXAMPLES

Organism

Human organism

Organ Systems

Respiratory system
Nervous system
Digestive system
Circulatory system

Organs

Lung
Brain
Stomach
Kidney

Tissues

Epithelial tissue
Nervous tissue
Muscle tissue
Connective tissue

Cells

Epithelial cell
Nerve cell
Muscle cell

Organelles

Mitochondrion
Nucleus
Ribosome

Molecules

Sugars
Proteins
Water

Atoms

Carbon
Hydrogen
Oxygen
Nitrogen

FIGURE 2–1

The human body: levels of organization.

Molecules

A **molecule** is a chemical combination of two or more atoms that form a specific chemical compound. In a water molecule (H_2O), oxygen forms polar covalent bonds with two hydrogen atoms. **Water** is a tasteless, clear, odorless liquid that makes up 65% of a male's body weight and 55% of a female's body weight. Water is the most important constituent of all body fluids, secretions, and excretions. It is an ideal transportation medium for inorganic and organic compounds.

Cells

The body consists of millions of cells working individually and with each other to sustain life. For the purposes of this book, **cells** are considered the basic building blocks for the various structures that together make up the human being. There are several types of cells, each specialized to perform specific functions. The size and shape of a cell are generally related directly to its function. See Figure 2–2. For example, cells forming the skin overlap each other to form a protective barrier, whereas nerve cells are usually elongated with branches connecting to other cells for the transmission of sensory impulses. Despite these differences, however, cells can generally be said to have a number of common components. The common parts of the cell are the **cell membrane** and the **protoplasm**.

THE CELL MEMBRANE

The outer covering of the cell is called the **cell membrane**. Cell membranes have the capability of allowing some substances to pass into and out of the cell while denying passage to other substances. This selectivity allows cells to receive nutrition and dispose of waste just as the human being eats food and disposes of waste.

PROTOPLASM

The substance within the cell membrane is called **protoplasm**. Protoplasm is composed of cytoplasm and karyoplasm. These substances and their functions are described below.

Karyoplasm.   Enclosed by its own membrane, **karyoplasm** is the substance of the cell's nucleus and contains the genetic matter necessary for cell reproduction as well as control over activity within the cell's cytoplasm.

Cytoplasm.   All protoplasm outside the nucleus is called **cytoplasm**. The cytoplasm provides storage and work areas for the cell. The work and storage elements of the cell, called organelles, are the endoplasmic reticulum, ribosomes, Golgi apparatus, mitochondria, lysosomes, and centrioles. See Figure 2–3 and Table 2–2.

Tissues

A **tissue** is a grouping of similar cells that together perform specialized functions. There are four basic types of tissue in the body: **epithelial**, **connective**, **muscle**, and **nerve**. Each of the four basic tissues has several subtypes named for their shape, appearance, arrangement, or function. The four basic types of tissue are described for you.

EPITHELIAL TISSUE

Epithelial tissue appears as sheet-like arrangements of cells, sometimes several layers thick, that form the outer layer of the skin, cover the surfaces of organs, line the walls of cavities, and form tubes, ducts, and portions of certain glands. The functions of epithelial tissues are protection, absorption, secretion, and excretion.

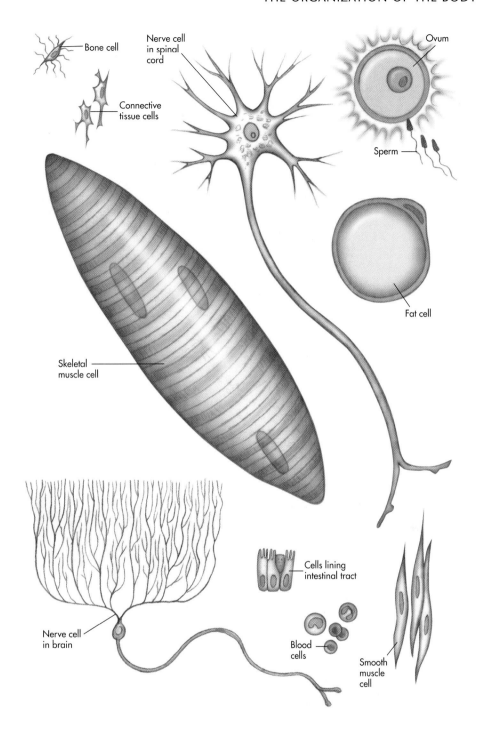

FIGURE 2–2

Cells may be described as the basic building blocks of the human body. They have many different shapes and vary in size and function. These examples show the range of forms and sizes with the dimensions they would have if magnified approximately 500 times.

CONNECTIVE TISSUE

The most widespread and abundant of the body tissues, **connective tissue** forms the supporting network for the organs of the body, sheaths the muscles, and connects muscles to bones and bones to joints. Bone is a dense form of connective tissue.

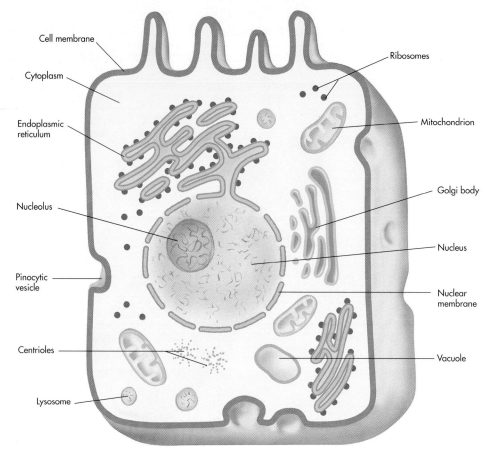

Cell membrane

Cytoplasm

Endoplasmic
reticulum

Nucleolus

Pinocytic
vesicle

Centrioles

Lysosome

Ribosomes

Mitochondrion

Golgi body

Nucleus

Nuclear
membrane

Vacuole

FIGURE 2–3

The major parts of a cell.

MUSCLE TISSUE

There are three types of **muscle tissue**: voluntary or striated, cardiac, and involuntary or smooth. Striated and smooth muscles are so described because of their appearance. Cardiac muscle is a specialized form of striated tissue under the control of the autonomic nervous system. Involuntary or smooth muscles are also controlled by this system. The striated or voluntary muscles are controlled by the person's will.

NERVE TISSUE

Nerve tissue consists of nerve cells (neurons) and interstitial tissue. It has the properties of excitability and conductivity, and functions to control and coordinate the activities of the body.

Organs

Tissues serving a common purpose or function make up structures called **organs**. Organs are specialized components of the body such as the brain, skin, or heart.

Systems

A group of organs functioning together for a common purpose is called a **system.** The various body systems function in support of the body as a whole. Listed in Figure 2–4 are the organ systems of the body.

TABLE 2–2 MAJOR CELL STRUCTURES AND PRIMARY FUNCTIONS

Cell Structures	Primary Functions
Cell membrane	Protects the cell; provides for communication via receptor proteins; surface proteins serve as positive identification tags; allow some substances to pass into and out of the cell while denying passage to other substances; this selectivity allows cells to receive nutrition and dispose of waste
Protoplasm	Composed of cytoplasm and karyoplasm
Karyoplasm	Substance of the cell's nucleus; contains the genetic matter necessary for cell reproduction as well as control over activity within the cell's cytoplasm
Cytoplasm	All protoplasm outside the nucleus. The cytoplasm provides storage and work areas for the cell:
Ribosomes	Make enzymes and other proteins; nicknamed "protein factories"
Endoplasmic reticulum (ER)	Carries proteins and other substances through the cytoplasm
Golgi apparatus	Chemically processes the molecules from the endoplasmic reticulum, then packages them into vesicles; nicknamed "chemical processing and packaging center"
Mitochondria	Complex, energy-releasing chemical reactions occur continuously; nicknamed "power plants"
Lysosomes	Contain enzymes that can digest food compounds; nicknamed "digestive bags"
Centrioles	Play an important role in cell reproduction
Cilia	Hair-like processes that project from epithelial cells; help propel mucus, dust particles, and other foreign substances from the respiratory tract
Flagellum	"Tail" of the sperm that makes it possible for the sperm to "swim" or move toward the ovum
Nucleus	Controls every organelle (little organ) in the cytoplasm; contains the genetic matter necessary for cell reproduction as well as control over activity within the cell's cytoplasm

ANATOMICAL LOCATIONS AND POSITIONS

Four primary reference systems have been adopted to provide uniformity to the anatomical description of the body. These reference systems are **direction, planes, cavities,** and **structural unit.** The standard anatomical position for the body is erect, head facing forward, arms by the sides with palms to the front. Left and right are from the subject's point of view, not the examiner's.

Direction

The following terms are used to describe direction:

- **Superior.** Above, in an upward direction
- **Anterior.** In front of or before
- **Posterior.** Toward the back
- **Cephalad.** Toward the head
- **Medial.** Nearest the midline
- **Lateral.** To the side

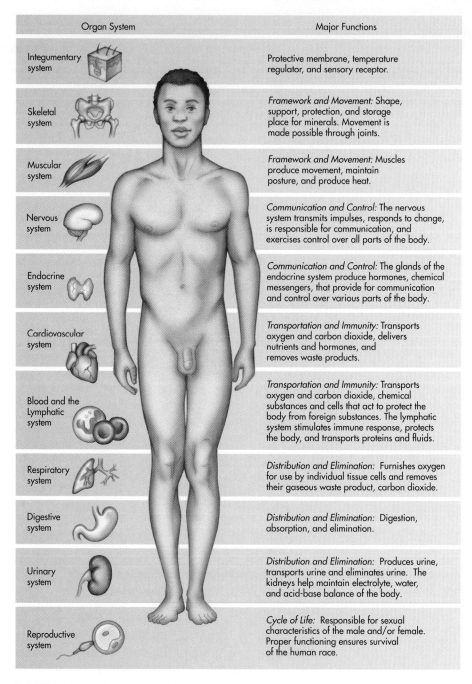

Organ System		Major Functions
Integumentary system		Protective membrane, temperature regulator, and sensory receptor.
Skeletal system		*Framework and Movement:* Shape, support, protection, and storage place for minerals. Movement is made possible through joints.
Muscular system		*Framework and Movement:* Muscles produce movement, maintain posture, and produce heat.
Nervous system		*Communication and Control:* The nervous system transmits impulses, responds to change, is responsible for communication, and exercises control over all parts of the body.
Endocrine system		*Communication and Control:* The glands of the endocrine system produce hormones, chemical messengers, that provide for communication and control over various parts of the body.
Cardiovascular system		*Transportation and Immunity:* Transports oxygen and carbon dioxide, delivers nutrients and hormones, and removes waste products.
Blood and the Lymphatic system		*Transportation and Immunity:* Transports oxygen and carbon dioxide, chemical substances and cells that act to protect the body from foreign substances. The lymphatic system stimulates immune response, protects the body, and transports proteins and fluids.
Respiratory system		*Distribution and Elimination:* Furnishes oxygen for use by individual tissue cells and removes their gaseous waste product, carbon dioxide.
Digestive system		*Distribution and Elimination:* Digestion, absorption, and elimination.
Urinary system		*Distribution and Elimination:* Produces urine, transports urine and eliminates urine. The kidneys help maintain electrolyte, water, and acid-base balance of the body.
Reproductive system		*Cycle of Life:* Responsible for sexual characteristics of the male and/or female. Proper functioning ensures survival of the human race.

FIGURE 2–4

Organ systems of the body with major functions.

- **Proximal.** Nearest the point of attachment
- **Distal.** Away from the point of attachment
- **Ventral.** The same as anterior, the front side
- **Dorsal.** The same as posterior, the back side

Planes

The terms defined below are used to describe the imaginary planes that are depicted in Figure 2–5 as passing through the body and dividing it into various sections.

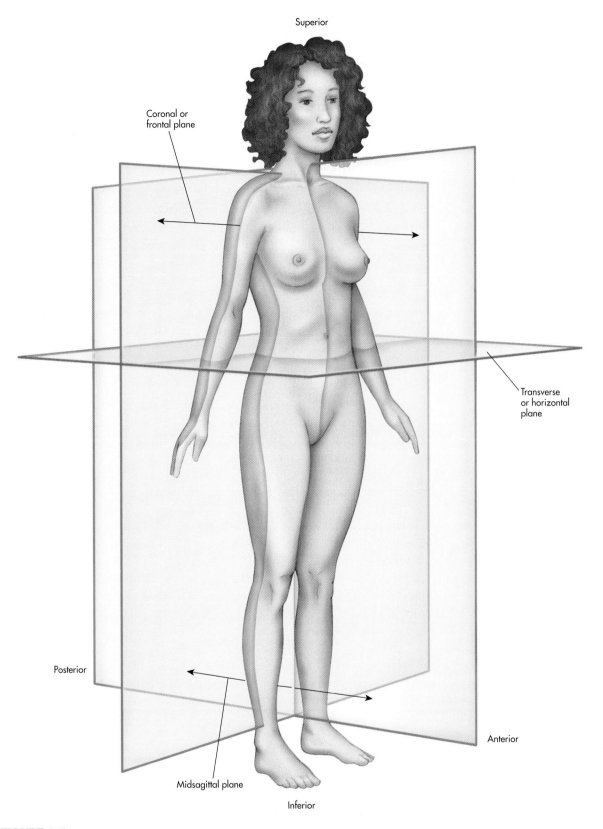

FIGURE 2–5

Planes of the body: coronal or frontal, transverse, and midsagittal.

MIDSAGITTAL PLANE

The **midsagittal plane** vertically divides the body as it passes through the midline to form a **right** and **left half**.

TRANSVERSE OR HORIZONTAL PLANE

A **transverse** or **horizontal plane** is any plane that divides the body into **superior** and **inferior** portions.

CORONAL OR FRONTAL PLANE

A **coronal** or **frontal plane** is any plane that divides the body at right angles to the midsagittal plane. The coronal plane divides the body into **anterior** (ventral) and **posterior** (dorsal) portions.

Cavities

A **cavity** is a hollow space containing body organs. Body cavities are classified into two groups according to their location. On the front are the **ventral** or **anterior cavities** and on the back are the **dorsal** or **posterior cavities**. The various cavities found in the human body are depicted in Figure 2–6.

THE VENTRAL CAVITY

The **ventral cavity** is the hollow portion of the human torso extending from the neck to the pelvis and containing the heart and the organs of respiration, digestion, reproduction, and elimination. The ventral cavity can be subdivided into three distinct areas: thoracic, abdominal, and pelvic.

The Thoracic Cavity.   The **thoracic cavity** is the area of the chest containing the heart and the lungs. Within this cavity, the space containing the **heart** is called the **pericardial** cavity and the spaces surrounding each **lung** are known as the **pleural** cavities. Other organs located in the thoracic cavity are the esophagus, trachea, thymus, and certain large blood and lymph vessels.

The Abdominal Cavity.   The **abdominal cavity** is the space below the diaphragm, commonly referred to as the belly. It contains the kidneys, stomach, intestines, and other organs of digestion.

The Pelvic Cavity.   The **pelvic cavity** is the space formed by the bones of the pelvic area and contains the organs of reproduction and elimination.

THE DORSAL CAVITY

Containing the structures of the nervous system, the **dorsal cavity** is subdivided into the cranial cavity and the spinal cavity.

The Cranial Cavity.   The **cranial cavity** is the space in the skull containing the brain.

The Spinal Cavity.   The **spinal cavity** is the space within the bony spinal column that contains the spinal cord and spinal fluid.

THE ABDOMINOPELVIC CAVITY

The **abdominopelvic cavity** is the combination of the abdominal and pelvic cavities. It is divided into nine regions.

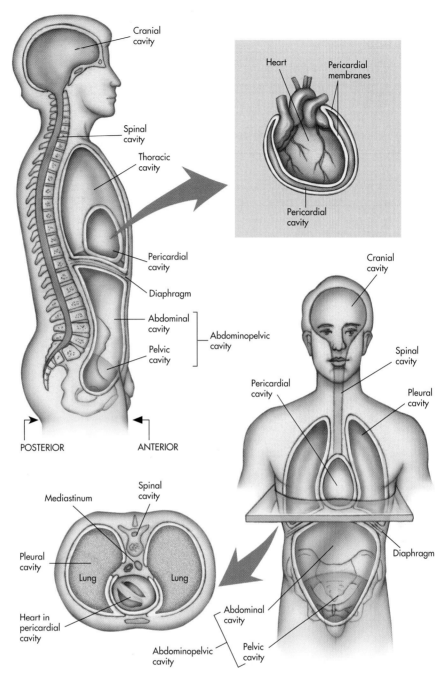

FIGURE 2–6

Body cavities.

Nine Regions of the Abdominopelvic Cavity

As a ready reference for locating visceral organs, anatomists divided the abdominopelvic cavity into nine regions. A tic-tac-toe pattern drawn across the abdominopelvic cavity (Fig. 2–7A) delineates these regions:

- **Right hypochondriac**—upper right region at the level of the ninth rib cartilage
- **Left hypochondriac**—upper left region at the level of the ninth rib cartilage
- **Epigastric**—region over the stomach
- **Right lumbar**—right middle lateral region

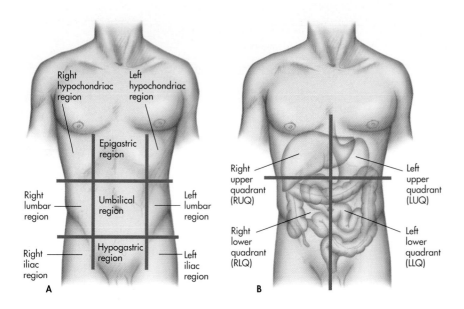

FIGURE 2–7

(A) The nine regions of the abdominopelvic cavity. **(B)** The four regions of the abdomen that are referred to as quadrants.

- **Left lumbar**—left middle lateral region
- **Umbilical**—in the center, between the right and left lumbar region; at the navel
- **Right iliac (inguinal)**—right lower lateral region
- **Left iliac (inguinal)**—left lower lateral region
- **Hypogastric**—lower middle region below the navel

Abdomen Divided into Quadrants

The **abdomen** is divided into four corresponding regions that are used for descriptive and diagnostic purposes. By using these regions one may describe the exact location of pain, a skin lesion, surgical incision, and/or abdominal tumor. The four **quadrants** are (Fig. 2–7B):

- **Right upper (RUQ)**
- **Left upper (LUQ)**
- **Right lower (RLQ)**
- **Left lower (LLQ)**

HEAD-TO-TOE ASSESSMENT

The terminology associated with head-to-toe assessment can be useful when studying the organization of the body. The following body areas, along with their word parts and/or related terminology, are provided for your study.

Body Area	Word Part/Terminology
abdomen (belly)	abdomin/o (ăb-dō′-mĭ-nō)
ankle	ankyl/o (ăn-kĭ′-lō)
arm	brach/i (bră′-chĭ)
back	poster/i; posterior (pŏs-tě-rĭ̌; pŏs-tě-rĭ-ōr)
bones	oste/o (ŏs-tē-ō)
breast	mast; mamm/o; mammary (măst; măm′-ō; măm′-ă-rē)
cheek	bucc/o; buccal (bŭk′-kō; bŭk′-ăl)
chest	thorac/o; thorax (thō-ră′-kō; thō′ raks)
ear	ot/o; otic (ō-tō; ō′ tĭk)
elbow	cubital (cū-bĭ-tăl′)
eye	ophthalm/o; ocul/o; opt/o (ŏp-thăl′-mō; ō-kū-lō; ōp-tō)
finger	dactyl/o; digit; phalanx (dăk′-tĭ-lō; dĭj′-ĭt; făl′-ănks)
foot	illus (il-lus)
gums	gingiv; gingiva (gĭn-gĭv-; gĭn-gĭv-vă)
hand	manus (mă-nūs)
head	cephal/o; cephalad (sě-fă-lō; sěf′ ă-lăd)
heart	cardi/o; cardiac (kăr-dĭ-ō; kăr′ dē-ăk)
hip	coxa (kŏk′-să)
leg	crural; femoral (crū-răl; fě-mō-răl)
liver	hepat/o; hepatic (hě-pă-tō; hě-păt ĭk)
lungs	pulm/o; pulmonary (pūl-mō; pŭl′ mō-ně-rē)
mouth	or/o; oral (ō-rō; or′ ăl)
muscles	muscul/o (mūs-cū-lō)
navel	umbilic; umbilicus (ŭm-bĭ-lĭ′-k; ŭm-bĭ-lĭ′-kŭs)
neck	cervic/o; cervical (sěr′-vĭ-cō; sěr′ vĭ-kă)
nerves	neur/o; neural (nū′-rō; nū′ răl)
nose	rhin/o; nas/o; nasal (rĭ′-nō; nă′-sō; nā′ zl)
ribs	cost/o; costal (cōs′-tō; cos′ tăl)
side	lateral (lă-tě-răl′)
skin	derm/a; dermad (děr′-mă; děr-măd)

Body Area	Word Part/Terminology
skull	crani/o; cranial (kră′-nĭ-ō; kră′-nē-ăl)
stomach	gastr/o; gastric (găs′-trō; găs′ trĭk)
teeth	dent; dental (dĕnt′; dĕn-tăl)
temples	tempora; temporal (tĕm-pō′-ră; tĕm′ pōr-ăl)
thigh	femoral; crural (fĕ-mō-răl; crŭ-răl)
throat	pharyng/o; pharyngeal (fă-rĭn′-hō; făr-ĭn′ jē-ăl)
thumb	pollex (pōl′-lĕx)
tongue	lingu/o; gloss/o; lingual; glossal (lĭn-gū-ō; glōs-sō; ling′ gwal; glŏs-săl)
wrist	carp/o; carpal (căr′-pō; căr-păl)

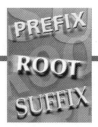

BUILDING YOUR MEDICAL VOCABULARY

This section provides the foundation for learning medical terminology. Medical words can be made up of four different types of word parts:

- Prefixes (P)
- Roots (R)
- Combining forms (CF)
- Suffixes (S)

By connecting various word parts in an organized sequence, thousands of words can be built and learned. In this text the word list is alphabetized so one can see the variety of meanings created when common prefixes and suffixes are repeatedly applied to certain word roots and/or combining forms. Words shown in pink are additional words related to the content of this chapter that are not built from word parts. These words are included to enhance your vocabulary.

MEDICAL WORD	WORD PARTS (WHEN APPLICABLE)			DEFINITION
	Part	**Type**	**Meaning**	
adipose (ăd″ ĭ-pōs)	adip	R	fat	Fatty tissue throughout the body
	-ose	S	like	
ambilateral (ăm″ bĭ-lăt′ ĕr-ăl)	ambi	P	both	Pertaining to both sides
	later	R	side	
	-al	S	pertaining to	

MEDICAL WORD	WORD PARTS (WHEN APPLICABLE)			DEFINITION
	Part	Type	Meaning	
anatomy (ăn-ăt′ ō-mē)	ana -tomy	P S	up incision	Literally means to cut up; the study of the structure of an organism such as humans
android (ăn′ droyd)	andr -oid	R S	man resemble	To resemble man
anterior (an-tĕr′ ē-ōr)	anter/i -or	CF S	toward the front a doer	In front of, before
apex (ā′ pĕks)				The pointed end of a cone-shaped structure
base (bās)				The lower part or foundation of a structure
bilateral (bī-lăt′ ĕr-ăl)	bi later -al	P R S	two side pertaining to	Pertaining to two sides
biology (bi-ŏl′ ō-jē)	bi/o -logy	CF S	life study of	The study of life
caudal (kŏd′ ăl)	caud -al	R S	tail pertaining to	Pertaining to the tail
center (sĕn′ tĕr)				The midpoint of a body or activity
cephalad (sĕf′ ă-lăd)	cephal -ad	R S	head pertaining to	Toward the head
chromosome (krō-mō-sōm)	chromo -some	P S	color body	Microscopic bodies that carry the genes that determine hereditary characteristics
cilia (sĭl′ ē-ă)				Hair-like processes that project from epithelial cells; they help propel mucus, dust particles, and other foreign substances from the respiratory tract
cytology (sī-tŏl′ ō-jē)	cyt/o -logy	CF S	cell study of	The study of cells
deep (dēp)				Far down from the surface
dehydrate (dē-hī′ drāt)	de hydr -ate	P R S	down, away from water use, action	To remove water away from the body

MEDICAL WORD	WORD PARTS (WHEN APPLICABLE)			DEFINITION
	Part	Type	Meaning	
diffusion (di-fū′ zhŭn)	dif fus -ion	P R S	apart to pour process	A process in which parts of a substance move from areas of high concentration to areas of lower concentration
distal (dĭs′ tăl)	dist -al	R S	away from the point of origin pertaining to	Farthest from the center or point of origin
dorsal (dōr′ săl)	dors -al	R S	backward pertaining to	Pertaining to the back side of the body
ectogenous (ĕk-tŏj′ ĕ-nŭs)	ecto gen -ous	P R S	outside formation, produce pertaining to	Pertaining to formation outside the organism or body
ectomorph (ĕk′ tō-morf)	ecto -morph	P S	outside form, shape	A slender physical body form
endomorph (ĕn″ dō-morf)	endo -morph	P S	within form, shape	A round physical body form
filtration (fĭl-trā′ shŭn)	filtrat -ion	R S	to strain through process	The process of filtering or straining particles from a solution
gene (jēn)				The hereditary unit that transmits and determines one's characteristics or hereditary traits
histology (hĭs-tŏl′ ō-jē)	hist/o -logy	CF S	tissue study of	The study of tissue
homeostasis (hō″ mē-ō-stā′ sĭs)	homeo -stasis	P S	similar, same control, stopping	The state of equilibrium maintained in the body's internal environment
horizontal (hŏr′ă-zŏn′ tăl)	horizont -al	R S	horizon pertaining to	Pertaining to the horizon, of or near the horizon, lying flat, even, level
human genome (hū′ măn jē′ nōm)				The complete set of genes and chromosomes tucked inside each of the body's trillions of cells
inferior (ĭn-fē′ rē-or)	infer/i -or	CF S	below a doer	Located below or in a downward direction
inguinal (ĭng′ gwĭ-năl)	inguin -al	R S	groin pertaining to	Pertaining to the groin, of or near the groin

MEDICAL WORD	WORD PARTS (WHEN APPLICABLE)			DEFINITION
	Part	**Type**	**Meaning**	
internal (ĭn-tĕr′ nal)	intern -al	R S	within pertaining to	Pertaining to within or the inside
karyogenesis (kăr″ i-ō-jĕn′ ĕ-sĭs)	kary/o -genesis	CF S	cell's nucleus formation, produce	Formation of a cell's nucleus
lateral (lăt′ ĕr-ăl)	later -al	R S	side pertaining to	Pertaining to the side
medial (mē′ dē al)	medi -al	R S	toward the middle pertaining to	Pertaining to the middle or midline
mesomorph (mĕs′ ō-morf)	meso -morph	P S	middle form, shape	A well-proportioned body form
organic (or-găn′ ĭk)	organ -ic	R S	organ pertaining to	Pertaining to an organ
pathology (pă-thŏl′ ō-jē)	path/o -logy	CF S	disease study of	The study of disease
perfusion (pur-fū′ zhŭn)	per fus -ion	P R S	through to pour process	The process of pouring through
phenotype (fē′ nō-tīp)	phen/o -type	CF S	to show type	The physical appearance or type of makeup of an individual
physiology (fiz″ i-ŏl′ ō-jē)	physi/o -logy	CF S	nature study of	The study of the nature of living organisms
posterior (pŏs-tē′ rĭ-ōr)	poster/i -or	CF S	behind, toward the back a doer	Toward the back
protoplasm (prō-tō-plăzm)	proto -plasm	P S	first a thing formed, plasma	The essential matter of a living cell
proximal (prŏk′ sĭm-ăl)	proxim -al	R S	near the point of origin pertaining to	Nearest the center or point of origin; nearest the point of attachment
somatotrophic (sō″ mă-tō-trŏf′ ĭk)	somat/o troph -ic	CF R S	body a turning pertaining to	Pertaining to stimulation of body growth
superficial (sū″ pĕr-fĭsh′ ăl)	superfic/i -al	CF S	near the surface pertaining to	Pertaining to the surface, on or near the surface

MEDICAL WORD	WORD PARTS (WHEN APPLICABLE)			DEFINITION
	Part	**Type**	**Meaning**	
superior (sū-pēr′ rĭ-ōr)	super/i -or	CF S	upper a doer	Located above or in an upward direction
systemic (sis-těm′ ĭk)	system -ic	R S	a composite whole pertaining to	Pertaining to the body as a whole
topical (tŏp′ ĭ-kăl)	topic -al	R S	place pertaining to	Pertaining to a place, definite locale
unilateral (ū″ nĭ-lăt′ ěr-ăl)	uni later -al	P R S	one side pertaining to	Pertaining to one side
ventral (věn′ trăl)	ventr -al	R S	near the belly side pertaining to	Pertaining to the front side of the body, abdomen, belly surface
vertex (věr′ těks)				The top or highest point; the top or crown of the head
visceral (vĭs′ ěr-ăl)	viscer -al	R S	body organs pertaining to	Pertaining to body organs enclosed within a cavity, especially abdominal organs

Terminology Translator

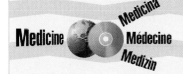

This feature, found on the accompanying CD-ROM, provides an innovative tool to translate medical words into Spanish, French, and German.

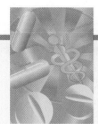

DRUG HIGHLIGHTS

A drug is a medicinal substance that may alter or modify the functions of a living organism. There are thousands of drugs that are available as over-the-counter (OTC) medicines and do not require a prescription. A prescription is a written legal document that gives directions for compounding, dispensing, and administering a medication to a patient.

In general, there are five medical uses for drugs. These are: therapeutic, diagnostic, curative, replacement, and preventive or prophylactic.

- **Therapeutic Use.** Used in the treatment of a disease or condition, such as an allergy, to relieve the symptoms or to sustain the patient until other measures are instituted.
- **Diagnostic Use.** Certain drugs are used in conjunction with radiology to allow the physician to pinpoint the location of a disease process.

- **Curative Use.** Certain drugs, such as antibiotics, kill or remove the causative agent of a disease.
- **Replacement Use.** Certain drugs, such as hormones and vitamins, are used to replace substances normally found in the body.
- **Preventive or Prophylactic Use.** Certain drugs, such as immunizing agents, are used to ward off or lessen the severity of a disease.

Drug Names

Most drugs may be cited by their chemical, generic, and trade or brand (proprietary) name. The chemical name is usually the formula that denotes the composition of the drug. It is made up of letters and numbers that represent the drug's molecular structure. The generic name is the drug's official name and is descriptive of its chemical structure. The generic name is written in lowercase letters. A generic drug can be manufactured by more than one pharmaceutical company. When this is the case, each company markets the drug under its own unique trade or brand name. A trade or brand name is registered by the US Patent Office as well as approved by the US Food and Drug Administration (FDA). A trade or brand name is written with a capital.

Undesirable Actions of Drugs

Most drugs have the potential for causing an action other than their intended action. For example, antibiotics that are administered orally may disrupt the normal bacterial flora of the gastrointestinal tract and cause gastric discomfort. This type of reaction is known as a side effect. An adverse reaction is an unfavorable or harmful unintended action of a drug. For example, the adverse reaction of Demerol may be lightheadedness, dizziness, sedation, nausea, and sweating. A drug interaction may occur when one drug potentiates or diminishes the action of another drug. These actions may be desirable or undesirable. Drugs may also interact with foods, alcohol, tobacco, and other substances.

Medication Order and Dosage

The medication order is given for a specific patient and denotes the name of the drug, the dosage, the form of the drug, the time for or frequency of administration, and the route by which the drug is to be given.

The dosage is the amount of medicine that is prescribed for administration. The form of the drug may be liquid, solid, semisolid, tablet, capsule, transdermal therapeutic patch, etc. The route of administration may be by mouth, by injection, into the eye(s), ear(s), nostril(s), rectum, vagina, etc.

It is important for the patient to know when and how to take a medication. See Terminology Translator for some hows, whens, and directions for taking medications. To assist you in communicating this information to a patient, English, Spanish, French, and German are provided for you to use.

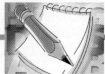

ABBREVIATIONS

ABBREVIATION	MEANING	ABBREVIATION	MEANING
abd	abdomen, abdominal	LAT, lat	lateral
A&P	anatomy and physiology	LLQ	left lower quadrant
AP	anteroposterior	LUQ	left upper quadrant
CNS	central nervous system	PA	posteroanterior
CV	cardiovascular	resp	respiratory
ER	endoplasmic reticulum	RLQ	right lower quadrant
GI	gastrointestinal	RUQ	right upper quadrant

STUDY AND REVIEW

Anatomy and Physiology

Write your answers to the following questions. Do not refer to the text.

1. The _____ consist of millions of _____ working individually and with each other to _____ life.

2. The outer covering of the cell is known as the _____, which has the capability of allowing some substances to pass into and out of the cell.

3. The substance within the cell is known as _____ and is composed of _____ and _____.

4. The cell's nucleus is composed of _____, which contains its genetic material.

5. The two primary functions of the cell's nucleus are _____ and _____.

6. List the four functions of epithelial tissue.

    a. _____   b. _____

    c. _____   d. _____

7. _____ tissue is the most widespread and abundant of the four body tissues.

8. Name the three types of muscle tissue.

    a. _____   b. _____   c. _____

9. Two properties of nerve tissue are _____ and _____.

10. Define organ. _____.

11. Define body system. _____.

12. Name the organ systems listed in this text.

    a. _____   b. _____

    c. _____   d. _____

    e. _____   f. _____

    g. _____   h. _____

    i. _____   j. _____

    k. _____

13. Define the following directional terms:

    a. superior _____   b. anterior _____

    c. posterior _____   d. cephalad _____

    e. medial _____   f. lateral _____

    g. proximal _____   h. distal _____

    i. ventral _____   j. dorsal _____

14. The _____ _____ vertically divides the body. It passes through the midline to form a right and left half.

15. The _____ plane is any plane that divides the body into superior and inferior portions.

16. The _____ plane is any plane that divides the body at right angles to the plane described in question 14.

17. List the three distinct cavities that are located in the ventral cavity.

    a. _____   b. _____   c. _____

18. Name the two distinct cavities located in the dorsal cavity.

    a. _____   b. _____

Word Parts

1. In the spaces provided, write the definition of these prefixes, roots, combining forms, and suffixes. Do not refer to the listings of medical words. Leave blank those words you cannot define.

2. After completing as many as you can, refer back to the medical word listings to check your work. For each word missed or left blank, write the word and its definition several times on the margins of these pages or on a separate sheet of paper.

3. To maximize the learning process, it is to your advantage to do the following exercises as directed. To refer to the word building section before completing these exercises invalidates the learning process.

PREFIXES

Give the definitions of the following prefixes:

    1. ambi- _____   2. ana- _____

    3. bi- _____   4. chromo- _____

    5. de- _____   6. dif- _____

7. ecto- _____

8. endo- _____

9. homeo- _____

10. meso- _____

11. per- _____

12. proto- _____

13. uni- _____

ROOTS AND COMBINING FORMS

Give the definitions of the following roots and combining forms:

1. adip _____

2. andr _____

3. bi/o _____

4. caud _____

5. cyt _____

6. cyt/o _____

7. fus _____

8. gen _____

9. hist/o _____

10. hydr _____

11. kary/o _____

12. later _____

13. path/o _____

14. physi/o _____

15. pin/o _____

16. somat/o _____

17. topic _____

18. troph _____

19. viscer _____

20. anter/i _____

21. cephal _____

22. dist _____

23. dors _____

24. filtrat _____

25. horizont _____

26. infer/i _____

27. inguin _____

28. intern _____

29. later _____

30. medi _____

31. organ _____

32. phen/o _____

33. poster/i _____

34. proxim _____

35. superfic/i _____

36. super/i _____

37. system _____

38. ventr _____

SUFFIXES

Give the definitions for the following suffixes:

1. -al _____

2. -ate _____

3. -genesis _____

4. -ic _____

5. -ion _____

6. -logy _____

7. -morph _____

8. -oid _____

9. -ose _____

10. -osis _____

11. -ous _____

12. -plasm _____

13. -some _____

14. -stasis _____

15. -tomy _____

16. -or _____

17. -ad _____

18. -type _____

Identifying Medical Terms

In the spaces provided, write the medical terms for the following meanings:

1. _____ To resemble man

2. _____ Pertaining to two sides

3. _____ The study of cells

4. _____ A slender physical body form

5. _____ Formation of a cell's nucleus

6. _____ Pertaining to the stimulation of body growth

7. _____ Pertaining to one side

Spelling

In the spaces provided, write the correct spelling of these misspelled terms:

1. adpose _____

2. caual _____

3. cytlogy _____

4. difusion _____

5. histlogy _____

6. mesmorph _____

7. prefusion _____

8. proxmal _____

9. somattrophic _____

10. unlateral _____

Matching

Select the appropriate lettered meaning for each word listed below.

_____ 1. ambilateral

_____ 2. anatomy

_____ 3. cephalad

_____ 4. chromosome

_____ 5. cilia

_____ 6. homeostasis

_____ 7. human genome

_____ 8. phenotype

_____ 9. physiology

_____10. vertex

a. Hair-like processes that project from epithelial cells
b. The top or highest point
c. Pertaining to both sides
d. The study of the structure of an organism such as humans
e. Toward the head
f. Microscopic bodies that carry the genes that determine hereditary characteristics
g. The complete set of genes and chromosomes
h. The physical appearance or type of makeup of an individual
i. The state of equilibrium maintained in the body's internal environment
j. The study of the nature of living organism
k. The study of disease

Abbreviations

Place the correct word, phrase, or abbreviation in the space provided.

1. abdomen _____

2. A&P _____

3. CNS _____

4. cardiovascular _____

5. gastrointestinal _____

6. LAT, lat _____

7. resp _____

8. ER _____

9. AP _____

10. PA _____

MedMedia
Wrap-Up
www.prenhall.com/rice

Additional interactive resources and activities for this chapter can be found on the Companion Website. For animations, videos, audio glossary, and review, access the accompanying CD-ROM in this book.

Audio Glossary
Medical Terminology Exercises & Activities
Terminology Translator
Animations
Videos

Objectives
Medical Terminology Exercises & Activities
Audio Glossary
Drug Updates
Medical Terminology in the News

THE INTEGUMENTARY SYSTEM

3

OUTLINE

OBJECTIVES

On completion of this chapter, you will be able to:

- Describe the integumentary system and its accessory structures.
- List the functions of the skin.
- Describe skin differences of the child and the older adult.
- Analyze, build, spell, and pronounce medical words.
- Describe each of the conditions presented in the Pathology Spotlights.
- Complete the Pathology Checkpoint.
- Review Drug Highlights presented in this chapter.
- Provide the description of diagnostic and laboratory tests related to the integumentary system.
- Identify and define selected abbreviations.
- Successfully complete the study and review section.

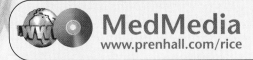

MedMedia
www.prenhall.com/rice

Additional interactive resources and activities for this chapter can be found on the Companion Website. For Terminology Translator, animations, videos, audio glossary, and review, access the accompanying CD-ROM in this book.

Anatomy and Physiology Overview

The integumentary system is composed of the **skin** and its accessory structures: **hair**, **nails**, **sebaceous glands**, and **sweat glands** (Table 3–1). This overview of the anatomy and physiology of the skin offers a general description of the integumentary system as an aid to those learning the terminology associated with its functions.

FUNCTIONS OF THE SKIN

The **skin** is the external covering of the body. In an average adult it covers more than 3000 square inches of surface area, weighs more than 6 pounds, and is the largest organ in the body. The skin is well supplied with blood vessels and nerves and has four main functions: **protection**, **regulation**, **sensation**, and **secretion**.

Protection

The skin serves as a **protective membrane** against invasion by bacteria and other potentially harmful agents that might try to penetrate to deeper tissues. It also protects against mechanical injury of delicate cells located beneath its epidermis or outer covering. The skin also serves to inhibit excessive loss of water and electrolytes and provides a reservoir for food and water storage. The skin guards the body against excessive exposure to the sun's ultraviolet rays by producing a protective pigmentation, and it helps to produce the body's supply of vitamin D.

TABLE 3–1 THE INTEGUMENTARY SYSTEM

Organ/Structure	Primary Functions
Skin	Protection, regulation, sensation, and secretion
Epidermis	The outer layer of the skin. It is divided into four strata:
Stratum corneum	Forms protective covering for the body
Stratum lucidum	Translucent layer that is frequently absent and not seen in thinner skin
Stratum granulosum	Active in the keratinization process, its cells become hard or horny
Stratum germinativum	Responsible for the regeneration of the epidermis
Dermis	Nourishes the epidermis, provides strength, and supports blood vessels
Papillae	Produce ridges that are one's fingerprints
Subcutaneous Tissue	Supports, nourishes, insulates, and cushions the skin
Hair	Provides sensation and some protection for the head. Hair around the eyes, in the nose, and in the ears serves to filter out foreign particles.
Nails	Protects ends of fingers and toes
Sebaceous Glands	Lubricates the hair and skin
Sweat (Sudoriferous) Glands	Secretes sweat or perspiration, which helps to cool the body by evaporation. Sweat also rids the body of waste.

Regulation

The skin serves to raise or lower body temperature as necessary. When the body needs to lose heat, the blood vessels in the skin dilate, bringing more blood to the surface for cooling by **radiation**. At the same time, the sweat glands are secreting more sweat for cooling by means of **evaporation**. Conversely, when the body needs to conserve heat, the reflex actions of the nervous system cause constriction of the skin's blood vessels, thereby allowing more heat-carrying blood to circulate to the muscles and vital organs.

Sensation

The skin contains millions of microscopic nerve endings that act as **sensory receptors** for pain, touch, heat, cold, and pressure. When stimulation occurs, nerve impulses are sent to the cerebral cortex of the brain. The nerve endings in the skin are specialized according to the type of sensory information transmitted and, once this information reaches the brain, any necessary response is triggered. For example, touching a hot surface with the hand causes the brain to recognize the senses of **touch**, **heat**, and **pain** and results in the immediate removal of the hand from the hot surface.

Secretion

The skin contains millions of sweat glands, which secrete **perspiration** or **sweat**, and sebaceous glands, which secrete **oil** for lubrication. Perspiration is largely water with a small amount of salt and other chemical compounds. This secretion, when left to accumulate, causes body odor, especially where it is trapped among hairs in the axillary region. Sebaceous glands produce **sebum**, which acts to protect the body from dehydration and possible absorption of harmful substances.

LAYERS OF THE SKIN

The skin is essentially composed of two layers, the **epidermis** and the **dermis**.

The Epidermis

The **epidermis** can be divided into four strata: the stratum corneum, the stratum lucidum, the stratum granulosum, and the stratum germinativum. See Figure 3–1 for the locations of these strata within the epidermis.

THE STRATUM CORNEUM

The **stratum corneum** is the outermost, horny layer, consisting of dead cells filled with a protein substance called **keratin**. It forms the protective covering for the body, and its thickness varies with the use made of the particular body part. Because of the pressure on their surfaces during use, the soles of the feet and palms of the hands have thicker layers of stratum corneum than do the eyelids or the forehead.

THE STRATUM LUCIDUM

The **stratum lucidum** is a translucent layer lying directly beneath the stratum corneum. It is frequently absent and is not seen in thinner skin. Cells in this layer are also dead or dying.

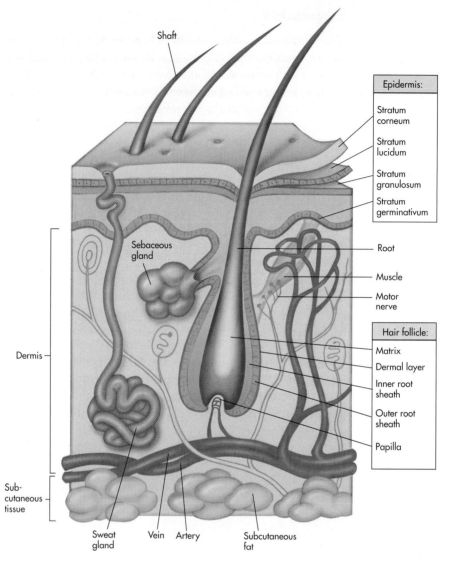

FIGURE 3–1

The integument: the epidermis, dermis, subcutaneous tissue, and its appendages.

THE STRATUM GRANULOSUM

The **stratum granulosum** consists of several layers of living cells that are in the process of becoming a part of the previously mentioned strata. Its cells are active in the **keratinization** process, during which they lose their nuclei and become hard or horny.

THE STRATUM GERMINATIVUM

The **stratum germinativum** is composed of several layers of living cells capable of **mitosis** or cell division. Sometimes called the **mucosum** or **Malpighii**, the stratum germinativum is the innermost layer and is responsible for the regeneration of the epidermis. Damage to this layer, as in severe burns, necessitates the use of skin grafts. **Melanin**, the pigment that gives color to the skin, is formed in this layer. The more abundant the melanin, the darker the color of the skin.

The Dermis

Sometimes called the **corium** or **true skin**, the dermis is composed of connective tissue containing lymphatics, nerves and nerve endings, blood vessels, sebaceous and sweat glands, elastic fibers, and hair follicles. It is divided into two layers: the **upper** or **papillary layer** and the **lower** or **reticular layer**. The papillary layer is arranged into parallel rows of microscopic structures called **papillae**. The papillae produce the ridges of the skin that are one's fingerprints or footprints. The reticular layer is composed of white fibrous tissue that supports the blood vessels. The dermis is attached to underlying structures by the **subcutaneous tissue**. This tissue supports, nourishes, insulates, and cushions the skin.

ACCESSORY STRUCTURES OF THE SKIN

The hair, nails, sebaceous glands, and sweat glands are the accessory structures of the skin.

Hair

A **hair** is a thin, thread-like structure formed by a group of cells that develop within a hair **follicle** or **socket**. Each hair is composed of a **shaft**, which is the visible portion, and a **root**, which is embedded within the follicle. At the base of each follicle is a loop of capillaries enclosed within connective tissue called the **hair papilla**. The **pilomotor muscle** attaches to the side of each follicle. When the skin is cooled or the individual has an emotional reaction, the skin often forms **"goose pimples"** as a result of contraction by these muscles. Hair is distributed over the whole body with the exception of the palms of the hands and soles of the feet. It is thicker on the scalp and thinner on the other parts of the body. Hair around the eyes, in the nose, and in the ears serves to filter out foreign particles. The color of one's hair is a product of genetic background and is determined by the amount of pigmentation within the hair shaft. Hair grows at approximately 0.5 inch a month, and its growth is not affected by cutting.

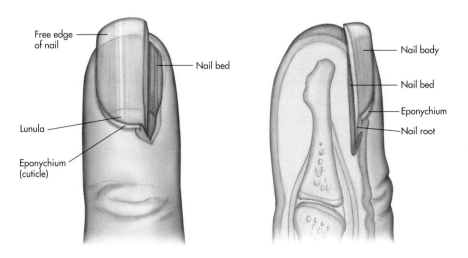

FIGURE 3–2

The fingernail, an appendage of the integument.

Nails

Finger- and **toenails** are horny cell structures of the epidermis and are composed of hard keratin. A nail consists of a **body**, a **root**, and a **matrix** or **nailbed** (Fig. 3–2). The crescent-shaped white area of the nail is the **lunula**. Nail growth may vary with age, disease, and hormone deficiency. Average growth is 1 mm per week, and a lost finger-nail usually regenerates in 3½ to 5½ months. A lost toenail may require 6 to 8 months for regeneration.

Sebaceous Glands

The oil-secreting glands of the skin are called **sebaceous glands**. They have tiny ducts that open into the hair follicles, and their secretion, **sebum**, lubricates the hair as well as the skin. The amount of secretion is controlled by the endocrine system and varies with age, puberty, pregnancy, and senility.

Sweat (Sudoriferous) Glands

There are approximately 2 million **sweat glands**. These coiled, tubular glands are distributed over the entire surface of the body with the exception of the margin of the lips, glans penis, and the inner surface of the prepuce. They are more numerous on the palms of the hands, soles of the feet, forehead, and axillae. Sweat glands secrete **sweat** or **perspiration**, which helps to cool the body by evaporation. Sweat also rids the body of waste through the pores of the skin. Left to accumulate, sweat becomes odorous by the action of bacteria. The body loses about 0.5 L of fluid per day through sweat.

LIFE SPAN
CONSIDERATIONS

■ THE CHILD

Vernix caseosa, a cheese-like substance, covers the fetus until birth. At first the fetal skin is transparent and blood vessels are clearly visible. In about 13 to 16 weeks downy lanugo hair begins to develop, especially on the head. At 21 to 24 weeks, the skin is reddish and wrinkled and has little subcutaneous fat. At birth, the subcutaneous glands are developed and the skin is smooth and pink. Preterm and term newborns have less subcutaneous fat than adults; therefore, they are more sensitive to heat and cold. Babies can blister easily.

Skin conditions may be acute or chronic, local or systemic, and some are congenital, such as strawberry nevi and Mongolian spots. Certain children's skin conditions may be associated with age, such as milia in babies and acne in adolescents. **Milia** are white pinhead-size papules occurring on the face, and sometimes the trunk, of a newborn. They usually disappear in several weeks. **Acne** is an inflammatory condition of the sebaceous glands and the hair follicles (**pimples**). See Figure 3–3.

Skin infections in children generally produce systemic symptoms, such as fever and malaise. Sebaceous glands do not produce sebum until about 8 to 10 years of age; therefore, a child's skin is more dry and chaps easily.

The hair of the child will vary according to race, texture, quality, and distribution. A newborn may have no hair on its head or a head covered with hair. Hair can become dry and brittle, due to improper nutrition. During a severe illness hair loss and color change may occur.

■ THE OLDER ADULT

With increasing years beyond reproductive maturity, the body begins the process of aging. By the year 2030 one in five people in the United States will be at least 65 years old. The process of aging varies with each individual. Aging is not a disease but rather a sequence of events regulated by complex processes.

The Integumentary System

As one ages, the skin becomes looser as the dermal papilla grows less dense. Collagen and elastic fibers of the upper dermis decrease and skin loses its elastic tone and wrinkles more easily. Skin conditions are common in the older adult. Dryness (**xerosis**) and itching (**pruritus**) are common. Premalignant and malignant skin lesions increase with aging. Carcinomas appear frequently on the nose, eyelid, or cheek. **Basal cell carcinomas** account for 80% of the skin cancers seen in the older adult. See Figure 3–4.

By age 50 approximately half of all people have some gray hair. Scalp hair thins in women and men. The hair becomes dry and often brittle. Older women may have an increase in facial hair. Men may have an increase in hair of the nares, eyebrows, or helix of the ear. In addition to the changes in the skin and hair, nails flatten and become discolored, dry, and brittle.

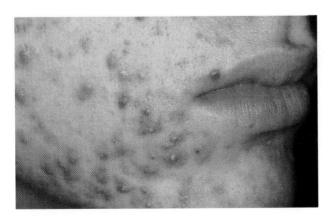

FIGURE 3–3

Acne. (Courtesy of Jason L. Smith, MD.)

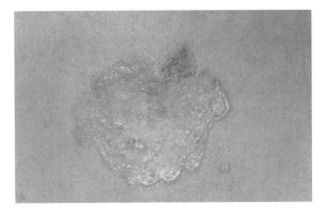

FIGURE 3–4

Basal cell carcinoma. (Courtesy of Jason L. Smith, MD.)

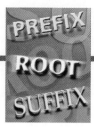

BUILDING YOUR MEDICAL VOCABULARY

This section provides the foundation for learning medical terminology. Medical words can be made up of four different types of word parts:

- Prefixes (P)
- Roots (R)
- Combining forms (CF)
- Suffixes (S)

By connecting various word parts in an organized sequence, thousands of words can be built and learned. In this text the word list is alphabetized so one can see the variety of meanings created when common prefixes and suffixes are repeatedly applied to certain word roots and/or combining forms. Words shown in pink are additional words related to the content of this chapter that are not built from word parts. These words are included to enhance your vocabulary. Note: an asterisk icon (✱) indicates terms that are covered in the Pathology Spotlights section in this chapter.

MEDICAL WORD	WORD PARTS (WHEN APPLICABLE)			DEFINITION
	Part	**Type**	**Meaning**	
acne (ăk′ nē)				An inflammatory condition of the sebaceous glands and the hair follicles; *pimples.* See Figure 3–3.
acrochordon (ăk″ rō-kor′ dŏn)	acr/o chord -on	CF R S	extremity cord pertaining to	A small outgrowth of epidermal and dermal tissue; *skin tags.* See Figure 3–5.
actinic dermatitis (ăk-tĭn′ ĭk dĕr″ mă-tī′ tĭs)	actin -ic dermat -itis	R S R S	ray pertaining to skin inflammation	Inflammation of the skin caused by exposure to radiant energy, such as x-rays, ultraviolet light, and sunlight. See Figure 3–6.
albinism (ăl′ bĭn-ĭsm)	albin -ism	R S	white condition of	Absence of pigment in the skin, hair, and eyes
alopecia (al″ ō-pē′ shĭ-ă)	a lopec -ia	P R S	without, lack of fox mange pertaining to	Loss of hair, baldness; *alopecia areata* is loss of hair in defined patches usually involving the scalp. See Figure 3–7. Male pattern alopecia begins in the frontal area and proceeds until only a horseshoe area of the hair remains in the back and temples. See Figure 3–8.

MEDICAL WORD	WORD PARTS (WHEN APPLICABLE)			DEFINITION
	Part	Type	Meaning	
anhidrosis (ăn″ hī-drō′ sĭs)	an	P	without, lack of	A condition in which there is a lack or complete absence of sweating
	hidr	R	sweat	
	-osis	S	condition of	
autograft (ŏ-tō-grăft)	auto	P	self	A graft taken from one part of the patient's body and transferred to another part
	-graft	S	pencil, grafting knife	
avulsion (ă-vŭl′ shŭn)	a	P	away from	The process of forcibly tearing off a part or structure of the body, such as a finger or toe.
	vuls	R	to pull	
	-ion	S	process	
basal cell carcinoma (bā′ săl sel kăr″ sĭ-nō′ mă)				An epithelial malignant tumor of the skin that rarely metastasizes. It usually begins as a small, shiny papule and enlarges to form a whitish border around a central depression. See Figure 3–4.
bite (bīt)				An injury in which a part of the body surface is torn by an insect, animal, or human, resulting in an abrasion, puncture, or laceration. See Figures 3–9, 3–10, 3–11, and 3–12.
boil (boil)				An acute, painful nodule formed in the subcutaneous layers of the skin, gland, or hair follicle; most often caused by the invasion of staphylococci; *furuncle.* See Figure 3–13.
bulla (bŭl′ lă)				A larger blister; *a bleb.* See Figure 3–14.
burn (burn) (bərn)				An injury to tissue caused by heat, fire, chemical agents, electricity, lightning, or radiation; burns are classified according to degree or depth of skin damage. See Figure 3–15.
callus (kăl′ ŭs)				Hardened skin
candidiasis (kăn″ dĭ-dī′ ă-sĭs)				An infection of the skin or mucous membranes with any species of *Candida,* but chiefly *Candida albicans. Candida* is a genus of yeasts and was formerly called *Monilia.* See Figure 3–16.

MEDICAL WORD	WORD PARTS (WHEN APPLICABLE)			DEFINITION
	Part	**Type**	**Meaning**	
carbuncle (kăr′ bŭng″ kl)				An infection of the subcutaneous tissue, usually composed of a cluster of boils. See Figure 3–17.
causalgia (kŏ-săl′ jĭ-ă)	caus -algia	R S	heat pain	Intense burning pain associated with trophic skin changes in the hand or foot after trauma to the part
cellulitis (sĕl-ū-lī′ tĭs)	cellul -itis	R S	little cell inflammation	Inflammation of cellular or connective tissue. See Figure 3–18.
cicatrix (sĭk′ ă-trĭks)				The scar left after the healing of a wound
comedo (kŏm′ ē-dō)				Blackhead
corn (korn) (ko(ə)rn)				A horny induration and thickening of the skin on the toes caused by ill-fitting shoes.
cutaneous (kū-tā′ nē-ŭs)	cutane -ous	R S	skin pertaining to	Pertaining to the skin
cyst (sĭst)				A bladder or sac; a closed sac that contains fluid, semifluid, or solid material
decubitus (dē-kū′ bĭ-tŭs)	de cubit -us	P R S	down to lie pertaining to	Literally means a lying down; *a bedsore.* ✱ See Pathology Spotlight: Decubitus Ulcer.
dehiscence (dē-hĭs′ ĕns)				The separation or bursting open of a surgical wound. See Figure 3–19.
dermatitis (dĕr″ mă-ti′ tĭs)	dermat -itis	R S	skin inflammation	Inflammation of the skin. See Figures 3–20 and 3–21.
dermatologist (dĕr′ mah-tol′ŏ-jĭst)	dermat/o log -ist	CF R S	skin study of one who specializes	One who specializes in the study of the skin
dermatology (dĕr″ mah-tol′ ŏ-jē)	dermat/o -logy	CF S	skin study of	The study of the skin
dermatome (dĕr″ mah-tōm)	derm/a -tome	CF S	skin instrument to cut	An instrument used to cut the skin for grafting
dermomycosis (dĕr′ mō-mī-kō′ sĭs)	derm/o myc -osis	CF R S	skin fungus condition of	A skin condition caused by a fungus

MEDICAL WORD	WORD PARTS (WHEN APPLICABLE)			DEFINITION
	Part	**Type**	**Meaning**	
ecchymosis (ĕk-ĭ-mō′ sĭs)	ec chym -osis	P R S	out juice condition of	A condition in which the blood seeps into the skin causing discolorations ranging from blue-black to greenish-yellow
eczema (ĕk′ zĕ-mă)				An inflammatory skin disease of the epidermis. ✳ See Pathology Spotlight: Eczema.
erythema (ĕr″ ĭ-thē′ mă)				A redness of the skin; may be caused by capillary congestion, inflammation, heat, sunlight, or cold temperature. *Erythema infectiosum* is known as Fifth disease, a mild, moderately contagious disease caused by the human parvovirus B-19. It is most commonly seen in school-age children and is thought to be spread via respiratory secretions from infected persons. See Figure 3–22.
erythroderma (ĕ-rĭth″ rō-dĕr′-mă)	erythr/o -derma	CF S	red skin	Abnormal redness of the skin occurring over widespread areas of the body. See Figure 3–23.
eschar (ĕs′ kăr)				A slough, scab
excoriation (ĕks-kō″ rē-ā′ shŭn)	ex coriat -ion	P R S	out corium process	Abrasion of the epidermis by scratching, trauma, chemicals, burns, etc.
exudate (ĕks′ ū-dāt)				The production of pus or serum
folliculitis (fō-lĭk″ ū-lī′ tĭs)	follicul -itis	R S	little bag inflammation	Inflammation of a follicle or follicles. See Figure 3–24.
herpes simplex (hĕr′ pēz sĭm′ plĕks)				An inflammatory skin disease caused by a herpes virus (Type I); *cold sore or fever blister.* See Figures 3–25 and 3–26.
hidradenitis (hī-drăd-ĕ-nī′ tĭs)	hidr aden -itis	R R S	sweat gland inflammation	Inflammation of the sweat glands
hives (hīvz)				Eruption of itching and burning swellings on the skin; *urticaria.* See Figure 3–27.

MEDICAL WORD	WORD PARTS (WHEN APPLICABLE)			DEFINITION
	Part	Type	Meaning	
hyperhidrosis (hī″ pĕr-hī-drō′ sĭs)	hyper hidr -osis	P R S	excessive sweat condition of	A condition of excessive sweating. See Figure 3–28.
hypodermic (hī″ pō-dĕr′ mĭk)	hypo derm -ic	P R S	under skin pertaining to	Pertaining to under the skin or inserted under the skin, as a hypodermic injection
icteric (ik-tĕr′ ik)	icter -ic	R S	jaundice pertaining to	Pertaining to jaundice
impetigo (ĭm″ pĕ-tī′ gō)				A skin infection marked by vesicles or bullae; usually caused by streptococci or staphylococci. See Figure 3–29.
integumentary (ĭn-tĕg″ ū-mĕn′ tă-rē)	integument -ary	R S	a covering pertaining to	A covering; the skin, consisting of the dermis and the epidermis
intradermal (in″ trăh-dĕr′ măl)	intra derm -al	P R S	within skin pertaining to	Pertaining to within the skin, as an intradermal injection
jaundice (jawn′ dĭs)	jaund -ic(e)	R S	yellow pertaining to	Yellow; a symptom of a disease in which there is excessive bile in the blood; the skin, whites of the eyes, and mucous membranes are yellow; *icterus*
keloid (kē′ lŏyd)	kel -oid	R S	tumor resemble	Overgrowth of scar tissue caused by excessive collagen formation. See Figure 3–30.
lentigo (lĕn-tī′ gō)				A flat, brownish spot on the skin sometimes caused by exposure to the sun and weather; *freckle*. See Figure 3–31.
leukoderma (lū″ kō-dĕr′ mă)	leuk/o -derma	CF S	white skin	Localized loss of pigmentation of the skin
leukoplakia (lū″ kō-plā′ kē-ă)	leuk/o plak -ia	CF R S	white plate pertaining to	White spots or patches formed on the mucous membrane of the tongue or cheek; the spots are smooth, hard, and irregular in shape and may become malignant
lupus (lū′ pŭs)				Originally used to describe a destructive type of skin lesion; current usage of the word is usually in combination with the words *vulgaris* or *erythematosus: lupus vulgaris* or *lupus erythematosus*

MEDICAL WORD	WORD PARTS (WHEN APPLICABLE)			DEFINITION
	Part	Type	Meaning	
melanocarcinoma (mĕl″ ă-nō-kar″ sĭn-ō′ mă)	melan/o carcin -oma	CF R S	black cancer tumor	A cancerous tumor that has black pigmentation
melanoma (mĕl″ ă-nō′ mă)	melan -oma	R S	black tumor	A malignant black mole or tumor. ✳ See Figures 3–50 and 3–51 in Pathology Spotlight: Skin Cancer.
miliaria (mĭl-ē-ā′ rē-ă)	miliar -ia	R S	millet (tiny) pertaining to	Is called *prickly heat* and is commonly seen in newborns and/or infants. It is caused by excessive body warmth. There is retention of sweat in the sweat glands, which have become blocked or inflamed, and then rupture or leak into the skin. *Miliaria* appears as a rash with tiny pinhead-sized papules, vesicles, and/or pustules. See Figure 3–32.
mole (mōl)				A pigmented, elevated spot above the surface of the skin; a *nevus*. See Figure 3–33.
onychitis (ŏn″ ĭ-kī′ tĭs)	onych -itis	R S	nail inflammation	Inflammation of the nail
onychomycosis (ŏn″ ĭ-kō-mī-kō′ sĭs)	onych/o myc -osis	CF R S	nail fungus condition of	A condition of the nail caused by a fungus. See Figure 3–34.
pachyderma (păk-ē-der′ mă)	pachy -derma	R S	thick skin	Thick skin
paronychia (păr″ ō-nĭk′ ĭ-ă)	par onych -ia	P R S	around nail condition	An infectious condition of the marginal structures around the nail
pediculosis (pĕ-dĭk″ ū-lō′ sĭs)	pedicul -osis	R S	a louse condition of	A condition of infestation with lice. See Figure 3–35.
petechiae (pē-tē′ kĭ-ē)				Small, pinpoint, purplish hemorrhagic spots on the skin
pruritus (proo-rī′ tŭs)	prurit -us	R S	itching pertaining to	A severe itching
psoriasis (sō-rī′ ă-sĭs)				A chronic skin disease characterized by pink or dull-red lesions surmounted by silvery scaling. ✳ See Figure 3–49 in Pathology Spotlight: Psoriasis.

MEDICAL WORD	WORD PARTS (WHEN APPLICABLE)			DEFINITION
	Part	**Type**	**Meaning**	
purpura (pur′ pū-ră)				A purplish discoloration of the skin caused by extravasation of blood into the tissues. See Figures 3–36 and 3–37.
rhytidoplasty (rĭt′ ĭ-dō-plăs″ tē)	rhytid/o -plasty	CF S	wrinkle surgical repair	Plastic surgery for the removal of wrinkles
roseola (rō-zē′ ō-lă)				Any rose-colored rash marked by *maculae* or red spots on the skin. See Figure 3–38.
rubella (roo-bĕl′ lă)				A systemic disease caused by a virus and characterized by a rash and fever; also called *German measles* and *three-day measles*
rubeola (roo-bē′ ō-lă)				A contagious disease characterized by fever, inflammation of the mucous membranes, and rose-colored spots on the skin; also called *measles*
scabies (skā′ bēz) or (skā′ bĭ-ēz)				A contagious skin disease characterized by papules, vesicles, pustules, burrows, and intense itching; it is caused by the itch mite and is also called "*the itch*" or the "*seven-year itch*." See Figure 3–39.
scar (skahr)				The mark left by the healing process of a wound, sore, or injury
scleroderma (skli rō-dĕr′ mă)	scler/o -derma	CF S	hard skin	A chronic condition with hardening of the skin and other connective tissues of the body
seborrhea (sĕb″ or-ē′ ă)	seb/o -rrhea	CF S	oil flow	Excessive flow of oil from the sebaceous glands
sebum (sē′ bŭm)				The fatty or oil secretion of sebaceous glands of the skin
senile keratosis (sĕn′ īl kĕr″ ă-tō′ sĭs)	senile kerat -osis	R R S	old horn condition of	A condition occurring in older people wherein there is dry skin and localized scaling caused by excessive exposure to the sun. See Figure 3–40.
striae (plural) (strī′ ē)				Streaks or lines on the breasts, thighs, abdomen, or buttocks caused by weakening of elastic tissue. See Figure 3–41.

MEDICAL WORD	WORD PARTS (WHEN APPLICABLE)			DEFINITION
	Part	Type	Meaning	
subcutaneous (sŭb″ kū-tā′ nē-ŭs)	sub cutane -ous	P R S	below skin pertaining to	Pertaining to below the skin, as a subcutaneous injection
subungual (sŭb-ŭng′ gwăl)	sub ungu -al	P R S	below nail pertaining to	Pertaining to below the nail
taut (tŏt)				Tight, firm; to pull or draw tight a surface, such as the skin
telangiectasia (tĕl-ăn″ jē-ĕk-tā′ zē-ă)	tel ang/i -ectasia	R CF S	end, distant vessel dilatation	Dilatation of small blood vessels that may appear as a "*birthmark*"
thermanesthesia (thĕrm″ ăn-ĕs-thē′ zē-ă)	therm an -esthesia	R P S	hot, heat without, lack of sensation	Inability to distinguish between the sensations of heat and cold
tinea (tĭn′ ē-ă)				Contagious skin diseases affecting both man and domestic animals, caused by certain fungi, and marked by the localized appearance of discolored, scaly patches on the skin; also called *ringworm*. See Figures 3–42 and 3–43.
trichomycosis (trĭk″ ō-mi-kō′ sĭs)	trich/o myc -osis	CF R S	hair fungus condition of	A fungus condition of the hair
ulcer (ŭl′ sĕr)				An open lesion or sore of the epidermis or mucous membrane. See Figure 3–44.
varicella (văr″ i-sĕl′ ă)				A contagious viral disease characterized by fever, headache, and a crop of red spots that become macules, papules, vesicles, and crusts; also called *chickenpox*. See Figure 3–45.
vitiligo (vĭt″ ĭl-ĭ′ gō)				A skin condition characterized by milk-white patches surrounded by areas of normal pigmentation. See Figure 3–46.
wart (wōrt)				An elevation of viral origin on the epidermis; *verruca*. See Figure 3–47. A plantar wart is known as *verruca plantaris*. It occurs on a pressure-bearing area, especially the sole of the foot. See Figure 3–48.

MEDICAL WORD	WORD PARTS (WHEN APPLICABLE)			DEFINITION
	Part	Type	Meaning	
wound (woond)				An injury to soft tissue caused by trauma; generally classified as open or closed
xanthoderma (zăn″ thō-dĕr′ mă)	xanth/o -derma	CF S	yellow skin	Yellow skin
xanthoma (zăn-thō′ mă)	xanth -oma	R S	yellow tumor	Yellow tumor
xeroderma (zē″ rō-dĕr′ mă)	xer/o -derma	CF S	dry skin	Dry skin
xerosis (zē-rō′ sĭs)	xer -osis	R S	dry condition of	Abnormal dryness of skin, mucous membranes, or the conjunctiva.

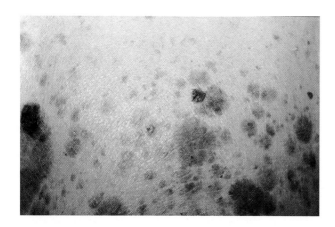

FIGURE 3–5

Acrochordon (skin tags). (Courtesy of Jason L. Smith, MD.)

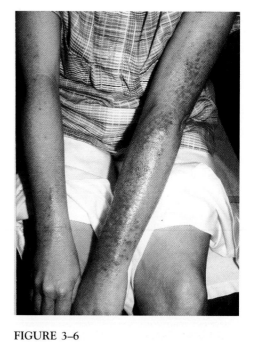

FIGURE 3–6

Photodermatitis. (Courtesy of Jason L. Smith, MD.)

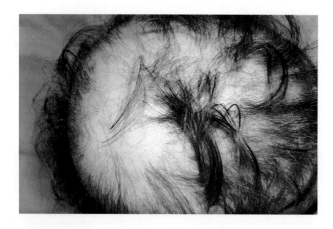

FIGURE 3–7

Alopecia areata. (Courtesy of Jason L. Smith, MD.)

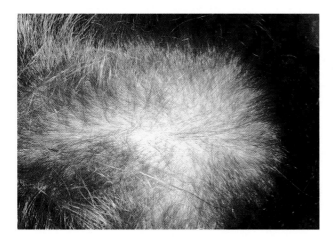

FIGURE 3–8

Male pattern alopecia. (Courtesy of Jason L. Smith, MD.)

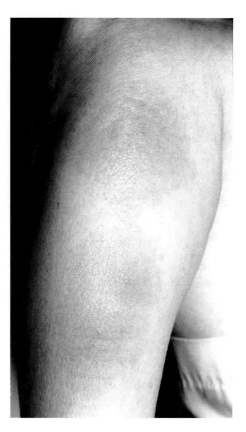

FIGURE 3–9

Fire ant bites. (Courtesy of Jason L. Smith, MD.)

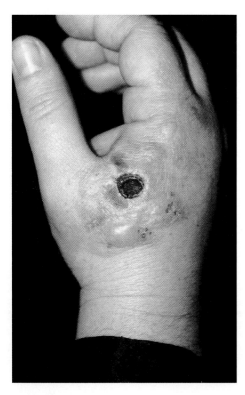

FIGURE 3–10

Brown recluse spider bites. (Courtesy of Jason L. Smith, MD.)

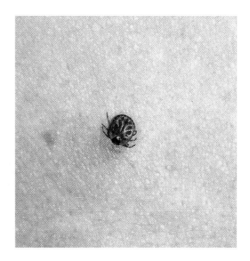

FIGURE 3–11

Tick bite. (Courtesy of Jason L. Smith, MD.)

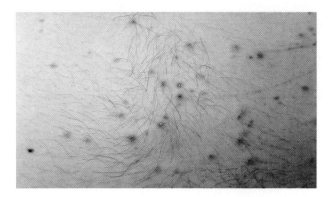

FIGURE 3–12

Flea bites. (Courtesy of Jason L. Smith, MD.)

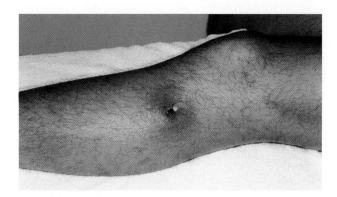

FIGURE 3–13

Furuncle. (Courtesy of Jason L. Smith, MD.)

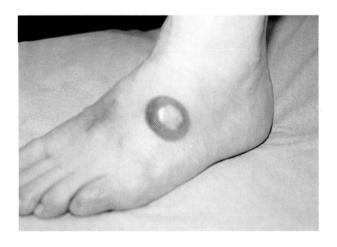

FIGURE 3–14

Bulla. (Courtesy of Jason L. Smith, MD.)

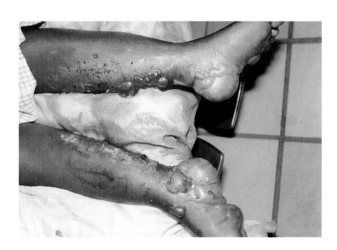

FIGURE 3–15

Burn, second degree. (Courtesy of Jason L. Smith, MD.)

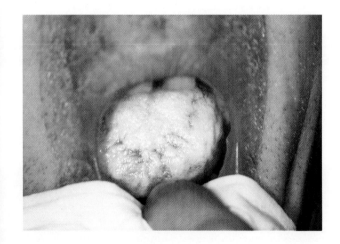

FIGURE 3–16

Candidiasis. (Courtesy of Jason L. Smith, MD.)

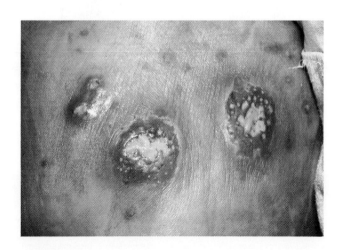

FIGURE 3–17

Carbuncles. (Courtesy of Jason L. Smith, MD.)

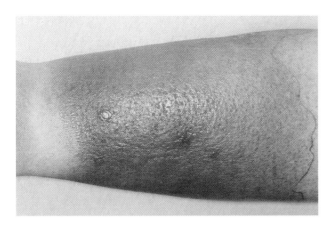

FIGURE 3–18

Cellulitis. (Courtesy of Jason L. Smith, MD.)

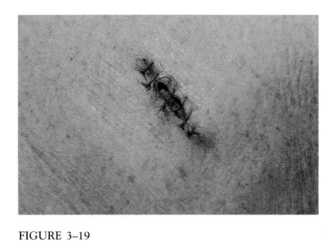

FIGURE 3–19

Wound dehiscence, back. (Courtesy of Jason L. Smith, MD.)

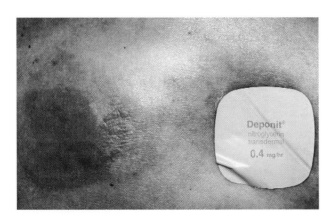

FIGURE 3–20

Contact dermatitis; adhesive reaction. (Courtesy of Jason L. Smith, MD.)

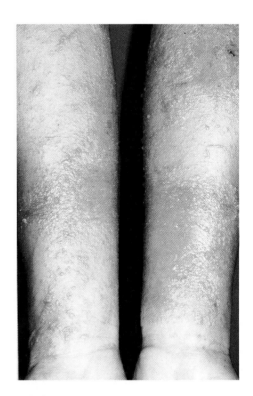

FIGURE 3–21

Dermatitis; poison ivy. (Courtesy of Jason L. Smith, MD.)

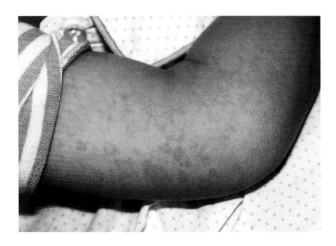

FIGURE 3–22

Erythema infectiosum (Fifth disease). (Courtesy of Jason L. Smith, MD.)

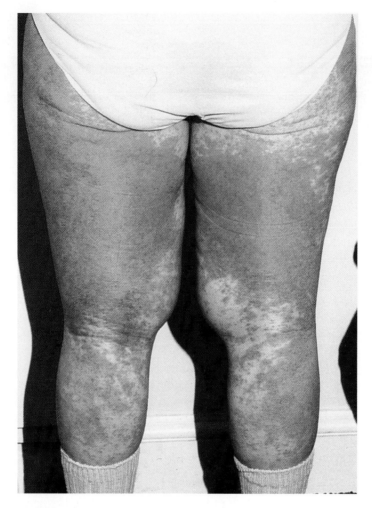

FIGURE 3–23

Erythroderma. (Courtesy of Jason L. Smith, MD.)

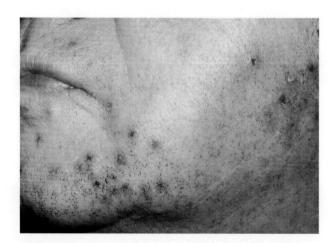

FIGURE 3–24

Staphylococcal folliculitis. (Courtesy of Jason L. Smith, MD.)

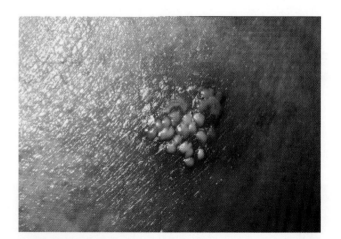

FIGURE 3–25

Herpes simplex. (Courtesy of Jason L. Smith, MD.)

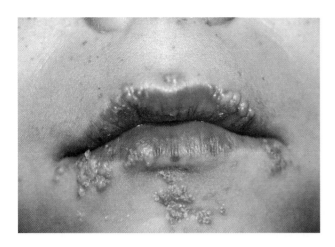

FIGURE 3–26

Herpes labialis. (Courtesy of Jason L. Smith, MD.)

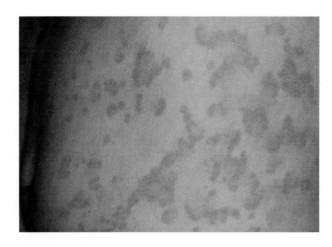

FIGURE 3–27

Urticaria (hives). (Courtesy of Jason L. Smith, MD.)

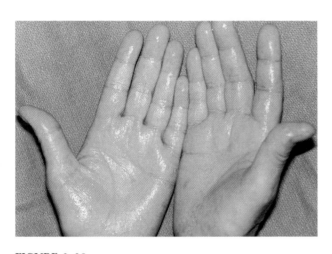

FIGURE 3–28

Hyperhidrosis. (Courtesy of Jason L. Smith, MD.)

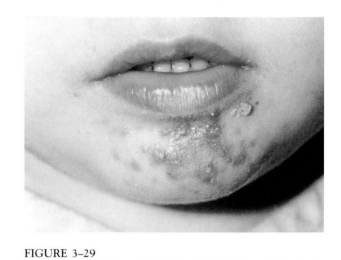

FIGURE 3–29

Impetigo. (Courtesy of Jason L. Smith, MD.)

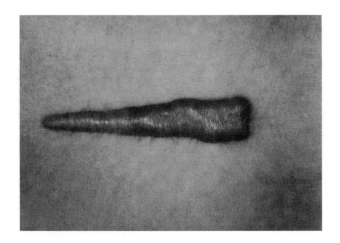

FIGURE 3–30

Keloid. (Courtesy of Jason L. Smith, MD.)

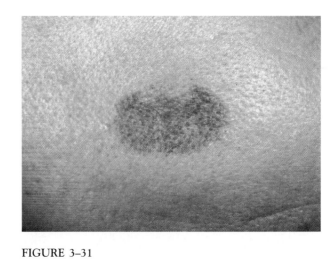

FIGURE 3–31

Lentigo. (Courtesy of Jason L. Smith, MD.)

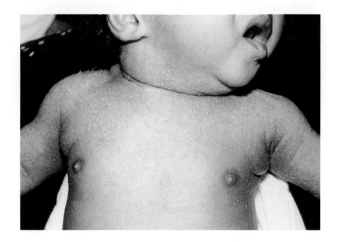

FIGURE 3–32

Miliaria. (Courtesy of Jason L. Smith, MD.)

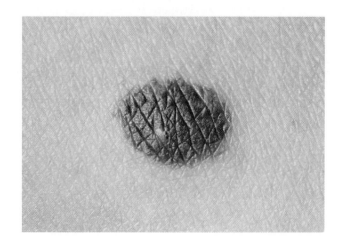

FIGURE 3–33

Nevus (mole). (Courtesy of Jason L. Smith, MD.)

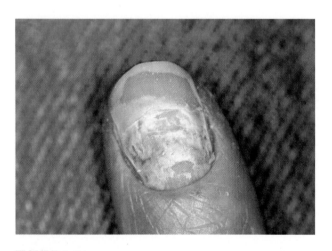

FIGURE 3–34

Onychomycosis. (Courtesy of Jason L. Smith, MD.)

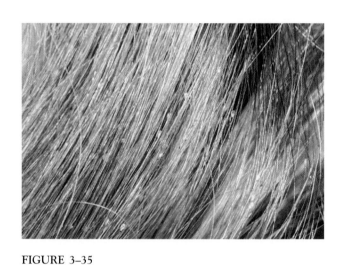

FIGURE 3–35

Pediculosis capitis. (Courtesy of Jason L. Smith, MD.)

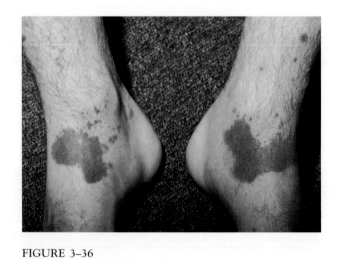

FIGURE 3–36

Purpura. (Courtesy of Jason L. Smith, MD.)

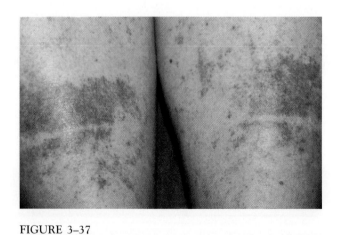

FIGURE 3–37

Benign pigmented purpura. (Courtesy of Jason L. Smith, MD.)

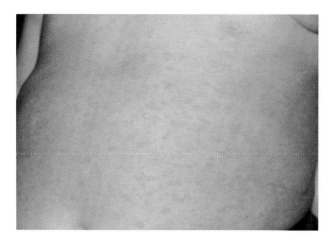

FIGURE 3–38

Roseola. (Courtesy of Jason L. Smith, MD.)

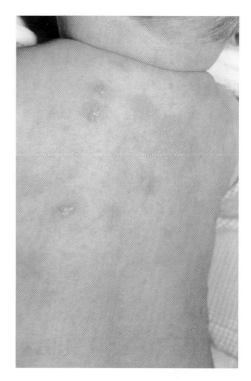

FIGURE 3–39

Scabies. (Courtesy of Jason L. Smith, MD.)

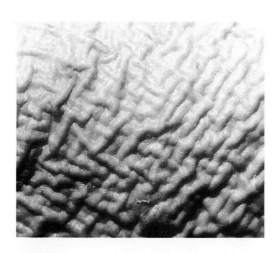

FIGURE 3–40

Photoaging solar elastosis; senile keratosis. (Courtesy of Jason L. Smith, MD.)

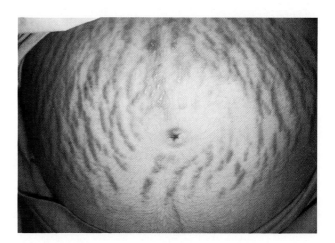

FIGURE 3–41

Striae. (Courtesy of Jason L. Smith, MD.)

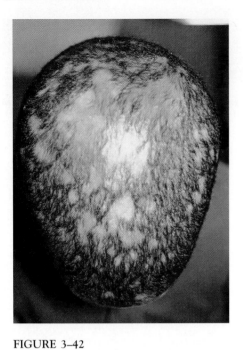

FIGURE 3–42

Tinea capitis. (Courtesy of Jason L. Smith, MD.)

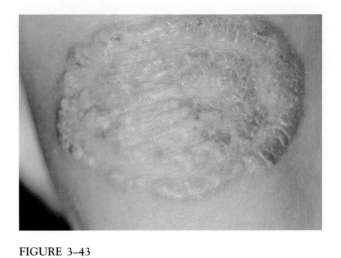

FIGURE 3–43

Tinea corporis. (Courtesy of Jason L. Smith, MD.)

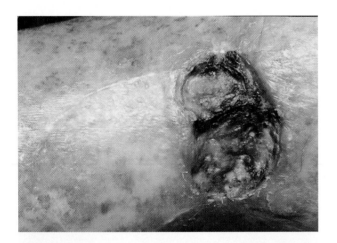

FIGURE 3–44

Leg ulcer radiation site. (Courtesy of Jason L. Smith, MD.)

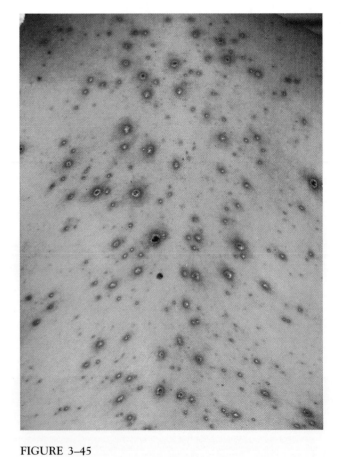

FIGURE 3–45

Varicella (chickenpox). (Courtesy of Jason L. Smith, MD.)

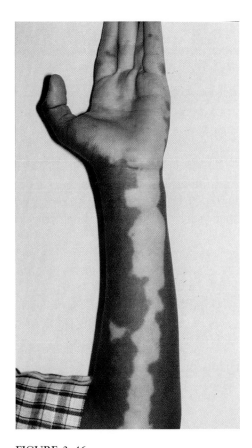

FIGURE 3–46

Vitiligo. (Courtesy of Jason L. Smith, MD.)

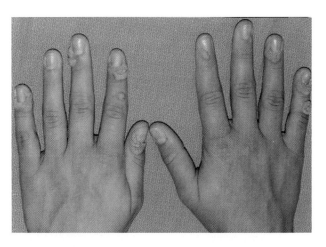

FIGURE 3–47

Verrucae (warts). (Courtesy of Jason L. Smith, MD.)

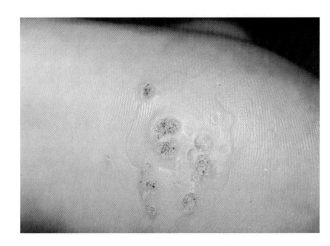

FIGURE 3–48

Plantar wart. (Courtesy of Jason L. Smith, MD.)

Terminology Translator

Medicine   Medicina   Médecine   Medizin

This feature, found on the accompanying CD-ROM, provides an innovative tool to translate medical words into Spanish, French, and German.

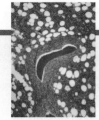

PATHOLOGY SPOTLIGHTS

PATHOLOGY SPOTLIGHTS

Decubitus Ulcer

Also known as a bedsore or pressure ulcer, a decubitus ulcer is an area of skin and tissue that becomes injured or broken down. See the "Skin Signs" section that follows, as well as Figure 3–52. The literal meaning of the word, decubitus, is a lying down. This meaning points to what causes a decubitus (pressure) ulcer: When a person is in a sitting or lying position for too long without shifting his or her weight, the constant pressure against the tissue causes a decreased blood supply to that area. Without a blood supply, the affected tissue dies. The most common places for pressure ulcers are over bony prominences such as the elbow, heels, hips, ankles, shoulders, back, and the back of the head.

Although it is more common for people to get pressure ulcers if they spend most of their time in bed or use a wheelchair, those who can walk can also get pressure ulcers when they are bedridden as a result of an illness or injury.

The National Pressure Ulcer Advisory Panel (NPUAP) created a system for evaluating pressure sores, which is based on a staging system from Stage I (earliest signs) to Stage IV (worst):

Stage I: A reddened area on the skin that, when pressed, is "non-blanchable" (does not turn white). This indicates that a pressure ulcer is starting to develop.

Stage II: The skin blisters or forms an open sore. The area around the sore may be red and irritated.

Stage III: The skin breakdown now looks like a crater where there is damage to the tissue below the skin.

Stage IV: The pressure ulcer has become so deep that there is damage to the muscle and bone, and sometimes tendons and joints.

Once a pressure ulcer is identified, certain basic steps are taken. This includes relieving the pressure to the affected area. Pillows, special foam cushions, and sheepskin are used to help reduce the pressure. Treating the sore is based on the stage of the ulcer. Pressure ulcers are rinsed with a salt-water rinse that removes the loose, dead tissue. The sore is then covered with special gauze dressing made for pressure ulcers. Avoiding further trauma or friction is important, and powdering the sheets lightly can help decrease friction in bed.

Infection may occur, and can lead to serious problems because the infection can become systemic.

Eczema

Eczema, which is also called atopic or contact dermatitis (see Figure 3–20), is a chronic skin disorder characterized by scaly and itching rashes. People with eczema often have a family history of eczema, or allergic conditions like asthma and hay fever. Eczema is most common in infants, and at least half of those cases clear by age 3. In adults, it is generally a chronic condition.

Eczema results from a hypersensitivity reaction (similar to an allergy) that occurs in the skin, causing chronic inflammation. The inflammation causes the skin to become itchy and scaly. Chronic irritation and scratching causes the skin to thicken and become a leathery texture. Symptoms can be worsened by exposure to environmental irritants, dryness of the skin, exposure to water, temperature changes, and stress.

Treatment depends on the appearance or stage of the lesions. For example, acute "weeping" lesions, dry scaly lesions, or chronic dry, thickened lesions are each treated differently. Weeping lesions may be treated with moisturizers, mild soaps, or wet dressings. Less severe cases and dry, scaly lesions may be treated with mild anti-itch lotions or low-potency topical corticosteroids. Chronic thickened areas may be treated with ointments or creams that contain tar compounds, medium to very high potency corticosteroids, and lubricating ingredients. In severe cases, systemic corticosteroids may be prescribed to reduce inflammation. The most promising treatment for eczema is a new class of nonsteroidal skin medications called topical immunomodulators (TIMs).

People who suffer from eczema should avoid anything that aggravates the symptoms, including any food allergens and irritants such as wool and lanolin. Dry skin often makes the condition worse, so patients are encouraged to use a mild soap when washing or bathing, and to use as little soap as possible. After bathing, it is important that patients trap the moisture in the skin by applying a moisturizer on the skin while it is damp. Temperature changes and stress may cause sweating and aggravate the condition.

Psoriasis

Psoriasis is a common skin condition that is characterized by frequent episodes of redness, itching, and thick, dry, scales on the skin (see Figure 3–49). It is a very common condition that affects approximately 3 million Americans. The condition may affect people of any age, but it most commonly begins between ages 15 and 35. It is believed be an inherited disorder, related to an inflammatory response in which the immune system targets the body's own cells. Normally, it takes about a month for new skin cells to move up from the lower layers to the surface. In psoriasis, this process takes only a few days, resulting in a build-up of dead skin cells and formation of thick scales. The condition is most commonly seen on the trunk, elbows, knees, scalp, skin folds, or fingernails, but it may affect any (or all) parts of the skin.

Psoriasis can appear suddenly or gradually. In many cases, it goes away and then flares up again repeatedly over time. Medications, viral or bacterial infections, excessive alcohol consumption, obesity, lack of sunlight, sunburn, stress, general poor health, cold climate, and frequent friction on the skin are also associated with psoriasis flare-ups. The condition is not contagious.

Treatment varies with the extent and severity of the disorder. Psoriasis lesions that cover all or most of the body may require hospitalization, and may be acutely painful. In such severe cases, the body loses vast quantities of fluid and is susceptible to severe secondary infections that can become systemic, involve internal organs, and can even progress to septic shock and death. Treatment includes analgesics, sedation, intravenous fluids, retinoids (such as Retin-A), and antibiotics (such as cyclosporine).

Mild cases are usually treated at home with topical medications such as prescription or nonprescription dandruff shampoos, cortisone or other corticosteroids, and antifungal medications.

Nonpharmacologic treatments may include moderate exposure to sunlight or phototherapy. In phototherapy, the skin is sensitized by the application of coal tar ointment or by taking

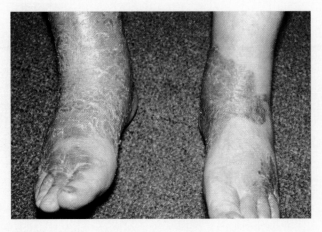

FIGURE 3–49

Psoriasis, lower extremities. (Courtesy of Jason L. Smith, MD.)

oral medications that cause the skin to become sensitive to light. The person is then exposed to ultraviolet light.

Skin Cancer

Skin cancer is a disease in which malignant cells are found in the epidermis. The epidermis contains three kinds of cells: flat, scaly cells on the surface called squamous cells; round cells called basal cells, and cells called melanocytes, which give the skin its color.

The most common types of skin cancer are basal cell cancer and squamous cell cancer. Skin cancer is more common in persons with light-colored skin who have spent a lot of time in the sunlight. Skin cancer can occur anywhere on the body, but it is most common in places that have been exposed to more sunlight, such as the face, neck, hands, and arms.

The most common sign of skin cancer is a change on the skin, such as a growth or a sore that will not heal. Sometimes there may be a small lump. This lump can be smooth, shiny and waxy looking, or it can be red or reddish brown. Skin cancer may also appear as a flat red spot that is rough or scaly. Not all changes in the skin are cancer, but it is very important to have a dermatologist evaluate any change that occurs in one's skin.

It is recommended that one check his/her skin on a regular basis and to have a skin examination every three years if between the ages of 20 and 40 and every year after age 40.

Cancer that develops in the pigment cells is called **melanoma** (see Figures 3–50 and 3–51). It usually occurs in adults, but may occasionally be found in children and adolescents. Melanoma strikes more than 50,000 Americans annually and causes an estimated 7,800 deaths.

Often the first sign of melanoma is change in the size, shape, or color of a mole. The ABCDs of melanoma describe the changes that can occur in a mole using the letters:

A—asymmetry; the shape of one half does not match the other.

B—border; the edges are ragged, notched, or blurred.

C—color; is uneven. Shades of black, brown, or tan are present. Areas of white, red, or blue may be seen.

D—diameter; there is a change in size.

Scientists have pinpointed a genetic marker that may serve as an early indicator for melanoma. Protein produced by the gene, known as Id1, was found in tissue samples of early-stage melanoma. If this research holds up, then a physician can biopsy a mole and if it is positive for Id1, it can be surgically removed. This is very important because the disease is curable if caught early, but is usually fatal if not.

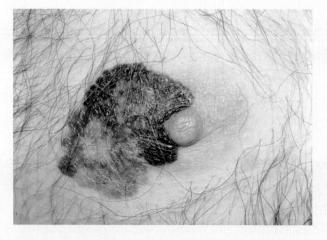

FIGURE 3–50

Melanoma. (Courtesy of Jason L. Smith, MD.)

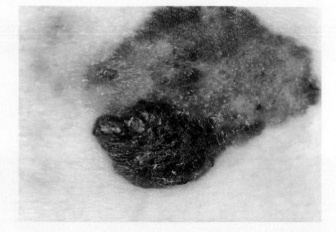

FIGURE 3–51

Melanoma, forearm. (Courtesy of Jason L. Smith, MD.)

Melanoma is a more serious type of cancer than basal cell or squamous cell cancers. Like most cancers, melanoma is best treated when it is found early. Melanoma can metastasize quickly to other parts of the body through the lymph system or through the blood.

Skin Signs

Skin signs are objective evidence of an illness or disorder. They can be seen, measured, or felt. They may be described as lesions that are circumscribed areas of pathologically altered tissue. Types of skin signs are shown and described in Figure 3–52.

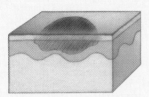

A macule is a discolored spot on the skin; freckle

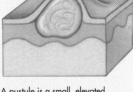

A pustule is a small, elevated, circumscribed lesion of the skin that is filled with pus; varicella (chickenpox)

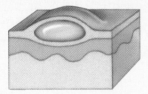

A wheal is a localized, evanescent elevation of the skin that is often accompanied by itching; urticaria

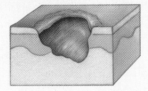

An erosion or ulcer is an eating or gnawing away of tissue; decubitus ulcer

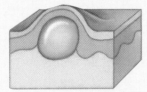

A papule is a solid, circumscribed, elevated area on the skin; pimple

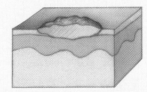

A crust is a dry, serous or seropurulent, brown, yellow, red, or green exudation that is seen in secondary lesions; eczema

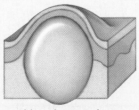

A nodule is a larger papule; acne vulgaris

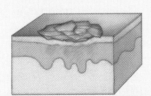

A scale is a thin, dry flake of cornified epithelial cells; psoriasis

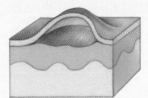

A vesicle is a small fluid filled sac; blister.
A bulla is a large vesicle.

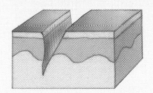

A fissure is a crack-like sore or slit that extends through the epidermis into the dermis; athlete's foot

FIGURE 3–52

Skin signs are objective evidence of an illness or disorder. They can be seen, measured, or felt.

✔PATHOLOGY CHECKPOINT

Following is a concise list of the pathology-related terms that you've seen in the chapter. Review this checklist to make sure that you are familiar with the meaning of each term before moving on to the next section.

Conditions and Symptoms

- ❏ acne
- ❏ acrochordon
- ❏ actinic dermatitis
- ❏ albinism
- ❏ alopecia
- ❏ anhidrosis
- ❏ avulsion
- ❏ basal cell carcinoma
- ❏ bite
- ❏ boil
- ❏ bulla
- ❏ burn
- ❏ callus
- ❏ candidiasis
- ❏ carbuncle
- ❏ causalgia
- ❏ cellulites
- ❏ cicatrix
- ❏ comedo
- ❏ corn
- ❏ cyst
- ❏ decubitus
- ❏ dehiscence
- ❏ dermatitis
- ❏ dermomycosis
- ❏ ecchymosis
- ❏ eczema
- ❏ erythema
- ❏ erythroderma
- ❏ eschar
- ❏ excoriation
- ❏ exudate
- ❏ folliculitis
- ❏ herpes simplex
- ❏ hidradenitis
- ❏ hives
- ❏ hyperhydrosis
- ❏ icteric
- ❏ impetigo
- ❏ jaundice
- ❏ keloid
- ❏ lentigo
- ❏ leukoderma
- ❏ leukoplakia
- ❏ lupus
- ❏ melanocarcinoma
- ❏ melanoma
- ❏ miliaria
- ❏ mole
- ❏ onychitis
- ❏ onychomycosis
- ❏ pachyderma
- ❏ paronychia
- ❏ pediculosis
- ❏ petechiae
- ❏ pruritus
- ❏ psoriasis
- ❏ purpura
- ❏ roseola
- ❏ rubella
- ❏ rubeola
- ❏ scabies
- ❏ scar
- ❏ scleroderma
- ❏ seborrhea
- ❏ senile keratosis
- ❏ striae
- ❏ telangiectasia
- ❏ thermanesthesia
- ❏ tinea
- ❏ trichomycosis
- ❏ ulcer
- ❏ varicella
- ❏ vitiligo
- ❏ wart
- ❏ wound
- ❏ xanthoderma
- ❏ xanthoma
- ❏ xeroderma
- ❏ xerosis

Diagnosis and Treatment

- ❏ autograft
- ❏ dermatome
- ❏ hypodermic (injection)
- ❏ intradermal (injection)
- ❏ subcutaneous (injection)
- ❏ subungual
- ❏ rhytidoplasty

DRUG HIGHLIGHTS

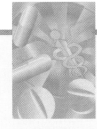

Drugs that are used for dermatologic diseases or disorders include emollient, keratolytic, local anesthetic, antipruritic, antibiotic, antifungal, antiviral, anti-inflammatory, and antiseptic agents. Other drugs include Retin-A, Rogaine, and Botulinum toxin type A.

Emollients

Substances that are generally oily in nature. These substances are used for dry skin caused by aging, excessive bathing, and psoriasis.

Examples: Dermassage and Desitin.

Keratolytics

Agents that cause or promote loosening of horny (keratin) layers of the skin. These agents may be used for acne, warts, psoriasis, corns, calluses, and fungal infections.

Examples: Duofilm, Keralyt, and Compound W.

Local Anesthetic Agents

Agents that inhibit the conduction of nerve impulses from sensory nerves and thereby reduce pain and discomfort. These agents may be used topically to reduce discomfort associated with insect bites, burns, and poison ivy.

Examples: Solarcaine, Xylocaine, and Dyclone.

Antipruritic Agents

Agents that prevent or relieve itching.

Examples: Topical—PBZ (tripelennamine HCl); Oral—Benadryl (diphenhydramine HCl) and Atarax (hydroxyzine HCl).

Antibiotic Agents

Agents that destroy or stop the growth of microorganisms. These agents are used to prevent infection associated with minor skin abrasions and to treat superficial skin infections and acne. Several antibiotic agents are combined in a single product to take advantage of the different antimicrobial spectrum of each drug.

Examples: Neosporin, Polysporin, and Mycitracin.

Antifungal Agents

Agents that destroy or inhibit the growth of fungi and yeast. These agents are used to treat fungus and/or yeast infection of the skin, nails, and scalp.

Examples: Fungizone (amphotericin B), Lotrimin (clotrimazole) and Lamisil (terbinafine).

Antiviral Agents

Agents that combat specific viral diseases. *Zovirax (acyclovir)* is used in the treatment of herpes simplex virus types 1 and 2, varicella-zoster, Epstein-Barr, and cytomegalovirus. *Relenza (zanamivir)* has antiviral activity against influenza A and B viruses.

Anti-inflammatory Agents

Agents used to relieve the swelling, tenderness, redness, and pain of inflammation. Topically applied corticosteroids are used in the treatment of dermatitis and psoriasis.

Examples: Hydrocortisone, Decadron (dexamethasone), and Temovate (clobetasol propionate).

Oral corticosteroids are used in the treatment of contact dermatitis, such as in poison ivy, when the symptoms are severe.

Example: Sterapred (prednisone) 12-day unipak.

Antiseptic Agents

Agents that prevent or inhibit the growth of pathogens. Antiseptics are generally applied to the surface of living tissue.

Examples: Isopropyl alcohol and Zephrian (benzalkonium chloride)

Other Drugs

Retin-A (tretinoin) is available as a cream, gel, or liquid. It is used in the treatment of acne vulgaris. *Rogaine (minoxidil)* is available as a topical solution to stimulate hair growth. It was first approved as a treatment of male pattern baldness.

Botulinum Toxin Type A (Botox Cosmetic) is approved by the FDA to temporarily improve the appearance of moderate to severe frown lines between the eyebrows (glabellar lines). Small doses of a sterile, purified botulinum toxin are injected into the affected muscles and block the release of the chemical acetylcholine that would otherwise signal the muscle to contract. The toxin thus paralyzes or weakens the injected muscle.

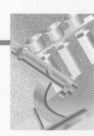

DIAGNOSTIC & LAB TESTS

TEST	DESCRIPTION
tuberculosis skin tests (tū-bĕr″ kū-lō′ sĭs)	Tests performed to identify the presence of the *Tubercle bacilli*. The tine, Heaf, or Mantoux test may be used. The tine test and Heaf test are intradermal tests performed using a sterile, disposable, multiple-puncture lancet. The tuberculin is on metal tines that are pressed into the skin. A hardened raised area at the test site 48 to 72 hours later indicates the presence of the pathogens in the blood.
	In the **Mantoux** test 0.1 mL of purified protein derivative (PPD) tuberculin is intradermally injected. Test results are read 48 to 72 hours after administration.
sweat test (chloride) (swĕt)	A test performed on **sweat** to determine the level of chloride concentration on the skin. In **cystic fibrosis**, there is an increase in skin chloride.
Tzanck test (tsănk)	A microscopic examination of a small piece of tissue that has been surgically scraped from a pustule. The specimen is placed on a slide and stained, and the type of viral infection can be identified.
wound culture (woond)	A test done on wound exudate to determine the presence of microorganisms. An effective antibiotic can be prescribed for identified microbes.
biopsy (skin) (bī′ ŏp-sē)	Any skin lesion that exhibits signs or characteristics of malignancy may be excised and examined microscopically to establish a diagnosis. Usually only a small piece of living tissue is needed for examination.

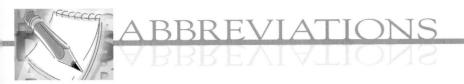

ABBREVIATIONS

ABBREVIATION	MEANING	ABBREVIATION	MEANING
decub	decubitus	SLE	systemic lupus erythematosus
derm	dermatology	staph	staphylococcus
FB	foreign body	STD	skin test done
FUO	fever of undetermined origin	strep	streptococcus
		STSG	split thickness skin graft
H	hypodermic	subcu, subq	subcutaneous
Hx	history		
ID	intradermal	T	temperature
I&D	incision and drainage	TIMS	topical immunomodulators
NPUAP	National Pressure Ulcer Advisory Panel	TTS	transdermal therapeutic system
		ung	ointment
PUVA	psoralen-ultraviolet light	UV	ultraviolet
SG	skin graft		

STUDY AND REVIEW

Anatomy and Physiology

Write your answers to the following questions. Do not refer to the text.

1. Name the primary organ of the integumentary system. _____

2. Name the four accessory structures of the integumentary system.

   a. _____   b. _____

   c. _____   d. _____

3. State the four main functions of the skin.

   a. _____   b. _____

   c. _____   d. _____

4. The skin is essentially composed of two layers, the _____ and the

   _____.

5. Name the four strata of the epidermis.

   a. _____   b. _____

   c. _____   d. _____

6. _____ is a protein substance found in the dead cells of the epidermis.

7. _____ is a pigment that gives color to the skin.

8. The _____ is known as the corium or true skin.

9. Name the two layers of the part of the skin described in question 8.

   a. _____   b. _____

10. The crescent-shaped white area of the nail is the _____.

Word Parts

1. In the spaces provided, write the definition of these prefixes, roots, combining forms, and suffixes. Do not refer to the listings of medical words. Leave blank those words you cannot define.

2. After completing as many as you can, refer back to the medical word listings to check your work. For each word missed or left blank, write the word and its

definition several times on the margins of these pages or on a separate sheet of paper.

3. To maximize the learning process, it is to your advantage to do the following exercises as directed. To refer to the word building section before completing these exercises invalidates the learning process.

PREFIXES

Give the definitions of the following prefixes:

1. a-, an- _____
2. auto- _____
3. ec- _____
4. de- _____
5. ex- _____
6. hyper- _____
7. hypo- _____
8. intra- _____
9. par- _____
10. sub- _____

ROOTS AND COMBINING FORMS

Give the definitions of the following roots and combining forms:

1. acr/o _____
2. actin _____
3. aden _____
4. albin _____
5. carcin _____
6. caus _____
7. chym _____
8. coriat _____
9. cutane _____
10. derm _____
11. derm/a _____
12. dermat _____
13. dermat/o _____
14. derm/o _____
15. lopec _____
16. erythr/o _____
17. hidr _____
18. icter _____
19. kel _____
20. kerat _____
21. leuk/o _____
22. log _____
23. melan _____
24. melan/o _____
25. myc _____
26. onych _____
27. cellul _____
28. onych/o _____
29. pachy _____
30. pedicul _____

31. chord _____

32. rhytid/o _____

33. scler/o _____

34. seb/o _____

35. senile _____

36. therm _____

37. vuls _____

38. trich/o _____

39. ungu _____

40. xanth/o _____

41. xer/o _____

42. cubit _____

43. follicul _____

44. integument _____

45. jaund _____

46. plak _____

47. miliar _____

48. prurit _____

49. tel _____

50. ang/i _____

SUFFIXES

Give the definitions of the following suffixes:

1. -al _____

2. -algia _____

3. -on _____

4. -us _____

5. -derma _____

6. -ary _____

7. -esthesia _____

8. -graft _____

9. -ia _____

10. -ic _____

11. -ion _____

12. -ism _____

13. -ist _____

14. -itis _____

15. -logy _____

16. -ectasia _____

17. -oid _____

18. -oma _____

19. -osis _____

20. -ous _____

21. -plasty _____

22. -rrhea _____

23. -tome _____

Identifying Medical Terms

In the spaces provided, write the medical terms for the following meanings:

1. _____ Inflammation of the skin caused by exposure to actinic rays

2. _____ Pertaining to the skin

3. _____ Inflammation of the skin

4. _____ The study of the skin

5. _____ Severe itching

6. _____ Condition of excessive sweating

7. _____ Pertaining to under the skin

8. _____ Pertaining to jaundice

9. _____ Inflammation of the nail

10. _____ Thick skin

11. _____ Inability to distinguish between the sensations of heat and cold

12. _____ Yellow skin

Spelling

In the spaces provided, write the correct spelling of these misspelled terms.

1. caualgia _____

2. dermomcosis _____

3. echymosis _____

4. exoriation _____

5. hyprhidrosis _____

6. melnoma _____

7. onychomyosis _____

8. rhytdoplasty _____

9. sleroderma _____

10. sebrrhea _____

Matching

Select the appropriate lettered meaning for each word listed below.

_____ 1. acne

_____ 2. alopecia

_____ 3. cicatrix

_____ 4. comedo

_____ 5. decubitus

_____ 6. dehiscence

_____ 7. exudate

_____ 8. leukoplakia

_____ 9. petechiae

_____ 10. pruritus

a. Small, pinpoint, purplish hemorrhagic spots on the skin

b. The production of pus or serum

c. A severe itching

d. An inflammatory condition of the sebaceous gland and the hair follicles

e. The scar left after the healing of a wound

f. Loss of hair, baldness

g. White spots or patches formed on the mucous membrane of the tongue or cheek

h. Blackhead

i. The separation or bursting open of a surgical wound

j. A bedsore

k. A slough, scab

Abbreviations

Place the correct word, phrase, or abbreviation in the space provided.

1. fever of undetermined origin _____

2. transdermal therapeutic system _____

3. H _____

4. incision and drainage _____

5. skin graft _____

6. ID _____

7. temperature _____

8. ultraviolet _____

9. FB _____

10. PUVA _____

Diagnostic and Laboratory Tests

Select the best answer to each multiple choice question. Circle the letter of your choice.

1. The _____ _____ is an intradermal test performed using a sterile, disposable, multiple puncture lancet.
   a. sweat test
   b. Mantoux test
   c. tine test
   d. Tzanck test

2. A test done on wound exudate to determine the presence of microorganisms is:
   a. sweat test
   b. biopsy
   c. Tzanck test
   d. wound culture

3. A microscopic examination of a small piece of tissue that has been surgically scraped from a pustule is:
   a. Tzanck test
   b. sweat test
   c. biopsy
   d. wound culture

4. Tests performed to identify the presence of the *Tubercle bacilli* include the:
   a. tine, Heaf, and sweat
   b. tine, Heaf, and Mantoux
   c. tine, Tzanck, and Mantoux
   d. tine, Mantoux, and sweat

5. The _____ test may be used to determine the level of chloride concentration on the skin.
   a. sweat
   b. Tzanck
   c. tine
   d. Mantoux

CASE STUDY — CONTACT DERMATITIS, POISON IVY

Read the following case study and then answer the questions that follow.

A 42-year-old male was seen by a dermatologist; the following is a synopsis of his visit.

Present History: The patient states that he apparently came into contact with poison ivy while working in the yard.

Signs and Symptoms: Moderate itching at first and then severe (pruritus); small blisters (vesicles) on right and left forearms; redness of skin (erythroderma) with moderate to severe swelling (edema) of surrounding tissue.

Diagnosis: Contact Dermatitis Poison Ivy. See Figure 3–21 and Figure 3–53.

Treatment: Antipruritic agent—hydroxyzine HCl 25 mg Tab; corticosteroid therapy—Temovate 0.05% cream—apply twice a day to affected area; and Sterapred 12 day unipak—take as directed.

Prevention: Stay away from poison ivy. When working outside in the yard, wear clothing that covers arms and legs. After working in the yard, immediately take a bath or shower to remove any possible contamination of skin with poison ivy.

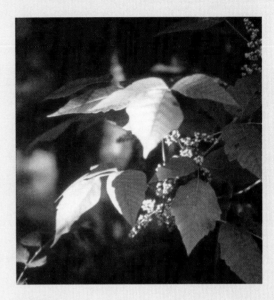

FIGURE 3–53

Poison ivy. (Source: Pearson Education/PH College.)

CASE STUDY QUESTIONS

1. When the patient states that his itching has become severe, you would note this in his chart as _____.

2. It is noted in the chart that small blisters appear on the right and left forearms. What is the medical term for blisters? _____

3. A person who is sensitive to poison ivy may develop what condition? _____

4. An _____ agent is used to help relieve itching.

5. Temovate 0.05% cream is a form of _____ therapy.

6. Prevention is a key concept in today's health care delivery system. List three preventive measures that this patient might have to use to help and/or prevent his condition.

   a. _____
   b. _____
   c. _____

7. What is the medical term for redness of the skin? _____

8. What medical term do you use to chart "moderate to severe swelling of surrounding tissue"? _____

MedMedia
Wrap-Up

www.prenhall.com/rice

Additional interactive resources and activities for this chapter can be found on the Companion Website. For animations, videos, audio glossary, and review, access the accompanying CD-ROM in this book.

Audio Glossary
Medical Terminology Exercises & Activities
Pathology Spotlights
Terminology Translator
Animations
Videos

Objectives
Medical Terminology Exercises & Activities
Audio Glossary
Drug Updates
Medical Terminology in the News

THE SKELETAL SYSTEM 4

OUTLINE

OBJECTIVES

On completion of this chapter, you will be able to:

- Describe the skeletal system.
- Describe various types of body movement.
- Describe the vertebral column.
- Identify abnormal curvatures of the spine.
- Describe the male and female pelvis.
- Describe various types of fractures.
- Describe skeletal differences of the child and the older adult.
- Analyze, build, spell, and pronounce medical words.
- Describe each of the conditions presented in the Pathology Spotlights.
- Complete the Pathology Checkpoint.
- Review Drug Highlights presented in this chapter.
- Provide the description of diagnostic and laboratory tests related to the skeletal system.
- Identify and define selected abbreviations.
- Successfully complete the study and review section.

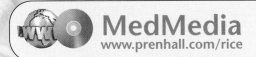

MedMedia
www.prenhall.com/rice

Additional interactive resources and activities for this chapter can be found on the Companion Website. For Terminology Translator, animations, videos, audio glossary, and review, access the accompanying CD-ROM in this book.

Anatomy and Physiology Overview

The skeletal system is composed of 206 **bones** that, together with **cartilage** and **ligaments**, make up the **framework** or skeleton of the body. The skeleton can be divided into two main groups of bones: the **axial skeleton** consisting of 80 bones and the **appendicular skeleton** with the remaining 126 bones (see Fig. 4–1). The principal bones of the axial skeleton are the skull, spine, ribs, and sternum. The shoulder girdle, arms, and hands and the pelvic girdle, legs, and feet are the primary bones of the appendicular skeleton.

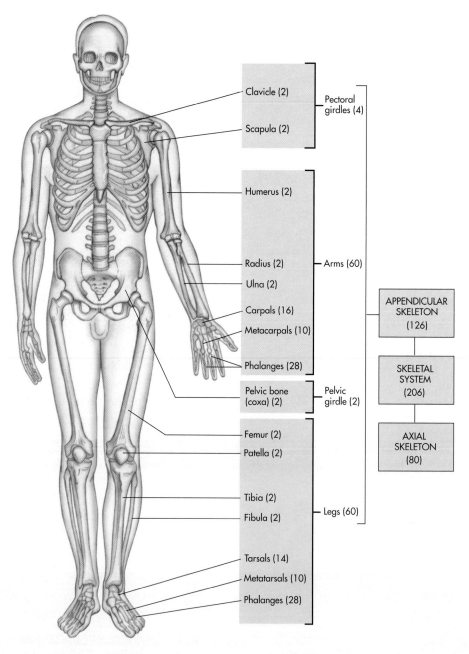

FIGURE 4–1

The principal bones of the appendicular skeleton.

THE SKELETAL SYSTEM

Organ/Structure	Primary Functions
Bones	Provide shape, support, protection, and the framework of the body
	Serve as a storage place for mineral salts, calcium, and phosphorus
	Play an important role in the formation of blood cells
	Provide areas for the attachment of skeletal muscles
	Help make movement possible
Cartilages	Form the major portion of the embryonic skeleton and part of the skeleton in adults
Ligaments	Connect the articular ends of bones, binding them together and facilitating or limiting motion
	Connect cartilage and other structures
	Serve to support or attach fascia or muscles

BONES

The **bones** are the primary organs of the skeletal system and are composed of about 50% water and 50% solid matter. The solid matter in bone is a calcified, rigid substance known as **osseous tissue**.

Classification of Bones

Bones are classified according to their shapes. See Figure 4–2. Table 4–1 classifies the bones and gives an example of each type.

Functions of Bones

The following are the main functions of bones:

1. Provide shape, support, and the framework of the body
2. Provide protection for internal organs
3. Serve as a storage place for mineral salts, calcium, and phosphorus
4. Play an important role in the formation of blood cells as **hemopoiesis** takes place in the bone marrow
5. Provide areas for the attachment of skeletal muscles
6. Help to make movement possible through **articulation**

The Structure of a Long Bone

Long bones, such as the tibia, femur, humerus, or radius, have most of the features found in all bones. These features are shown in Figure 4–3.

TABLE 4–1   CLASSIFICATIONS OF BONE

Shape	Example of This Classification
Flat	Ribs, scapula, parts of the pelvic girdle, bones of the skull
Long	Tibia, femur, humerus, radius
Short	Carpal, tarsal
Irregular	Vertebrae, ossicles of the ear
Sesamoid	Patella
Sutural or Wormian	Between the flat bones of the skull

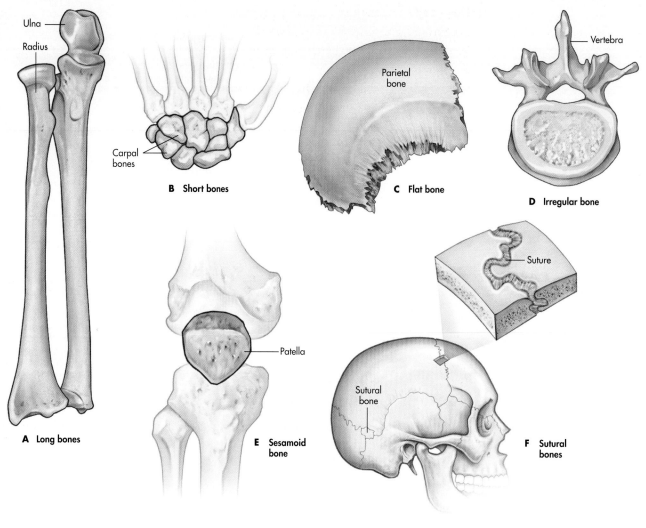

FIGURE 4–2

Classification of bones by shape.

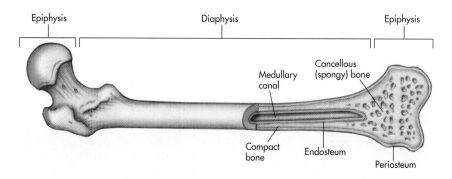

FIGURE 4–3

The features found in a long bone.

Epiphysis. The ends of a developing bone

Diaphysis. The shaft of a long bone

Periosteum. The membrane that forms the covering of bones except at their articular surfaces

Compact bone. The dense, hard layer of bone tissue

Medullary canal. A narrow space or cavity throughout the length of the diaphysis

Endosteum. A tough, connective tissue membrane lining the medullary canal and containing the bone marrow

Cancellous or spongy bone. The reticular tissue that makes up most of the volume of bone

Bone Markings

There are certain commonly used terms that describe the **markings of bones**. These markings are listed for your better understanding of their role in joining bones together, providing areas for muscle attachments, and serving as a passageway for blood vessels, ligaments, and nerves See Table 4–2.

JOINTS AND MOVEMENT

A **joint** is an articulation, a place where two or more bones connect. See Figure 4–4. The manner in which bones connect determines the type of movement allowed at the joint. Joints are classified as:

Synarthrosis. Does not permit movement. The bones are in close contact with each other and there is no joint cavity. An example is the *cranial sutures*.

Amphiarthrosis. Permits very slight movement. An example of this type of joint is the *vertebrae*.

Diarthrosis. Allows free movement in a variety of directions. Examples of this type of joint are the *knee*, *hip*, *elbow*, *wrist*, and *foot*.

TABLE 4–2 BONE MARKINGS

Marking	Description of the Bone Structure
Condyle	A rounded process that enters into the formation of a joint, articulation
Crest	A ridge on a bone
Fissure	A slit-like opening between two bones
Foramen	An opening in the bone for blood vessels, ligaments, and nerves
Fossa	A shallow depression in or on a bone
Head	The rounded end of a bone
Meatus	A tube-like passage or canal
Process	An enlargement or protrusion of a bone
Sinus	An air cavity within certain bones
Spine	A pointed, sharp, slender process
Sulcus	A groove, furrow, depression, or fissure
Trochanter	A very large process of the femur
Tubercle	A small, rounded process
Tuberosity	A large, rounded process

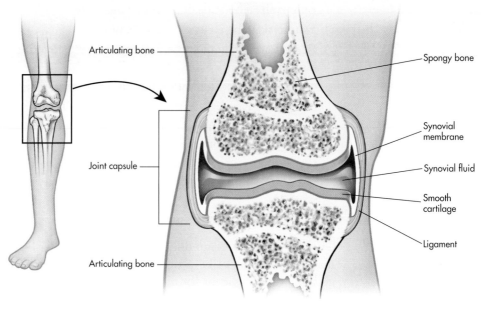

FIGURE 4–4

Typical joint.

The following terms describe types of body movement that occur at the **diarthrotic joints** (Fig. 4–5):

Abduction. The process of moving a body part away from the middle

Adduction. The process of moving a body part toward the middle

Circumduction. The process of moving a body part in a circular motion

Dorsiflexion. The process of bending a body part backward

Eversion. The process of turning outward

Extension. The process of straightening a flexed limb

Flexion. The process of bending a limb

Inversion. The process of turning inward

Pronation. The process of lying prone or face downward; also the process of turning the hand so the palm faces downward

Protraction. The process of moving a body part forward

Retraction. The process of moving a body part backward

Rotation. The process of moving a body part around a central axis

Supination. The process of lying supine or face upward; also the process of turning the palm or foot upward

THE VERTEBRAL COLUMN

The **vertebral column** is composed of a series of separate bones (**vertebrae**) connected in such a way as to form four spinal curves. These curves have been identified as the cervical, thoracic, lumbar, and sacral. The cervical curve consists of the first 7 verte-

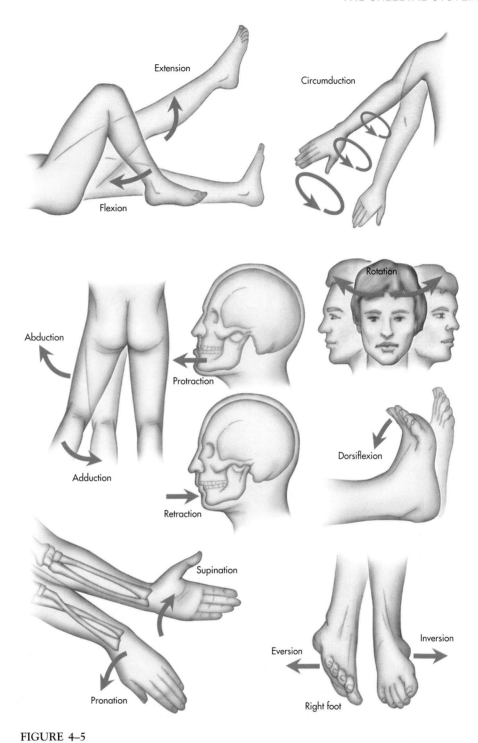

FIGURE 4–5

Types of body movements.

brae, the *thoracic curve* consists of the next 12 vertebrae, the *lumbar curve* consists of the next 5 vertebrae, and the *sacral curve* consists of the sacrum and coccyx (tailbone) (Fig. 4–6).

It is known that a curved structure has more strength than a straight structure. The spinal curves of the human body are most important, as they help support the weight of the body and provide the balance that is necessary to walk on two feet.

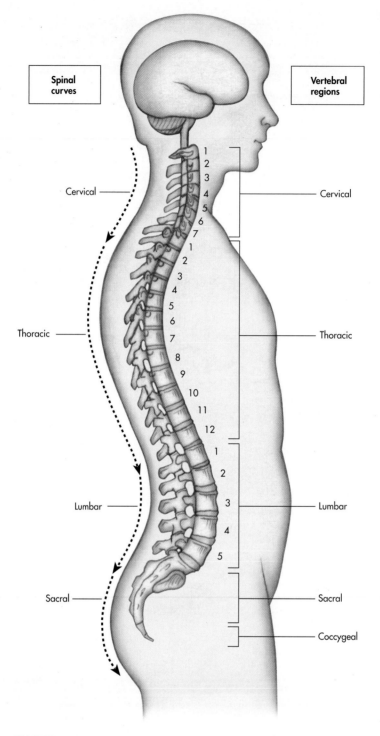

Spinal curves

Vertebral regions

Cervical

Cervical

1
2
3
4
5
6
7
1
2
3
4
5
6
7
8
9
10
11
12

Thoracic

Thoracic

1
2
3
4
5

Lumbar

Lumbar

Sacral

Sacral

Coccygeal

FIGURE 4–6

Vertebral regions, showing the four spinal curves.

THE MALE AND FEMALE PELVIS

The **pelvis** is the lower portion of the trunk of the body. It forms a basin bound anteriorly and laterally by the hip bones and posteriorly by the sacrum and coccyx.

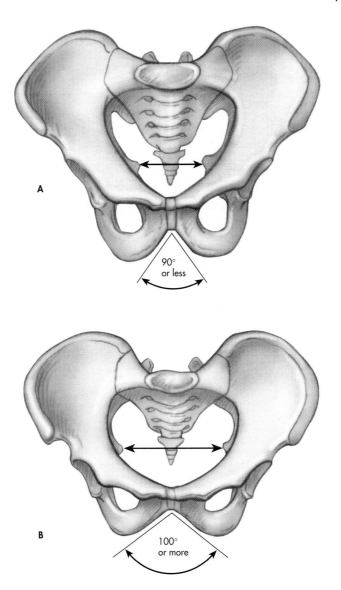

FIGURE 4–7

(A) The male pelvis is shaped like a funnel, forming a narrower outlet than the female. (B) The female pelvis is shaped like a basin.

The bony pelvis is formed by the sacrum, the coccyx, and the bones that form the hip and pubic arch, the ilium, pubis, and ischium. These bones are separate in the child, but become fused in adulthood.

The Male Pelvis

The **male pelvis** is shaped like a *funnel*, forming a narrower outlet than the female. It is heavier and stronger than the female pelvis; therefore, it is more suited for lifting and running. See Figure 4–7A.

The Female Pelvis

The **female pelvis** is shaped like a *basin*. It may be oval to round, and it is wider than the male pelvis. The female pelvis is constructed to accommodate the fetus during pregnancy and to facilitate its downward passage through the pelvic cavity in childbirth. In general the female pelvis is broader and lighter than the male pelvis. See Figure 4–7B.

LIFE SPAN CONSIDERATIONS

▓ THE CHILD

Bone begins to develop during the second month of fetal life as cartilage cells enlarge, break down, disappear, and are replaced by bone-forming cells called **osteoblasts**. Most bones of the body are formed by this process, known as **endochondral ossification**. In this process, the bone cells deposit organic substances in the spaces vacated by cartilage to form bone matrix. As this process proceeds, blood vessels form within the bone and deposit salts such as calcium and phosphorus that serve to harden the developing bone.

The **epiphyseal plate** is the center for longitudinal bone growth in children. See Figure 4–8. It is possible to determine the biological age of a child from the development of epiphyseal ossification centers as shown radiographically.

About 3 years from the onset of puberty the ends of the long bones (**epiphyses**) knit securely to their shafts (**diaphysis**), and further growth can no longer take place.

The bones of children are more resilient, tend to bend, and before breaking may become deformed. Fracture healing occurs more quickly in children because there is a rich blood supply to bones and their periosteum is thick and osteogenic activity is high.

Calcium is critical to the strength of bones. The daily recommendations of calcium by age group are:

1 to 3 years	500 mg
4 to 8 years	800 mg
9 to 13 years	1300 mg
14 to 18 years	1300 mg

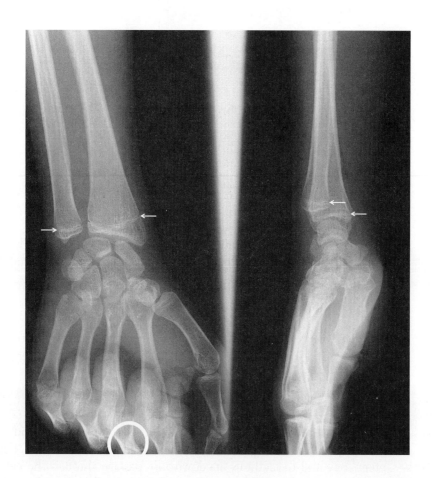

FIGURE 4–8

Epiphyseal plate (arrows). (Courtesy of Teresa Resch.)

■ THE OLDER ADULT

Women build bone until about age 35, then begin to lose about 1% of bone mass annually. Men usually start losing bone mass 10 to 20 years later. Most of the skeletal system changes that take place during the aging process involve changes in connective tissue. There is a loss of bone mass and bone strength due to the loss of bone mineral content during later life. Calcium salts may be deposited in the matrix and cartilage becomes hard and brittle.

Age-related **osteoporosis**, loss of bone mass, is often seen in older women and men. Other changes that may occur involve the joints as there is diminished viscosity of the synovial fluid, degeneration of collagen and elastin cells, outgrowth of cartilaginous clusters in response to continuous wear and tear, and formation of scar tissues and calcification in the joint capsules.

Low levels of calcium can make people more susceptible to osteoporosis and stress fractures, especially those that are commonly seen in the older adult. Bone healing in the older adult is slower and impaired due to osteoblasts being less able to use calcium to restructure bone tissue. The National Academy of Sciences suggests that people 51 and older consume 1200 mg of calcium per day to help strengthen their bones. See Table 4–3 for good sources of calcium.

TABLE 4–3 GOOD SOURCES OF CALCIUM

1 cup skim milk	300 mg
1 cup yogurt	450 mg
1 cup calcium-fortified orange juice	300 mg
1 ounce cheddar cheese	205 mg
1 ounce Swiss cheese	270 mg
1 cup tofu (processed with calcium sulfate)	520 mg
1 cup turnip greens, cooked	200 mg
3 ounces canned salmon (with bones)	205 mg
7-inch homemade waffle	179 mg
1 cup broccoli, cooked	90 mg

Dairy foods supply 75% of all the calcium in the U.S. food supply. People who get 2 to 3 servings of dairy products a day are most likely meeting the recommended requirements. For those who do not like milk or dairy products, there are other ways of getting enough calcium per day.

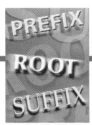

BUILDING YOUR MEDICAL VOCABULARY

This section provides the foundation for learning medical terminology. Medical words can be made up of four different types of word parts:

- Prefixes (P)
- Roots (R)
- Combining forms (CF)
- Suffixes (S)

By connecting various word parts in an organized sequence, thousands of words can be built and learned. In this text the word list is alphabetized so one can see the variety of meanings created when common prefixes and suffixes are repeatedly applied to certain word roots and/or combining forms. Words shown in pink are additional words related to the content of this chapter that are not built from word parts. These words are included to enhance your vocabulary. Note: an asterisk icon ✱ indicates terms that are covered in the Pathology Spotlights section in this chapter.

MEDICAL WORD	WORD PARTS (WHEN APPLICABLE)			DEFINITION
	Part	Type	Meaning	
acetabular (ăs″ ĕ-tăb′ ū-lăr)	acetabul -ar	R S	vinegar cup pertaining to	The cup-shaped socket of the hipbone into which the thighbone fits
achondroplasia (ă-kŏn″ drō-plā′ sĭ-ă)	a chondr/o -plasia	P CF S	without cartilage formation	A defect in the formation of cartilage at the epiphyses of long bones
acroarthritis (ăk″ rō-ăr-thrī′ tĭs)	acr/o arthr -itis	CF R S	extremity joint inflammation	Inflammation of the joints of the hands or feet
acromion (ă-krō′ mĭ-ŏn)	acr -omion	R S	extremity, point shoulder	The projection of the spine of the scapula that forms the point of the shoulder and articulates with the clavicle
ankylosis (ăng″ kĭ-lō′ sĭs)	ankyl -osis	R S	stiffening, crooked condition of	A condition of stiffening of a joint
arthralgia (ăr-thrăl′ jĭ-ă)	arthr -algia	R S	joint pain	Pain in a joint
arthritis (ăr-thrī′ tĭs)	arthr -itis	R S	joint inflammation	Inflammation of a joint. ✱ See Pathology Spotlight: Arthritis.
arthrocentesis (ăr″ thrō-sĕn-tē′ sĭs)	arthr/o -centesis	CF S	joint surgical puncture	Surgical puncture of a joint for removal of fluid
arthroplasty (ăr″ thrō-plăs′ tē)	arthr/o -plasty	CF S	joint surgical repair	Surgical repair of a joint
arthroscope (ăr-thrŏs′ kōp)	arthr/o -scope	CF S	joint instrument	An instrument used to examine the interior of a joint
bone marrow transplant (bōn măr′ ō trăns′ plănt)				The surgical process of transferring bone marrow from a donor to a patient
bursa (bŭr′ sah)				A small space between muscles, tendons, and bones that is lined with synovial membrane and contains a fluid, synovia
bursitis (bŭr-sī′ tĭs)	burs -itis	R S	a pouch inflammation	Inflammation of a bursa
calcaneal (kăl-kā′ nē-ăl)	calcan/e -al	CF S	heel bone pertaining to	Pertaining to the heel bone

MEDICAL WORD	WORD PARTS (WHEN APPLICABLE)			DEFINITION
	Part	Type	Meaning	
calcium (kăl′ sĭ-ŭm)				A mineral that is essential for bone growth, teeth development, blood coagulation, and many other functions
carpal (kär′ pəl)	carp -al	R S	wrist pertaining to	Pertaining to the wristbone
carpal tunnel syndrome (kär′ pĕl tŭn′ ĕl sĭn′ drōm)				A condition caused by compression of the median nerve by the carpal ligament; symptoms: soreness, tenderness, weakness, pain, tingling, and numbness at the wrist. ✳ See Figure 4–14 in Pathology Spotlight: Carpal Tunnel Syndrome.
cartilage (kär′ tĭ-lĭj)	cartil -age	R S	gristle related to	A specialized type of fibrous connective tissue present in adults, which forms the major portion of the embryonic skeleton
cast (kăst)				A type of material, made of plaster of paris, sodium silicate, starch, or dextrin used to immobilize a fractured bone, a dislocation, or a sprain
chondral (kŏn′ drăl)	chondr -al	R S	cartilage pertaining to	Pertaining to cartilage
chondrocostal (kŏn″ drō-kŏs′ tăl)	chondr/o cost -al	CF R S	cartilage rib pertaining to	Pertaining to the rib cartilage
clavicular (klă-vĭk′ ū-lăr)	clavicul -ar	R S	little key pertaining to	Pertaining to the clavicle
coccygeal (kŏk-sĭj′ ĭ-ăl)	coccyg/e -al	CF S	tailbone pertaining to	Pertaining to the coccyx
coccygodynia (kŏk-sĭ-gō-dĭn′ ĭ-ă)	coccyg/o -dynia	CF S	tailbone pain	Pain in the coccyx
collagen (kŏl′ă-jĕn)	coll/a -gen	CF S	glue formation, produce	A fibrous insoluble protein found in the connective tissue, skin, ligaments, and cartilage
connective (kə′ nĕk′ tĭv)	connect -ive	R S	to bind together nature of	That which connects or binds together
costal (kăst′ əl)	cost -al	R S	rib pertaining to	Pertaining to the rib

MEDICAL WORD	WORD PARTS (WHEN APPLICABLE)			DEFINITION
	Part	**Type**	**Meaning**	
costosternal (kŏs″ tō-stĕr′ năl)	cost/o stern -al	CF R S	rib sternum pertaining to	Pertaining to a rib and the sternum
craniectomy (krā″ nĭ-ĕk′ tŏ-mē)	cran/i -ectomy	CF S	skull excision	Surgical excision of a portion of the skull
craniotomy (krā″ nĭ-ŏt′ ō-mē)	crani/o -tomy	CF S	skull incision	Incision into the skull
dactylic (dăk′ tĭl′ ĭk)	dactyl -ic	R S	finger or toe pertaining to	Pertaining to the finger or toe
dactylogram (dăk-til′ə grăm)	dactyl/o -gram	CF S	finger or toe mark, record	A fingerprint
dislocation (dĭs″ lō-kā′ shŭn)	dis locat -ion	P R S	apart to place process	The displacement of a bone from a joint
femoral (fĕm′ ŏr-ăl)	femor -al	R S	femur pertaining to	Pertaining to the femur; the thighbone
fibular (fĭb′ ū-lăr)	fibul -ar	R S	fibula pertaining to	Pertaining to the fibula
fixation (fĭks-ā′ shŭn)	fixat -ion	R S	fastened process	The process of holding or fastening in a fixed position; making rigid, immobilizing
flatfoot (flăt fút)				An abnormal flatness of the sole and arch of the foot; also known as *pes planus*
genu valgum (jē′ nū văl gŭm)				Knock-knee
genu varum (jē′ nū vā′ rŭm)				Bowleg
gout (gowt)				A hereditary metabolic disease that is a form of acute arthritis; usually begins in the knee or foot but can affect any joint. ✳ See Pathology Spotlight: Arthritis.
hallux (hăl″ ŭks)				The big or great toe
hammertoe (hăm′ er-tō)				An acquired flexion deformity of the interphalangeal joint

MEDICAL WORD	WORD PARTS (WHEN APPLICABLE)			DEFINITION
	Part	**Type**	**Meaning**	
humeral (hū′ mĕr-ăl)	humer -al	R S	humerus pertaining to	Pertaining to the humerus
hydrarthrosis (hi″ drăr-thrō′ sĭs)	hydr arthr -osis	P R S	water joint condition of	Condition of fluid in a joint
iliac (ĭl′ ē-ăk)	ili -ac	R S	ilium pertaining to	Pertaining to the ilium
iliosacral (ĭl″ ĭ-ō-sā′ krăl)	ili/o sacr -al	CF R S	ilium sacrum pertaining to	Pertaining to the ilium and the sacrum
intercostal (ĭn″ tēr-kŏs′ tăl)	inter cost -al	R R S	between rib pertaining to	Pertaining to between the ribs
ischial (ĭs′ kĭ-al)	isch/i -al	CF S	ischium, hip pertaining to	Pertaining to the ischium, hip
ischialgia (ĭs″ kĭ-ăl′ jĭ-ă)	isch/i -algia	CF S	ischium, hip pain	Pain in the ischium, hip
kyphosis (kī-fō′ sĭs)	kyph -osis	R S	a hump condition of	Humpback
laminectomy (lăm″ ĭ-nĕk′ tō-mē)	lamin -ectomy	R S	lamina (thin plate) excision	Surgical excision of a vertebral posterior arch
ligament (lĭg′ ă-mĕnt)				A band of fibrous connective tissue that connects bones, cartilages, and other structures; also serves as a place for the attachment of fascia or muscle
lordosis (lŏr-dō′ sĭs)	lord -osis	R S	bending condition of	Abnormal anterior curvature of the spine
lumbar (lŭm′ băr)	lumb -ar	R S	loin pertaining to	Pertaining to the loins
lumbodynia (lŭm″ bō-dĭn′ ĭ-ă)	lumb/o -dynia	CF S	loin pain	Pain in the loins
mandibular (măn-dĭb′ ū-lăr)	mandibul -ar	R S	lower jawbone pertaining to	Pertaining to the lower jawbone
maxillary (măk′ sĭ-lĕr″ ē)	maxill -ary	R S	jawbone pertaining to	Pertaining to the upper jawbone

MEDICAL WORD	WORD PARTS (WHEN APPLICABLE)			DEFINITION
	Part	**Type**	**Meaning**	
meniscus (mĕn-ĭs′ kŭs)	menisc -us	R S	crescent pertaining to	Crescent-shaped interarticular fibrocartilage found in certain joints, especially the lateral and medial *menisci* (semilunar cartilages) of the knee joint
metacarpal (mĕt″ ă-kär′ pəl)	meta carp -al	P R S	beyond wrist pertaining to	Pertaining to the bones of the hand
metacarpectomy (mĕt″ ă-kăr-pĕk′ tō-mē)	meta carp -ectomy	P R S	beyond wrist excision	Surgical excision of one or more bones of the hand
myelitis (mī-ĕ-lī′ tĭs)	myel -itis	R S	marrow inflammation	Inflammation of the bone marrow
myeloma (mī-ē-lō′ mă)	myel -oma	R S	marrow tumor	A tumor of the bone marrow
myelopoiesis (mī′ ĕl-ō-poy-ē′ sĭs)	myel/o -poiesis	CF S	marrow formation	The formation of bone marrow
olecranal (ō-lĕk′ răn-ăl)	olecran -al	R S	elbow pertaining to	Pertaining to the elbow
osteoarthritis (ŏs″ tē-ō-ăr-thrī′ tĭs)	oste/o arthr -itis	CF R S	bone joint inflammation	Inflammation of the bone and joint. ✳ See Pathology Spotlight: Arthritis.
osteoblast (ŏs′ tē-ō-blăst″)	oste/o -blast	CF S	bone immature cell, germ cell	A bone-forming cell
osteocarcinoma (ŏs″ tē-ō-kăr″ sĭn-ō mă)	oste/o carcin -oma	CF R S	bone cancer tumor	A cancerous tumor of a bone; new growth of epithelial tissue
osteochondritis (ŏs″ tē-ō-kŏn-drī′ tĭs)	oste/o chondr -itis	CF R S	bone cartilage inflammation	Inflammation of the bone and cartilage
osteogenesis (ŏs″ tē-ō-jĕn′ ĕ-sĭs)	oste/o -genesis	CF S	bone formation, produce	The formation of bone
osteomalacia (ŏs″ tē-ō-măl-ā′ shĭ-ă)	oste/o -malacia	CF S	bone softening	Softening of the bones
osteomyelitis (ŏs″ tē-ō-mī″ ĕl-ī′ tĭs)	oste/o myel -itis	CF R S	bone marrow inflammation	Inflammation of the bone marrow. See Figure 4–9.

MEDICAL WORD	WORD PARTS (WHEN APPLICABLE)			DEFINITION
	Part	Type	Meaning	
osteopenia (ŏs″ tē-ō-pē′ nĭ-ă)	oste/o -penia	CF S	bone lack of	A lack of bone tissue
osteoporosis (ŏs″ tē-ō-por-ō′ sĭs)	oste/o por -osis	CF R S	bone a passage condition of	A condition that results in reduction of bone mass. ✶ See Figure 4–17 in Pathology Spotlight: Osteoporosis.
osteosarcoma (ŏs″ tē-ō-săr-kō′ mă)	oste/o sarc -oma	CF R S	bone flesh tumor	A malignant tumor of the bone; cancer arising from connective tissue
osteotome (ŏs′ tē-ō-tōm″)	oste/o -tome	CF S	bone instrument to cut	An instrument used for cutting bone
patellar (pă-tĕl′ ăr)	patell -ar	R S	kneecap pertaining to	Pertaining to the patella
pedal (pĕd′l)	ped -al	R S	foot pertaining to	Pertaining to the foot
periosteoedema (pĕr″ ĭ-ŏs″ tē-ō-ĕ-dē′ mă)	peri oste/o -edema	P CF S	around bone swelling	Swelling around a bone
phalangeal (fā-lăn′ jē-ăl)	phalang/e -al	CF S	closely knit row pertaining to	Pertaining to the bones of the fingers and the toes
phosphorus (fŏs′ fō-rŭs)	phos phor -us	R R S	light carrying pertaining to	A mineral that is essential in bone formation, muscle contraction, and many other functions
polyarthritis (pŏl″ ē-ăr-thrī′ tĭs)	poly arthr -itis	P R S	many, much joint inflammation	Inflammation of more than one joint
rachigraph (rā′ kĭ-grăf)	rach/i -graph	CF S	spine to write	An instrument used to measure the curvature of the spine
radial (rā′ dĭ-ăl)	rad/i -al	CF S	radius pertaining to	Pertaining to the radius
radiograph (rā′ dĭ-ō-grăf)	radi/o -graph	CF S	ray record	An x-ray photograph of a body part
reduction (rē-dŭk′ shŭn)	re duct -ion	P R S	back to lead process	The manipulative or surgical procedure used to correct a fracture or hernia

MEDICAL WORD	WORD PARTS (WHEN APPLICABLE)			DEFINITION
	Part	**Type**	**Meaning**	
rheumatoid arthritis (roo′ mă-toyd ăr-thrī′ tĭs)	rheumat -oid arthr -itis	R S R S	discharge resemble joint inflammation	A chronic systemic disease characterized by inflammation of the joints, stiffness, pain, and swelling that results in crippling deformities. ✱ See Pathology Spotlight: Arthritis.
rickets (rĭk′ ĕts)				A deficiency condition in children primarily caused by a lack of vitamin D; may also result from inadequate intake or excessive loss of calcium
scapular (skăp′ ū-lăr)	scapul -ar	R S	shoulder blade pertaining to	Pertaining to the shoulder blade
scoliosis (skō″ lĭ-ō′ sĭs)	scoli -osis	R S	curvature condition of	A condition of lateral curvature of the spine. ✱ See Pathology Spotlight: Abnormal Curvatures of the Spine.
spinal (spī′ năl)	spin -al	R S	spine pertaining to	Pertaining to the spine
splint (splĭnt)				An appliance used for fixation, support, and rest of an injured body part
spondylitis (spŏn-dĭl-ī′ tĭs)	spondyl -itis	R S	vertebra inflammation	Inflammation of one or more vertebrae
sprain (sprān)				Twisting of a joint that causes pain and disability
spur (spər)				A sharp or pointed projection, as on a bone
sternal (stēr′ năl)	stern -al	R S	sternum pertaining to	Pertaining to the sternum
sternotomy (stĕr-nŏt′ ō-mē)	stern/o -tomy	CF S	sternum incision	Surgical incision of the sternum
subclavicular (sŭb″ klă-vĭk′ ū-lăr)	sub clavicul -ar	P R S	under, beneath a little key pertaining to	Pertaining to beneath the clavicle
subcostal (sŭb-kŏs′ tăl)	sub cost -al	P R S	under, beneath rib pertaining to	Pertaining to beneath the ribs
submaxilla (sŭb″ măk-sĭl′ ă)	sub maxilla	P R	under, beneath jaw	The lower jaw or mandible

MEDICAL WORD	WORD PARTS (WHEN APPLICABLE)			DEFINITION
	Part	**Type**	**Meaning**	
symphysis (sĭm′ fĭ-sĭs)	sym -physis	P S	together growth	A growing together
tennis elbow (tĕn′ ĭs ĕl′ bō)				A chronic condition characterized by pain caused by excessive pronation and supination activities of the forearm; usually caused by strain, as in playing tennis
tenonitis (tĕn″ ō-nī′ tĭs)	tenon -itis	R S	tendon inflammation	Inflammation of a tendon
tibial (tĭb′ ĭ-ăl)	tibi -al	R S	tibia pertaining to	Pertaining to the tibia
traction (trăk′ shŭn)	tract -ion	P S	to draw process	The process of drawing or pulling on bones or muscles to relieve displacement and facilitate healing
ulnar (ŭl′ năr)	uln -ar	R S	elbow pertaining to	Pertaining to the elbow
ulnocarpal (ŭl″ nō-kăr′ păl)	uln/o carp -al	CF R S	elbow wrist pertaining to	Pertaining to the ulna side of the wrist
vertebral (vĕr′ tĕ-brăl)	vertebr -al	R S	vertebra pertaining to	Pertaining to a vertebra
vertebrosternal (vĕr″ tĕ-brō-ster′ năl)	vertebr/o stern -al	CF R S	vertebra sternum pertaining to	Pertaining to a vertebra and the sternum
xiphoid (zĭf′ oyd)	xiph -oid	R S	sword resemble	Resembling a sword

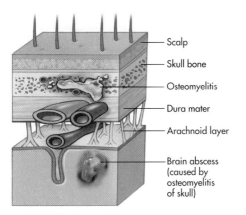
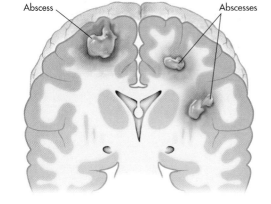

FIGURE 4–9

Abscess of the brain due to osteomyelitis.

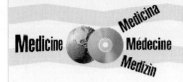

Terminology Translator

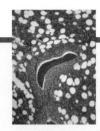

This feature, found on the accompanying CD-ROM, provides an innovative tool to translate medical words into Spanish, French, and German.

PATHOLOGY SPOTLIGHTS

Abnormal Curvatures of the Spine

Abnormal curvatures of the spine include scoliosis, lordosis, and kyphosis.

In scoliosis, there is an abnormal lateral curvature of the spine. This condition usually appears in adolescence, during periods of rapid growth. Treatment modalities may include the application of a cast, brace, traction, electrical stimulation, and/or surgery. See Figure 4–10C.

In lordosis, there is an abnormal anterior curvature of the spine. This condition may be referred to as "swayback" as the abdomen and buttocks protrude due to an exaggerated lumbar curvature. See Figure 4–10B.

In kyphosis, the normal thoracic curvature becomes exaggerated, producing a "humpback" appearance. This condition may be caused by a congenital defect, a disease process such as tuberculosis and/or syphilis, a malignancy, compression fracture, faulty posture, osteoarthritis, rheumatoid arthritis, rickets, osteoporosis, or other conditions. See Figure 4–10A.

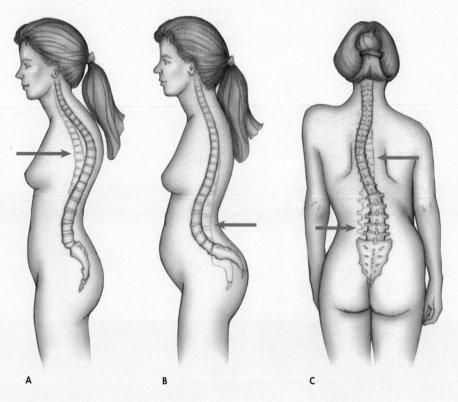

A   B   C

FIGURE 4–10

Abnormal curvatures of the spine: (A) kyphosis; (B) lordosis; and (C) scoliosis.

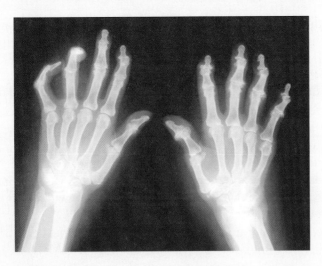

FIGURE 4–11

X-ray showing typical joint changes associated with osteoarthritis.
(Source: Getty Images/Stone Allstock.)

Arthritis

Arthritis is a disease that involves inflammation of one or more joints. Joint inflammation can result from various disease processes. Some of the most common include injury to a joint (including fracture), an attack on the joints by the body itself (an autoimmune disease), or "wear and tear" on joints.

Osteoarthritis is the most common type of arthritis in the United States. Osteoarthritis often results from years of accumulated "wear and tear" on joints, and tends to occur in the elderly in hips, knees, and finger joints. See Figure 4–11. In people over 55 years of age, women are more likely to suffer from osteoarthritis. Obesity, a history of trauma, and various genetic and metabolic diseases also increase the risk of osteoarthritis.

Gout, which is seen most often in men over 40 years of age, is caused by the formation of crystals in the joints, which leads to inflammation. See Figure 4–12. Autoimmune disorders, such as **rheumatoid arthritis** (see Figure 4–13), lupus, and scleroderma, can cause arthritis as well. In these diseases, the immune system attacks the joints.

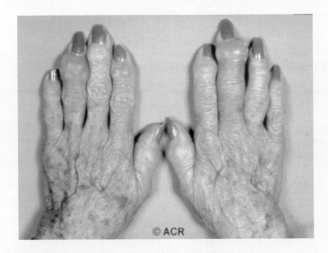

FIGURE 4–12

Gout of the finger joint. (Source: Reprinted from the Clinical Slide Collection on the Rheumatic Diseases, © 1991, 1995. Used by permission of the American College of Rheumatology.)

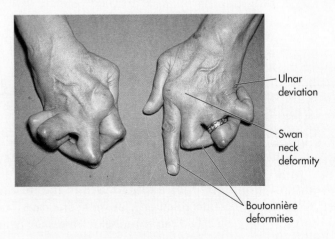

FIGURE 4–13

Typical hand deformities associated with rheumatoid arthritis.
(Source: Biophoto Associates/Photo Researchers, Inc.)

Arthritis can occur in both males and females of all ages. About 37 million people in America, almost 1 in 7 people, have arthritis of some kind. Symptoms of arthritis may include joint pain and swelling, morning stiffness, warmth around a joint, redness of the skin around a joint, and reduced ability to move a joint.

Arthritis treatment varies, depending on the particular cause, how severe the disease is, which joints are affected, to what degree the patient is affected, and the person's age, occupation, and daily activities. Treatment aims at reducing pain and discomfort and preventing further disability. Simple modifications in daily activities, along with adequate rest and appropriate forms of exercise may help to relieve some of the symptoms. For example, low impact aerobic exercise (such as swimming) can relieve joint strain. In other cases, more extensive therapies are needed. Treatment usually consists of exercise, heat or cold treatments, methods to protect the joints, various medications, and possibly surgery.

Medications to reduce joint pain and joint swelling in all types of arthritis may include acetaminophen, aspirin, nonsteroidal anti-inflammatory drugs (NSAIDs), corticosteroids, and other immunosuppressive drugs (drugs that suppress the immune system). The most recent breakthrough in rheumatoid arthritis treatment has been the development of "anti-biologic" medications that target individual molecules to reduce inflammation. These medications, which include etanercept (Enbrel) and infliximab (Remicade), are administered by injection or intravenously.

Carpal Tunnel Syndrome

Bounded by bones and ligaments, the carpal tunnel is a narrow passageway about as big around as one's thumb and located on the palm side of the wrist. This tunnel protects a main nerve to the hand and nine tendons that bend the fingers. When pressure is put on the median nerve it produces the numbness, pain and, eventually, hand weakness that characterize carpal tunnel syndrome. See Figure 4–14.

Injury or trauma to the area, including repetitive movement of the wrists, can cause swelling of the tissues and carpal tunnel syndrome. This type of repetitive-action injury may be caused by sports such as tennis and racquetball, or may occur during sewing, keyboarding, driving, assembly-line work, painting, writing, use of tools (especially hand tools or tools that vibrate), or similar activities. Some of the jobs associated with carpal tunnel syndrome include those that involve data entry or use of vibrating tools; mining; and professional musicians.

The condition occurs most often in people 30 to 60 years old, and is five times more common in women than men. Certain conditions, such as obesity, diabetes, and rheumatoid arthritis, have been associated with an increased risk of carpal tunnel syndrome.

Fortunately, for most people who develop carpal tunnel syndrome, proper treatment usually can relieve the pain and numbness and restore normal use of the wrists and hand. Treatment may include having the patient wear night splints for the wrist for several weeks. If unsuccessful, the splints are worn during the day and heat or cold compresses may be added. Other types of treatment include modifications in the work area. This may include ensuring that the keyboard is low enough so that the wrists aren't bent upwards during keyboarding, and modifying work duties or recreational activities. There are many specialized devices designed for the workplace to reduce the stress placed on the wrist and improve carpal tunnel syndrome.

Medications used in the treatment of carpal tunnel syndrome include NSAIDs such as ibuprofen or naproxen. The carpal tunnel may also be injected with corticosteroids. Surgery, called carpal tunnel release, may help those with carpal tunnel syndrome. This procedure cuts into the ligament to relieve pressure on the median nerve. Surgery has about an 85 percent success rate, depending on the severity of the problem. Surgery reduces the pressure on the nerve, but the damaged nerve must heal for the symptoms to improve. This can take months and in some cases the nerve may not fully heal. In severe cases, electromyography or nerve conduction studies may be used to follow the recovery of the nerve.

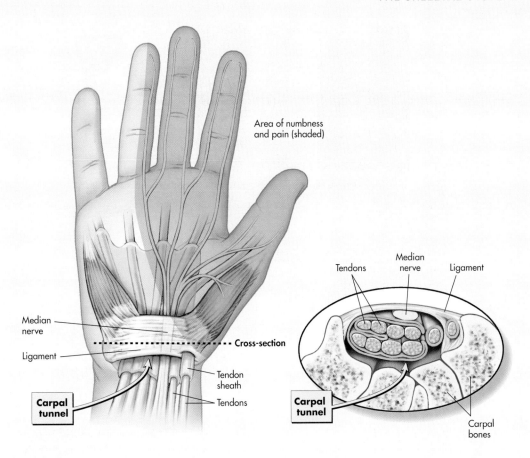

Area of numbness
and pain (shaded)

Median
nerve

Ligament

Cross-section

Carpal
tunnel

Tendon
sheath

Tendons

Tendons

Median
nerve

Ligament

Carpal
tunnel

Carpal
bones

FIGURE 4–14

Cross-section of wrist showing tendons and nerves involved in carpal tunnel syndrome.

Fractures

Fractures are classified according to their external appearance, the site of the fracture, and the nature of the crack or break in the bone. Important fracture types are indicated in Figure 4–15 and several have been paired with representative x-rays. Many fractures fall in more than one category. For example, Colles' fracture is a transverse fracture, but depending on the injury it may also be a comminuted fracture that can be either open or closed. The following list provides a summary of the types of fractures:

- **Closed,** or **simple,** fractures do not involve a break in the skin; they are completely internal.
- **Open,** or **compound,** fractures are more dangerous because the fracture projects through the skin and there is a possibility of infection or hemorrhage. See Figure 4–16.
- **Comminuted** fractures shatter the affected part into a multitude of bony fragments.
- **Transverse** fractures break the shaft of a bone across its longitudinal axis.
- **Greenstick** fractures usually occur in children whose long bones have not fully ossified; only one side of the shaft is broken, and the other is bent (like a greenstick).
- **Spiral** fractures are spread along the length of a bone and are produced by twisting stresses.
- **Colles'** fracture is often the result of reaching out to cushion a fall; there is a break in the distal portion of the radius.
- **Pott's** fracture occurs at the ankle and affects both bones of the lower leg (fibula and tibia).

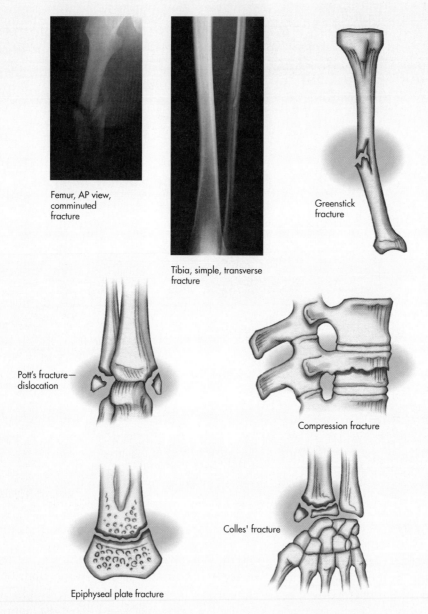

Femur, AP view, comminuted fracture

Tibia, simple, transverse fracture

Greenstick fracture

Pott's fracture—dislocation

Compression fracture

Colles' fracture

Epiphyseal plate fracture

FIGURE 4–15

Various types of fractures.

- **Compression** fractures occur in vertebrae subjected to extreme stresses, as when one falls and lands on his/her bottom.
- **Epiphyseal** fractures usually occur where the matrix is undergoing calcification and chondrocytes (cartilage cells) are dying; this type of fracture is seen in children.

Osteoporosis

Osteoporosis is a condition characterized by the progressive loss of bone density and thinning of bone tissue. See Figure 4–17. Osteoporosis occurs when the body fails to form enough new bone, or when too much old bone is reabsorbed by the body, or both. Osteoporosis frequently occurs when there is not enough calcium in the diet. The body then uses calcium stored in bones, weakening them and making them vulnerable to breaking. See Table 4–2 for good sources of calcium. Sufficient intake of vitamin D is also important for calcium absorption.

Vitamin D is absorbed through the skin from sunlight, and is also found in fatty fish, fish oils, and eggs from hens that have been fed vitamin D. Older adults are more prone to vitamin D deficiency.

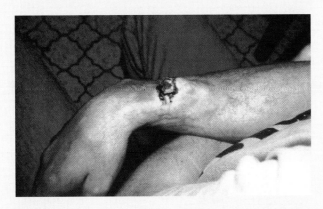

FIGURE 4–16

An open fracture of the wrist. (Source: Pearson Education/PH College.)

Osteoporosis affects more than 25 million Americans, most of them women 50 to 70 years of age. Each year, the disease leads to 1.4 million bone fractures, including more than 500,000 vertebral fractures, 300,000 hip fractures, and 200,000 wrist fractures.

There are some risk factors involved in developing osteoporosis and these are:

- Family history of osteoporosis
- Lack of exercise, especially weight-bearing exercise, which stimulates bone growth

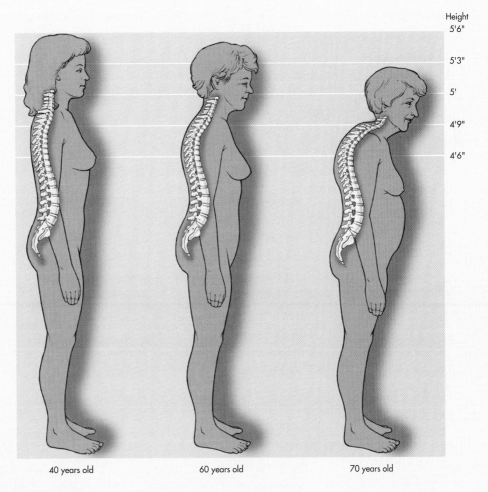

FIGURE 4–17

Spinal changes caused by osteoporosis.

- Thin, petite build
- Never been pregnant
- Early menopause (before 45 years)
- Prone to fractures, and loss of height in the past few years
- Avoided dairy products as a child
- Smoking, drinking alcoholic beverages
- Diet high in salt, caffeine, or fat
- Insufficient intake of vitamin D

Tests such as bone mineral density (BMD) testing are most frequently used for diagnosis and evaluation of osteoporosis. Treatments for osteoporosis focus on slowing down or stopping bone loss, preventing bone fractures by minimizing the risk of falls, and controlling pain associated with the disease. Hormone deficiencies (estrogen in women and testosterone in men) are the leading cause of osteoporosis. For this reason, estrogen replacement therapy is frequently used as a treatment for osteoporosis in women. Other drug treatments include biphosphonates such as alendronate (Fosamax).

✓PATHOLOGY CHECKPOINT

Following is a concise list of the pathology-related terms that you've seen in the chapter. Review this checklist to make sure that you are familiar with the meaning of each term before moving on to the next section.

Conditions and Symptoms

- ❏ achondroplasia
- ❏ acroarthritis
- ❏ ankylosis
- ❏ arthralgia
- ❏ arthritis
- ❏ bursitis
- ❏ carpal tunnel syndrome
- ❏ coccygodynia
- ❏ dislocation
- ❏ flatfoot
- ❏ genu valgum
- ❏ genu varum
- ❏ gout
- ❏ hammertoe
- ❏ hydrarthrosis
- ❏ ischialgia
- ❏ kyphosis
- ❏ lordosis
- ❏ lumbodynia

- ❏ myelitis
- ❏ myeloma
- ❏ osteoarthritis
- ❏ osteocarcinoma
- ❏ osteochondritis
- ❏ osteomalacia
- ❏ osteomyelitis
- ❏ osteopenia
- ❏ osteoporosis
- ❏ osteosarcoma
- ❏ periosteoedema
- ❏ polyarthritis
- ❏ rheumatoid arthritis
- ❏ rickets
- ❏ scoliosis
- ❏ spondylitis
- ❏ sprain
- ❏ spur
- ❏ tenonitis
- ❏ tennis elbow

Diagnosis and Treatment

- ❏ arthrocentesis
- ❏ arthroplasty
- ❏ arthroscope
- ❏ bone marrow transplant
- ❏ cast
- ❏ craniectomy
- ❏ craniotomy
- ❏ fixation
- ❏ laminectomy
- ❏ metacarpectomy
- ❏ osteotome
- ❏ rachigraph
- ❏ radiograph
- ❏ reduction
- ❏ splint
- ❏ sternotomy
- ❏ traction

DRUG HIGHLIGHTS

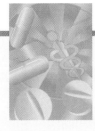

Drugs that are generally used for skeletal system diseases and disorders include anti-inflammatory agents, disease-modifying antirheumatic drugs (DMARDs), COX-2 inhibitors, antitumor necrosis factor drugs, agents used to treat gout, agents used to treat or prevent postmenopausal osteoporosis, and analgesics. Fractures, arthritis, rheumatoid arthritis, bursitis, carpal tunnel syndrome, dislocation, osteoporosis, and pain are some of the conditions involving the skeletal system and the need for pharmacologic therapy.

Anti-inflammatory Agents

Relieve the swelling, tenderness, redness, and pain of inflammation. These agents may be classified as steroidal (corticosteroids) and nonsteroidal.

Corticosteroids (Glucocorticoids)

Steroid substance with potent anti-inflammatory effects.

Examples: Depo-Medrol (methylprednisolone acetate), Aristocort (triamcinolone), Celestone (betamethasone), and Decadron (dexamethasone).

Nonsteroidal (NSAIDs)

Agents that are used in the treatment of arthritis and related disorders.

Examples: Bayer Aspirin (acetylsalicylic acid), Motrin (ibuprofen), Feldene (piroxicam), Orudis (ketoprofen), and Naprosyn (naproxen).

Disease-modifying Antirheumatic Drugs (DMARDs)

May influence the course of the disease progression; therefore, their introduction in early rheumatoid arthritis is recommended to limit irreversible joint damage.

Examples: gold preparations Ridaura (auranofin) and Solganol (aurothioglucose); antimalarial Plaquenil Sulfate (hydroxychloroquine sulfate); a chelating agent Cuprimine (penicillamine) and the immunosuppressants Rheumatrex (methotrexate), Imuran (azathioprine), and Cytoxan (cyclophosphamide).

COX-2 Inhibitors

Cyclooxygenase (COX) is an enzyme involved in many aspects of normal cellular function and also in the inflammatory response. COX-2 is found in joints and other areas affected by inflammation, such as occurs with osteoarthritis and rheumatoid arthritis. Inhibition of COX-2 reduces the production of compounds associated with inflammation and pain.

Examples: Celebrex (celecoxib), Vioxx (rofecoxib), and Mobic (meloxicam).

Antitumor Necrosis Factor (Anti-TNF) Drugs

These drugs have evolved out of the biotechnology industry and seem to slow, if not halt altogether, the destruction of the joints by disrupting the activity of tumor necrosis factor (TNF), a substance involved in the body's immune response.

Example: Enbrel (etanercept).

Agents Used to Treat Gout

Acute attacks of gout are treated with colchicine. Once the acute attack of gout has been controlled, drug therapy to control hyperuricemia can be initiated.

Example: Benemid (probenecid), Anturane (sulfinpyrazone), and Zyloprim (allopurinol).

Agents Used to Treat or Prevent Postmenopausal Osteoporosis

Include *Fosamax (alendronate sodium)* and *Actonel (risedronate)*. Fosamax reduces the activity of the cells that cause bone loss and increases the amount of bone in most patients. Actonel inhibits osteoclast-mediated bone resorption and modulates bone metabolism. To receive the clinical benefits of either of these drugs the patient must be informed and follow the prescribed drug regimen.

Analgesics

Agents that relieve pain without causing loss of consciousness. They are classified as narcotic or non-narcotic.

Narcotic

Examples: Demerol (meperidine HCl) and morphine sulfate.

Non-narcotic

Examples: Tylenol (acetaminophen), aspirin, ibuprofen (Advil, Motrin, Nuprin), and Naprosyn (naproxen).

DIAGNOSTIC & LAB TESTS

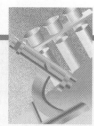

TEST	DESCRIPTION
arthrography (ăr-thrŏg′ ră-fē)	A diagnostic examination of a joint (usually the knee) in which air and then a radiopaque contrast medium are injected into the joint space, x-rays are taken, and internal injuries of the meniscus, cartilage, and ligaments may be seen, if present.
arthroscopy (ăr-thrŏs′ kō-pē)	The process of examining internal structures of a joint via an arthroscope; usually done after an arthrography and before joint surgery.
goniometry (gō″ nē-ŏm′ ĕt-rē)	The measurement of joint movements and angles via a goniometer.
photon absorptiometry (fō′ tŏn ăb-sorp′ shē-ŏm′ ĕt-rĕ)	A bone scan that uses a low beam of radiation to measure bone-mineral density and bone loss in the lumbar vertebrae; useful in monitoring osteoporosis.
thermography (thĕr-mŏg′ ră-fē)	The process of recording heat patterns of the body's surface; can be used to investigate the pathophysiology of rheumatoid arthritis.
x-ray (ĕks′ rā)	The examination of bones by use of an electromagnetic wave of high energy produced by the collision of a beam of electrons with a target in a vacuum tube; used to identify fractures and pathologic conditions of the bones and joints such as rheumatoid arthritis, spondylitis, and tumors.
alkaline phosphatase blood test (ăl′ kă-līn fŏs′ fă-tās)	A blood test to determine the level of alkaline phosphatase; increased in osteoblastic bone tumors, rickets, osteomalacia, and during fracture healing.
antinuclear antibodies (ANA) (ăn″ tĭ-nū′ klē-ăr ăn′ tĭ-bŏd″ ēs)	Present in a variety of immunologic diseases; positive result may indicate rheumatoid arthritis.
calcium (Ca) blood test (kăl′ sē-ŭm)	The calcium level of the blood may be increased in metastatic bone cancer, acute osteoporosis, prolonged immobilization, and during fracture healing; may be decreased in osteomalacia and rickets.
C-Reactive protein blood test (sē-rē-ăk″ tĭv prō′ tē-in)	Positive result may indicate rheumatoid arthritis, acute inflammatory change, and widespread metastasis.
phosphorus (P) blood test (fŏs′ fō-rŭs)	Phosphorus level of the blood may be increased in osteoporosis and fracture healing.
serum rheumatoid factor (RF) (sē′ rŭm roo′ mă-toyd făk′ tōr)	An immunoglobulin present in the serum of 50 to 95% of adults with rheumatoid arthritis.
uric acid blood test (ū′ rĭk ăs′ ĭd)	Uric acid is increased in gout, arthritis, multiple myeloma, and rheumatism.

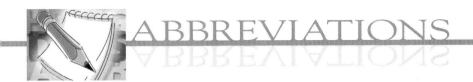

ABBREVIATIONS

ABBREVIATION	MEANING
ACL	anterior cruciate ligament
AP	anteroposterior
BMD	bone mineral density (test)
CDH	congenital dislocation of hip
C 1	cervical vertebra, first
C 2	cervical vertebra, second
C 3	cervical vertebra, third
Ca	calcium
DJD	degenerative joint disease
Fx	fracture
JRA	juvenile rheumatoid arthritis
jt	joint
KJ	knee jerk
L 1	lumbar vertebra, first
L 2	lumbar vertebra, second
L 3	lumbar vertebra, third
LAC	long arm cast
lig	ligament

ABBREVIATION	MEANING
LLC	long leg cast
LLCC	long leg cylinder cast
OA	osteoarthritis
ORTHO	orthopedics, orthopaedics
PCL	posterior cruciate ligament
PEMFs	pulsing electromagnetic fields
PWB	partial weight bearing
RA	rheumatoid arthritis
SAC	short arm cast
SLC	short leg cast
SPECT	single photon emission computed tomography
T 1	thoracic vertebra, first
T 2	thoracic vertebra, second
T 3	thoracic vertebra, third
TMJ	temporomandibular joint
Tx	traction

STUDY AND REVIEW

Anatomy and Physiology

Write your answers to the following questions. Do not refer to the text.

1. The skeletal system is composed of _____ bones.

2. Name the two main divisions of the skeletal system.

   a. _____   b. _____

3. Name five classifications of bone and give an example of each.

   a. _____   Example _____

   b. _____   Example _____

   c. _____   Example _____

   d. _____   Example _____

   e. _____   Example _____

4. State the six main functions of the skeletal system.

   a. _____   b. _____

   c. _____   d. _____

   e. _____   f. _____

5. Define the following features of a long bone:

   a. Epiphysis _____

   b. Diaphysis _____

   c. Periosteum _____

   d. Compact bone _____

   e. Medullary canal _____

   f. Endosteum _____

   g. Cancellous or spongy bone _____

6. Match the term in column one with its definition from column two. Place the
   correct number from column two in the space provided in column one.

_____ a. Meatus

_____ b. Head

_____ c. Tuberosity

_____ d. Process

_____ e. Condyle

_____ f. Tubercle

_____ g. Crest

_____ h. Trochanter

_____ i. Sinus

_____ j. Fissure

_____ k. Fossa

_____ l. Spine

_____ m. Foramen

_____ n. Sulcus

1. An air cavity within certain bones
2. A shallow depression in or on a bone
3. A pointed, sharp, slender process
4. A large, rounded process
5. A groove, furrow, depression, or fissure
6. A tube-like passage or canal
7. An opening in the bone for blood vessels, ligaments, and nerves
8. A rounded process that enters into the formation of a joint, articulation
9. A ridge on a bone
10. A small, rounded process
11. The rounded end of a bone
12. A slit-like opening between two bones
13. An enlargement or protrusion of a bone
14. A very large process of the femur

7. Name the three classifications of joints.

   a. _____   b. _____

   c. _____

8. _____ is the process of moving a body part away from the middle.

9. Adduction is _____.

10. _____ is the process of moving a body part in a circular motion.

11. Dorsiflexion is _____.

12. _____ is the process of turning outward.

13. Extension is _____.

14. _____ is the process of bending a limb.

15. Inversion is _____.

16. _____ is the process of lying face downward.

17. Protraction is _____.

18. _____ is the process of moving a body part backward.

19. Rotation is _____.

20. _____ is the process of lying face upward.

Word Parts

1. In the spaces provided, write the definition of these prefixes, roots, combining forms, and suffixes. Do not refer to the listings of medical words. Leave blank those words you cannot define.

2. After completing as many as you can, refer back to the medical word listings to check your work. For each word missed or left blank, write the word and its definition several times on the margins of these pages or on a separate sheet of paper.

3. To maximize the learning process, it is to your advantage to do the following exercises as directed. To refer to the word building section before completing these exercises invalidates the learning process.

PREFIXES

Give the definitions of the following prefixes:

1. a- _____

2. dis- _____

3. hydr- _____

4. inter- _____

5. meta- _____

6. peri- _____

7. poly- _____

8. sub- _____

9. sym- _____

10. re- _____

ROOTS AND COMBINING FORMS

Give the definitions of the following roots and combining forms:

1. acetabul _____

2. cartil _____

3. acr _____

4. acr/o _____

5. ankyl _____

6. arthr _____

7. arthr/o _____

8. burs _____

9. calcan/e _____

10. locat _____

11. carcin _____

12. carp _____

13. carp/o _____

14. chondr _____

15. chondr/o _____

16. clavicul _____

17. fixat _____

18. coccyg/e _____

19. coccyg/o _____

20. coll/a _____

21. duct _____

22. connect _____

23. cost _____

24. cost/o _____

25. menisc _____

26. phos _____

27. cran/i _____

28. crani/o _____

29. dactyl _____

30. dactyl/o _____

31. femor _____

32. phor _____

33. fibul _____

34. radi/o _____

35. humer _____

36. ili _____

37. ili/o _____

38. isch/i _____

39. kyph _____

40. lamin _____

41. lord _____

42. lumb _____

43. lumb/o _____

44. mandibul _____

45. maxill _____

46. maxilla _____

47. myel _____

48. myel/o _____

49. rheumat _____

50. olecran _____

51. oste/o _____

52. patell _____

53. tract _____

54. ped _____

55. phalang/e _____

56. por _____

57. rachi _____

58. radi _____

59. sacr _____

60. sarc _____

61. scapul _____

62. scoli _____

63. scoli/o _____

64. spin _____

65. spondyl _____

66. stern _____

67. stern/o _____

68. tenon _____

69. tibi _____

70. uln _____

71. uln/o _____

72. vertebr _____

73. vertebr/o _____

74. xiph _____

SUFFIXES

Give the definitions of the following suffixes:

1. -ac _____   2. -al _____

3. -algia _____   4. -ar _____

5. -ary _____   6. -blast _____

7. -centesis _____   8. -age _____

9. -ion _____   10. -dynia _____

11. -ectomy _____   12. -edema _____

13. -gen _____   14. -genesis _____

15. -gram _____   16. -graph _____

17. -ic _____   18. -itis _____

19. -ive _____   20. -scope _____

21. -malacia _____   22. -us _____

23. -oid _____   24. -oma _____

25. -omion _____   26. -osis _____

27. -penia _____   28. -physis _____

29. -plasia _____   30. -plasty _____

31. -poiesis _____   32. -tome _____

33. -tomy _____

Identifying Medical Terms

In the spaces provided, write the medical terms for the following meanings:

1. _____ Inflammation of the joints of the hands or feet

2. _____ The condition of stiffening of a joint

3. _____ Inflammation of a joint

4. _____ Pertaining to the heel bone

5. _____ Pertaining to cartilage

6. _____ Pain in the coccyx

7. _____ Pertaining to the rib

8. _____ Surgical excision of a portion of the skull

9. _____ Pertaining to the finger or toe

10. _____ Condition of fluid in a joint

11. _____ Pertaining to between the ribs

12. _____ Pain in the hip

13. _____ Pertaining to the loins

14. _____ A tumor of the bone marrow

15. _____ Inflammation of the joint and bone

16. _____ Inflammation of the bone marrow

17. _____ A lack of bone tissue

18. _____ Pertaining to the foot

19. _____ Resembling a sword

Spelling

In the spaces provided, write the correct spelling of these misspelled terms:

1. acrmoin _____

2. arthrscope _____

3. buritis _____

4. chondblast _____

5. conective _____

6. cranplasty _____

7. dislocaton _____

8. ischal _____

9. melyitis _____

10. ostchonditis _____

11. phosphous _____

12. patelar _____

13. phalangal _____

14. rachgraph _____

15. scolosis _____

16. spondlitis _____

17. symphsis _____

18. tenonis _____

19. ulncarpal _____

20. vertbral _____

Matching

Select the appropriate lettered meaning for each word listed below.

_____ 1. arthroscope

_____ 2. carpal tunnel syndrome

_____ 3. fixation

_____ 4. gout

_____ 5. hammertoe

_____ 6. kyphosis

_____ 7. metacarpal

_____ 8. rickets

_____ 9. tennis elbow

_____ 10. ulnar

a. A deficiency condition in children primarily caused by a lack of vitamin D

b. An acquired flexion deformity of the interphalangeal joint

c. A hereditary metabolic disease that is a form of acute arthritis

d. A chronic condition characterized by pain that is caused by excessive pronation and supination activities of the forearm

e. Making rigid, immobilizing

f. Pertaining to the elbow

g. Pertaining to the bones of the hand

h. Humpback

i. An instrument used to examine the interior of a joint

j. A condition caused by compression of the median nerve by the carpal ligament

k. Pertaining to the knee

Abbreviations

Place the correct word, phrase, or abbreviation in the space provided.

1. congenital dislocation of hip _____

2. degenerative joint disease _____

3. LLC _____

4. OA _____

5. pulsing electromagnetic fields _____

6. RA _____

7. single photon emission computed tomography _____

8. T1 _____

9. TMJ _____

10. traction _____

Diagnostic and Laboratory Test

Select the best answer to each multiple choice question. Circle the letter of your choice.

1. _____ is a diagnostic examination of a joint in which air and, then, a radiopaque contrast medium are injected into the joint space, x-rays are taken, and internal injuries of the meniscus, cartilage, and ligaments may be seen, if present.
   a. Arthroscopy
   b. Goniometry
   c. Arthrography
   d. Thermography

2. The process of recording heat patterns of the body's surface is:
   a. arthrography
   b. arthroscopy
   c. goniometry
   d. thermography

3. _____ is increased in gout, arthritis, multiple myeloma, and rheumatism.
   a. Calcium
   b. Phosphorus
   c. Uric acid
   d. Alkaline phosphatase

4. _____ level of the blood may be increased in osteoporosis and fracture healing.
   a. Antinuclear antibodies
   b. Phosphorus
   c. Uric acid
   d. Alkaline phosphatase

5. _____ is/are present in a variety of immunologic diseases.
   a. Alkaline phosphatase
   b. Antinuclear antibodies
   c. C-Reactive protein
   d. Uric acid

CASE STUDY   OSTEOPOROSIS

Read the following case study and then answer the questions that follow.

A 62-year-old female was seen by a physician; the following is a synopsis of her visit.

Present History: The patient states that she seems to be shorter, her back "hurts" all the time, and she has developed a humpback.

Signs and Symptoms: Loss of height, kyphosis, and pain in the back.

Diagnosis: Osteoporosis (postmenopausal)

Treatment: Actonel (risedronate sodium); one 5mg tablet orally, taken daily. Begin a regular exercise program, a diet rich in calcium, phosphorus, magnesium, and vitamins A, C, D, the B-complex vitamins, and analgesics for pain.

Prevention: Know the risk factors involved in developing osteoporosis, follow a regular exercise program, and include a diet rich in calcium, phosphorus, magnesium, and vitamins A, C, D, and the B-complex vitamins. For more information on osteoporosis you can call the National Osteoporosis Foundation at 1–202–223–2226.

Good sources of **vitamin A** are dairy products, fish liver oils, animal liver, green and yellow vegetables. Good sources of **vitamin D** are ultraviolet rays, dairy products, and commercial foods that contain supplemental vitamin D (milk and cereals). Good sources of **vitamin C** are citrus fruits, tomatoes,

melons, fresh berries, raw vegetables, and sweet potatoes. Good sources of the **B-complex vitamins** are organ meats, dried beans, poultry, eggs, yeast, fish, whole grains, and dark-green vegetables. Good sources of **calcium** are dairy products, beans, cauliflower, egg yolk, molasses, leafy green vegetables, tofu, sardines, clams, and oysters. Good sources of **phosphorus** are dairy products, eggs, fish, poultry, meats, dried peas and beans, whole grain cereals, and nuts. Good sources of **magnesium** are whole grain cereals, fruits, milk, nuts, vegetables, seafood, and meats.

CASE STUDY QUESTIONS

1. Signs and symptoms of osteoporosis include loss of height, kyphosis, and pain in the back. What is kyphosis? _____

2. What is the prescribed dosage of Actonel (risedronate sodium)? _____

3. Good sources of _____ are dairy products, fish liver oils, animal liver, and green and yellow vegetables.

4. Good sources of _____ are citrus fruits, tomatoes, melons, fresh berries, raw vegetables, and sweet potatoes.

5. Milk, yogurt, cheese, tofu, turnip greens, canned salmon, sardines, beans, egg yolk, molasses, and broccoli are examples of good sources of _____.

 MedMedia— Wrap-Up

www.prenhall.com/rice

Additional interactive resources and activities for this chapter can be found on the Companion Website. For animations, videos, audio glossary, and review, access the accompanying CD-ROM in this book.

Audio Glossary
Medical Terminology Exercises & Activities
Pathology Spotlights
Terminology Translator
Animations
Videos

 Objectives
Medical Terminology Exercises & Activities
Audio Glossary
Drug Updates
Medical Terminology in the News

THE MUSCULAR SYSTEM

5

OBJECTIVES

On completion of this chapter, you will be able to:

- Describe the muscular system.
- Describe types of muscle tissue.
- Provide the functions of muscles.
- Describe muscular differences of the child and the older adult.
- Analyze, build, spell, and pronounce medical words.
- Describe each of the conditions presented in the Pathology Spotlights.
- Complete the Pathology Checkpoint.
- Review Drug Highlights presented in this chapter.
- Provide the description of diagnostic and laboratory tests related to the muscular system.
- Identify and define selected abbreviations.
- Successfully complete the study and review section.

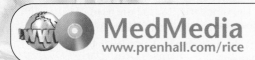

MedMedia
www.prenhall.com/rice

Additional interactive resources and activities for this chapter can be found on the Companion Website. For Terminology Translator, animations, videos, audio glossary, and review, access the accompanying CD-ROM in this book.

Anatomy and Physiology Overview

The muscular system is composed of all the **muscles** in the body. This overview will describe the three basic types of muscles and some of their functions. The muscles are the primary tissues of the system. They make up approximately 42% of a person's body weight and are composed of long, slender cells known as **fibers**. Muscle fibers are of different lengths and shapes and vary in color from white to deep red. Each muscle consists of a group of fibers held together by connective tissue and enclosed in a fibrous sheath or **fascia**. See Figure 5–1. Each fiber within a muscle receives its own nerve impulses and has its own stored supply of glycogen, which it uses as fuel for energy. Muscle has to be supplied with proper nutrition and oxygen to perform properly; therefore, blood and lymphatic vessels permeate its tissues.

TYPES OF MUSCLE TISSUE

Skeletal muscle, smooth muscle, and cardiac muscle are the three basic types of muscle tissue classed according to their functions and appearance (Fig. 5–2).

Skeletal Muscle

Also known as **voluntary** or **striated** muscles, **skeletal muscles** are controlled by the conscious part of the brain and attach to the bones. There are 600 skeletal muscles that, through contractility, extensibility, and elasticity, are responsible for the movement of the body. These muscles have a cross-striped appearance and thus are known as striated muscles. They vary in size, shape, arrangement of fibers, and means of attachment to bones. Selected skeletal muscles are listed with their functions in Tables 5–1 and 5–2 and shown in Figures 5–3 and 5–4.

Skeletal muscles have two or more attachments. The more fixed attachment is known as the **origin**, and the point of attachment of a muscle to the part that it moves is the **insertion**. The means of attachment is called a **tendon**, which can vary in length from less than 1 inch to more than 1 foot. A wide, thin, sheet-like tendon is known as an **aponeurosis**.

THE MUSCULAR SYSTEM

Organ/ Structure	Primary Functions
Muscles	Responsible for movement, help to maintain posture, and produce heat
Skeletal	Through contractility, extensibility, and elasticity, are responsible for the movement of the body
Smooth	Produce relatively slow contraction with greater degree of extensibility in the internal organs, especially organs of the digestive, respiratory, and urinary tract, plus certain muscles of the eye and skin, and walls of blood vessels
Cardiac	Muscle of the heart, controlled by the autonomic nervous system and specialized neuromuscular tissue located within the right atrium that is capable of causing cardiac muscle to contract rhythmically. The neuromuscular tissue of the heart comprises the sinoatrial node, the atrioventricular node, and the atrioventricular bundle
Tendons	A band of connective tissue serving for the attachment of muscles to bones

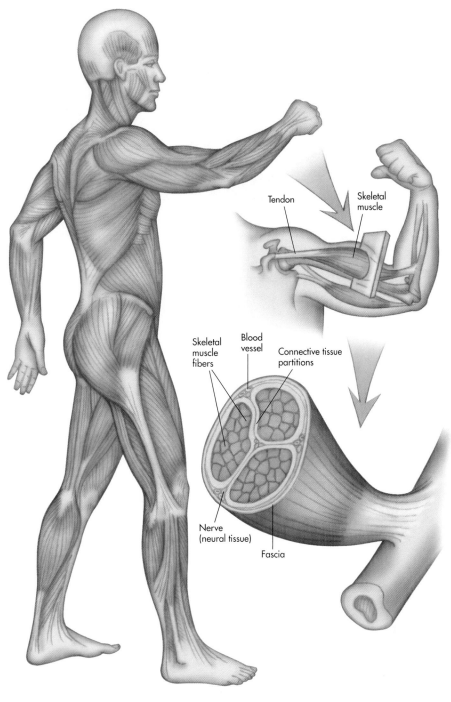

FIGURE 5–1

A skeletal muscle consists of a group of fibers held together by connective tissue. It is enclosed in a fibrous sheath (fascia).

A muscle has three distinguishable parts: the **body** or main portion, an **origin**, and an **insertion**. The skeletal muscles move body parts by pulling from one bone across its joint to another bone with movement occurring at the diarthrotic joint. The types of body movement occurring at the diarthrotic joints are described in Chapter 4, The Skeletal System.

Muscles and nerves function together as a motor unit. For skeletal muscles to contract, it is necessary to have stimulation by impulses from motor nerves. Muscles perform in groups and are classified as:

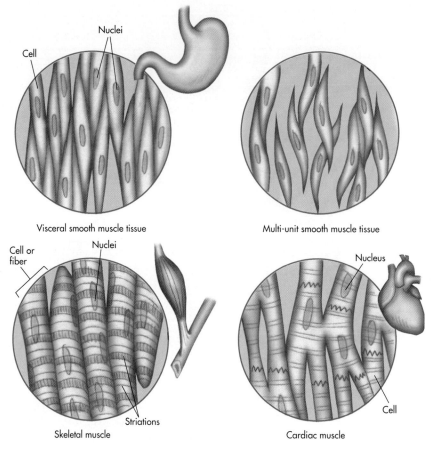

FIGURE 5–2

Types of muscle tissue.

- **Antagonist**—a muscle that counteracts the action of another muscle
- **Prime mover**—a muscle that is primary in a given movement. Its contraction produces the movement.
- **Synergist**—a muscle that acts with another muscle to produce movement

TABLE 5–1 SELECTED SKELETAL MUSCLES (ANTERIOR VIEW)

Muscle	Action
Sternocleidomastoid	Rotates and laterally flexes neck
Trapezius	Draws head back and to the side, rotates scapula
Deltoid	Raises and rotates arm
Rectus femoris	Extends leg and assists flexion of thigh
Sartorius	Flexes and rotates the thigh and leg
Tibialis anterior	Dorsiflexes foot and increases the arch in the beginning process of walking
Pectoralis major	Flexes, adducts, and rotates arm
Biceps brachii	Flexes arm and forearm and supinates forearm
Rectus abdominis	Compresses or flattens abdomen
Gastrocnemius	Plantar flexes foot and flexes knee
Soleus	Plantar flexes foot

TABLE 5–2 SELECTED SKELETAL MUSCLES (POSTERIOR VIEW)

Muscle	Action
Trapezius	Draws head back and to the side, rotates scapula
Deltoid	Raises and rotates arm
Triceps	Extends forearm
Latissimus dorsi	Adducts, extends, and rotates arm. Used during swimming
Gluteus maximus	Extends and rotates thigh
Biceps femoris	Flexes knee and rotates it outward
Gastrocnemius	Plantar flexes foot and flexes knee
Semitendinosus	Flexes and rotates leg, extends thigh

Smooth Muscle

Also called *involuntary*, *visceral*, or *unstriated*, **smooth muscles** are not controlled by the conscious part of the brain. They are under the control of the autonomic nervous system and, in most cases, produce relatively slow contraction with greater degree of extensibility. These muscles lack the cross-striped appearance of skeletal muscle and are smooth. Included in this type are the muscles of internal organs of the digestive, respiratory, and urinary tract, plus certain muscles of the eye and skin.

Cardiac Muscle

The muscle of the heart (**myocardium**) is *involuntary* but *striated* in appearance. It is controlled by the autonomic nervous system and specialized neuromuscular tissue located within the right atrium.

FUNCTIONS OF MUSCLES

The following is a list of the primary functions of muscles:

1. Muscles are responsible for movement. The types of movement are locomotion, propulsion of substances through tubes as in circulation and digestion, and changes in the size of openings as in the contraction and relaxation of the iris of the eye.
2. Muscles help to maintain posture through a continual partial contraction of skeletal muscles. This process is known as **tonicity**.
3. Muscles help to produce heat through the chemical changes involved in muscular action.

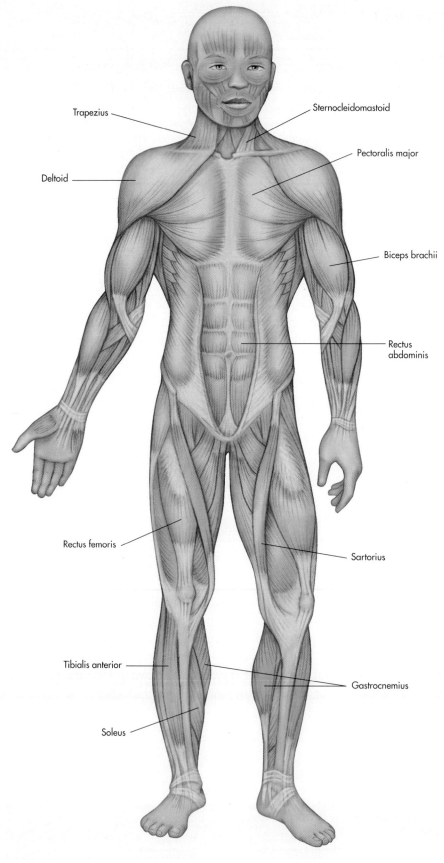

FIGURE 5–3

Selected skeletal muscles (anterior view).

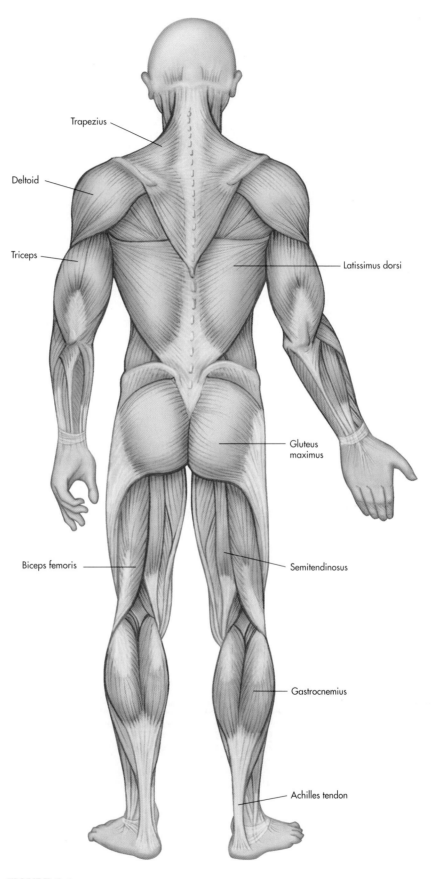

FIGURE 5–4

Selected skeletal muscles and the Achilles tendon (posterior view).

LIFE SPAN CONSIDERATIONS

■ THE CHILD

At about 6 weeks the size of the embryo is 12 mm (0.5 inch). The limb buds are extending and the skeletal and muscular systems are developing. At about 7 weeks the **diaphragm**, a partition of muscles and membranes that separates the chest cavity and the abdominal cavity, is completely developed. At the end of 8 weeks, the embryo is now known as the **fetus**. Fetal growth proceeds from head to tail (**cephalo** to **caudal**), with the head being larger in comparison to the rest of the body.

During fetal development the bones and muscles continue growing and developing. At about 32 weeks the developed skeletal system is soft and flexible. Muscle and fat accumulate and the fetus weighs approximately 2000 g (4 lb, 7 oz). At about 40 weeks the fetus is ready for birth and extrauterine life.

The movements of the newborn are uncoordinated and random. Muscular development proceeds from head to foot and from the center of the body to the periphery. Head and neck muscles are the first ones that can be controlled by the baby. A baby can hold his head up before he can sit erect. The baby needs freedom of movement. The bath is an excellent time for the newborn to exercise.

■ THE OLDER ADULT

With aging, changes related to mobility are most significant. There is a decrease in muscle strength, endurance, range of motion, coordination and elasticity, and flexibility of connective tissue. There is an actual loss in the number of muscle fibers due to **myofibril atrophy** with fibrous tissue replacement, which begins in the fourth decade of life.

To prevent loss of strength, muscles need to be exercised. Regular exercise strengthens muscles and keeps joints, tendons, and ligaments more flexible, allowing active people to move freely and carry out routine activities easily. Exercises such as aerobic dance, brisk walking, and bicycling improve muscle tone and heart and lung function. To maintain aerobic fitness one needs to participate in such activities for 20 minutes or more at least three times a week and work at one's target heart rate. The target range declines with age; the following table shows the correct range during exercise for women between 45 and 65 years old.

Age	Target Heart Rate (Beats per Minute)
45 years old	108 to 135
50 years old	102 to 127
55 years old	99 to 123
60 years old	96 to 120
65 years old	93 to 116

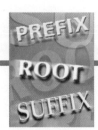

BUILDING YOUR MEDICAL VOCABULARY

This section provides the foundation for learning medical terminology. Medical words can be made up of four different types of word parts:

- Prefixes (P)
- Roots (R)
- Combining forms (CF)
- Suffixes (S)

By connecting various word parts in an organized sequence, thousands of words can be built and learned. In this text the word list is alphabetized so one can see the variety of meanings created when common prefixes and suffixes are repeatedly applied to certain word roots and/or combining forms. Words shown in pink are additional words related to the content of this chapter that are not built from word parts. These words are included to enhance your vocabulary. Note: an asterisk icon * indicates words that are covered in the Pathology Spotlights section in this chapter.

MEDICAL WORD	WORD PARTS (WHEN APPLICABLE)			DEFINITION
	Part	**Type**	**Meaning**	
abductor (ăb-dŭk′tōr)	ab duct -or	P R S	away from to lead a doer	A muscle that, on contraction, draws away from the middle
adductor (ă-dŭk′tōr)	ad duct -or	P R S	toward to lead a doer	A muscle that draws a part toward the middle
amputation (ăm″ pū-tā′shŭn)	amputat -ion	R S	to cut through process	The removal of a limb, part, or other appendage. See Figure 5–5.
antagonist (ăn-tăg′ō-nĭst)	ant agon -ist	P R S	against agony, a contest agent	A muscle that counteracts the action of another muscle
aponeurosis (ăp″ ō-nū-rō′sĭs)	apo neur -osis	P R S	separation nerve condition of	A fibrous sheet of connective tissue that serves to attach muscle to bone or to other tissues
ataxia (ă-tăks′ĭ-ă)	a -taxia	P S	lack of order	A lack of muscular coordination
atonic (ă-tŏn′ĭk)	a ton -ic	P R S	lack of tone, tension pertaining to	Pertaining to a lack of normal tone or tension
atrophy (ăt′rō-fē)	a -trophy	P S	lack of nourishment, development	A lack of nourishment; a wasting of muscular tissue that may be caused by lack of use. * See Pathology Spotlight: Atrophy.
biceps (bī′sĕps)	bi -ceps	P S	two head	A muscle with two heads or points of origin
brachialgia (brā″ ki-ăl′jĭ-ă)	brach/i -algia	CF S	arm pain	Pain in the arm
bradykinesia (brăd″ ĭ-kĭ-nē′sĭ-ă)	brady -kinesia	P S	slow motion	Slowness of motion or movement
clonic (klŏn′ĭk)	clon -ic	R S	turmoil pertaining to	Pertaining to alternate contraction and relaxation of muscles

MEDICAL WORD	WORD PARTS (WHEN APPLICABLE)			DEFINITION
	Part	**Type**	**Meaning**	
contraction (kŏn-trăk′shŭn)	con	P	with, together	The process of drawing up and thickening of a muscle fiber
	tract	R	to draw	
	-ion	S	process	
contracture (kŏn-trăk′chūr)	con	P	with, together	A condition in which a muscle shortens and renders the muscle resistant to the normal stretching process. See Figure 5–6.
	tract	R	to draw	
	-ure	S	process	
dactylospasm (dăk′tĭ-lō-spăzm)	dactyl/o	CF	finger or toe	Cramp of a finger or toe
	-spasm	S	tension, spasm	
dermatomyositis (dĕr″ mă-tō-mī″ ō-sī′tĭs)	dermat/o	CF	skin	Inflammation of the muscles and the skin; a connective tissue disease characterized by edema, dermatitis, and inflammation of the muscles. See Figure 5–7.
	my/os	CF	muscle	
	-itis	S	inflammation	
diaphragm (dī′ă-frăm)	dia	P	through	The partition of muscles and membranes that separates the chest cavity and the abdominal cavity
	-phragm	S	a fence, partition	
diathermy (dī′ă-thĕr″ mē)	dia	P	through	Treatment using high-frequency current to produce heat within a part of the body; used to increase blood flow and should not be used in acute stage of recovery from trauma. Types: **Microwave.** Electromagnetic radiation is directed to specified tissues **Short-wave.** High-frequency electric current (wavelength of 3–30 m) is directed to specified tissues **Ultrasound.** High-frequency sound waves (20,000–10 billion cycles/sec) are directed to specified tissues
	therm	R	hot, heat	
	-y	S	pertaining to	
dystonia (dĭs′tō′nĭ-ă)	dys	P	difficult	A condition of impaired muscle tone
	ton	R	tone, tension	
	-ia	S	condition	
dystrophin (dĭs-trōf′ĭn)	dys	P	difficult	A protein found in muscle cells; when the gene that is responsible for this protein is defective and sufficient dystrophin is not produced, muscle wasting occurs
	troph	R	a turning	
	-in	S	chemical	
dystrophy (dĭs′trō-fē)	dys	P	difficult	Faulty muscular development caused by lack of nourishment
	-trophy	S	nourishment, development	

MEDICAL WORD	WORD PARTS (WHEN APPLICABLE)			DEFINITION
	Part	**Type**	**Meaning**	
exercise (ĕk′sĕr-sīz)				Performed activity of the muscles for improvement of health or correction of deformity. Types: **Active.** The patient contracts and relaxes his or her muscles **Assistive.** The patient contracts and relaxes his or her muscles with the assistance of a therapist **Isometric.** Active muscular contraction performed against stable resistance, thereby not shortening the muscle length **Passive.** Exercise is performed by another individual without the assistance of the patient **Range of Motion.** Movement of each joint through its full range of motion. Used to prevent loss of motility or to regain usage after an injury or fracture **Relief of Tension.** Technique used to promote relaxation of the muscles and provide relief from tension
fascia (făsh′ĭ-ă)	fasc -ia	R S	a band condition	A thin layer of connective tissue covering, supporting, or connecting the muscles or inner organs of the body
fascitis (fă-sī′tĭs)	fasc -itis	R S	a band inflammation	Inflammation of a fascia
fatigue (fă-tēg′)				A state of tiredness or weariness occurring in a muscle as a result of repeated contractions
fibromyalgia (fī″ brō-mī-ăl′jē-ă)	fibr/o my -algia	CF R S	fiber muscle pain	A condition with widespread muscular pain and debilitating fatigue. ✱ See Pathology Spotlight: Fibromyalgia.
fibromyitis (fī″ brō-mī-ī′tĭs)	fibr/o my -itis	CF R S	fiber muscle inflammation	Inflammation of muscle and fibrous tissue
First Aid Treatment—RICE **Rest** **Ice** **Compression** **Elevation**				**Cryotherapy** (use of cold) is the treatment of choice for soft tissue injuries and muscle injuries. It causes vasoconstriction of blood vessels and is effective in diminishing bleeding and edema. Ice should not be placed directly onto the skin.

MEDICAL WORD	WORD PARTS (WHEN APPLICABLE)			DEFINITION
	Part	**Type**	**Meaning**	
				Compression by an elastic bandage is generally determined by the type of injury and the preference of the physician. Some experts disagree on the use of elastic bandages. When used, the bandage should be 3 to 4 inches wide and applied firmly, and toes or fingers should be periodically checked for blue or white discoloration, indicating that the bandage is too tight. **Elevation** is used to reduce swelling. The injured part should be elevated on two or three pillows.
flaccid (flăk′sĭd)				Lacking muscle tone; *weak, soft,* and *flabby*
heat (hēt)				**Thermotherapy.** The treatment using scientific application of heat may be used 48 to 72 hours after the injury. Types: heating pad, hot water bottle, hot packs, infrared light, and immersion of body part in warm water. Extreme care should be followed when using or applying heat.
hydrotherapy (hī-drō-thĕr′ă-pē)	hydro -therapy	P S	water treatment	Treatment using scientific application of water; types: hot tub, cold bath, whirlpool, and vapor bath
insertion (ĭn″ sûr′shŭn)	in sert -ion	P R S	into to gain process	The point of attachment of a muscle to the part that it moves
intramuscular (ĭn″ tră-mŭs′kū-lər)	intra muscul -ar	P R S	within muscle pertaining to	Pertaining to within a muscle
isometric (ī″ sō-mĕt′rĭk)	is/o metr -ic	CF R S	equal to measure pertaining to	Pertaining to having equal measure
isotonic (ī″ sō-tŏn′ĭk)	is/o ton -ic	CF R S	equal tone, tension pertaining to	Pertaining to having the same tone or tension
levator (lē-vā′tər)	levat -or	R S	lifter a doer	A muscle that raises or elevates a part

MEDICAL WORD	WORD PARTS (WHEN APPLICABLE)			DEFINITION
	Part	Type	Meaning	
massage (măh-săhzh)				To knead, apply pressure and friction to external body tissues
muscular dystrophy (mŭs′kū-lăr dĭs′trō-fē)				A chronic, progressive wasting and weakening of muscles. ✷ See Pathology Spotlight: Muscular Dystrophy.
myalgia (mī-ăl′jĭ-ă)	my -algia	R S	muscle pain	Pain in the muscle
myasthenia gravis (mī-ăs-thē′nĭ-ă gră vĭs)	my -asthenia gravis	R S R	muscle weakness grave	A chronic disease characterized by progressive muscular weakness
myitis (mī-ī′tĭs)	my -itis	R S	muscle inflammation	Inflammation of a muscle
myoblast (mī′ō blăst)	my/o -blast	CF S	muscle immature cell, germ cell	An embryonic cell that develops into a cell of muscle fiber
myofibroma (mī″ ō fī-brō′mă)	my/o fibr -oma	CF R S	muscle fiber tumor	A tumor that contains muscle and fiber
myograph (mī′ō-grăf)	my/o -graph	CF S	muscle to write, record	An instrument used to record muscular contractions
myokinesis (mī″ ō-kĭn-ē′sĭs)	my/o -kinesis	CF S	muscle motion	Muscular motion or activity
myology (mĭ-ŏl ō-jē)	my/o -logy	CF S	muscle study of	The study of muscles
myoma (mī-ō′ mă)	my -oma	R S	muscle tumor	A tumor containing muscle tissue
myomalacia (mī″ ō-mă-lā′sĭ-ă)	my/o -malacia	CF S	muscle softening	Softening of muscle tissue
myoparesis (mī″ ō-păr′ ĕ-sĭs)	my/o -paresis	CF S	muscle weakness	Weakness or slight paralysis of a muscle
myopathy (mī-ŏp′ ă-thē)	my/o -pathy	CF S	muscle disease	Muscle disease
myoplasty (mī′ ŏ-plăs″ tē)	my/o -plasty	CF S	muscle surgical repair	Surgical repair of a muscle
myorrhaphy (mī-ŏr′ ă-fē)	my/o -rrhaphy	CF S	muscle suture	Suture of a muscle wound

MEDICAL WORD	WORD PARTS (WHEN APPLICABLE)			DEFINITION
	Part	Type	Meaning	
myosarcoma (mī″ ō-sar-kō′ mă)	my/o sarc -oma	CF R S	muscle flesh tumor	A malignant tumor derived from muscle tissue
myosclerosis (mī″ ō-sklĕr-ō′ sĭs)	my/o scler -osis	CF R S	muscle hardening condition of	A condition of hardening of muscle
myospasm (mī″ ō-spăzm)	my/o -spasm	CF S	muscle tension, spasm	Spasmodic contraction of a muscle
myotome (mī′ ō-tōm)	my/o -tome	CF S	muscle instrument to cut	An instrument used to cut muscle
myotomy (mī″ ŏt′ ō-mē)	my/o -tomy	CF S	muscle incision	Incision into a muscle
neuromuscular (nū″ rō-mŭs′ kū-lăr)	neur/o muscul -ar	CF R S	nerve muscle pertaining to	Pertaining to both nerves and muscles
neuromyopathic (nū″ rō-mī″ ō-păth′ ĭk)	neur/o my/o path -ic	CF CF R S	nerve muscle disease pertaining to	Pertaining to disease of both nerves and muscles
polyplegia (pŏl″ ē-plē′ jĭ-ă)	poly -plegia	P S	many stroke, paralysis	Paralysis affecting many muscles
position (pō-zĭsh′ ŭn)				Bodily posture or attitude; the manner in which a patient's body may be arranged for examination. See Table 5–3.
prosthesis (prŏs′ thē-sĭs)	prosth/e -sis	CF S	an addition condition of	An artificial device, organ, or part such as a hand, arm, leg, or tooth
quadriceps (kwŏd′ rĭ-sĕps)	quadri -ceps	P S	four head	A muscle that has four heads or points of origin
relaxation (rē-lăk-sā′ shŭn)	relaxat -ion	R S	to loosen process	The process in which a muscle loosens and returns to a resting stage
rhabdomyoma (răb″ dō-mī-ō′ mă)	rhabd/o my -oma	CF R S	rod muscle tumor	A tumor of striated muscle tissue
rheumatism (roo′mă-tĭzm)	rheumat -ism	R S	discharge condition of	A general term used to describe conditions characterized by inflammation, soreness, and stiffness of muscles, and pain in joints

MEDICAL WORD	WORD PARTS (WHEN APPLICABLE)			DEFINITION
	Part	**Type**	**Meaning**	
rigor mortis (rĭg′ ur mór tĭs)				Stiffness of skeletal muscles seen in death
rotation (rō-tā′ shŭn)	rotat -ion	R S	to turn process	The process of moving a body part around a central axis
rotator cuff (rō-tā′ tor kŭf)				A term used to describe the muscles immediately surrounding the shoulder joint. They stabilize the shoulder joint while the entire arm is moved.
sarcolemma (sar″ kō-lĕm′ ă)	sarc/o lemma	CF R	flesh a rind	A plasma membrane surrounding each striated muscle fiber
spasticity (spăs-tĭs′ ĭ-tē)	spastic -ity	R S	convulsive condition	A condition of increased muscular tone causing stiff and awkward movements
sternocleidomastoid (stur″ nō-klī″ dō-măs′ toyd)	stern/o cleid/o mast -oid	CF CF R S	sternum clavicle breast resemble	Muscle arising from the sternum and clavicle with its insertion in the mastoid process
strain (strān)				Excessive, forcible stretching of a muscle or the musculotendinous unit
synergetic (sin″ ĕr-jĕt′ ĭk)	syn erget -ic	P R S	with, together work pertaining to	Pertaining to certain muscles that work together
synovitis (sĭn″ ȯ-vī′ tĭs)	synov -itis	R S	joint fluid inflammation	Inflammation of a synovial membrane
tendon (tĕn′ dŭn)				A band of fibrous connective tissue serving for the attachment of muscles to bones; a giant cell tumor of a tendon sheath is a benign, small, yellow, tumor-like nodule. See Figure 5–8.
tenodesis (tĕn-ōd′ ĕ-sĭs)	ten/o -desis	CF S	tendon binding	Surgical binding of a tendon
tenodynia (tĕn″ ō-dĭn-ĭ-ă)	ten/o -dynia	CF S	tendon pain	Pain in a tendon
tonic (tŏn′ ĭk)	ton -ic	R S	tone, tension pertaining to	Pertaining to tone, especially muscular tension

MEDICAL WORD	WORD PARTS (WHEN APPLICABLE)			DEFINITION
	Part	**Type**	**Meaning**	
torsion (tòr′ shŭn)	tors -ion	R S	twisted process	The process of being twisted
torticollis (tòr″ tĭ-kŏl′ ĭs)	tort/i -collis	CF R	twisted neck	Stiff neck caused by spasmodic contraction of the muscles of the neck; wryneck
triceps (trī′ sĕps)	tri -ceps	P S	three head	A muscle having three heads with a single insertion
voluntary (vŏl′ ŭn-tĕr″ ē)	volunt -ary	R S	will pertaining to	Pertaining to under the control of one's will

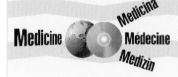

Terminology Translator

This feature, found on the accompanying CD-ROM, provides an innovative tool to translate medical words into Spanish, French, and German.

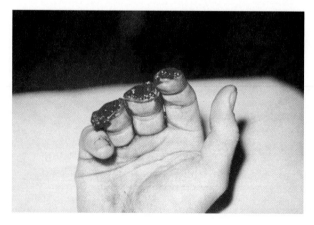

FIGURE 5–5

Amputation of three fingers. (Source: Pearson Education/PH College.)

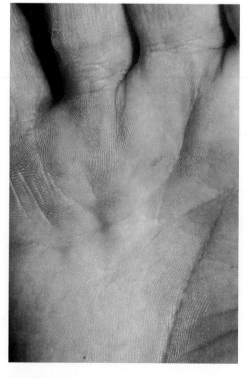

FIGURE 5–6

Dupuytren's contracture. (Courtesy of Jason L. Smith, MD.)

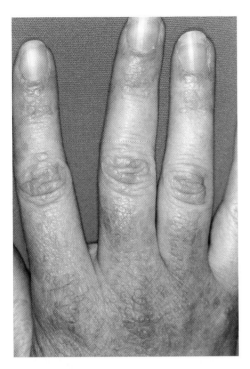

FIGURE 5–7

Dermatomyositis. (Courtesy of Jason L. Smith, MD.)

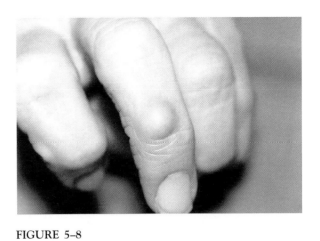

FIGURE 5–8

Giant cell tumor of tendon sheath. (Courtesy of Jason L. Smith, MD.)

TABLE 5–3 TYPES OF POSITIONS

Position	Description
Anatomic	Body is erect, head facing forward, arms by the sides with palms to the front; used as the position of reference in designating the site or direction of a body structure
Dorsal recumbent	Patient is on back with lower extremities flexed and rotated outward; used in application of obstetric forceps, vaginal and rectal examination, and bimanual palpation
Fowler's	The head of the bed or examining table is raised about 18 inches or 46 cm, and the patient sits up with knees also elevated
Knee-chest	Patient on knees, thighs upright, head and upper part of chest resting on bed or examining table, arms crossed and above head; used in sigmoidoscopy, displacement of prolapsed uterus, rectal exams, and flushing of intestinal canal
Lithotomy	Patient is on back with lower extremities flexed and feet placed in stirrups; used in vaginal examination; Pap smear, vaginal operations, and diagnosis and treatment of diseases of the urethra and bladder
Orthopneic	Patient sits upright or erect; used for patients with dyspnea
Prone	Patient lying face downward; used in examination of the back, injections, and massage
Sims'	Patient is lying on left side, right knee and thigh flexed well up above left leg that is slightly flexed, left arm behind the body, and right arm forward, flexed at elbow; used in examination of rectum, sigmoidoscopy, enema, and intrauterine irrigation after labor
Supine	Patient lying flat on back with face upward and arms at the sides; used in examining the head, neck, chest, abdomen, and extremities and in assessing vital signs
Trendelenburg	Patient's body is supine on a bed or examining table that is tilted at about 45° angle with the head lower than the feet; used to displace abdominal organs during surgery and in treating cardiovascular shock; also called the "shock position"

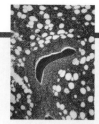

PATHOLOGY SPOTLIGHTS

Atrophy

Atrophy occurs with the disuse of muscles over a long period of time. Bedrest and immobility can cause loss of muscle mass and strength. When immobility is due to a treatment mode, such as casting or traction, one can decrease the effects of immobility by isometric exercise of the muscles of the immobilized part. Isometric exercise involves active muscular contraction performed against stable resistance, such as tightening the muscles of the thigh and/or tightening the muscles of the buttocks. Active exercise of uninjured parts of the body helps prevent muscle atrophy.

Other benefits of exercise:

- It may slow down the progression of osteoporosis.
- It reduces the levels of triglycerides and raises the "good" cholesterol (high-density lipoproteins).
- It can lower systolic and diastolic blood pressure.
- It may improve blood glucose levels in the diabetic person.
- Combined with a low-fat, low-calorie diet, it is effective in preventing obesity and helping individuals maintain a proper body weight.
- It can elevate one's mood and reduce anxiety and tension.

Lipoatrophy is atrophy of fat tissue. This condition may occur at the site of an insulin and/or corticosteroid injection. It is also known as lipodystrophy. See Figure 5–9.

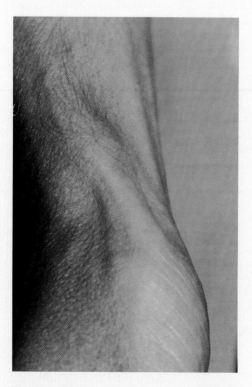

FIGURE 5–9

Lipoatrophy, wrist. (Courtesy of Jason L. Smith, MD.)

Fibromyalgia

Fibromyalgia, or fibromyalgia syndrome (FMS), is a widespread musculoskeletal pain and fatigue disorder. An estimated 3 million are affected in the United States. It affects women more than men, but occurs in those of all ages.

Symptoms include mild to severe muscle pain and fatigue, sleep disorders, irritable bowel syndrome, depression, and chronic headaches. Although the exact cause is still unknown, fibromyalgia is often traced to an injury or physical or emotional trauma. Some doctors feel that many causes contribute to the development of the syndrome, including bacterial, fungal, or viral infection, and hormonal changes. Researchers have found that people with fibromyalgia may have abnormal levels of several chemicals, such as substance P and serotonin, used by the body to transmit and respond to pain signals.

The American College of Rheumatology (ACR) has identified specific criteria for fibromyalgia. The ACR classifies a patient with fibromyalgia if at least 11 of 18 specific areas of the body are painful under pressure. These specific areas are often called "trigger points." See Figure 5–10. Another criterion is that the patient must have had widespread pain lasting at least three months. The location of some of these trigger points includes the inside of the elbow joint, the front of the collarbone, and the base of the skull.

Treatments are geared toward improving the quality of sleep, as well as reducing pain. Because deep sleep is so crucial for many body functions, such as tissue repair and antibody

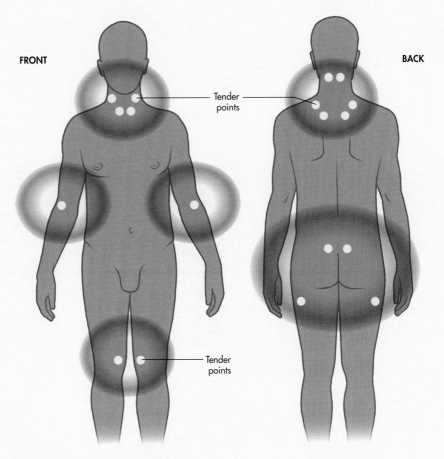

FIGURE 5–10

The 18 tender points of fibromyalgia.

production, the sleep disorders that frequently occur in fibromyalgia are thought to be a major contributing factor to the symptoms. Medications that boost the body's level of serotonin and norepinephrine—neurotransmitters that modulate sleep, pain, and immune system function— are commonly prescribed. Examples of drugs in this category would include cyclobenzaprine (Flexeril), paroxetine (Paxil), and alprazolam (Xanax). In addition, nonsteroidal, anti-inflammatory drugs (NSAIDs) like ibuprofen may also be beneficial. Most patients will probably need to use other treatment methods as well, such as trigger point injections with lidocaine, physical therapy, acupuncture, acupressure, relaxation techniques, chiropractic care, therapeutic massage, or a gentle exercise program.

Myasthenia Gravis

Myasthenia gravis (MG) is a chronic autoimmune neuromuscular disease characterized by varying degrees of weakness of the skeletal (voluntary) muscles of the body. The name *myasthenia gravis*, which is Latin and Greek in origin, literally means "grave muscle weakness." With current therapies, however, most cases of myasthenia gravis are not as "grave" as the name implies. For the majority of individuals with myasthenia gravis, life expectancy is not lessened by the disorder.

The primary symptom of myasthenia gravis is muscle weakness that increases during periods of activity and improves after periods of rest. Certain muscles such as those that control eye and eyelid movement, facial expression, chewing, talking, and swallowing are often, but not always, involved in the disorder. The muscles that control breathing and neck and limb movements may also be affected.

Myasthenia gravis is caused by a defect in the transmission of nerve impulses to muscles. It occurs when normal communication between the nerve and muscle is interrupted at the neuromuscular junction—the place where nerve cells connect with the muscles they control.

Normally when impulses travel down the nerve, the nerve endings release a neurotransmitter substance called acetylcholine. Acetylcholine travels through the neuromuscular junction and binds to acetylcholine receptors which are activated and generate a muscle contraction.

In myasthenia gravis, antibodies block, alter, or destroy the receptors for acetylcholine at the neuromuscular junction, which prevents the muscle contraction from occurring. These antibodies are produced by the body's own immune system. Thus, myasthenia gravis is an autoimmune disease because the immune system—which normally protects the body from foreign organisms—mistakenly attacks itself.

Myasthenia gravis occurs in all ethnic groups and both genders. It most commonly affects young adult women (under 40) and older men (over 60), but it can occur at any age.

Treatment may include lifestyle adjustments that may enable continuation of many activities, including planning activity to allow for scheduled rest periods, and avoiding stress and excessive heat exposure. Some medications, such as neostigmine or pyridostigmine, improve the communication between the nerve and the muscle. Prednisone and other medications that suppress the immune response (such as azathioprine or cyclosporine) may be used if symptoms are severe and there is inadequate response to other medications.

Muscular Dystrophy

Muscular dystrophy (MD) refers to a group of genetic diseases characterized by progressive weakness and degeneration of the skeletal or voluntary muscles which control movement. The muscles of the heart and some other involuntary muscles are also affected in some forms of MD, and a few forms involve other organs as well.

The major forms of MD include myotonic, Duchenne, Becker, limb-girdle, facioscapulohumeral, congenital, oculopharyngeal, distal and Emery-Dreifuss. Duchenne is the most common form of MD affecting children, and myotonic MD is the most common form affecting adults. MD can affect people of all ages. Although some forms first become apparent in infancy or childhood, others may not appear until middle age or later.

The prognosis of MD varies according to the type of MD and the progression of the disorder. Some cases may be mild and very slowly progressive, with normal lifespan, while other cases may have more marked progression of muscle weakness, functional disability and loss of ambulation. Life expectancy may depend on the degree of progression and late respiratory deficit. In Duchenne MD, death usually occurs in the late teens to early twenties.

There is no specific treatment for any of the forms of MD. Physical therapy to prevent contractures (a condition in which shortened muscles around joints cause abnormal and sometimes painful positioning of the joints), orthoses (orthopedic appliances used for support) and corrective orthopedic surgery may be needed to improve the quality of life in some cases. The cardiac problems that occur with Emery-Dreifuss MD and myotonic MD may require a pacemaker. The myotonia (delayed relaxation of a muscle after a strong contraction) occurring in myotonic MD may be treated with medications such as phenytoin or quinine.

✓ PATHOLOGY CHECKPOINT

Following is a concise list of the pathology-related terms that you've seen in the chapter. Review this checklist to make sure that you are familiar with the meaning of each term before moving on to the next section.

Conditions and Symptoms

- ❏ amputation
- ❏ ataxia
- ❏ atonic
- ❏ atrophy
- ❏ brachialgia
- ❏ bradykinesia
- ❏ contracture
- ❏ dactylospasm
- ❏ dermatomyositis
- ❏ dystonia
- ❏ dystrophy
- ❏ fascitis
- ❏ fatigue
- ❏ fibromyalgia
- ❏ fibromyitis
- ❏ flaccid
- ❏ muscular dystrophy
- ❏ myalgia
- ❏ myasthenia

- ❏ myasthenia gravis
- ❏ myitis
- ❏ myofibroma
- ❏ myokinesis
- ❏ myoma
- ❏ myomalacia
- ❏ myoparesis
- ❏ myopathy
- ❏ myosarcoma
- ❏ myosclerosis
- ❏ myospasm
- ❏ neuromyopathic
- ❏ polyplegia
- ❏ rhabdomyoma
- ❏ rheumatism
- ❏ rigor mortis
- ❏ spasticity
- ❏ strain
- ❏ synovitis
- ❏ tenodynia

- ❏ torsion
- ❏ torticollis

Diagnosis and Treatment

- ❏ diathermy
- ❏ exercise
- ❏ First Aid—RICE
- ❏ heat
- ❏ hydrotherapy
- ❏ massage
- ❏ myograph
- ❏ myoplasty
- ❏ myorrhaphy
- ❏ myotome
- ❏ myotomy
- ❏ position
- ❏ prosthesis
- ❏ tenodesis

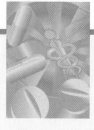

DRUG HIGHLIGHTS

DRUG HIGHLIGHTS

Drugs that are generally used for muscular system diseases and disorders include skeletal muscle relaxants and stimulants, neuromuscular blocking agents, anti-inflammatory agents, and analgesics. See Chapter 4, The Skeletal System, Drug Highlights for a description of anti-inflammatory agents and analgesics.

Skeletal Muscle Relaxants

Used to treat painful muscle spasms that may result from strains, sprains, and musculo-skeletal trauma or disease. Centrally acting muscle relaxants act by depressing the central nervous system (CNS) and can be administered either orally or by injection. The patient must be informed of the sedative effect produced by these drugs. Drowsiness, dizziness, and blurred vision may diminish the patient's ability to drive a vehicle, operate equipment, or climb stairs.

Examples: Lioresal (baclofen), Flexeril (cyclobenzaprine HCl), and Robaxin (methocarbamol).

Skeletal Muscle Stimulants

Used in the treatment of myasthenia gravis. This disease is characterized by progressive weakness of skeletal muscles and their rapid fatiguing. Skeletal muscle stimulants act by inhibiting the action of acetylcholinesterase, the enzyme that halts the action of acetylcholine at the neuromuscular junction. By slowing the destruction of acetylcholine, these drugs foster accumulation of higher concentrations of this neurotransmitter and increase the number of interactions between acetylcholine and the available receptors on muscle fibers.

Examples: Tensilon (edrophonium chloride), Prostigmin Bromide (neostigmine bromide), and Mestinon (pyridostigmine bromide).

Neuromuscular Blocking Agents

Used to provide muscle relaxation. These agents are used in patients undergoing surgery and/or electroconvulsive therapy, endotracheal intubation, and to relieve laryngospasm.

Examples: Tracrium (atracurium besylate), Flaxedil (gallamine triethiodide), and Norcuron (vecuronium).

DIAGNOSTIC & LAB TESTS

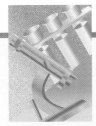

TEST	DESCRIPTION
aldolase (ALD) blood test (ăl′ dō-lāz blod test)	A test performed on serum that measures ALD enzyme present in skeletal and heart muscle. It is helpful in the diagnosis of Duchenne's muscular dystrophy before symptoms appear.
calcium blood test (kăl′ sē-ŭm blod test)	A test performed on serum to determine levels of calcium. Calcium is essential for muscular contraction, nerve transmission, and blood clotting.
creatine phosphokinase (CPK) (krē′ ă-tĭn fŏs″ fō-kīn′ āz)	A blood test to determine the level of CPK. It is increased in necrosis or atrophy of skeletal muscle, traumatic muscle injury, strenuous exercise, and progressive muscular dystrophy.
electromyography (EMG) (ē-lĕk″ trō-mī-ŏg′ ră-fē)	A test to measure electrical activity across muscle membranes by means of electrodes that are attached to a needle that is inserted into the muscle. Electrical activity can be heard over a loudspeaker, viewed on an oscilloscope, or printed on a graph (electromyogram). Abnormal results may indicate myasthenia gravis, amyotrophic lateral sclerosis, muscular dystrophy, peripheral neuropathy, and anterior poliomyelitis.
lactic dehydrogenase (LDH) (lăk′ tĭk dē-hī-drŏj′ ě-nāz)	A blood test to determine the level of LDH enzyme. It is increased in muscular dystrophy, damage to skeletal muscles, after a pulmonary embolism, and during skeletal muscle malignancy.
muscle biopsy (mŭs′ ĕl bī′ ŏp-sē)	An operative procedure in which a small piece of muscle tissue is excised and then stained for microscopic examination. Lower motor neuron disease, degeneration, inflammatory reactions, or involvement of specific muscle fibers may indicate myopathic disease.
serum glutamic oxaloacetic transaminase (SGOT) (sē′ rŭm gloo-tăm′ ĭk ŏks″ ăl-ō-ă-sē′ tĭk trăns ăm′ ĭn-āz)	A blood test to determine the level of SGOT enzyme. It is increased in skeletal muscle damage and muscular dystrophy. This test is also called aspartate aminotransferase (AST).
serum glutamic pyruvic transaminase (SGPT) (sē′ rŭm gloo-tăm′ ĭk pī-roo′ vĭk trăns-ăm′ ĭn-āz)	A blood test to determine the level of SGPT enzyme. It is increased in skeletal muscle damage. This test is also called alanine aminotransferase (ALT).

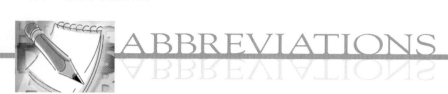

ABBREVIATIONS

ABBREVIATION	MEANING
ACR	American College of Rheumatology
ADP	adenosine diphosphate
AE	above elbow
AK	above knee
ALD	aldolase
AST	aspartate aminotransferase
ATP	adenosine triphosphate
BE	below elbow
BK	below knee
Ca	calcium
CPK	creatine phosphokinase
CPM	continuous passive motion
DTRs	deep tendon reflexes
EMG	electromyography
FMS	fibromyalgia syndrome
FROM	full range of motion
Ht	height
IM	intramuscular

ABBREVIATION	MEANING
LDH	lactic dehydrogenase
LOM	limitation or loss of motion
MD	muscular dystrophy
MG	myasthenia gravis
MS	musculoskeletal
NSAIDs	nonsteroidal anti-inflammatory drugs
PM	physical medicine
PMR	physical medicine and rehabilitation
ROM	range of motion
SGOT	serum glutamic oxaloacetic transaminase
SGPT	serum glutamic pyruvic transaminase
sh	shoulder
TBW	total body weight
TJ	triceps jerk
wt	weight

STUDY AND REVIEW

Anatomy and Physiology

Write your answers to the following questions. Do not refer to the text.

1. The muscular system is made up of three types of muscle tissue. Name the three types.

   a. _____   b. _____

   c. _____

2. Muscles make up approximately _____ percent of a person's body weight.

3. Name the two essential ingredients that are needed for a muscle to perform properly.

   a. _____   b. _____

4. Name the two points of attachment for a skeletal muscle.

   a. _____   b. _____

5. Skeletal muscle is also known as _____ or _____.

6. A wide, thin, sheet-like tendon is known as an _____.

7. Name the three distinguishable parts of a muscle.

   a. _____   b. _____

   c. _____

8. Define the following:

   a. Antagonist _____

   b. Prime mover _____

   c. Synergist _____

9. Smooth muscle is also called _____, _____, or

   _____.

10. Smooth muscles are found in the internal organs. Name five examples of these locations.

   a. _____   b. _____

   c. _____   d. _____

   e. _____

11. _____ is the muscle of the heart.

12. Name the three primary functions of the muscular system.

   a. _____   b. _____

   c. _____

Word Parts

1. In the spaces provided, write the definition of these prefixes, roots, combining forms, and suffixes. Do not refer to the listings of medical words. Leave blank those words you cannot define.

2. After completing as many as you can, refer to the medical word listings to check your work. For each word missed or left blank, write the word and its definition several times on the margins of these pages or on a separate sheet of paper.

3. To maximize the learning process, it is to your advantage to do the following exercises as directed. To refer to the word building section before completing these exercises invalidates the learning process.

PREFIXES

Give the definitions of the following prefixes:

1. a- _____   2. ab- _____

3. ad- _____   4. ant- _____

5. apo- _____   6. bi- _____

7. brady- _____   8. con- _____

9. dia- _____   10. dys- _____

11. in- _____   12. intra- _____

13. hydro- _____   14. quadri- _____

15. syn- _____   16. tri- _____

ROOTS AND COMBINING FORMS

Give the definitions of the following roots and combining forms:

1. agon _____

2. brach\i _____

3. cleid/o _____

4. amputat _____

5. collis _____

6. dactyl/o _____

7. duct _____

8. erget _____

9. fasc _____

10. dermat/o _____

11. rheumat _____

12. fibr _____

13. fibr/o _____

14. is/o _____

15. lemma _____

16. levat _____

17. prosth/e _____

18. mast _____

19. therm _____

20. metr _____

21. muscul _____

22. my _____

23. my/o _____

24. my/os _____

25. neur _____

26. neur/o _____

27. path _____

28. relaxat _____

29. rhabd/o _____

30. rotat _____

31. troph _____

32. sarc/o _____

33. scler _____

34. sert _____

35. spastic _____

36. stern/o _____

37. teno _____

38. ton _____

39. torti _____

40. tract _____

41. volunt _____

42. synov _____

43. tors _____

SUFFIXES

Give the definitions of the following suffixes:

1. -algia _____

2. -ar _____

3. -ary _____

4. -asthenia _____

5. -blast _____

6. -ceps _____

7. -desis _____

8. -dynia _____

9. -in _____

10. -therapy _____

11. -graph _____

12. -ia _____

13. -ic _____

14. -ion _____

15. -ist _____

16. -itis _____

17. -ity _____

18. -kinesia _____

19. -kinesis _____

20. -logy _____

21. -ure _____

22. -malacia _____

23. -oid _____

24. -oma _____

25. -or _____

26. -osis _____

27. -paresis _____

28. -pathy _____

29. -phragm _____

30. -plasty _____

31. -plegia _____

32. -rrhaphy _____

33. -y _____

34. -spasm _____

35. -taxia _____

36. -tome _____

37. -tomy _____

38. -trophy _____

39. -sis _____

40. -ism _____

Identifying Medical Terms

In the spaces provided, write the medical terms for the following meanings:

1. _____ Pertaining to a lack of normal tone or tension

2. _____ Slowness of motion or movement

3. _____ Cramp of a finger or toe

4. _____ Faulty muscular development caused by lack of nourishment

5. _____ Pertaining to within a muscle

6. _____ A muscle that raises or elevates a part

7. _____ Muscle weakness

8. _____ Study of muscles

9. _____ Weakness or slight paralysis of a muscle

10. _____ Surgical repair of a muscle

11. _____ A malignant tumor derived from muscle tissue

12. _____ Incision into a muscle

13. _____ Paralysis affecting many muscles

14. _____ Surgical binding of a tendon

15. _____ Pertaining to certain muscles that work together

16. _____ A muscle having three heads with a single insertion

Spelling

In the spaces provided, write the correct spelling of these misspelled terms:

1. facia _____

2. mykinesis _____

3. dermatomyoitis _____

4. rhadomyoma _____

5. sarclemma _____

6. sterncleidomastoid _____

7. dystropin _____

8. torticolis _____

Matching

Select the appropriate lettered meaning for each ward listed below.

_____ 1. dermatomyositis

_____ 2. fibromyalgia

_____ 3. muscular dystrophy

_____ 4. flaccid

_____ 5. prosthesis

_____ 6. rotator cuff

_____ 7. strain

_____ 8. tenodynia

_____ 9. torsion

_____ 10. voluntary

a. A term used to describe the muscles immediately surrounding the shoulder joint

b. The process of being twisted

c. Pain in a tendon

d. Inflammation of the muscles and the skin

e. Lacking muscle tone

f. Pertaining to under the control of one's will

g. A chronic, progressive wasting and weakening of muscles

h. Excessive, forcible stretching of a muscle or the musculotendinous unit

i. A condition with widespread muscular pain and debilitating fatigue

j. An artificial device, organ, or part

k. Pain in a joint

Abbreviations

Place the correct word, phrase, or abbreviation in the space provided.

1. AE _____

2. AST _____

3. calcium _____

4. electromyography _____

5. FROM _____

6. MS _____

7. range of motion _____

8. shoulder _____

9. TBW _____

10. TJ _____

Diagnostic and Laboratory Tests

Select the best answer to each multiple choice question. Circle the letter of your choice.

1. A diagnostic test to help diagnose Duchenne's muscular dystrophy before symptoms appear.
   a. creatine phosphokinase
   b. aldolase blood test
   c. calcium blood test
   d. muscle biopsy

2. A test to measure electrical activity across muscle membranes by means of electrodes that are attached to a needle that is inserted into the muscle.
   a. muscle biopsy
   b. lactic dehydrogenase
   c. creatine phosphokinase
   d. electromyography

3. This test is also called aspartate aminotransferase.
   a. lactic dehydrogenase
   b. serum glutamic oxaloacetic transaminase
   c. serum glutamic pyruvic transaminase
   d. creatine phosphokinase

4. This test is also called alanine aminotransferase.
   a. lactic dehydrogenase
   b. serum glutamic oxaloacetic transaminase
   c. serum glutamic pyruvic transaminase
   d. creatine phosphokinase

5. For a/an _____, a small piece of muscle tissue is excised and then stained for microscopic examination.
   a. muscle biopsy
   b. electromyography
   c. bone biopsy
   d. electrocardiography

CASE STUDY

DUCHENNE'S MUSCULAR DYSTROPHY

Read the following case study and then answer the questions that follow.

A 3-year-old male child was seen by a physician; the following is a synopsis of the visit.

Present History: The mother states that she noticed that her son has been falling a lot and seems to be very clumsy. She says that he has a waddling gait, is very slow in running and climbing, and walks on his toes. She is most concerned as she is at risk for carrying the gene that causes muscular dystrophy.

Signs and Symptoms: A waddling gait, very slow in running and climbing, walks on his toes, frequent falling, clumsy.

Diagnosis: Duchenne's muscular dystrophy. The diagnosis was determined by the characteristic symptoms, family history, a muscle biopsy, an electromyography, and an elevated serum creatine kinase level.

Treatment: Physical therapy, deep breathing exercises to help delay muscular weakness, supportive measures such as splints and braces to help minimize deformities and to preserve mobility. Counseling and referral services are essential. For more information you may contact the Muscular Dystrophy Association at: 3561 E. Sunrise Drive, Tucson, AZ 85718. Telephone: 1-602-529-2000 or 1-800-572-1717. E-mail: mda@mdausa.org

CASE STUDY QUESTIONS

1. Signs and symptoms of Duchenne's muscular dystrophy include a _____ gait, frequent falls, clumsiness, slowness in running and climbing, and walking on toes.

2. The diagnosis was determined by the characteristic symptoms, family history, a muscle biopsy, an _____, and an elevated serum creatine kinase level.

3. As part of the treatment for Duchenne's muscular dystrophy, the use of splints and braces help to: a. _____ and b. _____.

 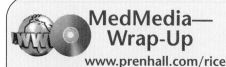

MedMedia— Wrap-Up

www.prenhall.com/rice

Additional interactive resources and activities for this chapter can be found on the Companion Website. For animations, videos, audio glossary, and review, access the accompanying CD-ROM in this book.

Audio Glossary
Pathology Spotlights
Medical Terminology Exercises & Activities
Terminology Translator
Animations
Videos

Objectives
Medical Terminology Exercises & Activities
Audio Glossary
Drug Updates
Medical Terminology in the News

THE DIGESTIVE SYSTEM 6

OBJECTIVES

On completion of this chapter, you will be able to:

- Describe the digestive system.
- Describe the primary organs of the digestive system and state their functions.
- Describe the two sets of teeth that man is provided with.
- Describe the three main portions of a tooth.
- Describe the accessory organs of the digestive system and state their functions.
- Describe digestive differences of the child and the older adult.
- Analyze, build, spell, and pronounce medical words.
- Describe each of the conditions presented in the Pathology Spotlights.
- Complete the Pathology Checkpoint.
- Review Drug Highlights presented in this chapter.
- Provide the description of diagnostic and laboratory tests related to the digestive system.
- Identify and define selected abbreviations.
- Successfully complete the study and review section.

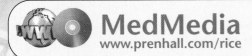

MedMedia
www.prenhall.com/rice

Additional interactive resources and activities for this chapter can be found on the Companion Website. For Terminology Translator, animations, videos, audio glossary, and review, access the accompanying CD-ROM in this book.

Anatomy and Physiology Overview

Ageneral description of the digestive system is that of a continuous tube beginning with the mouth and ending at the anus. This tube is known as the **alimentary canal** and/or **gastrointestinal tract**. It measures about 30 feet in adults and contains both primary and accessory organs for the conversion of food and fluids into a semiliquid that can be absorbed for use by the body. The three main functions of the digestive system are **digestion, absorption,** and **elimination**. Each of the various organs commonly associated with digestion is described in this chapter. The organs of digestion are shown in Figure 6–1.

THE MOUTH

The **mouth** is the cavity formed by the palate or roof, the lips and cheeks on the sides, and the tongue at its floor. Contained within are the teeth and salivary glands. The cheeks form the lateral walls and are continuous with the lips. The vestibule includes the space between the cheeks and the teeth. The **gingivae** (gums) surround the necks of the teeth. The hard and soft palates provide a roof for the oral cavity, with the tongue at its floor. The free portion of the tongue is connected to the underlying epithelium by a thin fold of mucous membrane, the **lingual frenulum**. The **tongue** is made of skeletal muscle and is covered with mucous membrane. The tongue can be divided into a blunt rear portion called the **root**, a pointed **tip**, and a central **body**. Located on the surface of the tongue are **papillae** (elevations) and **taste buds** (sweet,

THE DIGESTIVE SYSTEM

Organ	Functions
Mouth	Breaks food apart by the action of the teeth, moistens and lubricates food with saliva; food formed into a bolus
Teeth	Serve as organs of mastication
Pharynx	Common passageway for both respiration and digestion; muscular constrictions move the bolus into the esophagus
Esophagus	Peristalsis moves the food down the esophagus into the stomach
Stomach	Reduces food to a digestible state, converts the food to a semiliquid form
Small Intestine	Digestion and absorption take place. Nutrients are absorbed into tiny capillaries and lymph vessels in the walls of the small intestine and transmitted to body cells by the circulatory system
Large Intestine	Removes water from the fecal material, stores, and then eliminates waste from the body via the rectum and anus
Salivary Glands	Secrete saliva to moisten and lubricate food
Liver	Changes glucose to glycogen and stores it until needed; changes glycogen back to glucose; desaturates fats, assists in protein catabolism, manufactures bile, fibrinogen, prothrombin, heparin, and blood proteins, stores vitamins, produces heat, and detoxifies substances
Gallbladder	Stores and concentrates bile
Pancreas	Secretes pancreatic juice into the small intestine, contains cells that produce digestive enzymes, secretes insulin and glucagon

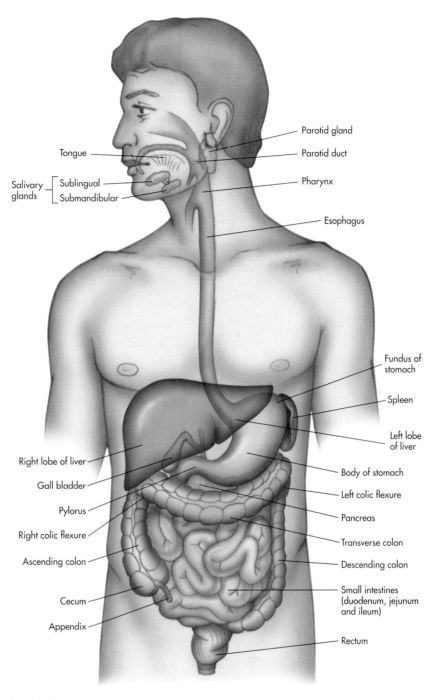

FIGURE 6–1

The digestive system.

salt, sour, and bitter). Three pairs of salivary glands secrete fluids into the oral cavity. These glands are the **parotid**, **sublingual**, and **submandibular**. The posterior margin of the soft palate supports the dangling uvula and two pairs of muscular pharyngeal arches. On either side, a palatine tonsil lies between an anterior palatoglossal arch and a posterior palatopharyngeal arch. A curving line that connects the palatoglossal arches and uvula forms the boundaries of the fauces, the passageway between the oral cavity and the pharynx (Fig. 6–2). Digestion begins as food is broken apart by the action of the teeth, moistened and lubricated by saliva, and formed into a **bolus**. A bolus is a small mass of masticated food ready to be swallowed.

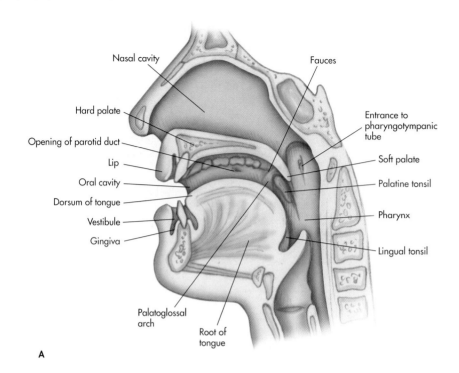

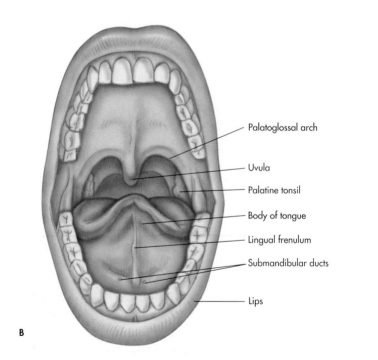

FIGURE 6–2

The oral cavity: (A) sagittal section; (B) anterior view as seen through the open mouth.

THE TEETH

Man is provided with two sets of teeth. There are twenty **deciduous** teeth: eight incisors, four canines (cuspids), and eight molars. There are thirty-two **permanent** teeth: eight incisors, four canines, eight premolars, and twelve molars. See Figure 6–3.

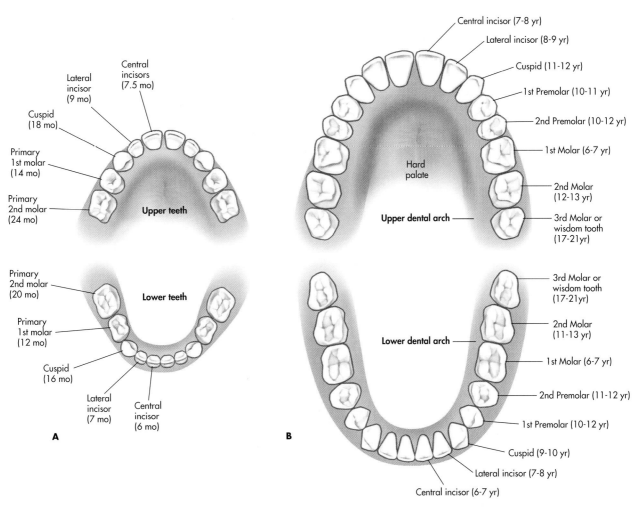

FIGURE 6–3

Deciduous and permanent teeth. (A) The deciduous teeth, with the age of eruption given in months; (B) the permanent teeth, with the age at eruption given in years.

The **incisors** are so named from their presenting a sharp cutting edge, adapted for biting the food. They form the four front teeth in each dental arch. The upper incisors are larger and stronger than the lower.

The **canine** or **cuspid** teeth are larger and stronger than the incisors, and their roots sink deeply into the bones, and cause well-marked prominences upon the surface. The upper canine teeth are called "eye teeth" and are larger and longer than the lower. The lower canine teeth, called "stomach teeth," are placed nearer the middle line than the upper.

The **premolars** or **bicuspid** teeth are situated lateral to and behind the canine teeth. They are eight in number, four in each arch and are smaller and shorter than the canine teeth.

The **molar** teeth are the largest of the permanent set, and their broad crowns are adapted for grinding and pounding the food. They are twelve in number: six in each arch, three being placed posterior to each of the second premolars.

The deciduous teeth are smaller than, but generally resemble in form, the teeth which bear the same names in the permanent set.

Each tooth consists of three main portions: the **crown**, projecting above the gum; the **root**, imbedded in the alveolus; and the **neck**, the constricted portion between the crown and root. The roots of the teeth are firmly implanted in depressions within the alveoli; these depressions are lined with periosteum, which invests the tooth as far as the neck. At the margins of the alveoli, the periosteum is continuous with the fibrous structure of the gums.

On making a vertical section of a tooth, a cavity will be found in the interior of the crown and the center of each root; it opens by a minute orifice at the extremity of the latter. See Figure 6–4. This is called the **pulp cavity**, and contains the dental pulp, a loose connective tissue richly supplied with vessels and nerves, which enter the cavity through the small aperture at the point of each root. The pulp cavity receives blood vessels and nerves from the **root canal**, a narrow tunnel located at the **root**, or base, of the tooth. Blood vessels and nerves enter the root canal through an opening called the **apical foramen** to supply the pulp cavity.

The root of each tooth sits in a bony socket called an alveolus. Collagen fibers of the **periodontal ligament** extend from the dentin of the root to the bone of the alveolus, creating a strong articulation known as a gomphosis (that binds the teeth to bony sockets in the maxillary bone and mandible). A layer of **cementum** covers the dentin of the root, providing protection and firmly anchoring the periodontal ligament.

The solid portion of the tooth consists of the **dentin**, which forms the bulk of the tooth; the **enamel**, which covers the exposed part of the crown and is the hardest and most compact part of a tooth; and a thin layer of bone, the **cementum**, which is disposed on the surface of the root.

The neck of the tooth marks the boundary between the root and the crown, the exposed portion of the tooth that projects above the soft tissue of the **gingiva**. A shallow groove called the **gingival sulcus** surrounds the neck of each tooth.

When the calcification of the different tissues of the tooth is sufficiently advanced to enable it to bear the pressure to which it will be afterward subjected, eruption takes place, the tooth making its way through the gums. The eruption of the deciduous teeth commences about the seventh month after birth, and is completed about the end of the second year, the teeth of the lower jaw preceding those of the upper. At the age of 2½ years a child should have 20 teeth.

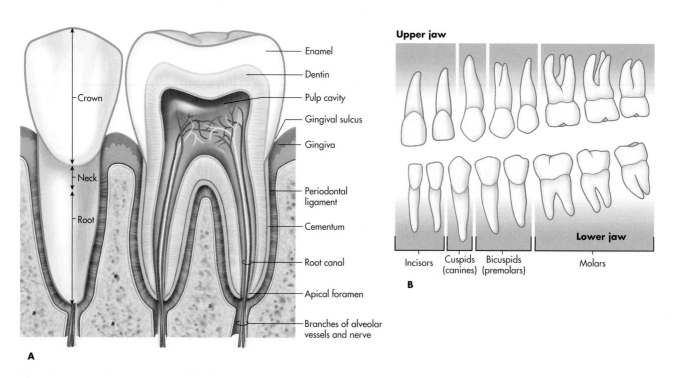

FIGURE 6–4

Teeth. (A) A diagrammatic section through a typical adult tooth; (B) the adult teeth.

The eruption of the permanent teeth takes place around the following time periods:

Upper Dental Arch

First molars	6th to 7th year
Two central incisors	7th to 8th year
Two lateral incisors	8th to 9th year
First premolars	10th to 11th year
Second premolars	10th to 12th year
Canines	11th to 12th year
Second molars	12th to 13th year
Third molars	17th to 21st year

THE PHARYNX

Just beyond the mouth, at the beginning of the tube leading to the stomach, is the **pharynx**. Simply put, the pharynx is a common passageway for both respiration and digestion. Both the **larynx**, or voicebox, and the esophagus begin in the pharynx. Food that is swallowed passes through the pharynx into the esophagus reflexively. Muscular constrictions move the ball of food into the esophagus while, at the same time, blocking the opening to the larynx and preventing the food from entering the airway leading to the trachea or windpipe.

THE ESOPHAGUS

The **esophagus** is a collapsible tube about 10 inches long that leads from the pharynx to the stomach. Food passes down the esophagus and into the stomach. Food is carried along the esophagus by a series of wave-like muscular contractions called **peristalsis**.

THE STOMACH

The **stomach** is a large sac-like organ into which food passes from the esophagus for storage while undergoing the early processes of digestion. In the stomach, food is further reduced to a digestible state. Hydrochloric acid and gastric juices convert the food to a semiliquid state, which is passed, at intervals, into the small intestine.

THE SMALL INTESTINE

The **small intestine** is about 21 feet long and 1 inch in diameter. It extends from the pyloric orifice at the base of the stomach to the entrance of the large intestine. The small intestine is considered to have three parts: the **duodenum**, the **jejunum**, and the

ileum. The duodenum is the first 12 inches just beyond the stomach. The jejunum is the next 8 feet or so, and the ileum is the remaining 12 feet of the tube. Semiliquid food (called **chyme**) is received from the stomach through the pylorus and mixed with bile from the liver and gallbladder along with pancreatic juice from the pancreas. Digestion and absorption take place chiefly in the small intestine. Nutrients are absorbed into tiny capillaries and lymph vessels in the walls of the small intestine and transmitted to body cells by the circulatory system.

THE LARGE INTESTINE

The **large intestine** is about 5 feet long and 2.5 inches in diameter. It extends from the ileocecal orifice at the small intestine to the anus. The large intestine may be divided into the **cecum**, the **colon**, the **rectum**, and the **anal canal**. The cecum is a pouch-like structure forming the beginning of the large intestine. It is about 3 inches long and has the appendix attached to it. The **colon** makes up the bulk of the large intestine and is divided into several parts—the ascending colon, the transverse colon, the descending colon, and, at its end, the sigmoid colon. Digestion and absorption continue in the large intestine on a reduced scale. The waste products of digestion are eliminated from the body via the rectum and the anus.

ACCESSORY ORGANS

The **salivary glands**, the **liver**, the **gallbladder**, and the **pancreas** are not actually part of the digestive tube; however, they are closely related to it in their functions.

The Salivary Glands

Located in or near the mouth, the **salivary glands** secrete **saliva** in response to the sight, smell, taste, or mental image of food. The various salivary glands are the **parotid**, located on either side of the face slightly below the ear; the **submandibular**, located in the floor of the mouth; and the **sublingual**, located below the tongue. All salivary glands secrete through openings into the mouth to moisten and lubricate food.

The Liver

The largest glandular organ in the body, the **liver** weighs about 3½ lb and is located in the upper right part of the abdomen. The liver plays an essential role in the normal metabolism of carbohydrates, fats, and proteins. In carbohydrate metabolism, it changes glucose to glycogen and stores it until needed by body cells. It also changes glycogen back to glucose. In fat metabolism, the liver serves as a storage place and acts to desaturate fats before releasing them into the bloodstream. In protein metabolism, the liver acts as a storage place and assists in protein catabolism.

The liver manufactures the following important substances:

- **Bile**—a digestive juice
- **Fibrinogen and prothrombin**—coagulants essential for blood clotting
- **Heparin**—an anticoagulant that helps to prevent the clotting of blood
- **Blood proteins**—albumin, gamma globulin

Additionally, the liver stores iron and vitamins B_{12}, A, D, E, and K. It also produces body heat and detoxifies many harmful substances such as drugs and alcohol.

The Gallbladder

The **gallbladder** is a membranous sac attached to the liver in which excess bile is stored and concentrated. Bile leaving the gallbladder is 6 to 10 times as concentrated as that which comes to it from the liver. Concentration is accomplished by absorption of water from the bile into the mucosa of the gallbladder.

The Pancreas

The **pancreas** is a large, elongated gland situated behind the stomach and secreting pancreatic juice into the small intestine. The pancreas is 6 to 9 inches long and contains cells that produce digestive **enzymes**. Other cells in the pancreas secrete the hormones insulin and glucagon directly into the bloodstream.

LIFE SPAN CONSIDERATIONS

■ THE CHILD

The primitive digestive tract is formed by the embryonic membrane (yolk sac) and is divided into three sections. The **foregut** evolves into the pharynx, lower respiratory tract, esophagus, stomach, duodenum, and beginning of the common bile duct. The **midgut** elongates in the fifth week to form the primary intestinal loop. The remainder of the large colon is derived from the primitive **hindgut**. The liver, pancreas, and biliary tract evolve from the **foregut**. At 8 weeks, the anal membrane ruptures, forming the anal canal and opening.

Normally the functioning of the gastrointestinal tract begins after birth. Food is prepared for absorption and absorbed, and waste products are eliminated. **Meconium**, the first stool, is a mixture of amniotic fluid and secretions of the intestinal glands. It is thick and sticky, and dark green in color. It is usually passed 8 to 24 hours following birth. The stools change during the first week and become loose and greenish-yellow. The stools of a breast-fed baby are bright yellow, soft, and pasty. The stools of a bottle-fed baby are more solid than those of the breast-fed baby and they vary from yellow to brown in color.

The infant's stomach is small and empties rapidly. Newborns produce very little saliva until they are 3 months of age. Swallowing is a reflex action for the first 3 months. The hepatic efficiency of the newborn is often immature, thereby, causing **jaundice**. Fat absorption is poor because of a decreased level of bile production.

■ THE OLDER ADULT

With aging, the digestive system becomes less motile, as muscle contractions become weaker. Glandular secretions decrease, thus causing a drier mouth and a lower volume of gastric juices. Nutrient absorption is mildly reduced due to **atrophy** of the mucosal lining. The teeth are mechanically worn down with age and begin to recede from the gums. There is a loss of tastebuds, and food preferences change. Gastric motor activity slows; as a result, gastric emptying is delayed and hunger contractions diminish. There are no significant changes in the small intestine, but in the large intestine, the muscle layer and mucosa atrophy. Smooth muscle tone and blood flow decrease, and connective tissue increases.

Constipation is a frequent problem among older adults. It is believed that constipation is not a normal age-related change, but is caused by low fluid intake, lack of dietary fiber, inactivity, medicines, depression, and other health-related conditions.

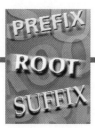

BUILDING YOUR MEDICAL VOCABULARY

This section provides the foundation for learning medical terminology. Medical words can be made up of four different types of word parts:

- Prefixes (P)
- Roots (R)
- Combining forms (CF)
- Suffixes (S)

By connecting various word parts in an organized sequence, thousands of words can be built and learned. In this text the word list is alphabetized so one can see the variety of meanings created when common prefixes and suffixes are repeatedly applied to certain word roots and/or combining forms. Words shown in pink are additional words related to the content of this chapter that are not built from word parts. These words are included to enhance your vocabulary. Note: an asterisk icon ✱ indicates words that are covered in the Pathology Spotlights section in this chapter.

MEDICAL WORD	WORD PARTS (WHEN APPLICABLE)			DEFINITION
	Part	Type	Meaning	
absorption (ăb-sōrp′ shŭn)	absorpt -ion	R S	to suck in process	The process whereby nutrient material is taken into the bloodstream or lymph
amylase (ăm′ ĭ-lās)	amyl -ase	R S	starch enzyme	An enzyme that breaks down starch
anabolism (ă-năb′ ō-lĭzm)	ana bol -ism	P R S	up to cast, throw condition of	Literally "a throwing upward"; the building up of the body substance
anorexia (ăn″ ō-rĕks′ ĭ-ă)	an -orexia	P S	lack of appetite	Lack of appetite
appendectomy (ăp″ ĕn-dĕk′ tō-mē)	append -ectomy	R S	appendix excision	Surgical excision of the appendix
appendicitis (ă-pĕn″ dĭ-sī′ tĭs)	appendic -itis	R S	appendix inflammation	Inflammation of the appendix
ascites (ă-sī′ tēz)				An accumulation of serous fluid in the peritoneal cavity
biliary (bĭl′ ĭ-ār″ ē)	bil/i -ary	CF S	gall, bile pertaining to	Pertaining to or conveying bile

MEDICAL WORD	WORD PARTS (WHEN APPLICABLE)			DEFINITION
	Part	**Type**	**Meaning**	
bilirubin (bĭl″ ĭ-rōō′ bĭn)				The orange-colored bile pigment produced by the separation of hemoglobin into parts that are excreted by the liver cells
black hairy tongue				A condition in which the tongue is covered by hair-like papillae, entangled with threads produced by *Aspergillus niger* or *Candida albicans* fungi. This condition may be caused by poor oral hygiene and/or overgrowth of fungi due to antibiotic therapy. See Figure 6–5.
bowel (bou′əl)				The intestine, gut, entrail
buccal (bək′ əl)	bucc -al	R S	cheek pertaining to	Pertaining to the cheek
bulimia (bū-lĭm′ē-ă)				A condition of episodic binge eating with or without self-induced vomiting. ✱ See Pathology Spotlight: Eating Disorders.
catabolism (kă-tăb′ ō-lĭzm)	cata bol -ism	P R S	down to cast, throw condition of	Literally "a throwing down"; a breaking of complex substances into more basic elements
celiac (sē′ lĭ-ăk)	celi -ac	R S	abdomen, belly pertaining to	Pertaining to the abdomen
cheilosis (kī-lō′ sĭs)	cheil -osis	R S	lip condition of	An abnormal condition of the lip as seen in riboflavin and other B-complex deficiencies
cholecystectomy (kō″ lē-sĭs-tĕk′ tō-mē)	chol/e cyst -ectomy	CF R S	gall, bile bladder excision	Surgical excision of the gallbladder; with laparoscopic cholecystectomy, the gallbladder is removed through a small incision near the navel
cholecystitis (kō″ lē-sĭs-tī′ tĭs)	chol/e cyst -itis	CF R S	gall, bile bladder inflammation	Inflammation of the gallbladder
choledochotomy (kō-lĕd″ ō-kŏt′ ō-mē)	choledoch/o -tomy	CF S	common bile duct incision	Surgical incision of the common bile duct
chyle (kīl)				The milky fluid of intestinal digestion, composed of lymph and emulsified fats

MEDICAL WORD	WORD PARTS (WHEN APPLICABLE)			DEFINITION
	Part	**Type**	**Meaning**	
cirrhosis (sĭ-rō′ sĭs)	cirrh -osis	R S	orange-yellow condition of	A chronic degenerative liver disease characterized by changes in the lobes; parenchymal cells and the lobules are infiltrated with fat. See Figure 6–6.
colectomy (kō-lĕk′ tō-mē)	col -ectomy	R S	colon excision	Surgical excision of part of the colon
colon cancer (kō-lŏn kăn′ ser)				A malignancy of the colon; sometimes called "colorectal cancer"
colonic (kō-lŏn′ ĭk)	colon -ic	R S	colon pertaining to	Pertaining to the colon
colonoscopy (kō-lŏn-ŏs′ kō-pē)	colon/o -scopy	CF S	colon to view, examine	Examination of the upper portion of the colon
colostomy (kō-lŏs′ tō-mē)	col/o -stomy	CF S	colon new opening	The creation of a new opening into the colon
constipation (kon″ stĭ-pā′ shŭn)	constipat -ion	R S	to press together process	Infrequent passage of unduly hard and dry feces; *difficult defecation*
Crohn's disease (krōnz dĭ-zez′)				A chronic autoimmune disease that can affect any part of the gastrointestinal tract but most commonly occurs in the ileum
defecation (dĕf-ĕ-kā′ shŭn)	defecat -ion	R S	to remove dregs process	The evacuation of the bowel
deglutition (dē″ glo͞o-tĭsh′ ŭn)				The act or process of swallowing
dentalgia (dĕn-tăl′ jĭ-ă)	dent -algia	R S	tooth pain	Pain in a tooth; *toothache*
dentist (dĕn′ təst)	dent -ist	R S	tooth one who specializes	One who specializes in dentistry
diarrhea (dī′ ă-rē′ ă)	dia -rrhea	P S	through flow	Frequent passage of unformed watery stools
digestion (dī-jĕst′ chŭn)	di gest -ion	P R S	through to carry process	The process by which food is changed in the mouth, stomach, and intestines by chemical, mechanical, and physical action so that it can be absorbed by the body

MEDICAL WORD	WORD PARTS (WHEN APPLICABLE)			DEFINITION
	Part	**Type**	**Meaning**	
diverticulitis (dī″ vĕr-tĭk″ ū-lī′ tĭs)	diverticul -itis	R S	diverticula inflammation	Inflammation of the diverticula in the colon. ✱ See Figure 6–10 in Pathology Spotlight: Diverticulitis.
duodenal (dū″ ō-dē′ năl)	duoden -al	R S	duodenum pertaining to	Pertaining to the duodenum; the first part of the small intestine
dysentery (dĭs′ ĕn-tĕr″ ē)	dys enter -y	P R S	difficult intestine pertaining to	An intestinal disease characterized by inflammation of the mucous membrane
dyspepsia (dĭs-pĕp′ sĭ-ă)	dys -pepsia	P S	difficult to digest	Difficulty in digestion; *indigestion*
dysphagia (dĭs-fā′ jĭ-ă)	dys -phagia	P S	difficult to eat	Difficulty in swallowing
eating disorder (ē′ tĭng dĭs-ōr′ dĕr)				A health condition characterized by a preoccupation with weight that results in severe disturbances in eating behavior; anorexia nervosa and bulimia are the most common types. ✱ See Pathology Spotlight: Eating Disorders.
emesis (ĕm′ ĕ-sĭs)	eme -sis	R S	to vomit condition of	Vomiting
enteric (ĕn-tĕr′ ĭk)	enter -ic	R S	intestine pertaining to	Pertaining to the intestine
enteritis (ĕn″ tĕr-ī′ tĭs)	enter -itis	R S	intestine inflammation	Inflammation of the intestine
enzyme (ĕn′ zīm)				A protein substance capable of causing chemical changes in other substances without being changed itself
epigastric (ĕp′ ĭ-găs′ trĭc)	epi gastr -ic	P R S	above stomach pertaining to	Pertaining to the region above the stomach
eructation (ē-rk-tā′ shŭn)	eructat -ion	R S	a breaking out process	Belching
esophageal (ē-sŏf″ ă-jē′ ăl)	esophag/e -al	CF S	esophagus pertaining to	Pertaining to the esophagus
feces (fē′ sēz)				Body waste expelled from the bowels; *stools, excreta*

MEDICAL WORD	WORD PARTS (WHEN APPLICABLE)			DEFINITION
	Part	Type	Meaning	
fibroma (fĭ-brō' mă)	fibr -oma	R S	fibrous tissue tumor	A fibrous, encapsulated connective tissue tumor. See Figure 6–7.
flatus (flā' tŭs)				Gas in the stomach or intestines
gastrectomy (găs-trĕk' tō-mē)	gastr -ectomy	R S	stomach excision	Surgical excision of a part or the whole stomach
gastric (găs' trĭk)	gastr -ic	R S	stomach pertaining to	Pertaining to the stomach
gastroenterology (găs″ trō-ĕn″ tĕr-ŏl' ō-jē)	gastr/o enter/o -logy	CF CF S	stomach intestine study of	Study of the stomach and the intestines
gastroesophageal (găs' trō ē-sŏf″ ă-jē-ăl)	gastr/o esophag/e -al	CF CF S	stomach esophagus pertaining to	Pertaining to the stomach and esophagus
gastroesophageal reflux (găs' trō ē-sŏf″ ă-jē-ăl rē' flŭcks)				Occurs when the muscle between the esophagus and the stomach, the lower esophageal sphincter, is weak or relaxes inappropriately, allowing the stomach's contents to back up ("reflux") into the esophagus. ✱ See Pathology Spotlight: Gastroesophageal Reflux Disease.
gavage (gă-văzh')				To feed liquid or semiliquid food via a tube (stomach or nasogastric)
gingivitis (jĭn″ jĭ-vī' tĭs)	gingiv -itis	R S	gums inflammation	Inflammation of the gums
glossotomy (glŏ-sŏt' ō-mē)	gloss/o -tomy	CF S	tongue incision	Surgical incision into the tongue
glycogenesis (glī″ kŏ-jĕn' ĕ-sĭs)	glyc/o -genesis	CF S	sweet, sugar formation, produce	The formation of glycogen from glucose
halitosis (hăl″ ĭ-tō' sĭs)	halit -osis	R S	breath condition of	Bad breath
hematemesis (hĕm″ ăt-ēm' ĕ-sĭs)	hemat -emesis	R S	blood vomiting	Vomiting of blood
hemorrhoid (hĕm' ō-royd)	hemorrh -oid	R S	vein liable to bleed resemble	A mass of dilated, tortuous veins in the anorectum; may be internal or external

MEDICAL WORD	WORD PARTS (WHEN APPLICABLE)			DEFINITION
	Part	Type	Meaning	
hepatitis (hĕp″ă-tī′ tĭs)	hepat -itis	R S	liver inflammation	Inflammation of the liver
hepatoma (hĕp″ă-tŏ′ mă)	hepat -oma	R S	liver tumor	A tumor of the liver
hernia (hĕr′ nē-ă)				The abnormal protrusion of an organ or a part of an organ through the wall of the body cavity that normally contains it. ✱ See Figure 6–12 in Pathology Spotlight: Hernia.
herniotomy (hĕr″ nĭ-ŏt′ ō-mē)	herni/o -tomy	CF S	hernia incision	Surgical incision for the repair of a hernia
hyperalimentation (hī″ pĕr-ăl″ ĭ mĕn- tā′ shŭn)	hyper alimentat -ion	P R S	excessive nourishment process	An intravenous infusion of a hypertonic solution to sustain life; used in patients whose gastrointestinal tracts are not functioning properly
hyperemesis (hī″ pĕr-ĕm′ ĕ-sĭs)	hyper -emesis	P S	excessive, above vomiting	Excessive vomiting
hypogastric (hī″ pō-găs′ trĭk)	hypo gastr -ic	P R S	deficient, below stomach pertaining to	Pertaining to below the stomach
ileitis (ĭl″ ē-ī′ tis)	ile -itis	R S	ileum inflammation	Inflammation of the ileum
ileostomy (ĭl″ ē-ŏs′ tō-mē)	ile/o -stomy	CF S	ileum new opening	The creation of a new opening through the abdominal wall into the ileum
irritable bowel syndrome (IBS) (ĭr′ ă-tă-bl bŏu′ ĕl sĭn′ drōm)				A disorder that interferes with the normal functions of the large intestine (colon). It is characterized by a group of symptoms, including crampy abdominal pain, bloating, constipation, and diarrhea. ✱ See Pathology Spotlight: Irritable Bowel Syndrome.
labial (lā′ bĭ-ăl)	labi -al	R S	lip pertaining to	Pertaining to the lip
laparotomy (lăp″ ăr-ŏt′ ō-mē)	lapar/o -tomy	CF S	flank, abdomen incision	Surgical incision into the abdomen
lavage (lă-văzh′)				To wash out a cavity

MEDICAL WORD	WORD PARTS (WHEN APPLICABLE)			DEFINITION
	Part	**Type**	**Meaning**	
laxative (lăk′ să-tĭv)	laxat -ive	R S	to loosen nature of, quality of	A substance that acts to loosen the bowels
lingual (lĭng′ gwal)	lingu -al	R S	tongue pertaining to	Pertaining to the tongue
lipolysis (lĭp-ŏl′ ĭ-sĭs)	lip/o -lysis	CF S	fat destruction, to separate	The destruction of fat
liver transplant (lĭv′ ĕr trăns′ plănt)				The surgical process of transferring the liver from a donor to a patient
malabsorption (măl″ ăb-sōrp′ shŭn)	mal absorpt -ion	P R S	bad to suck in process	The process of bad or inadequate absorption of nutrients from the intestinal tract
mastication (măs″ tĭ-kā′ shŭn)	masticat -ion	R S	to chew process	Chewing
melena (mĕl′ ĕ-nă)				Black feces caused by the action of intestinal juices on blood
mesentery (mĕs′ ĕn-tĕr″ ē)	mes enter -y	R R S	middle intestine pertaining to	Pertaining to the peritoneal fold encircling the small intestines and connecting the intestines to the abdominal wall
nausea (naw′ sē-ă)				The feeling of the inclination to vomit
pancreas transplant (păn′ krē-ăs trăns plănt)				The surgical process of transferring the pancreas from a donor to a patient
pancreatitis (păn″ krē-ă-tī′ tĭs)	pancreat -itis	R S	pancreas inflammation	Inflammation of the pancreas
paralytic ileus (păr″ ă-lĭt′ ĭk ĭl′ ē-ŭs)	paralyt -ic ile -us	R S R S	to disable; paralysis pertaining to a twisting pertaining to	A paralysis of the intestines that causes distention and symptoms of acute obstruction and prostration
peptic (pĕp′ tĭk)	pept -ic	R S	to digest pertaining to	Pertaining to gastric digestion
periodontal (pĕr″ ē-ō-dŏn′ tăl)	peri odont -al	P R S	around tooth pertaining to	Pertaining to the area around the tooth

MEDICAL WORD	WORD PARTS (WHEN APPLICABLE)			DEFINITION
	Part	**Type**	**Meaning**	
periodontal disease (pĕr″ ē-ō-dŏn′ tăl dĭ-zēz′)				Inflammation and degeneration of the gums and surrounding bone, which frequently causes loss of the teeth
peristalsis (pĕr″ ĭ-stăl′ sĭs)	peri -stalsis	P S	around contraction	A wave-like contraction that occurs involuntarily in hollow tubes of the body, especially the alimentary canal
pharyngeal (făr-ĭn′ jē-ăl)	pharyng/e -al	CF S	pharynx pertaining to	Pertaining to the pharynx
pilonidal cyst (pī″ lō-nī′ dăl sĭst)	pil/o nid -al cyst	CF R S R	hair nest pertaining to sac	A closed sac in the crease of the sacrococcygeal region caused by a developmental defect that permits epithelial tissue and hair to be trapped below the skin
postprandial (pōst-prăn′ dĭ-ăl)	post prand/i -al	P CF S	after meal pertaining to	Pertaining to after a meal
proctologist (prŏk-tŏl′ ō-jĭst)	proct/o log -ist	CF R S	rectum, anus study of one who specializes	One who specializes in the study of the anus and the rectum
proctoscope (prŏk′ tō-scōp)	proct/o -scope	CF S	rectum, anus instrument	An instrument used to view the anus and rectum
pyloric (pī-lōr′ ĭk)	pylor -ic	R S	pylorus, gatekeeper pertaining to	Pertaining to the gatekeeper, the opening between the stomach and the duodenum
rectocele (rĕk′ tō-sēl)	rect/o -cele	CF S	rectum hernia	A hernia of part of the rectum into the vagina
sialadenitis (sī″ ăl-ăd″ ĕ-nī′ tĭs)	sial aden -itis	R R S	saliva gland inflammation	Inflammation of the salivary gland
sigmoidoscope (sĭg-moy′ dō-skōp)	sigmoid/o -scope	CF S	sigmoid instrument	An instrument used to view the sigmoid
splenomegaly (splē″ nō-mĕg′ ă-lē)	splen/o -megaly	CF S	spleen enlargement, large	Enlargement of the spleen
stomatitis (stō″ mă-tī′ tĭs)	stomat -itis	R S	mouth inflammation	Inflammation of the mouth

MEDICAL WORD	WORD PARTS (WHEN APPLICABLE)			DEFINITION
	Part	Type	Meaning	
sublingual (sŭb-lĭng′ gwăl)	sub lingu -al	P R S	below tongue pertaining to	Pertaining to below the tongue. See Figure 6–8.
ulcer (ŭl′ sĕr)				An open lesion or sore of the epidermis or mucous membrane. A peptic ulcer forms in the mucosal wall of the stomach, the pylorus, the duodenum, or the esophagus. It is referred to as a *gastric, duodenal,* or *esophageal ulcer,* depending on the location. ✱ See Figure 6–13 in Pathology Spotlight: Peptic Ulcer Disease.
ulcerative colitis (ŭl′ sĕr-ă-tĭv kō-lī′ tĭs)				A disease that causes inflammation and ulcers in the lining of the large intestine. The inflammation usually occurs in the rectum and lower part of the colon, but it may affect the entire colon. May also be called colitis or proctitis.
vermiform (vēr′ mĭ-form)	verm/i -form	CF S	worm shape	Shaped like a worm
volvulus (vŏl′ vū-lŭs)	volvul -us	R S	to roll pertaining to	A twisting of the bowel on itself that causes an obstruction. See Figure 6–9.
vomit (vŏm′ ĭt)				To eject stomach contents through the mouth

Terminology Translator

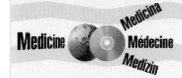

This feature, found on the accompanying CD-ROM, provides an innovative tool to translate medical words into Spanish, French, and German.

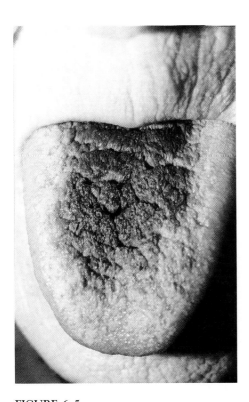

FIGURE 6–5

Black hairy tongue. (Courtesy of Jason L. Smith, MD.)

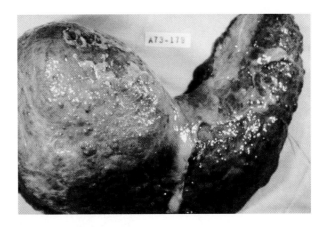

FIGURE 6–6

Cirrhosis of the liver. (Source: Pearson Education/PH College.)

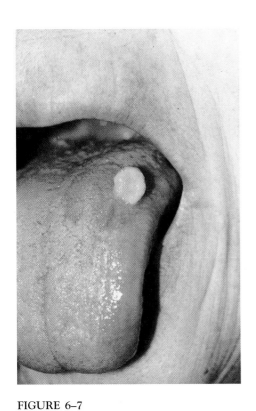

FIGURE 6–7

Fibroma. (Courtesy of Jason L. Smith, MD.)

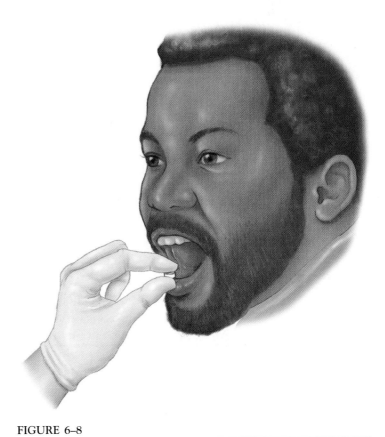

FIGURE 6–8

Sublingual drug administration. (Source: Pearson Education/PH College.)

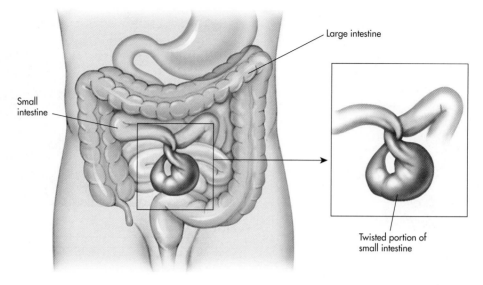

Small intestine

Large intestine

Twisted portion of small intestine

FIGURE 6-9

Volvulus.

PATHOLOGY SPOTLIGHTS

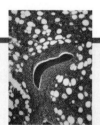

Diverticulitis

Diverticulitis is an inflammation of the diverticula in the colon. Pain is a common symptom of diverticulitis. Diverticulitis occurs when a **diverticulum** (a pouch or sac in the walls of an organ or canal) becomes inflamed or infected. See Figure 6–10. The exact cause of this condition is unknown, but it generally begins when stool lodges in the diverticula. Infection can lead to complications such as swelling or rupturing of the diverticula. Symptoms include pain, fever, chills, cramping, bloating, constipation, or diarrhea. Treatment depends upon the severity of the condition. A liquid diet and oral antibiotics are used for mild conditions, generally, followed by a high-fiber diet (see Table 6–1). If the condition is severe, hospitalization, bedrest, IV antibiotics and fluids, and/or surgery are recommended.

Eating Disorders

Eating disorders are health conditions characterized by a preoccupation with weight that results in severe disturbances in eating behavior. These disorders include anorexia nervosa and bulimia.

Anorexia nervosa essentially is self-starvation, in which a person refuses to maintain a normal body weight. It is a complex psychological disorder in which the individual refuses to eat or has an aberrant eating pattern. People with eating disorders may engage in self-induced vomiting and abuse of laxatives, diuretics or exercise in order to control their weight. The condition may lead them to become thin or even emaciated. In severe cases, anorexia can be life-threatening. See Figure 6–11.

Bulimia involves repeated episodes of binge eating, followed by inappropriate ways of trying to rid the body of the food or of the expected weight gain. A person with bulimia may consume large, high-calorie meals, and then induce vomiting or take laxatives to try to rid the body of the food before the body absorbs calories and weight gain occurs. People may have this condition and be of normal weight.

The incidence of anorexia and bulimia is higher among teenage girls and young women than in other groups of Americans. Males can develop either disorder, and the disorders may be more common among males than previously thought. Females account for about 90 percent

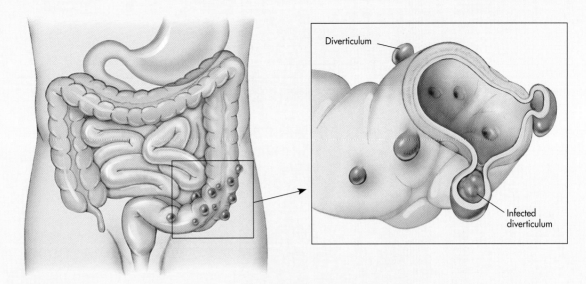

FIGURE 6–10

Diverticulitis.

of eating disorders in the United States. According to the American Psychiatric Association, between 0.5 percent and 3.7 percent of females experience anorexia, and between 1.1 and 4.2 percent of females experience bulimia in their lifetime.

Gastroesophageal Reflux Disease (GERD)

Gastroesophageal reflux disease (GERD) occurs when the muscle between the esophagus and the stomach, the lower esophageal sphincter, is weak or relaxes inappropriately. This allows the stomach's contents to back up ("reflux") into the esophagus. It is also called esophageal reflux or reflux esophagitis. Symptoms include heartburn, belching, and regurgitation of food.

TABLE 6–1 GOOD CHOICES OF HIGH-FIBER FOODS

One needs 25 to 30 grams of fiber each day to keep the colon working at its best. The following are selected good choices of high-fiber foods.

Fruits		*Whole-Grain Cereals*	
1 medium apple	4 grams	$^1/_3$ cup all-bran cereal	10 grams
1 medium pear	4 grams	$^1/_3$ cup wheat flakes	3 grams
1 medium orange	3 grams	$^1/_3$ cup shredded wheat	3 grams
1 cup strawberries	3 grams		
5 dried prunes (uncooked)	3 grams	*Whole-Bran Breads and Rice*	
		2 slices whole-wheat bread	4 grams
Vegetables		2 slices rye bread	4 grams
1 baked potato (with skin)	5 grams	$^1/_2$ cup cooked brown rice	2 grams
$^1/_2$ cup cooked frozen peas	4 grams		
$^1/_2$ cup cooked fresh spinach	3 grams	*Pure Bran*	
$^1/_2$ cup cooked frozen corn	2 grams		
		3 T unprocessed wheat bran	6 grams
Beans		3 T unprocessed oat bran	3 grams
$^1/_2$ cup cooked lentils	8 grams		
$^1/_2$ cup cooked kidney beans	6 grams		
$^1/_2$ cup cooked green beans	2 grams		

T = tablespoon

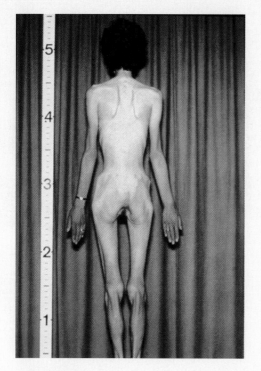

FIGURE 6–11

An emaciated young woman with anorexia nervosa.
(Source: Custom Medical Stock Photo, Inc.)

Most GERD sufferers have frequent, severe heartburn. This tears down and damages the cell wall lining of the esophagus. Without treatment, GERD can lead to the following conditions: Barrett's esophagus, a precancerous change in the cells lining the esophagus; esophageal cancer; esophageal perforation, or a hole in the esophagus; esophageal ulcers, which damage the lining further; esophagitis, inflammation of the esophagus and/or esophageal stricture, or narrowing of the esophagus that interferes with eating. When deemed necessary, a surgical procedure known as **dilation** is done to correct esophageal stricture. The surgeon passes a series of dilators down the esophagus. The dilators gently stretch the narrowed opening apart.

Dietary and lifestyle choices may contribute to GERD. Certain foods and beverages, such as chocolate, peppermint, fried or fatty foods, coffee, or alcoholic beverages, may weaken the lower esophageal sphincter (LES) and cause reflux and heartburn. Studies show that cigarette smoking relaxes the lower esophageal sphincter. Obesity and pregnancy can also cause GERD. Some doctors believe a **hiatal hernia** may weaken the LES and cause reflux.

Decreasing the size of portions at mealtime may help control symptoms. Eating meals at least 2 to 3 hours before bedtime may lessen reflux by allowing the acid in the stomach to decrease and the stomach to empty partially. In addition, being overweight often worsens symptoms. Many overweight people find relief when they lose weight.

Some of the medical and surgical treatments for GERD include: **fundoplication**, a surgical reduction of the opening into the fundus of the stomach, and suturing of the previously removed end of the esophagus to the opening; medications: H$_2$ blockers, such as cimetidine (Tagamet), ranitidine (Zantac), famotidine (Pepcid), and nizatidine (Axid) and proton-pump inhibitors, such as esomeprazole (Nexium), omeprazole (Prilosec), lansoprazole (Prevacid), rabeprazole (Aciphex), or pantoprazole (Protonix).

Hernia

A **hernia** is the abnormal protrusion of an organ or a part of an organ through the wall of the body cavity that normally contains it. Most often, the term hernia refers to an abdominal hernia. The two most common types of abdominal hernia are hiatal and inguinal.

Hiatal hernia occurs when the upper part of the stomach moves up into the chest through a small opening in the diaphragm. See Figure 6–12. Studies show that the opening in the diaphragm acts as an additional sphincter around the lower end of the esophagus. Studies also show that hiatal hernia results in retention of acid and other contents above this opening. These substances can reflux easily into the esophagus.

Coughing, vomiting, straining, or sudden physical exertion can cause increased pressure in the abdomen that results in hiatal hernia. Obesity and pregnancy also contribute to this condition. Many otherwise healthy people age 50 and over have a small hiatal hernia. Although considered a condition of middle age, hiatal hernias affect people of all ages.

Hiatal hernias usually do not require treatment. However, treatment may be necessary if the hernia is in danger of becoming strangulated (twisted in a way that cuts off blood supply) or is complicated by severe GERD or esophagitis. The physician may perform surgery to reduce the size of the hernia or to prevent strangulation.

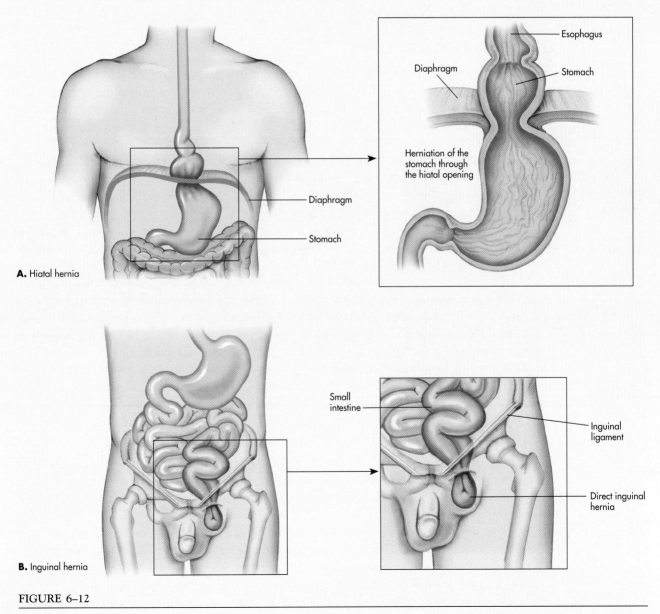

A. Hiatal hernia

B. Inguinal hernia

FIGURE 6–12

Hernias.

An **inguinal hernia** occurs when a loop of intestine enters the inguinal canal, a tubular passage through the lower layers of the abdominal wall. Symptoms include groin discomfort or pain, and in the male, a scrotum lump.

This type of hernia is sometimes associated with heavy lifting. In men, an inguinal hernia can develop in the groin near the scrotum. A direct inguinal hernia creates a bulge in the groin area, and an indirect hernia descends into the scrotum. Inguinal hernias occur more often in men than in women. A family history of hernias increases the risk.

Infants and children may also develop inguinal hernias. In these populations, hernias can occur when a portion of the peritoneum (the lining around all the organs in the abdomen) does not close properly before birth. This causes a small portion of the intestine to push out into the opening (a bulge might be seen in the groin or scrotum). According to the American Academy of Pediatrics, 5 out of 100 children have inguinal hernias (more boys than girls). Some may not have symptoms until adulthood.

Diagnosis is typically made through a physical examination in which the hernia mass is palpated, and may increase in size when coughing, bending, lifting, or straining. The hernia (bulge) may not be obvious in infants and children, except when the child is crying or coughing. Treatment is usually done through a hernia repair surgery, in which the hernia is pushed back into the abdominal cavity.

Irritable Bowel Syndrome (IBS)

Irritable bowel syndrome (IBS) is a disorder that interferes with the normal functions of the large intestine (colon). It is characterized by a group of symptoms, including crampy abdominal pain, bloating, constipation, and diarrhea. The cause is not known, but the symptoms are often worsened by emotional stress.

Symptoms of irritable bowel syndrome may include: abdominal distress that is often relieved with a bowel movement; bloating, or feeling like the stomach is inflated; excess gas and changes in stool. Some people with IBS may have painful, loose stools, or diarrhea, while others may have painful hard stools, or constipation. Some people may alternate between diarrhea and constipation.

One in five Americans has IBS, making it one of the most common disorders diagnosed by doctors. It occurs more often in women than in men, and it usually begins between the ages of 20 and 30. Predisposing factors may include a low-fiber diet, emotional stress, and use of laxatives.

IBS causes a great deal of discomfort and distress, but it does not permanently harm the intestines and does not lead to intestinal bleeding or to any serious disease such as cancer. Treatment of irritable bowel syndrome often focuses on treating the symptoms and preventing flare-ups. Most people can control their symptoms with diet, stress management, and medications prescribed by their physician. Increasing dietary fiber and eliminating stimulants such as caffeine may be beneficial. See Table 6–1. Exercise and counseling for anxiety may be helpful, as well. But for some people, IBS can be disabling. They may be unable to work, go to social events, or travel even short distances.

Peptic Ulcer Disease

Peptic ulcer disease occurs when the lining of the esophagus, stomach, or duodenum is worn away. See Figure 6–13. Peptic ulcer disease most commonly occurs in the upper part of the small intestine, called the duodenum. It also occurs in the stomach. Ulcers less commonly occur in the esophagus.

Symptoms of peptic ulcer disease include abdominal pain, nausea, vomiting, and weight loss. Peptic ulcers may also cause no symptoms. An esophageal ulcer may also cause chest pain. Other common symptoms include: black, tarlike, or maroon-colored stools; blood in the stool; and/or burning or gnawing pain in the stomach, the chest, or the back.

Peptic ulcers are caused by an imbalance between acid and pepsin (an enzyme) secretion and the defenses of the mucosal lining. This leads to inflammation, which may also be caused

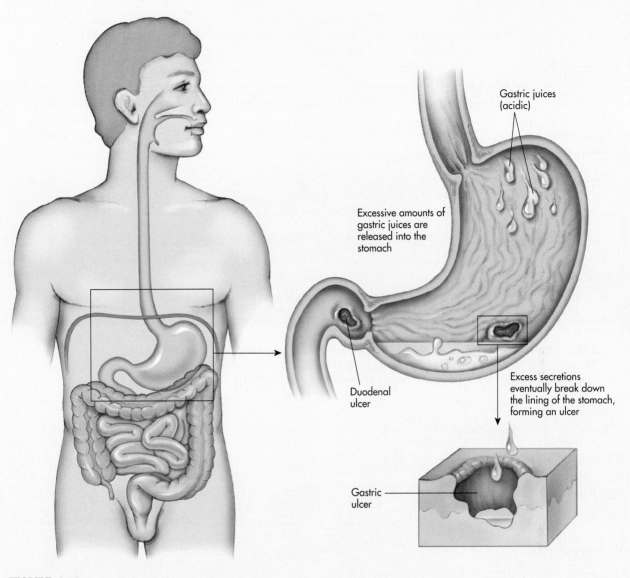

Gastric juices
(acidic)

Excessive amounts of
gastric juices are
released into the
stomach

Duodenal
ulcer

Excess secretions
eventually break down
the lining of the stomach,
forming an ulcer

Gastric
ulcer

FIGURE 6–13

Peptic ulcer disease (PUD).

by aspirin and nonsteroidal anti-inflammatory medications (NSAIDs). Contrary to popular belief, ulcers are not caused by spicy foods or stress but rather are aggravated by them. The erosion of the mucosa that characterizes peptic ulcers is often caused by infection with a bacterium called *Helicobacter pylori*. Approximately 90 percent of duodenal ulcers and 70 percent of peptic ulcers are associated with *Helicobacter pylori*. The bacteria settle in the lining of the duodenum or stomach, opening a wound that is then made worse by digestive juices and stomach acids. The wound is said to resemble a flattened volcano or a white-centered, red-rimmed, painful canker sore. By killing the bacteria with antibiotics, it is estimated that 90 percent of the ulcers caused by *H. pylori* can be cured.

Prevention of peptic ulcer disease includes avoiding alcohol and tobacco; avoiding or limiting use of aspirin and nonsteroidal anti-inflammatory drugs (NSAIDs); taking enteric-coated aspirin with meals, if aspirin is needed daily.

The medical history and physical examination may be sufficient for diagnosis. X-ray tests or endoscopy can confirm the diagnosis. **Endoscopy** is a procedure that involves putting a thin telescope into the mouth. This telescope can be moved down into the stomach and intestines. This procedure allows the physician to directly see any ulcers. The physician may take samples of the stomach contents to test for *H. pylori* infection.

Untreated peptic ulcer disease may cause a hole in the digestive tract. It may also cause bleeding, inflammation, or abnormal connections between abdominal organs.

Treatment of peptic ulcer disease depends on the cause. If aspirin or other medications are the cause, then these medications must be stopped. Smoking and drinking alcohol should be stopped as well, because they can delay healing. Medications are given to help protect the stomach lining and allow faster healing. Most of these medications work by neutralizing stomach acid or preventing its production. If an infection with *H. pylori* is present, antibiotics are given. Surgery may be needed for severe ulcers that bleed, are unresponsive to medication, or that cause a hole in the stomach.

✔ PATHOLOGY CHECKPOINT

Following is a concise list of the pathology-related terms that you've seen in the chapter. Review this checklist to make sure that you are familiar with the meaning of each term before moving on to the next section.

Conditions and Symptoms

- ❏ anorexia
- ❏ appendicitis
- ❏ ascites
- ❏ bulimia
- ❏ cheilosis
- ❏ cholecystitis
- ❏ cirrhosis
- ❏ colon cancer
- ❏ constipation
- ❏ Crohn's disease
- ❏ dentalgia
- ❏ diarrhea
- ❏ diverticulitis
- ❏ dysentery
- ❏ dyspepsia
- ❏ dysphagia
- ❏ eating disorder
- ❏ emesis
- ❏ enteritis
- ❏ eructation
- ❏ flatus
- ❏ gastroesophageal reflux
- ❏ gastroesophageal reflux disease (GERD)

- ❏ gingivitis
- ❏ halitosis
- ❏ hematemesis
- ❏ hemorrhoid
- ❏ hepatitis
- ❏ hepatoma
- ❏ hernia
- ❏ hiatal hernia
- ❏ hyperemesis
- ❏ ileitis
- ❏ inguinal hernia
- ❏ irritable bowel syndrome (IBS)
- ❏ malabsorption
- ❏ melena
- ❏ nausea
- ❏ pancreatitis
- ❏ paralytic ileus
- ❏ peptic ulcer disease
- ❏ periodontal disease
- ❏ pilonidal cyst
- ❏ rectocele
- ❏ sialadentitis
- ❏ splenomegaly
- ❏ stomatitis

- ❏ ulcer
- ❏ ulcerative colitis
- ❏ volvulus
- ❏ vomit

Diagnosis and Treatment

- ❏ appendectomy
- ❏ cholecystectomy
- ❏ choledochotomy
- ❏ colectomy
- ❏ colonoscopy
- ❏ colostomy
- ❏ gastrectomy
- ❏ gavage
- ❏ glossotomy
- ❏ herniotomy
- ❏ hyperalimentation
- ❏ ileostomy
- ❏ laparotomy
- ❏ lavage
- ❏ laxative
- ❏ liver transplant
- ❏ pancreas transplant
- ❏ proctoscope
- ❏ sigmoidscope

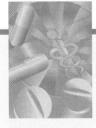

DRUG HIGHLIGHTS

DRUG HIGHLIGHTS

Drugs that are generally used for digestive system diseases and disorders include antacids, antacid mixtures, histamine H_2-receptor antagonists, mucosal protective medications, gastric acid pump inhibitors (proton pump inhibitor), other ulcer medications, laxatives, antidiarrheal agents, antiemetics, and emetics. See Figure 6–14.

Antacids
Neutralize hydrochloric acid in the stomach. Antacids are classified as nonsystemic and systemic.

Nonsystemic
Examples: Amphojel (aluminum hydroxide), Tums (calcium carbonate), Riopan (magaldrate), and Milk of Magnesia (magnesium hydroxide).

Systemic
Example: sodium bicarbonate.

Antacid Mixtures
Products that combine aluminum (may cause constipation) and/or calcium compounds with magnesium (may cause diarrhea) salts. By combining the antacid properties of two single-entity agents, these products provide the antacid action of both, yet tend to counter the adverse effects of each other.

Examples: Gaviscon, Gelusil, Maalox Plus, and Mylanta.

Histamine H_2-Receptor Antagonists
Inhibit both daytime and nocturnal basal gastric acid secretion and inhibit gastric acid stimulated by food, histamines, caffeine, insulin, and pentagastrin. These drugs are used in the treatment of active duodenal ulcer.

Examples: Tagamet (cimetidine), Pepcid (famotidine), Axid (nizatidine), and Zantac (ranitidine).

Mucosal Protective Medications
These medicines protect the stomach's mucosal lining from acids, but they do not inhibit the release of acid.

Examples: Carafate (sucralfate) and Cytotec (misoprostol).

Gastric Acid Pump Inhibitors (Proton Pump Inhibitor—PPI)
These are antiulcer agents that suppress gastric acid secretion by specific inhibition of the H + /K + ATPase enzyme at the secretory surface of the gastric parietal cell. Because this enzyme system is regarded as the acid (proton) pump within the gastric mucosa, gastric acid pump inhibitors are so classified, as they block the final step of acid production.

Examples: Prilosec (omeprazole), Aciphex (rabeprazole sodium), Prevacid (lansoprazole), and Protonix (pantoprazole).

Other Ulcer Medications
The treatment regimen for active duodenal ulcers associated with *H. pylori* may involve a two- or three-drug program.

Examples: a two-drug program—Biaxin (clarithromycin) and Prilosec (omeprazole); and a three-drug program—Flagyl (metronidazole) and either tetracycline or amoxicillin and Pepto Bismol.

Note: For the treatment program to be effective, the patient has to complete the full treatment program that involves taking 15 pills a day for a total of at least 2 weeks.

Laxatives
Used to relieve constipation and to facilitate the passage of feces through the lower gastrointestinal tract.

Examples: Dulcolax (bisacodyl), Milk of Magnesia (magnesium hydroxide), Metamucil (psyllium hydrophilic muciloid), and Ex-Lax (phenolphthalein).

Antidiarrheal Agents
Used to treat diarrhea.

Examples: Pepto-Bismol (bismuth subsalicylate), Kaopectate (kaolin mixture with pectin), and Imodium (loperamide HCl).

Antiemetics   Prevent or arrest vomiting. These drugs are also used in the treatment of vertigo, motion sickness, and nausea.

Examples: Dramamine (dimenhydrinate), Phenergan (promethazine HCl), Tigan (trimethobenzamide HCl), and Transderm Scop (scopolamine).

Emetics   Are used to induce vomiting in people who have taken an overdose of oral drugs or who have ingested certain poisons. An emetic agent should not be given to a person who is unconscious, in shock, or in a semicomatose state. Emetics are also contraindicated in individuals who have ingested strongly caustic substances, such as lye or acid, since their use could result in additional injury to the person's esophagus.

Example: Ipecac syrup.

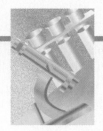

DIAGNOSTIC & LAB TESTS

TEST	DESCRIPTION
alcohol toxicology (ethanol and ethyl) (ăl′ kō-hōl tŏks″ ĭ-kŏl′ ō-jē)	A test performed on blood serum or plasma to determine levels of alcohol. Legally, 0.05% or 50 mg/dL is considered not under the influence. Increased values indicate alcohol consumption that may lead to cirrhosis of the liver, gastritis, malnutrition, vitamin deficiencies, and other gastrointestinal disorders.
ammonia (NH$_4$) (ă-mō′ nē-ă)	A test performed on blood plasma to determine the level of ammonia (end product of protein breakdown). Increased values may indicate hepatic failure, hepatic encephalopathy, portacaval anastomosis, high protein diet in hepatic failure, and Reye's syndrome.
barium enema (BE) (bă′ rē-ūm ĕn′ ĕ-mă)	A test performed by administering barium via the rectum to determine the condition of the colon. X-rays are taken to ascertain the structure and to check the filling of the colon. Abnormal results may indicate cancer of the colon, polyps, fistulas, ulcerative colitis, diverticulitis, hernias, and intussusception.
bilirubin blood test (total) (bĭl-ĭ-roo′ bĭn blod test)	A test done on blood serum to determine if bilirubin is conjugated and excreted in the bile. Abnormal results may indicate obstructive jaundice, hepatitis, and cirrhosis.
carcinoembryonic antigen (CEA) (kăr″ sĭn-ō-ĕm″ brē-ōn′ ĭk ăn′ tĭ-jĕn)	A test performed on whole blood or plasma to determine the presence of CEA (antigens originally isolated from colon tumors). Increased values may indicate stomach, intestinal, rectal, and various other cancers and conditions. This test is nonspecific and must be combined with other tests for a final diagnosis. It is being used to monitor the course of cancer therapy.
cholangiography (kō-lăn″ jē-ŏg′ ră-fē)	X-ray examination of the common bile duct, cystic duct, and hepatic ducts. A radiopaque dye is injected, and then films are taken. Abnormal results may indicate obstruction, stones, and tumors.
cholecystography (kō″ lē-sĭs-tŏg′ ră-fē)	X-ray examination of the gallbladder. A radiopaque dye is injected, and then films are taken. Abnormal results may indicate cholecystitis, cholelithiasis, and tumors.

TEST	DESCRIPTION
colonofiberoscopy (kŏ′ lō-nŏ-fī″ běr-ŏs′ kō-pē)	Fiberoptic colonoscopy. The direct visual examination of the colon via a flexible colonoscope; used as a diagnostic aid, for removal of foreign bodies, polyps, and tissue.
endoscopic retrograde cholangiopancreatography (ERCP) (ĕn′ dō-skōp-ĭk rĕt′ rō-grād kō-lăn″ jē-ō-păn″ krē-ă-tŏg′ ră-fē)	X-ray examination of the biliary and pancreatic ducts. A contrast medium is injected, and then films are taken. Abnormal results may indicate fibrosis, biliary or pancreatic cysts, strictures, stones, and chronic pancreatitis.
esophagogastroduodenoscopy (ĕ-sŏf″ ă-gō′ găs″ trō-dū″ ō-dĕ-nŏs′ kō-pē)	An endoscopic examination of the esophagus, stomach, and small intestine. During the procedure, photographs, biopsy, or brushings may be done.
gamma-glutamyl transferase (GGT) (găm′ ă glōō-tăm′ ĭl trăns′ fĕr-ās)	A test performed on blood serum to determine the level of GGT (enzyme found in the liver, kidney, prostate, heart, and spleen). Increased values may indicate cirrhosis, liver necrosis, hepatitis, alcoholism, neoplasms, acute pancreatitis, acute myocardial infarction, nephrosis, and acute cholecystitis.
gastric analysis (găs′ trĭk ă-năl′ ĭ sĭs)	A test performed to determine quality of secretion, amount of free and combined HCl, and absence or presence of blood, bacteria, bile, and fatty acids. Increased level of HCl may indicate peptic ulcer disease, Zollinger-Ellison syndrome, and hypergastremia. Decreased level of HCl may indicate stomach cancer, pernicious anemia, and atrophic gastritis.
gastrointestinal (GI) series (găs″ trō-ĭn-tes′ tĭn″ ăl sēr′ ēz)	Fluoroscopic examination of the esophagus, stomach, and small intestine. Barium is given orally, and it is observed as it flows through the GI system. See Figure 6–15. Abnormal results may indicate esophageal varices, ulcers, gastric polyps, malabsorption syndrome, hiatal hernias, diverticuli, pyloric stenosis, and foreign bodies.
hepatitis-associated antigen (HAA) (hĕp″ ă-tī-tĭs ă-sō′ shē-āt′ ĕd ăn′ tĭ-jĕn)	A test performed to determine the presence of the hepatitis B virus.
liver biopsy (lĭv′ ĕr bī-ŏp-sē)	Microscopic examination of liver tissue. Abnormal results may indicate cirrhosis, hepatitis, and tumors
occult blood (ŭ-kŭlt blod)	A test performed on feces to determine gastrointestinal bleeding that is invisible (hidden). Positive results may indicate gastritis, stomach cancer, peptic ulcer, ulcerative colitis, bowel cancer, bleeding esophageal varices, portal hypertension, pancreatitis, and diverticulitis.
ova and parasites (O & P) (o′ vă păr′ ă-sīts)	A test performed on stool to identify ova and parasites. Positive results indicate protozoa infestation.
stool culture (stool kŭl′ tūr)	A test performed on stool to identify the presence of organisms.
ultrasonography, gallbladder (ŭl-tră-sŏn-ŏg′ ră-fē găl″ blăd′ dĕr)	A test to visualize the gallbladder by using high-frequency sound waves. The echoes are recorded on an oscilloscope and film. See Figure 6–16. Abnormal results may indicate biliary obstruction, cholelithiasis, and acute cholecystitis.

ultrasonography, liver
(ŭl-tră-sŏn-ŏg′ ră-fē
lĭv′ ēr)

A test to visualize the liver by using high-frequency sound waves. The echoes are recorded on an oscilloscope and film. See Figure 6–17. Abnormal results may indicate hepatic tumors, cysts, abscess, and cirrhosis.

upper gastrointestinal fiberoscopy
(ŭp′ ir găs′ trō-ĭn-tĕs′ tĭn″ ăl
fī′ bĕr-ŏs′ kō-pē)

The direct visual examination of the gastric mucosa via a flexible fiberscope. Colored photographs or motion pictures can be taken during the procedure; used when gastric neoplasm is suspected.

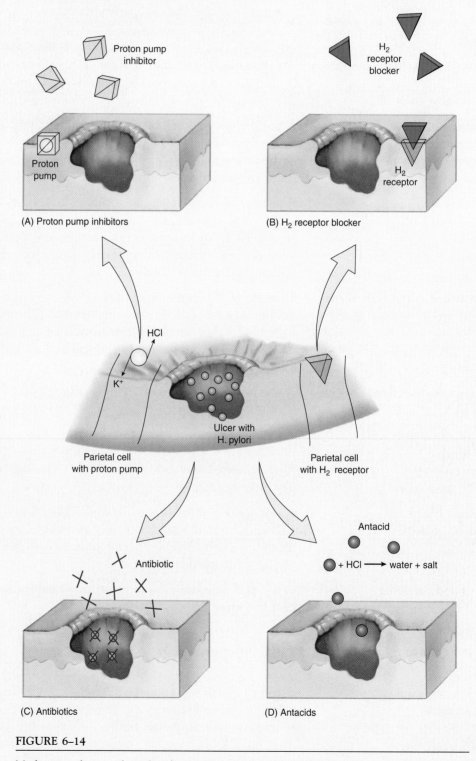

FIGURE 6–14

Mechanisms of action of antiulcer drugs. (Source: Pearson Education/PH College.)

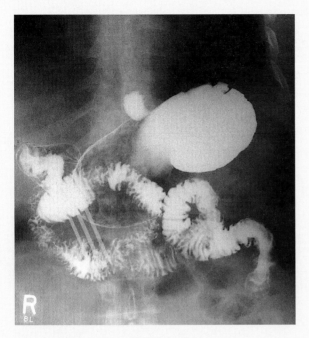

FIGURE 6–15

Upper GI series. (Courtesy of Teresa Resch.)

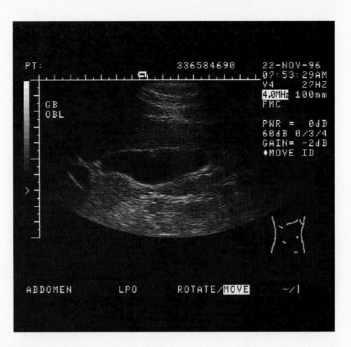

FIGURE 6–16

Gallbladder ultrasound. (Courtesy of Teresa Resch.)

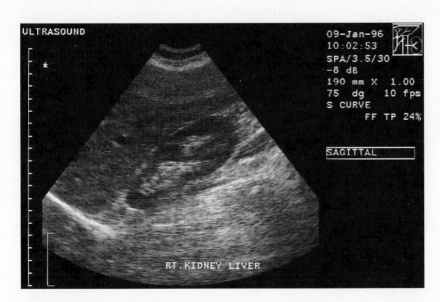

FIGURE 6–17

Ultrasound liver and right kidney. (Courtesy of Teresa Resch.)

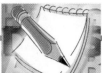 ABBREVIATIONS

ABBREVIATION	MEANING	ABBREVIATION	MEANING
ac	before meals (ante cibum)	HBV	hepatitis B virus
A/G	albumin/globulin (ratio)	HCl	hydrochloric acid
Ba	barium	*H. pylori*	*Helicobacter pylori*
BE	barium enema	IBS	irritable bowel syndrome
BM	bowel movement	LES	lower esophageal sphincter
BRP	bathroom privileges	NANBH	non-A, non-B hepatitis virus
BS	bowel sounds	NG	nasogastric (tube)
BSP	bromsulphalein	NH_4	ammonia
CEA	carcinoembryonic antigen	npo, NPO	nil per os (nothing by mouth)
CHO	carbohydrate	N&V	nausea and vomiting
chol	cholesterol	O & P	ova and parasites
cib	food (cibus)	pc	after meals (post cibum)
CUC	chronic ulcerative colitis	PEG	percutaneous endoscopic gastrostomy
E. coli	*Escherichia coli*		
ERCP	endoscopic retrograde cholangiopancreatography	po, PO	per os (by mouth)
		PP	postprandial (after meals)
GB	gallbladder	PTC	percutaneous transhepatic cholangiography
GERD	gastroesophageal reflux disease		
GGT	gamma-glutamyl transferase	PPI	proton pump inhibitor
GI	gastrointestinal	PUD	peptic ulcer disease
GTT	glucose tolerance test	RDA	recommended dietary or daily allowance
HAA	hepatitis-associated antigen		
HAV	hepatitis A virus	TPN	total parenteral nutrition
HBIG	hepatitis B immune globulin	UGI	upper gastrointestinal

STUDY AND REVIEW

Anatomy and Physiology

Write your answers to the following questions. Do not refer to the text.

1. Name the primary organs commonly associated with digestion.

   a. _____ b. _____

   c. _____ d. _____

   e. _____ f. _____

2. Name four accessory organs of digestion.

   a. _____ b. _____

   c. _____ d. _____

3. State the three main functions of the digestive system.

   a. _____

   b. _____

   c. _____

4. Define bolus. _____

   _____

5. Define peristalsis. _____

   _____

6. _____ _____ and _____ _____ convert the food into a semiliquid state.

7. The _____ is the first portion of the small intestine.

8. Semiliquid food is called _____.

9. The _____ _____ transports nutrients to body cells.

10. The large intestine can be divided into four distinct sections called the

    _____, the _____, the _____, and the

    _____.

11. The _____ is the largest glandular organ in the body.

12. State the function of the gallbladder. _____

13. Name an important function of the pancreas. _____

14. State three functions of the liver.

a. _____ b. _____

c. _____

15. Where does digestion and absorption chiefly take place? _____

16. The salivary glands located in and about the mouth are called the

_____, the _____, and the _____.

17. Name the two hormones secreted into the bloodstream by the pancreas.

a. _____ b. _____

Word Parts

1. In the spaces provided, write the definition of these prefixes, roots, combining forms, and suffixes. Do not refer to the listings of medical words. Leave blank those words you cannot define.

2. After completing as many as you can, refer to the medical word listings to check your work. For each word missed or left blank, write the word and its definition several times on the margins of these pages or on a separate sheet of paper.

3. To maximize the learning process, it is to your advantage to do the following exercises as directed. To refer to the word building section before completing these exercises invalidates the learning process.

PREFIXES

Give the definitions of the following prefixes:

1. an- _____ 2. ana- _____

3. cata- _____ 4. dys- _____

5. epi- _____ 6. hyper- _____

7. hypo- _____ 8. mal- _____

9. di- _____ 10. peri- _____

11. post- _____ 12. dia- _____

13. sub- _____

ROOTS AND COMBINING FORMS

Give the definitions of the following roots and combining forms:

1. absorpt _____

2. aden _____

3. amyl _____

4. cirrh _____

5. append _____

6. appendic _____

7. bil/i _____

8. bol _____

9. bucc _____

10. celi _____

11. cheil _____

12. chol/e _____

13. choledoch/o _____

14. col _____

15. col/o _____

16. colon _____

17. colon/o _____

18. cyst _____

19. dent _____

20. constipat _____

21. diverticul _____

22. duoden _____

23. enter _____

24. defecat _____

25. esophag/e _____

26. gest _____

27. gastr _____

28. gastr/o _____

29. gingiv _____

30. gloss/o _____

31. glyc/o _____

32. hemat _____

33. hepat _____

34. hepat/o _____

35. herni/o _____

36. ile _____

37. ile/o _____

38. labi _____

39. lapar/o _____

40. laxat _____

41. lingu _____

42. lip/o _____

43. log _____

44. mes _____

45. pancreat _____

46. pept _____

47. pharyng/e _____

48. prand/i _____

49. eme _____

50. proct/o _____

51. pylor _____

52. rect/o _____

53. sial _____

54. sigmoid/o _____

55. splen/o _____

56. stomat _____

57. tox _____

58. eructat _____

59. verm/i _____

60. halit _____

61. hemorrh _____

62. alimentat _____

63. masticat _____

64. paralyt _____

65. pil/o _____

66. nid _____

67. volvul _____

68. odont _____

SUFFIXES

Give the definitions of the following suffixes:

1. -ac _____

2. -al _____

3. -algia _____

4. -ary _____

5. -ase _____

6. -cele _____

7. -oid _____

8. -sis _____

9. -ectomy _____

10. -emesis _____

11. -form _____

12. -genesis _____

13. -ic _____

14. -in _____

15. -ion _____

16. -ism _____

17. -ist _____

18. -itis _____

19. -ive _____

20. -logy _____

21. -lysis _____

22. -megaly _____

23. -oma _____

24. -orexia _____

25. -osis _____

26. -rrhea _____

27. -pepsia _____

28. -us _____

29. -phagia _____

30. -scope _____

31. -scopy _____

32. -stalsis _____

33. -stomy _____

34. -tomy _____

35. -y _____

Identifying Medical Terms

In the spaces provided, write the medical terms for the following meanings:

1. _____ An enzyme that breaks down starch

2. _____ The building up of the body substances

3. _____ Lack of appetite

4. _____ Surgical excision of the appendix

5. _____ Inflammation of the appendix

6. _____ Pertaining to or conveying bile

7. _____ Pertaining to the abdomen

8. _____ Difficulty in swallowing

9. _____ Inflammation of the liver

10. _____ Surgical incision for the repair of a hernia

11. _____ Pertaining to after meals

12. _____ Enlargement of the spleen

13. _____ Instrument used to view the sigmoid

Spelling

In the spaces provided, write the correct spelling of these misspelled terms:

1. bilery _____

2. colonscopy _____

3. degultition _____

4. gastorentreology _____

5. haltosis _____

6. laxtive _____

7. persitalsis _____

8. salademitis _____

9. peridontal _____

10. verimform _____

Matching

Select the appropriate lettered meaning for each word listed below.

_____ 1. cirrhosis

_____ 2. constipation

_____ 3. diarrhea

_____ 4. gavage

_____ 5. hemorrhoid

_____ 6. hernia

_____ 7. hyperalimentation

_____ 8. lavage

_____ 9. pilonidal cyst

_____ 10. volvulus

a. To wash out a cavity
b. To feed liquid or semiliquid food via a tube
c. A twisting of the bowel on itself
d. Frequent passage of unformed watery stools
e. A chronic degenerative liver disease
f. Infrequent passage of unduly hard and dry feces
g. A closed sac in the crease of the sacrococcygeal region
h. The abnormal protrusion of an organ or a part of an organ through the wall of the body cavity that normally contains it
i. A mass of dilated, tortuous veins in the anorectum
j. An intravenous infusion of a hypertonic solution to sustain life
k. The evacuation of the bowel

Abbreviations

Place the correct word, phrase, or abbreviation in the space provided.

1. before meals _____

2. BM _____

3. BS _____

4. food _____

5. gallbladder _____

6. hepatitis A virus _____

7. NG _____

8. NPO, npo _____

9. after meals _____

10. total parenteral nutrition _____

Diagnostic and Laboratory Tests

Select the best answer to each multiple choice question. Circle the letter of your choice.

1. X-ray examination of the common bile duct, cystic duct, and hepatic ducts.
   a. cholangiography
   b. cholecystography
   c. cholangiopancreatography
   d. ultrasonography

2. The direct visual examination of the colon via a flexible colonoscope.
   a. cholangiography
   b. ultrasonography
   c. colonofiberoscopy
   d. cholecystography

3. Fluoroscopic examination of the esophagus, stomach, and small intestine.
   a. barium enema
   b. ultrasonography
   c. cholangiography
   d. gastrointestinal series

4. An endoscopic examination of the esophagus, stomach, and small intestine.
   a. cholangiography
   b. gastroduodenoesophagoscopy
   c. esophagogastroduodenoscopy
   d. gastric analysis

5. A test performed to determine the presence of the hepatitis B virus.
   a. occult blood test
   b. stool culture
   c. hepatic antigen
   d. ova and parasites test

CASE STUDY

PEPTIC ULCER DISEASE (PUD)

Read the following case study and then answer the questions that follow.

A 35-year-old male was seen by a physician; the following is a synopsis of the visit.

Present History: The patient states that he has been under a lot of pressure at work lately and has noticed a dull, aching pain in his stomach and back. He states that he has heartburn and "belches" a lot.

Signs and Symptoms: Dull, gnawing pain and a burning sensation in the midepigastrium. Pyrosis (heartburn) and sour eructation (belching).

Diagnosis: Acute gastric ulcer; peptic ulcer disease. Diagnosis determined by a gastrointestinal (GI) series, gastric analysis, and histology with culture to determine presence of *Helicobacter pylori*. No *H. pylori* were found in the culture.

Treatment: Goal is to manage and reduce gastric acidity. This may be accomplished through various treatment regimens such as stress management, rest, diet, avoidance of tobacco, caffeine, and alcohol, and medication. The patient is placed on Mylanta 2 tablets every 2 to 4 hours between meals and at bedtime, and Zantac 300 mg at bedtime.

Prevention: Avoid substances that produce gastric acidity. Stress management, rest, diet, avoidance of tobacco, caffeine, and alcohol are recommended.

CASE STUDY QUESTIONS

1. Signs and symptoms of a gastric ulcer include a dull, gnawing pain and a burning sensation in the midepigastrium. Other indications are: _____, which is heartburn, and sour eructation.
2. The diagnosis of acute gastric ulcer was determined by a gastric analysis and a _____ series.
3. The goal of treatment for acute gastric ulcer is to manage and reduce gastric _____.
4. The medication regimen prescribed included _____ 2 tablets every 2 to 4 hours between meals and at bedtime and,
5. Zantac _____ mg at bedtime.

MedMedia Wrap-Up

www.prenhall.com/rice

Additional interactive resources and activities for this chapter can be found on the Companion Website. For animations, videos, audio glossary, and review, access the accompanying CD-ROM in this book.

Audio Glossary
Medical Terminology Exercises & Activities
Pathology Spotlights
Terminology Translator
Animations
Videos

Objectives
Medical Terminology Exercises & Activities
Audio Glossary
Drug Updates
Medical Terminology in the News

THE CARDIOVASCULAR SYSTEM

7

OBJECTIVES

On completion of this chapter, you will be able to:

- Describe the cardiovascular system.
- Describe and state the functions of arteries, veins, and capillaries.
- Describe cardiovascular differences of the child and the older adult.
- Identify the commonly used pulse checkpoints of the body.
- Describe blood pressure.
- Analyze, build, spell, and pronounce medical words.
- Describe each of the conditions presented in the Pathology Spotlights.
- Complete the Pathology Checkpoint.
- Review Drug Highlights presented in this chapter.
- Provide the description of diagnostic and laboratory tests related to the cardiovascular system.
- Identify and define selected abbreviations.
- Successfully complete the study and review section.

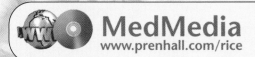

MedMedia
www.prenhall.com/rice

Additional interactive resources and activities for this chapter can be found on the Companion Website. For Terminology Translator, animations, videos, audio glossary, and review, access the accompanying CD-ROM in this book.

Anatomy and Physiology Overview

Through the cardiovascular system, blood is circulated to all parts of the body by the action of the heart. This process provides the body's cells with oxygen and nutritive elements and removes waste materials and carbon dioxide. The **heart**, a muscular pump, is the central organ of the system, which also includes **arteries**, **veins**, and **capillaries**. The various organs and components of the cardiovascular system are described in this chapter, along with some of their functions.

THE HEART

The **heart** is a four-chambered, hollow muscular pump that circulates blood throughout the cardiovascular system. The heart is the center of the cardiovascular system from which the various blood vessels originate and later return. It is slightly larger than a man's fist and weighs approximately 300 g in the average adult male. It lies slightly to the left of the midline of the body and is shaped like an inverted cone with its apex downward. The heart has three layers or linings; see Figure 7–1.

Endocardium. The inner lining of the heart

Myocardium. The muscular middle layer of the heart

Pericardium. The outer membranous sac surrounding the heart

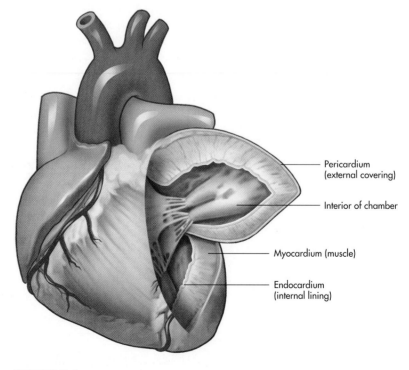

Pericardium (external covering)

Interior of chamber

Myocardium (muscle)

Endocardium (internal lining)

FIGURE 7–1

Tissues of the heart.

Chambers of the Heart

The human heart acts as a double pump and is divided into the right and left heart by a partition called the **septum**. Each side contains an upper and lower chamber. The **atria** or upper chambers are separated by the interatrial septum. The **ventricles** or lower chambers are separated by the interventricular septum. The atria receive blood from the various parts of the body, whereas the ventricles pump blood to body parts. A description of the heart's four chambers and some of their functions is given below.

THE RIGHT ATRIUM

The right upper portion of the heart is called the **right atrium**. It is a thin-walled space that receives blood from all body parts except the lungs. Two large veins bring the blood into the right atrium and are known as the superior and inferior vena cavae.

THE CARDIOVASCULAR SYSTEM

Organ/Structure	Primary Functions
Heart	Hollow muscular pump that circulates blood throughout the cardiovascular system
Arteries	Branching system of vessels that transports blood from the right and left ventricles of the heart to all body parts
Veins	Vessels that transport blood from peripheral tissues to the heart
Capillaries	Microscopic blood vessels that connect arterioles with venules; facilitate passage of life-sustaining fluids containing oxygen and nutrients to cell bodies and the removal of accumulated waste and carbon dioxide

THE RIGHT VENTRICLE

The right lower portion of the heart is called the **right ventricle**. It receives blood from the right atrium through the atrioventricular valve and pumps it through a semilunar valve to the lungs.

THE LEFT ATRIUM

The left upper portion of the heart is called the **left atrium**. It receives blood rich in oxygen as it returns from the lungs via the left and right pulmonary veins.

THE LEFT VENTRICLE

The left lower portion of the heart is called the **left ventricle**. It receives blood from the left atrium through an atrioventricular valve and pumps it through a semilunar valve to a large artery known as the aorta and from there to all parts of the body except the lungs.

Heart Valves

The **valves** of the heart are located at the entrance and exit of each ventricle. See Figure 7–2. The functions of each of the four heart valves are described in the following section.

THE TRICUSPID VALVE

The **right atrioventricular** or **tricuspid valve** guards the opening between the atrium and the right ventricle. The tricuspid valve allows the flow of blood into the ventricle and prevents its return to the right atrium.

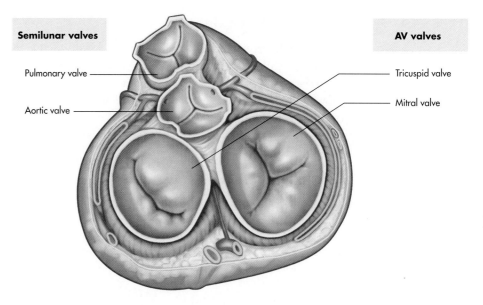

Semilunar valves

Pulmonary valve ——————

Aortic valve ——————

AV valves

—————— Tricuspid valve

—————— Mitral valve

FIGURE 7–2

Heart valves in closed position viewed from the top.

THE PULMONARY SEMILUNAR VALVE

The exit point for blood leaving the right ventricle is called the **pulmonary semilunar valve**. Located between the right ventricle and the pulmonary artery, it allows blood to flow from the right ventricle through the pulmonary artery to the lungs.

THE BICUSPID OR MITRAL VALVE

The left atrioventricular valve between the left atrium and ventricle is called the **bicuspid** or **mitral valve**. It allows blood to flow to the left ventricle and closes to prevent its return to the left atrium.

THE AORTIC SEMILUNAR VALVE

Blood exits from the left ventricle through the **aortic semilunar valve**. Located between the left ventricle and the aorta, it allows blood to flow into the aorta and prevents its return to the ventricle.

Vascular System of the Heart

Due to the membranous lining of the heart (**endocardium**) and the thickness of the myocardium, it is essential that the heart have its own vascular system. The coronary arteries supply the heart with blood, and the cardiac veins, draining into the coronary sinus, collect the blood and return it to the right atrium (Fig. 7–3).

THE FLOW OF BLOOD

Blood flows through the heart, to the lungs, back to the heart, and on to the various body parts as indicated in Figure 7–4. Blood from the superior and inferior vena cavae enters the right atrium and subsequently passes through the tricuspid valve and into

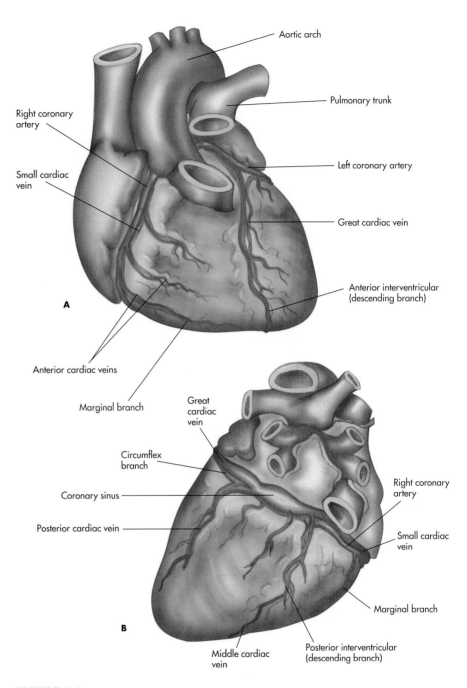

Aortic arch

Pulmonary trunk

Right coronary
artery

Small cardiac
vein

Left coronary artery

Great cardiac vein

Anterior interventricular
(descending branch)

A

Anterior cardiac veins

Marginal branch

Great
cardiac
vein

Circumflex
branch

Coronary sinus

Posterior cardiac vein

Right coronary
artery

Small cardiac
vein

Marginal branch

Middle cardiac
vein

Posterior interventricular
(descending branch)

B

FIGURE 7–3

Coronary circulation. (A) Coronary vessels portraying the complexity and extent of the coronary circulation.
(B) Coronary vessels that supply the anterior surface of the heart.

the right ventricle, which pumps it through the pulmonary semilunar valve into the
left and right pulmonary arteries, which carry it to the lungs. In the lungs, the blood
gives up wastes and takes on oxygen as it passes through capillaries into veins. Blood
leaves the lungs through the left and right pulmonary veins, which carry it to the
heart's left atrium. The oxygenated blood then passes through the bicuspid or mitral
valve into the left ventricle, which pumps it out through the aortic valve and into the
aorta. This large artery supplies a branching system of smaller arteries that connect to
tiny capillaries throughout the body.

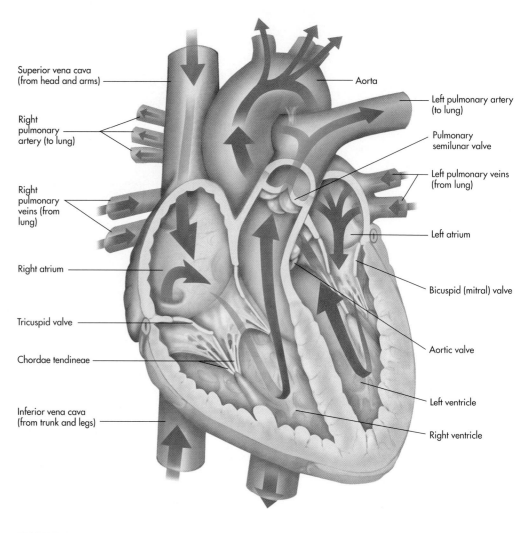

FIGURE 7–4

The flow of blood through the heart.

Capillaries are microscopic blood vessels with thin walls that allow the passage of oxygen and nutrients to the body and let the blood pick up waste and carbon dioxide. Veins lead away from the capillaries as tiny vessels and increase in size until they join the superior and inferior vena cavae as they return to the heart.

The Heartbeat

The **heartbeat** is controlled by the autonomic nervous system. It is normally generated by specialized neuromuscular tissue of the heart that is capable of causing cardiac muscle to contract rhythmically. The neuromuscular tissue of the heart comprises the **sinoatrial node**, the **atrioventricular node**, and the **atrioventricular bundle** (Fig. 7–5).

SINOATRIAL NODE (SA NODE)

Often called the **pacemaker of the heart**, the **SA node** is located in the upper wall of the right atrium, just below the opening of the superior vena cava. It consists of a dense network of **Purkinje fibers** (*atypical muscle fibers*) considered to be the source of impulses initiating the heartbeat. Electrical impulses discharged by the SA node are distributed to the right and left atria and cause them to contract.

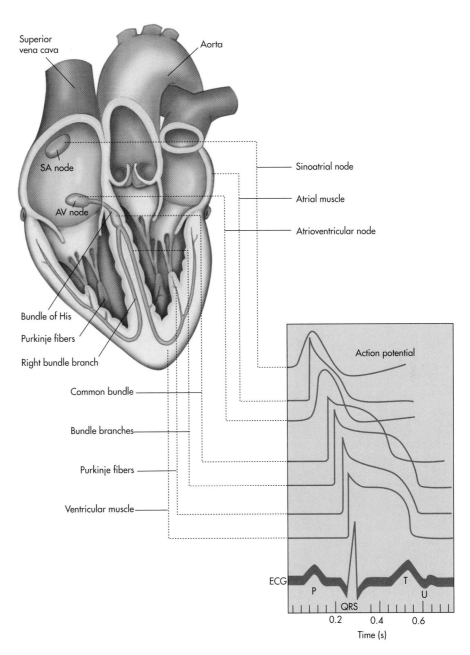

FIGURE 7–5

The conduction system of the heart. Action potentials for the SA and AV nodes, other parts of the conduction system, and the atrial and ventricular muscles are shown along with the correlation to recorded electrical activity (electrocardiogram ECG [EKG]).

ATRIOVENTRICULAR NODE (AV NODE)

Located beneath the endocardium of the right atrium, the **AV node** transmits electrical impulses to the **bundle of His** (*atrioventricular bundle*).

ATRIOVENTRICULAR BUNDLE (BUNDLE OF HIS)

The **bundle of His** forms a part of the conducting system of the heart. It extends from the AV node into the intraventricular septum, where it divides into two branches within the two ventricles. The **Purkinje system** includes the bundle of His and the peripheral fibers. These fibers end in the ventricular muscles, where the excitation of muscle is initiated, causing contraction. The average heartbeat (*pulse*) is between 60 and 100 beats per minute for the average adult. The rate of heartbeat may be affected by emotions, smoking, disease, body size, age, stress, the environment, and many other factors.

Electrocardiogram

An **electrocardiogram** (ECG, EKG) records the electrical activity of the heart. A standard electrocardiogram consists of 12 different leads. With electrodes placed on the patient's arms, legs, and six positions on the chest, a 12-lead ECG can be recorded. There are six unipolar chest leads that record electrical activity of different parts of the heart. An ECG provides valuable information in the diagnosing of cardiac abnormalities, such as myocardial damage and arrhythmias (Fig. 7–6).

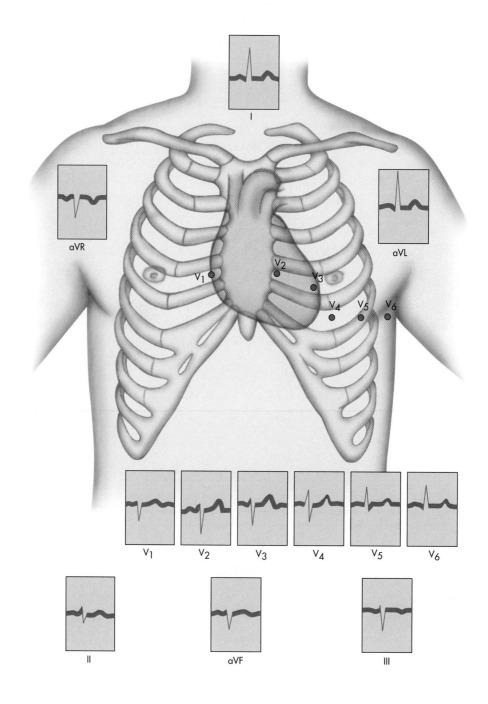

FIGURE 7–6

A normal electrocardiogram (ECG [EKG]).

ARTERIES

The **arteries** constitute a branching system of vessels that transports blood from the right and left ventricles of the heart to all body parts (Table 7–1, and Fig. 7–7). In a normal state, arteries are elastic tubes that recoil and carry blood in pulsating waves. See Figure 7–8. All arteries have a pulse, reflecting the rhythmical beating of the heart; however, certain points are commonly used to check the rate, rhythm, and condition of the arterial wall. These checkpoints are listed below and shown in Figure 7–9.

> **Radial**. Located on the radial (*thumb side*) of the wrist. This is the most common site for taking a pulse.
>
> **Brachial**. Located in the antecubital space of the elbow. This is the most common site used to check blood pressure.
>
> **Carotid**. Located in the neck. In an emergency (*cardiac arrest*), this site is the most readily accessible.
>
> **Temporal**. Located at the temple.
>
> **Femoral**. Located in the groin.
>
> **Popliteal**. Located behind the knee.
>
> **Dorsalis Pedis**. Located on the upper surface of the foot.

BLOOD PRESSURE

Blood pressure, generally speaking, is the pressure exerted by the blood on the walls of the vessels. The term most commonly refers to the pressure exerted in large arteries at the peak of the pulse wave. This pressure is measured with a **sphygmomanometer** used

TABLE 7–1 SELECTED ARTERIES

Artery	Tissue Supplied
Right common carotid	Right side of the head and neck
Left common carotid	Left side of the head and neck
Left subclavian	Left upper extremity
Brachiocephalic	Head and arm
Aortic arch	Branches to head, neck, and upper extremities
Celiac	Stomach, spleen, and liver
Renal	Kidneys
Superior mesenteric	Lower half of large intestine
Inferior mesenteric	Small intestines and first half of the large intestine
Axillary	Axilla
Brachial	Arm
Radial	Lateral side of the hand
Ulnar	Medial side of the hand
Internal iliac	Pelvic viscera and rectum
External iliac	Genitalia and lower trunk muscles
Deep femoral	Deep thigh muscles
Femoral	Thigh
Popliteal	Leg and foot
Anterior tibial	Leg
Dorsalis pedis	Foot

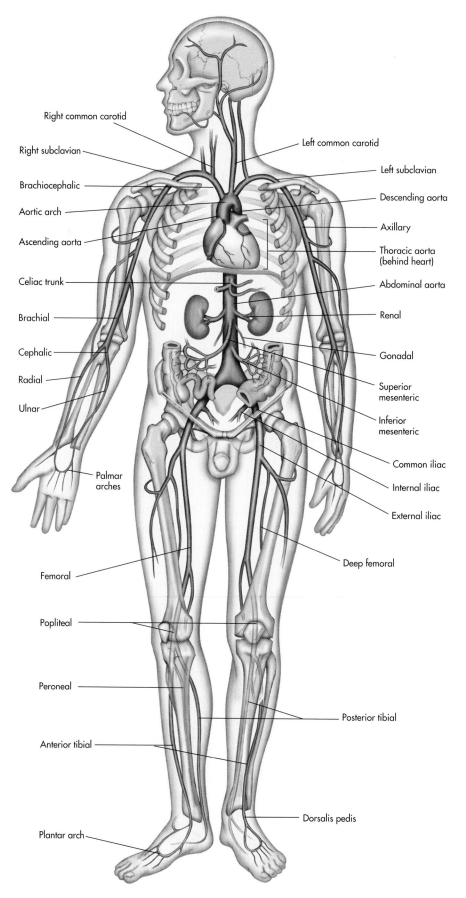

FIGURE 7–7

An overview of the arterial system.

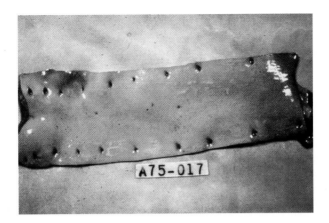

FIGURE 7–8

Inside surface of a normal artery. (Source: Pearson Education/PH College.)

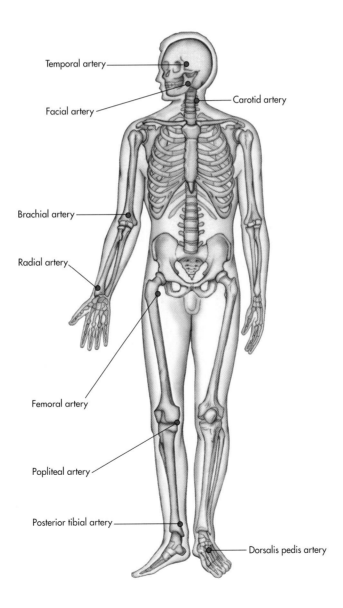

FIGURE 7–9

The primary pulse points of the body.

in concert with a **stethoscope**. Pressure is reported in millimeters of mercury as observed on a graduated column. With the use of a pressure cuff, circulation is interrupted in the brachial artery just above the elbow. Pressure from the cuff is shown on the graduated column of the sphygmomanometer, and as the pressure is released, blood again flows past the cuff. At this point, using a stethoscope, one hears a heartbeat and records the systolic pressure. Continued release of pressure results in a change in the heartbeat sound from loud to soft, at which point one records the diastolic pressure. This method results in a ratio of systolic over diastolic readings expressed in millimeters of mercury (mm Hg). In the average adult, the systolic pressure usually ranges from 100 to 140 mm Hg and the diastolic from 60 to 90 mm Hg. A typical blood pressure showing systolic over diastolic readings might be expressed as 120/80. Two types of sphygmomanometers are shown in Figure 7–10.

Pulse Pressure

The **pulse pressure** is the difference between the systolic and diastolic readings. This reading is an indication of the tone of the arterial walls. The normal pulse pressure is found when the systolic pressure is about 40 points higher than the diastolic reading. For example, if the blood pressure is 120/80, the pulse pressure would be 40. A pulse pressure over 50 points or under 30 points is considered abnormal.

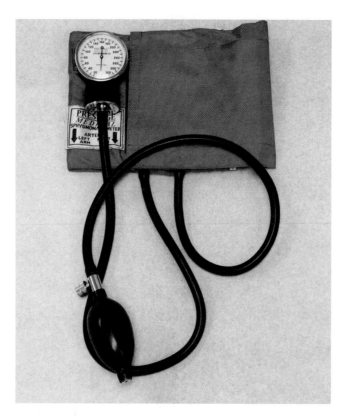
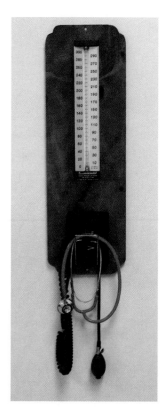

A **B**

FIGURE 7–10

Sphygmomanometers: (A) aneroid type, (B) mercury type.

VEINS

The vessels that transport blood from peripheral tissues to the heart are the *veins* (see Table 7–2, and Fig. 7–11). In a normal state, veins have thin walls and valves that prevent the backflow of blood. Veins are the vessels used when blood is removed for analysis. The process of removing blood from a vein is called **venipuncture**.

CAPILLARIES

The **capillaries** are microscopic blood vessels with single-celled walls that connect **arterioles** (*small arteries*) with **venules** (*small veins*). Blood, passing through capillaries, gives up the oxygen and nutrients carried to this point by the arteries and picks up waste and carbon dioxide as it enters veins. The extremely thin walls of capillaries facilitate passage of life-sustaining fluids containing oxygen and nutrients to cell bodies and the removal of accumulated waste and carbon dioxide.

TABLE 7–2 SELECTED VEINS

Vein	Tissue Drained
External jugular	Superficial tissues of the head and neck
Internal jugular	Sinuses of the brain
Subclavian	Upper extremities
Superior vena cava	Head, neck, and upper extremities
Inferior vena cava	Lower body
Hepatic	Liver
Hepatic portal	Liver and gallbladder
Superior mesenteric	Small intestine and most of the colon
Inferior mesenteric	Descending colon and rectum
Cephalic	Lateral arm
Axillary	Axilla and arm
Basilic	Medial arm
External iliac	Lower limb
Internal iliac	Pelvic viscera
Femoral	Thigh
Great saphenous	Leg
Popliteal	Lower leg
Peroneal	Foot
Anterior tibial	Deep anterior leg and dorsal foot

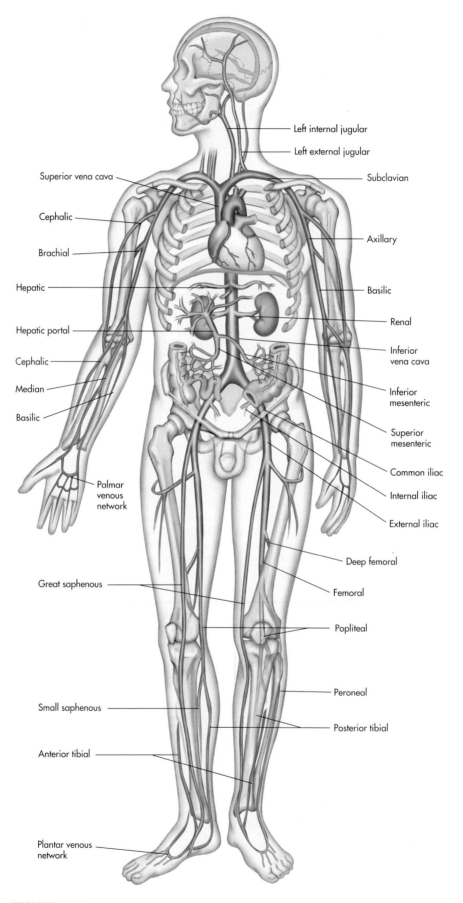

FIGURE 7–11

An overview of the venous system.

■ THE CHILD

The development of the fetal heart is usually completed during the first 2 months of intrauterine life. It is completely formed and functioning by 10 weeks. At 16 weeks fetal heart tones can be heard with a **fetoscope**. Oxygenated blood is transported by the umbilical vein from the placenta to the fetus. Fetal circulation is terminated at birth when the umbilical cord is clamped. The newborn's circulation begins to function shortly after birth and if proper adaptations do not take place, congenital heart disease may occur. Most congenital heart defects develop before the 10th week of pregnancy. Pediatric cardiologists have recognized more than 50 congenital heart defects. If the left side of the heart is not completely separated from the right side, various septal defects develop. If the four chambers of the heart do not occur normally, complex anomalies form, such as tetralogy of Fallot, a congenital heart defect involving pulmonary stenosis, ventricular septal defect, dextroposition of the aorta, and hypertrophy of the right ventricle.

The **pulse**, **blood pressure**, and **respirations** will vary according to the age of the child. A newborn's pulse rate is irregular and rapid, varying from 120 to 140 beats/minute. Blood pressure is low and may vary with the size of the cuff used. The average blood pressure at birth is 80/46. The respirations are approximately 35 to 50 per minute.

■ THE OLDER ADULT

Current evidence indicates that cardiac changes that were once attributed to the aging process may be minimized by modifying lifestyle and personal habits, such

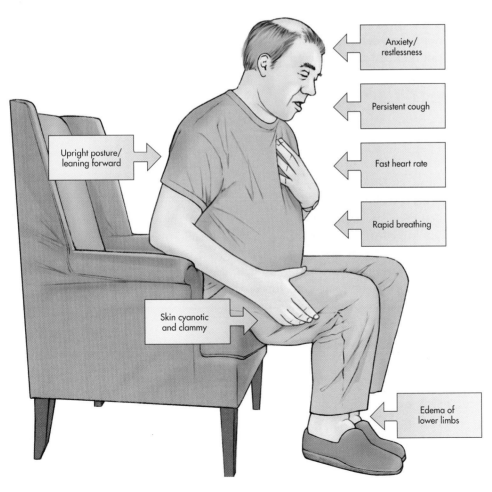

Anxiety/restlessness

Persistent cough

Fast heart rate

Rapid breathing

Upright posture/leaning forward

Skin cyanotic and clammy

Edema of lower limbs

FIGURE 7–12

Signs and symptoms of the patient with heart failure.

as following a low-sodium, low-fat diet, not smoking, drinking in moderation, managing stress, and exercising regularly. Studies have shown that the normal aging heart is able to provide an adequate cardiac output. But in some older adults, the heart must work harder to pump blood because of hardening of the arteries (**arteriosclerosis**) and a buildup of fatty plaques in the arterial walls (**atherosclerosis**). Arteries may gradually become stiff and lose their elastic recoil. The aorta and arteries supplying the heart and brain are generally affected first. Reduced blood flow, elevated blood lipids, and defective endothelial repair that can be seen in aging accelerate the course of cardiovascular disease.

Heart failure (HF) is one of the most common types of cardiovascular disease seen in the older adult.

It is the inability of the ventricles to pump enough blood to meet the needs of the body and may involve either the left or right side of the heart or both sides. Left-sided failure leads to a buildup of fluid in the lungs, or **pulmonary edema**, which causes **dyspnea** and shortness of breath. Right-sided failure is a result of a buildup of blood flowing into the right side of the heart which causes edema of the ankles, distention of the neck veins, and enlargement of the spleen and/or liver.

Heart failure may be caused by coronary artery disease, diabetes, chronic hypertension, myocardial infarction, infection, and valvular disorders such as mitral stenosis. Left-sided heart failure is commonly called congestive heart failure (CHF). See Figure 7–12 for some signs and symptoms of a patient with heart failure.

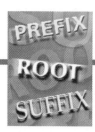

BUILDING YOUR MEDICAL VOCABULARY

This section provides the foundation for learning medical terminology. Medical words can be made up of four different types of word parts:

- Prefixes (P)
- Roots (R)
- Combining forms (CF)
- Suffixes (S)

By connecting various word parts in an organized sequence, thousands of words can be built and learned. In this text the word list is alphabetized so one can see the variety of meanings created when common prefixes and suffixes are repeatedly applied to certain word roots and/or combining forms. Words shown in pink are additional words related to the content of this chapter that are not built from word parts. These words are included to enhance your vocabulary. Note: an asterisk (✱) indicates words that are covered in the Pathology Spotlights section in this chapter.

MEDICAL WORD	WORD PARTS (WHEN APPLICABLE)			DEFINITION
	Part	**Type**	**Meaning**	
anastomosis (ă-năs″ tō-mō′ sĭs)	anastom -osis	R S	opening condition of	A surgical connection between blood vessels or the joining of one hollow or tubular organ to another
aneurysm (ăn′ ū-rĭzm)				A sac formed by a local widening of the wall of an artery or a vein; usually caused by injury or disease

MEDICAL WORD	WORD PARTS (WHEN APPLICABLE)			DEFINITION
	Part	**Type**	**Meaning**	
anginal (ăn′ jĭ-năl)	angin -al	R S	to choke, quinsy pertaining to	Pertaining to attacks of choking or suffocative pain
angioblast (ăn′ jĭ-ō-blăst)	angi/o -blast	CF S	vessel immature cell, germ cell	The germ cell from which blood vessels develop
angiocardiography (ăn″ jĭ-ō-kăr″ dĭ-ŏg′ ră-fē)	angi/o cardi/o -graphy	CF CF S	vessel heart recording	The process of recording the heart and vessels after an intravenous injection of a radiopaque solution
angiocarditis (ăn″ jĭ-ō-kăr-dī′ tĭs)	angi/o card -itis	CF R S	vessel heart inflammation	Inflammation of the heart and its great vessels
angioma (ăn″ jĭ-ō′ mă)	ang/i -oma	CF S	vessel tumor	A tumor of a blood vessel. See Figure 7–13.
angioplasty (ăn′ jĭ-ō-plăs″ tē)	angi/o -plasty	CF S	vessel surgical repair	Surgical repair of a blood vessel or vessels
angiostenosis (ăn″ jĭ-ō-stĕ-nō′ sĭs)	angi/o sten -osis	CF R S	vessel narrowing condition of	A condition of narrowing of a blood vessel
aortomalacia (ā-ōr″ tō-mă-lā′ shĭ-ă)	aort/o -malacia	CF S	aorta softening	Softening of the walls of the aorta
arrhythmia (ă-rĭth′ mĭ-ă)	a rrhythm -ia	P R S	lack of rhythm condition	A condition in which there is a lack of rhythm of the heartbeat
arterial (ăr-tē′ rĭ-ăl)	arter/i -al	CF S	artery pertaining to	Pertaining to an artery
arteriosclerosis (ăr-tē″ rĭ-ō-sklĕ-rō′ sĭs)	arteri/o scler -osis	CF R S	artery hardening condition of	A condition of hardening of an artery
arteritis (ăr″ tĕ-rī′ tĭs)	arter -itis	R S	artery inflammation	Inflammation of an artery. See Figure 7–14.
artificial pacemaker (ăr tĭ-fĭsh′ ăl pās′ māk-ĕr)				An electronic device that stimulates impulse initiation within the heart
atheroma (ăth″ ĕr-ō mă)	ather -oma	R S	fatty substance, porridge tumor	Tumor of an artery containing a fatty substance

MEDICAL WORD	WORD PARTS (WHEN APPLICABLE)			DEFINITION
	Part	Type	Meaning	
atherosclerosis (ăth″ ĕr-ō-sklĕ-rō′ sĭs)	ather/o	CF	fatty substance, porridge	A condition of the arteries characterized by the buildup of fatty substances and hardening of the walls. ✱ See Pathology Spotlight: Coronary Heart Disease, and Figures 7–27—7–29.
	scler	R	hardening	
	-osis	S	condition of	
atrioventricular (ăt″ rĭ-ō-vĕn-trĭk′ ū-lăr)	atri/o	CF	atrium	Pertaining to the atrium and the ventricle
	ventricul	R	ventricle	
	-ar	S	pertaining to	
auscultation (ŏs″ kool-tā′ shŭn)	auscultat	R	listen to	A method of physical assessment using a stethoscope to listen to sounds within the chest, abdomen, and other parts of the body
	-ion	S	process	
bicuspid (bī-kŭs′ pĭd)	bi	P	two	Having two points or cusps; pertaining to the mitral valve
	-cuspid	S	point	
bradycardia (brăd″ ĭ-kăr′ dĭ-ă)	brady	P	slow	A condition of slow heartbeat
	card	R	heart	
	-ia	S	condition	
bruit (broot)				Noise; a sound of venous or arterial origin heard on auscultation
cardiac (kăr′ dĭ-ăk)	card/i	CF	heart	Pertaining to the heart
	-ac	S	pertaining to	
cardiocentesis (kăr″ dĭ-ō-sĕn-tē′ sĭs)	cardi/o	CF	heart	Surgical puncture of the heart
	-centesis	S	surgical puncture	
cardiologist (kăr-dē-ŏl′ ō-jĭst)	cardi/o	CF	heart	One who specializes in the study of the heart
	log	R	study of	
	-ist	S	one who specializes	
cardiology (kăr″ dĭ-ōl′ ō-jē)	cardi/o	CF	heart	The study of the heart
	-logy	S	study of	
cardiomegaly (kăr″ dĭ-ō-mĕg′ ă-lē)	cardi/o	CF	heart	Enlargement of the heart
	-megaly	S	enlargement, large	
cardiometer (kăr″ dĭ-ōm′ ĕ-tĕr)	cardi/o	CF	heart	An instrument used to measure the action of the heart
	-meter	S	instrument to measure	

MEDICAL WORD	WORD PARTS (WHEN APPLICABLE)			DEFINITION
	Part	**Type**	**Meaning**	
cardiomyopathy (kăr″ dē-ō-mī-ŏp′ ă-thē)	cardi/o my/o -pathy	CF CF S	heart muscle disease	Disease of the heart muscle that may be caused by a viral infection, a parasitic infection, or overconsumption of alcohol. See Figure 7–15.
cardiopathy (kăr″ dĭ-ŏp′ ă-thē)	cardi/o -pathy	CF S	heart disease	Heart disease
cardiopulmonary (kăr″ dĭ-ō-pŭl′ mō-nĕr-ē)	cardi/o pulmonar -y	CF R S	heart lung pertaining to	Pertaining to the heart and lungs
cardiotonic (kăr″ dĭ-ō-tŏn′ ĭk)	cardi/o ton -ic	CF R S	heart tone pertaining to	Pertaining to increasing the tone of the heart; a type of medication
cardiovascular (kăr″ dĭ-ō-văs′ kū-lar)	cardi/o vascul -ar	CF R S	heart small vessel pertaining to	Pertaining to the heart and small blood vessels
carditis (kăr-dī′ tĭs)	card -itis	R S	heart inflammation	Inflammation of the heart
catheterization (kăth″ ĕ-tĕr-ĭ-zā′ shŭn)				The process of inserting a catheter into the heart or the urinary bladder
cholesterol (kō-lĕs′ tĕr-ŏl)	chol/e sterol	CF R	bile solid (fat)	A waxy, fat-like substance in the bloodstream of all animals. It is believed to be dangerous when it builds up on arterial walls and contributes to the risk of coronary heart disease.
circulation (sər″ -kyə lā′ shŭn)	circulat -ion	R S	circular process	The process of moving the blood in the veins and arteries throughout the body
claudication (klaw-dĭ-kā′ shŭn)	claudicat -ion	R S	to limp process	The process of lameness, limping; may result from inadequate blood supply to the muscles in the leg
constriction (kən-strĭk′ shŭn)	con strict -ion	P R S	together, with to draw, to bind process	The process of drawing together, as in the narrowing of a vessel
coronary bypass (kŏr′ ō-nă-rē bī′ păs)				A surgical procedure performed to increase blood flow to the myocardium by using a section of a saphenous vein or internal mammary artery to bypass the obstructed or occluded coronary artery

MEDICAL WORD	WORD PARTS (WHEN APPLICABLE)			DEFINITION
	Part	Type	Meaning	
coronary heart disease (CHD) (kŏr′ ō-nă-rē hart dĭ-zēz′)				Coronary heart disease (CHD), also referred to as coronary artery disease (CAD), refers to the narrowing of the coronary arteries sufficient to prevent adequate blood supply to the myocardium. ✱ See Pathology Spotlight: Coronary Heart Disease.
cyanosis (sī-ă n-ō′ sĭs)	cyan -osis	R S	dark blue condition of	A dark blue condition of the skin and mucous membranes caused by oxygen deficiency
diastole (dī-ăs′ tō-lē)	diast -ole	R S	to expand small	The relaxation phase of the heart cycle during which the heart muscle relaxes and the heart chambers fill with blood
dysrhythmia (dĭs-rĭth′ mē-ă)	dys rhythm -ia	P R S	difficult rhythm condition	An abnormal, difficult, or bad rhythm. ✱ See Pathology Spotlight: Dysrythmias.
echocardiography (ĕk″ ō-kăr″ dē-ŏg′ rah-fē)	ech/o cardi/o -graphy	CF CF S	echo heart recording	A noninvasive ultrasound method for evaluating the heart for valvular or structural defects and coronary artery disease
electrocardiograph (ē-lĕk″ trō-kăr′ dĭ-ō-grăf)	electr/o cardi/o -graph	CF CF S	electricity heart to write, record	A device used for recording the electrical impulses of the heart muscle
electrocardio-phonograph (ē-lĕk″ trō-kăr″ dĭ-ō-fō′ nō-grăf)	electr/o cardi/o phon/o -graph	CF CF CF S	electricity heart sound to write, record	A device used to record heart sounds
embolism (ĕm′ bō-lĭzm)	embol -ism	R S	a throwing in condition of	A condition in which a blood clot obstructs a blood vessel; *a moving blood clot*
endarterectomy (ĕn″ dăr-tĕr-ĕk′ tō-mē)	end arter -ectomy	P R S	within artery excision	Surgical excision of the inner portion of an artery
endocarditis (ĕn″ dō-kăr-dī′ tĭs)	endo card -itis	P R S	within heart inflammation	Inflammation of the endocardium. See Figure 7–16.
endocardium (ĕn″ dō-kăr′ dē-ŭm)	endo card/i -um	P CF S	within heart tissue	The inner lining of the heart

MEDICAL WORD	WORD PARTS (WHEN APPLICABLE)			DEFINITION
	Part	**Type**	**Meaning**	
extracorporeal circulation (ĕks-tră-kor-pōr′ ē-ăl sər″ -kyə lā′ shŭn)	extra	P	outside	Pertaining to the circulation of the blood outside the body via a heart–lung machine or hemodialyzer
	corpor/e	CF	body	
	-al	S	pertaining to	
	circulat	R	circular	
	-ion	S	process	
fibrillation (fĭ″ brĭl-ā′ shŭn)	fibrillat	R	fibrils (small fibers)	Quivering of muscle fiber; may be atrial or ventricular
	-ion	S	process	
flutter (flŭt′ ər)				A condition of the heartbeat in which the contractions become extremely rapid
heart failure				A disorder in which the heart loses its ability to pump blood efficiently. See Fig. 7–12.
heart–lung transplant (hart-lŭng trăns′ plănt)				The surgical process of transferring the heart and lungs from a donor to a patient
heart transplant (hart trăns′ plănt)				The surgical process of transferring the heart from a donor to a patient
hemangiectasis (hē″ măn-jĭ-ĕk′ tă-sĭs)	hem	R	blood	Dilatation of a blood vessel
	ang/i	CF	vessel	
	-ectasis	S	dilatation	
hemangioma (hē-măn″ jĭ-ō′ mă)	hem	R	blood	A benign tumor of a blood vessel. See Figures 7–17 and 7–18.
	ang/i	CF	vessel	
	-oma	S	tumor	
hemodynamic (hē″ mō-dī-năm′ ĭk)	hem/o	CF	blood	Pertaining to the study of the heart's ability to function as a pump; the movement of the blood and its pressure
	dynam	R	power	
	-ic	S	pertaining to	
hypertension (hī″ pĕr-tĕn′ shŭn)	hyper	P	excessive, above	High blood pressure; a disease of the arteries caused by such pressure. ✱ See Pathology Spotlight: Hypertension.
	tens	R	pressure	
	-ion	S	process	
hypotension (hī″ pō-tĕn′ shŭn)	hypo	P	deficient, below	Low blood pressure
	tens	R	pressure	
	-ion	S	process	
infarction (ĭn-fărk′ shŭn)	infarct	R	infarct (necrosis of an area)	Process of development of an infarct, which is necrosis of tissue resulting from obstruction of blood flow
	-ion	S	process	

MEDICAL WORD	WORD PARTS (WHEN APPLICABLE)			DEFINITION
	Part	**Type**	**Meaning**	
ischemia (ĭs-kē′ mĭ-ă)	isch -emia	R S	to hold back blood condition	A condition in which there is a lack of blood supply to a part caused by constriction or obstruction of a blood vessel
lipoprotein (lĭp-ō-prō′ tēn)	lip/o prot/e -in	CF CF S	fat first chemical	*Fat (lipid)* and *protein molecules* that are bound together. They are classified as: **VLDL**—very-low-density lipoproteins; **LDL**—low-density lipoproteins; and **HDL**—high-density lipoproteins. High levels of VLDL and LDL are associated with cholesterol and triglyceride deposits in arteries, which could lead to coronary heart disease, hypertension, and atherosclerosis.
lubb-dupp (lŭb-dŭp)				The two separate heart sounds that can be heard with the use of a stethoscope
mitral stenosis (mī′ trăl stě-nō′ sĭs)	mitr -al sten -osis	R S R S	mitral valve pertaining to narrowing condition of	A condition of narrowing of the mitral valve
murmur (mər′ mər)				A soft blowing or rasping sound heard by auscultation of various parts of the body, especially in the region of the heart
myocardial (mī″ ō-kăr′ dĭ-ăl)	my/o card/i -al	CF CF S	muscle heart pertaining to	Pertaining to the heart muscle
myocardial infarction (MI) (mī″ ō-kăr′ dē-ăl ĭn-fărk′ shŭn)	my/o card/i -al infarct -ion	CF CF S R S	muscle heart pertaining to infarct (necrosis of an area) process	Occurs when an area of heart muscle dies or is permanently damaged because of an inadequate supply of oxygen to that area; also known as a heart attack. ✱ See Pathology Spotlight: Heart Attack.
myocarditis (mī″ ō-kăr-dī′ tĭs)	my/o card -itis	CF R S	muscle heart inflammation	Inflammation of the heart muscle
occlusion (ŏ-kloo′ zhŭn)	occlus -ion	R S	to shut up process	The process or state of being closed

MEDICAL WORD	WORD PARTS (WHEN APPLICABLE)			DEFINITION
	Part	**Type**	**Meaning**	
oximetry (ŏk-sĭm′ ĕ-trē)	ox/i -metry	CF S	oxygen measurement	The process of measuring the oxygen saturation of blood. A photoelectric device (oximeter) measures oxygen saturation of the blood by recording the amount of light transmitted or reflected by deoxygenated versus oxygenated hemoglobin. A pulse oximetry is a noninvasive method of indicating the arterial oxygen saturation of functional hemoglobin. See Figure 7–19.
oxygen (ŏk′ sĭ-jĕn)	oxy -gen	R S	sour, sharp, acid formation, produce	A colorless, odorless, tasteless gas essential to respiration in animals
palpitation (păl-pĭ-tā′ shŭn)	palpitat -ion	R S	throbbing process	Rapid throbbing or fluttering of the heart
percutaneous transluminal coronary angioplasty (pĕr″ kū-tā′ nē-ŭs trăns-lū′ mĭ-năl kŏr′ ō-nă-rē ăn′ jĭ-ō-plăs″ tē)				The use of a balloon-tipped catheter to compress fatty plaques against an artery wall. When successful, the plaques remain compressed, and this permits more blood to flow through the artery, thereby relieving the symptoms of heart disease.
pericardial (pĕr″ ĭ-kăr′ dĭ-ăl)	peri card/i -al	P CF S	around heart pertaining to	Pertaining to the pericardium, the sac surrounding the heart
pericarditis (pĕr″ ĭ-kăr-dī′ tĭs)	peri card -itis	P R S	around heart inflammation	Inflammation of the pericardium
phlebitis (flĕ-bī′ tĭs)	phleb -itis	R S	vein inflammation	Inflammation of a vein
phlebotomy (flĕ-bŏt′ ō-mē)	phleb/o -tomy	CF S	vein incision	Incision into a vein
Raynaud's phenomenon (rā-nōz fĕ-nŏm′ ĕ-nŏn)				A disorder that generally affects the blood vessels in the fingers and toes; it is characterized by intermittent attacks that cause the blood vessels in the digits to narrow. The attack is usually due to exposure to cold or occurs during emotional stress. Once the attack begins, the patient may experience pallor, cyanosis, and/or rubor in the affected part. See Figure 7–20.

MEDICAL WORD	WORD PARTS (WHEN APPLICABLE)			DEFINITION
	Part	Type	Meaning	
rheumatic heart disease (rōo-măt′ ĭk hart dĭ-zēz′)				Endocarditis or valvular heart disease as a result of complications of acute rheumatic fever
semilunar (sĕm″ ĭ-lū′ năr)	semi lun -ar	P R S	half moon pertaining to	Valves of the aorta and pulmonary artery
septum (sĕp′ tŭm)	sept -um	R S	a partition tissue	A wall or partition that divides or separates a body space or cavity
shock (shŏk)				A state of disruption of oxygen supply to the tissues and a return of blood to the heart. See Figure 7–21.
sinoatrial (sīn″ ō-ā ′ trĭ-ăl)	sin/o atri -al	CF R S	a curve atrium pertaining to	Pertaining to the sinus venosus and the atrium
sphygmomano-meter (sfĭg″ mō-măn-ŏm ĕt-ĕr)	sphygm/o man/o -meter	CF CF S	pulse thin instrument to measure	An instrument used to measure the arterial blood pressure. See Figure 7–10.
spider veins (spī′ dĕr vāns)				Hemangioma in which numerous telangiectatic vessels radiate from a central point. See Figure 7–22.
stethoscope (stĕth′ ō-skōp)	steth/o -scope	CF S	chest instrument	An instrument used to listen to the sounds of the heart, lungs, and other internal organs
systole (sĭs′ tō-lē)	syst -ole	R S	contraction small	The contractive phase of the heart cycle during which blood is forced into the aorta and the pulmonary artery
tachycardia (tăk″ ĭ-kăr′ dĭ-ă)	tachy card -ia	P R S	fast heart condition	A fast heartbeat
telangiectasis (tĕl-ăn″ jĕ-ĕk-tă′ sĭs)	tel ang/i -ectasis	R CF S	end vessel dilatation	A vascular lesion formed by dilatation of a group of small blood vessels; it may appear as a birthmark or be caused by long-term exposure to the sun. See Figure 7–23.
thrombophlebitis (thrŏm″ bō-flē-bī′ tĭs)	thromb/o phleb -itis	CF R S	clot of blood vein inflammation	Inflammation of a vein associated with the formation of a thrombus. See Figure 7–24.

MEDICAL WORD	WORD PARTS (WHEN APPLICABLE)			DEFINITION
	Part	Type	Meaning	
thrombosis (thrŏm-bō′ sĭs)	thromb -osis	R S	clot of blood condition of	A condition in which there is a blood clot within the vascular system; *a stationary blood clot.* See Figure 7–25.
tricuspid (trī-kŭs′ pĭd)	tri -cuspid	P S	three a point	Having three points; pertaining to the tricuspid valve
triglyceride (trī-glĭs′ ĕr-īd)	tri glyc -er -ide	P R S S	three sweet, sugar relating to having a particular quality	Pertaining to a compound consisting of three molecules of fatty acids
varicose veins (văr′ ĭ-kōs vāns)				Swollen, distended, and knotted veins which usually occur in the lower leg(s). They result from a stagnated or sluggish flow of blood in combination with defective valves and weakened walls of the veins. See Figure 7–26.
vasoconstrictive (văs″ ō-kŏn-strĭk′ tĭv)	vas/o con strict -ive	CF P R S	vessel together to draw, to bind nature of, quality of	The drawing together, as in the narrowing of a blood vessel
vasodilator (văs″ ō-dī-lā′ tor)	vas/o dilat -or	CF R S	vessel to widen one who, a doer	A nerve or agent that causes dilation of blood vessels
vasospasm (văs′ ō-spăzm)	vas/o -spasm	CF S	vessel contraction, spasm	Contraction of a blood vessel
venipuncture (věn′ ĭ-pŭnk″ chūr)	ven/i -puncture	CF S	vein to pierce	To pierce a vein
ventricular (věn-trĭk′ ū-lăr)	ventricul -ar	R S	ventricle pertaining to	Pertaining to a ventricle

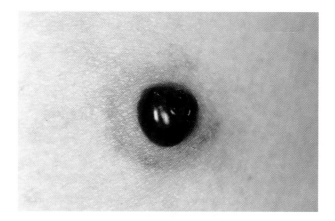

FIGURE 7–13

Infarction angioma. (Courtesy of Jason L. Smith, MD.)

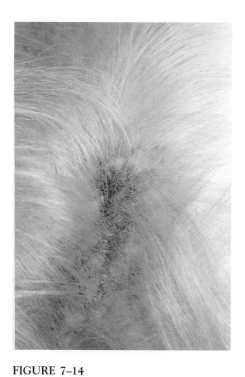

FIGURE 7–14

Temporal arteritis. (Courtesy of Jason L. Smith, MD.)

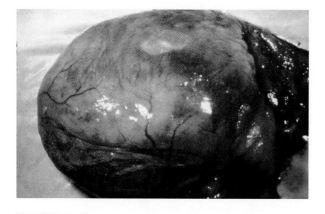

FIGURE 7–15

Cardiomyopathy. (Source: Pearson Education/PH College.)

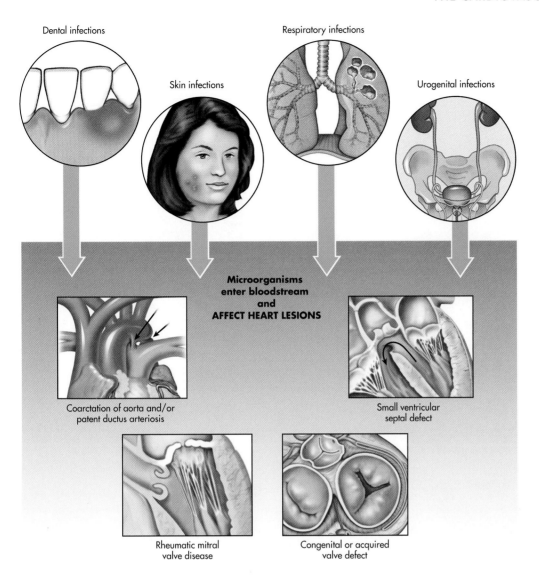

Dental infections

Skin infections

Respiratory infections

Urogenital infections

Microorganisms enter bloodstream and AFFECT HEART LESIONS

Coarctation of aorta and/or patent ductus arteriosis

Small ventricular septal defect

Rheumatic mitral valve disease

Congenital or acquired valve defect

FIGURE 7–16

Infections resulting in bacterial endocarditis.

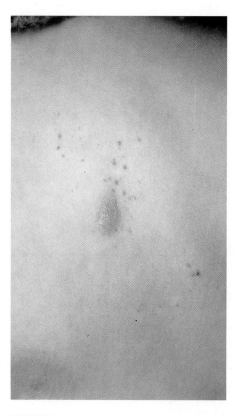

FIGURE 7–17

Hemangioma. (Courtesy of Jason L. Smith, MD.)

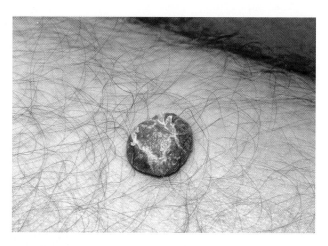

FIGURE 7–18

Sclerosing hemangioma. (Courtesy of Jason L. Smith, MD.)

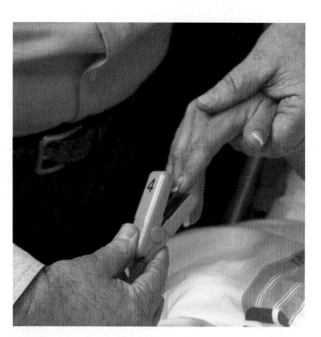

FIGURE 7–19

Pulse oximetry: the sensor probe is applied securely, flush with skin, making sure that both sensor probes are aligned directly opposite each other.

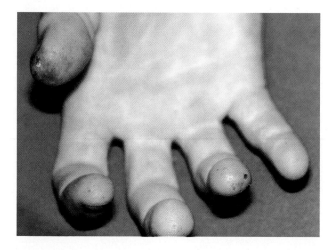

FIGURE 7–20

Raynaud's phenomenon. (Courtesy of Jason L. Smith, MD.)

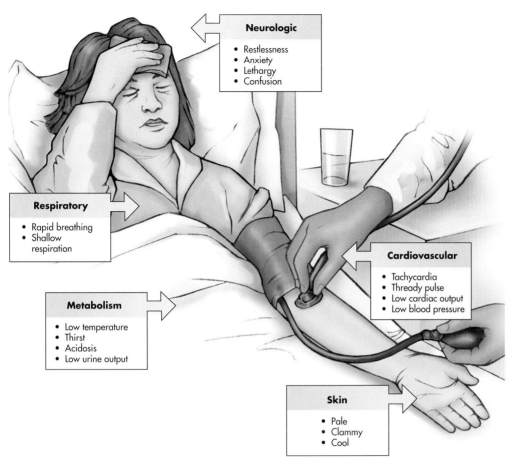

Neurologic
- Restlessness
- Anxiety
- Lethargy
- Confusion

Respiratory
- Rapid breathing
- Shallow respiration

Metabolism
- Low temperature
- Thirst
- Acidosis
- Low urine output

Cardiovascular
- Tachycardia
- Thready pulse
- Low cardiac output
- Low blood pressure

Skin
- Pale
- Clammy
- Cool

FIGURE 7–21

Symptoms of a patient in shock.

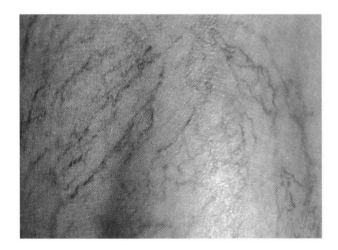

FIGURE 7–22

Spider veins. (Courtesy of Jason L. Smith, MD.)

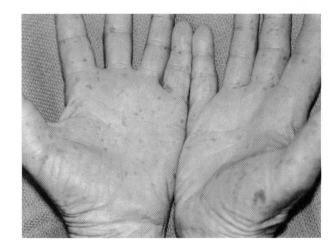

FIGURE 7–23

Telangiectasis. (Courtesy of Jason L. Smith, MD.)

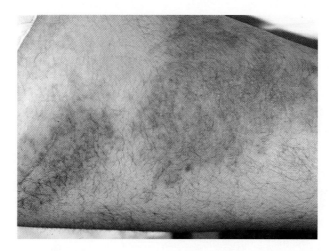

FIGURE 7–24

Thrombophlebitis. (Courtesy of Jason L. Smith, MD.)

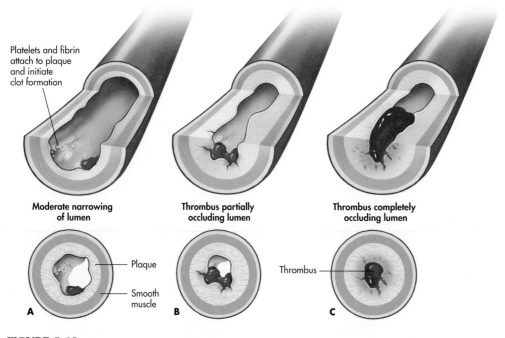

FIGURE 7–25

Thrombus formation in an atherosclerotic vessel. Depicted are the initial clot formation (A) and the varying degrees of occlusion (B) and (C).

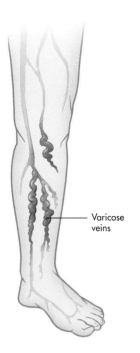

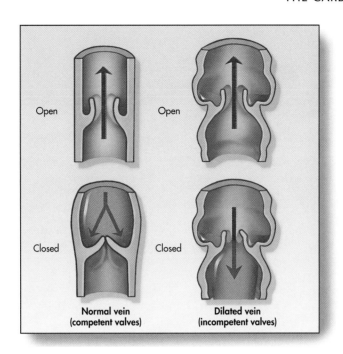

Varicose veins

Open   Open

Closed   Closed

Normal vein   Dilated vein
(competent valves)   (incompetent valves)

FIGURE 7–26

Development of varicose veins.

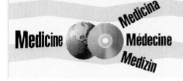

TERMINOLOGY TRANSLATOR

This feature, found on the accompanying CD-ROM, provides an innovative tool to translate medical words into Spanish, French, and German.

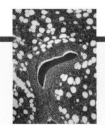

PATHOLOGY SPOTLIGHTS

Coronary Heart Disease (CHD)

Coronary heart disease (CHD) is the most common form of heart disease. It is also referred to as coronary artery disease (CAD) and refers to the narrowing of the coronary arteries that supply blood to the heart. It is a progressive disease that increases the risk of myocardial infarction (heart attack) and sudden death.

CHD usually results from the buildup of fatty material and plaque (**atherosclerosis**). See Figures 7–27, 7–28, and 7–29. As the coronary arteries narrow, the flow of blood to the heart can slow or stop. Blockage can occur in one or many coronary arteries.

Small blockages may not always affect the heart's performance. The person may not have symptoms until the heart needs more oxygen-rich blood than the arteries can supply. This commonly occurs during exercise or other activity. The pain that results is called stable angina.

If a blockage is large, angina pain can occur with little or no activity. This is known as unstable angina. In this case, the flow of blood to the heart is so limited that the person cannot

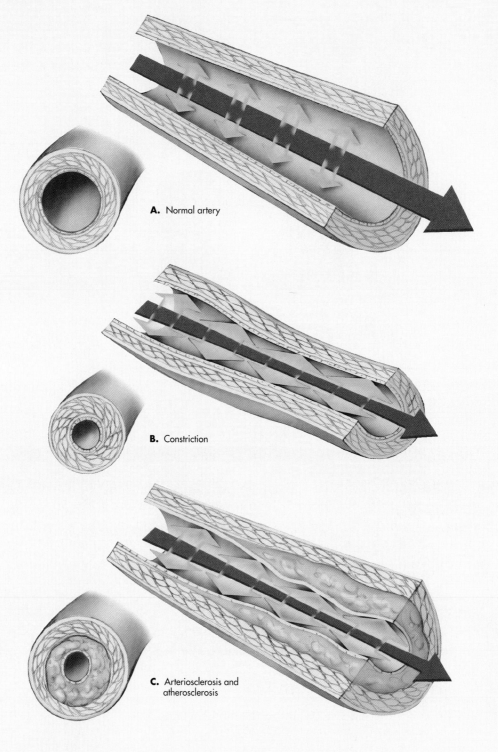

FIGURE 7–27

Blood vessels: (A) normal artery, (B) constriction, and (C) arteriosclerosis and atherosclerosis.

do daily tasks without bringing on an angina attack. When the blood flow to an area of the heart is completely blocked, a myocardial infarction (heart attack) occurs.

Symptoms of CHD vary widely. The classic indicator of CHD is angina, or chest pain. The pain may radiate to the neck, jaw, or left arm. It is often described as a crushing, burning, or squeezing sensation. The person may also have shortness of breath. This is usually a symptom of **heart failure**. The heart at this point is weak because of the long-term lack of blood and

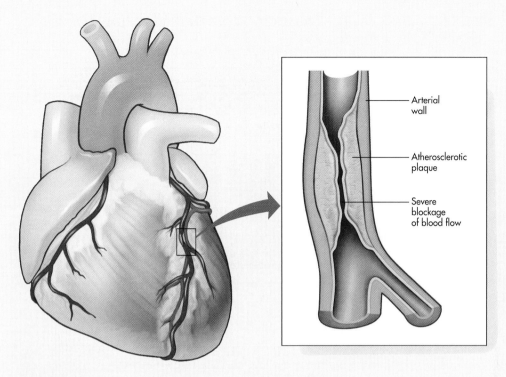

FIGURE 7–28

An atherosclerotic artery.

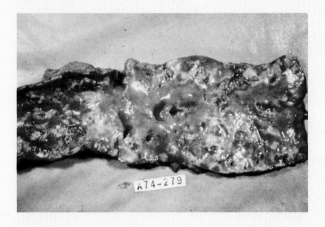

FIGURE 7–29

Inside surface of a diseased artery showing atherosclerosis.
(Source: Pearson Education/PH College.)

oxygen, or sometimes from a recent or past heart attack. If the heart is not pumping enough blood to circulate in the body, shortness of breath may be accompanied by swollen feet and ankles. Sometimes, a person may have no symptoms at all until he or she suffers a heart attack.

CHD is the leading cause of death in the United States for men and women. According to the American Heart Association, about every 29 seconds someone in the United States suffers from a CHD-related event, and about every minute someone dies from such an event. The lifetime risk of having coronary heart disease after age 40 is 49 percent for men and 32 percent for women. As women get older, the risk increases almost to that of men.

One in ten American women 45 to 64 years of age has some form of heart disease, and this increases to one in four women over 65. The common misconception that heart disease is

TABLE 7–3 RISK FACTORS ASSOCIATED WITH DEVELOPING CORONARY HEART DISEASE

Male age 45 or older	Diabetes mellitus
Female age 55 or older	High-density lipoprotein (HDL) below 35 mg/dL
Female under age 55 with premature menopause	Family history of early heart disease (parent or sibling; male less than 55, female less than 65)
Smoker	Obesity
Hypertension	

Note: To help lower cholesterol one should limit intake of foods that are high in saturated fat:

Whole milk	Bacon
Dairy cream	Ribs
Cheese	Ground red meat
Butter	Cold cuts
Red meat, heavily marbled with fat	Poultry skin
Prime cuts	Coconut or palm oil
Sausage	Hydrogenated vegetable oil

a man's disease may cause many women to be misinformed about heart disease, the risk factors associated with developing heart disease, and lifestyle changes.

CHD affects people of all races. It can be caused by a combination of unhealthy lifestyle choices and genetics. High levels of VLDL and LDL lipoproteins are associated with cholesterol and **triglyceride** deposits in arteries, which could lead to coronary heart disease, hypertension, and atherosclerosis. One's total cholesterol level should be below 200 mg/dL and HDL (good cholesterol) above 35 mg/dL. See Table 7–3 for risk factors that increase the risk of CHD. The more risk factors that one has, the greater the possibility of developing coronary artery disease, a major cause of myocardial infarction.

Dysrhythmias

A **dysrhythmia** of the heart is an abnormality of the rhythm or rate of the heartbeat. The dysrhythmia is caused by a disturbance of the normal electrical activity within the heart. Dysrhythmias can be divided into 2 main groups: **tachycardias** and **bradycardias**. Tachycardias cause a rapid heartbeat, with over 100 beats per minute. Bradycardias cause a slow heartbeat, with less than 60 beats per minute. The rhythm of the heart may be regular during a dysrhythmia: each beat of the atria, or upper chambers of the heart, is followed by one beat of the ventricles, or lower chambers of the heart. The beat may also be irregular and may begin in an abnormal area of the heart.

TABLE 7–4 CONTRIBUTING FACTORS TO HYPERTENSION

Those That One Can Control:	
Smoking	Avoid the use of tobacco products
Overweight	Maintain a proper weight for age and body size
Lack of Exercise	Exercise regularly
Stress	Learn to manage stress
Alcohol	Limit intake of alcohol

Other Contributing Factors:	
Heredity	Family history of high blood pressure, heart attack, stroke, or diabetes
Race	There is a greater incidence of hypertension among African-Americans
Sex	Males have a greater chance of developing hypertension
Age	The likelihood of hypertension increases with age

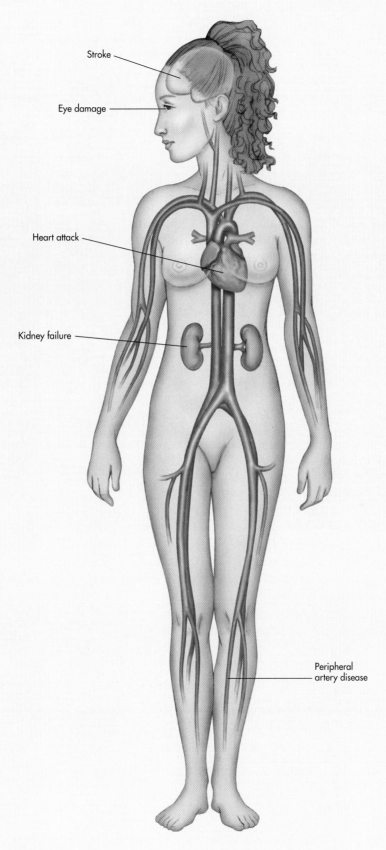

FIGURE 7–30

Uncontrolled hypertension can lead to kidney failure, stroke, heart attack, peripheral artery disease, and eye damage.

Symptoms vary depending on the type of dysrhythmia, but may include: dizziness, or light-headedness, palpitations, shortness of breath, fatigue, weakness, **angina**, and fainting. Most dysrhythmias are caused by heart disease, including coronary heart disease, disease of the heart valves, including infections such as **endocarditis**, and **heart failure**.

Dysrhythmias can be life-threatening if they cause a severe decrease in the pumping function of the heart. When the pumping function is severely decreased for more than a few seconds, blood circulation is essentially stopped, and organ damage (such as brain damage) may occur within a few minutes.

Hypertension

Hypertension is a medical term that is used to describe a blood pressure higher than normal. Approximately 50 million adults in the United States are believed to have hypertension, a number expected to climb as the population ages. With hypertension (high blood pressure: HBP), the blood vessels can become tight and constricted. These changes can cause the blood to press on the vessel walls with extra force. When this force exceeds a certain level and remains there, one has high blood pressure. Hypertension often has no symptoms and is frequently called "the silent killer" because, if left untreated, it can lead to kidney failure, stroke, heart attack, peripheral artery disease, and eye damage. See Figure 7–29. There are various factors that can contribute to developing hypertension and it is important to know these factors (see Table 7–4).

Hypertension can be controlled by a variety of methods, such as taking blood pressure medications as prescribed, seeing a physician on a regular basis, establishing healthy eating habits, exercising, avoiding stress, and making lifestyle changes.

Prehypertension

Individuals aged 18 years and over with blood pressure ranging from 120/80 to 139/89 mm Hg belong to a new category designated as prehypertension, a high-risk precursor to hypertension, according to the Joint National Committee (JNC) seventh report. Because of this report, recently released by the National Heart, Lung, and Blood Institute (NHLBI), part of the National Institutes of Health (NIH), new blood pressure categories have become a part of the guidelines for the prevention and treatment of hypertension.

According to the report, adults at the upper end of the prehypertension blood pressure range (130/80 to 139/89 mm Hg) are twice as likely to progress to hypertension than those with lower blood pressure levels. The reporting panel of experts recommended lifestyle modification for patients with prehypertension. Therapeutic behavior changes identified as critical in the prevention of high blood pressure included reducing dietary fat and sodium, increasing exercise, and limiting alcohol consumption.

Other changes were made to the blood pressure classification system. While stage 1 hypertension (blood pressure range 140/90 to 159/99 mm Hg) remained a category, therapeutic recommendations were altered, identifying thiazide-type diuretics as treatment of choice for uncomplicated cases. The focus on diuretics for initial treatment of stage 1 hypertension is primarily associated with recently published results of the Antihypertensive and Lipid-Lowering Treatment to Prevent Heart Attack Trial (ALLHAT), suggesting that diuretics are as or more effective than other single drug therapies in the treatment of hypertension.

Former stages 2 and 3 hypertension were combined as stage 2, including patients with blood pressure above 160/100 mm Hg. Multi-drug therapy is recommended for these patients, in which a diuretic is combined with an angiotensin-converting enzyme (ACE) inhibitor, a beta-blocker, or calcium channel blocker. Public health, community, and school programs were identified as opportunities to promote public awareness and encourage healthy lifestyle behaviors. "The JNC 7th endorses the American Public Health Association resolution that the food manufacturers and restaurants reduce sodium in the food supply by 50% during the next decade," the report stated.

Heart Attack (Myocardial Infarction)

A **heart attack** (or **myocardial infarction**) occurs when the blood supply to part of the heart muscle (myocardium) is severely reduced or stopped. This occurs when one of the coronary arteries that supplies blood to the heart muscle is blocked. The blockage is usually from the buildup of plaque (deposits of fat-like substances) due to atherosclerosis. The plaque can eventually tear or rupture, triggering a blood clot that blocks the artery and leads to a heart attack. Such an event is called a coronary thrombosis or coronary occlusion.

If the blood supply is cut off severely or for a long time, muscle cells suffer irreversible injury and die. Disability or death can result, depending on how much heart muscle is damaged.

A recent study indicates that having a large "pot belly" or "spare tire" around the middle is associated with an increased risk for atherosclerosis. Experts explain that in addition to the fat one can see bulging around the middle, there are also fat deposits deep within the abdomen tucked around abdominal organs. The presence of this fat further increases the risk of having high cholesterol and insulin resistance, a precursor to diabetes.

The most common symptom of a heart attack is chest pain (angina). This pain is often described as a feeling of crushing, pressure, fullness, heaviness, or aching in the center of the chest. These sensations may extend into the neck, the jaw, and down the left arm. Angina is often associated with excessive sweating, feelings of apprehension, nausea, shortness of breath, and weakness.

Some heart attacks are sudden and intense, but most heart attacks start slowly, with mild pain or discomfort. Often the people affected are not sure of what is happening and wait too long before getting help. Heart attack and stroke are life-and-death emergencies; every second counts.

The American Heart Association lists the following as warning signs of heart attack:

- Pressure, fullness, squeezing pain in the center of the chest that lasts 2 minutes or longer
- Pain that spreads to the shoulders, neck, or arms
- Dizziness, fainting, sweating, nausea, or shortness of breath

Today heart attack and stroke victims can benefit from new medications and treatments. Clot-busting drugs can stop some heart attacks and strokes in progress, reducing disability and saving lives. But to be effective, these drugs must be given relatively quickly after heart attack or stroke symptoms first appear. It is said that the average heart attack victim waits 3 hours after symptoms occur to seek help. Many times they try to ignore the symptoms or say "it's just indigestion." It is imperative to seek medical help immediately. Calling 911 is almost always the fastest way to get lifesaving treatment.

✓ PATHOLOGY CHECKPOINT

Following is a concise list of the pathology-related terms that you've seen in the chapter. Review this checklist to make sure that you are familiar with the meaning of each term before moving on to the next section.

Conditions and Symptoms

- ❏ aneurysm
- ❏ anginal
- ❏ angiocarditis
- ❏ angioma
- ❏ angiostenosis
- ❏ aortomalacia
- ❏ arrhythmia
- ❏ arteriosclerosis
- ❏ arteritis
- ❏ atheroma
- ❏ atherosclerosis
- ❏ bradycardia
- ❏ bruit
- ❏ cardiomegaly
- ❏ cardiomyopathy
- ❏ cardiopathy
- ❏ carditis
- ❏ claudication
- ❏ constriction
- ❏ coronary heart disease (CHD)
- ❏ cyanosis
- ❏ dysrhythmia
- ❏ embolism
- ❏ endocarditis
- ❏ fibrillation
- ❏ flutter

- ❏ heart failure (HF)
- ❏ hemangiectasis
- ❏ hemangioma
- ❏ hypertension
- ❏ hypotension
- ❏ infarction
- ❏ ischemia
- ❏ mitral stenosis
- ❏ murmur
- ❏ myocardial infarction (MI)
- ❏ myocarditis
- ❏ occlusion
- ❏ palpitation
- ❏ pericarditis
- ❏ phlebitis
- ❏ Raynaud's phenomenon
- ❏ rheumatic heart disease
- ❏ shock
- ❏ spider veins
- ❏ tachycardia
- ❏ telangiectasis
- ❏ thrombophlebitis
- ❏ thrombosis
- ❏ vasoconstrictive
- ❏ vasospasm
- ❏ varicose veins

Diagnosis and Treatment

- ❏ anastomosis
- ❏ angiocardiography
- ❏ artificial pacemaker
- ❏ auscultation
- ❏ cardiocentesis
- ❏ cardiometer
- ❏ cardiotonic
- ❏ catheterization
- ❏ coronary bypass
- ❏ echocardiography
- ❏ electrocardiograph
- ❏ electrocardiophonograph
- ❏ endarterectomy
- ❏ extracorporeal circulation
- ❏ heart-lung transplant
- ❏ heart transplant
- ❏ oximetry
- ❏ percutaneous transluminal coronary angioplasty
- ❏ phlebotomy
- ❏ sphygmomanometer
- ❏ stethoscope
- ❏ vasodilator
- ❏ venipuncture

DRUG HIGHLIGHTS

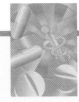

Drugs that are generally used for cardiovascular diseases and disorders include digitalis preparations, antiarrhythmic agents, vasopressors, vasodilators, antihypertensive agents, antihyperlipidemic, antiplatelet drugs, and thrombolytic agents.

Digitalis Drugs

Strengthen the heart muscle, increase the force and velocity of myocardial systolic contraction, slow the heart rate, and decrease conduction velocity through the atrioventricular (AV) node. These drugs are used in the treatment of congestive heart failure, atrial fibrillation, atrial flutter, and paroxysmal atrial tachycardia. With the administration of digitalis, toxicity may occur. The most common early symptoms of digitalis toxicity are anorexia, nausea, vomiting, and arrhythmias.

Examples: Crystodigin (digitoxin), Lanoxin (digoxin), and Digitaline (digitoxin).

Antiarrhythmic Agents

Used in the treatment of cardiac arrhythmias.

Examples: Tambocor (flecainide acetate), Tonocard (tocainide HCl), Inderal (propranolol HCl), and Calan (verapamil).

Vasopressors

Cause contraction of the muscles associated with capillaries and arteries, thereby narrowing the space through which the blood circulates. This narrowing results in an elevation of blood pressure. Vasopressors are useful in the treatment of patients suffering from shock.

Examples: Intropin (dopamine HCl), Aramine (metaraminol bitartrate), and Levophed Bitartrate (norepinephrine).

Vasodilators

Cause relaxation of blood vessels and lower blood pressure. Coronary vasodilators are used for the treatment of angina pectoris.

Examples: Sorbitrate (isosorbide dinitrate), nitroglycerin, amyl nitrate, and Peritrate (pentaerythritol tetranitrate).

Antihypertensive Agents

Used in the treatment of hypertension.

Examples: Catapres (clonidine HCl), Aldomet (methyldopa), Lopressor (metoprolol tartrate), and Capoten (captopril).

Antihyperlipidemic Agents

Used to lower abnormally high blood levels of fatty substances (lipids) when other treatment regimens fail.

Examples: Nicolar or Nicobid (niacin), Mevacor (lovastatin), Lopid (gemfibrozil), Lipitor (atorvastatin calcium), Pravachol (pravastatin), and Zocor (simvastatin).

Antiplatelet Drugs

Help reduce the occurrence of and death from vascular events such as heart attacks and strokes. *Aspirin* is considered to be the reference standard antiplatelet drug and is recommended by the American Heart Association for use in patients with a wide range of cardiovascular disease. Aspirin helps keep platelets from sticking together to form clots. *Plavix (clopidogrel)* is approved by the Food and Drug Administration for many of the same indications as aspirin. It is recommended for patients for whom aspirin fails to achieve a therapeutic benefit.

Thrombolytic Agents

Act to dissolve an existing thrombus when administered soon after its occurrence. They are often referred to as **tissue plasminogen activators** (tPA, TPA) and may reduce the chance of dying after a myocardial infarction by 50 percent. Unless contraindicated, the drug should be administered within 6 hours of the onset of chest pain. In some hospitals the time period for administering thrombolytic agents has been extended to 12 and 24 hours. These agents dissolve the clot, reopen the artery, restore blood flow to the heart, and prevent further damage to the myocardium. Bleeding is the most common complication encountered during thrombolytic therapy.

Examples: Kabikinase and Streptase (streptokinase), Eminase (anistreplase), Activase (alteplase), and Abbokinase (urokinase).

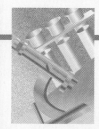

DIAGNOSTIC & LAB TESTS

TEST	DESCRIPTION
angiogram (ăn′ jē-ō-grăm)	A test used to determine the size and shape of arteries and veins of organs and tissues. A radiopaque substance is injected into the blood vessel, and x-rays are taken.
angiography (ăn″ jē-ŏg′ ră-fē)	The x-ray recording of a blood vessel after the injection of a radiopaque substance. Used to determine the condition of the blood vessels, organ, or tissue being studied. Types: aortic, cardiac, cerebral, coronary, digital subtraction (use of a computer technique), peripheral, pulmonary, selective, and vertebral.
cardiac catheterization (kăr′ dĭ-ăk kăth″ ĕ-tĕr-ĭ-zā′ shŭn)	A test used in diagnosis of heart disorders. A tiny catheter is inserted into an artery in the arm or leg of the patient and is fed through this artery to the heart. Dye is then pumped through the catheter, enabling the physician to locate by x-ray any blockages in the arteries supplying the heart. See Figure 7–31.
cardiac enzymes (kar′ dĭ-ăk ĕn′-zīmz)	Blood tests performed to determine cardiac damage in an acute myocardial infarction.
alanine aminotransferase (ALT)	Levels begin to rise 6 to 10 hours after an MI and peak at 24 to 48 hours.
aspartate aminotransferase (AST)	Levels begin to rise 6 to 10 hours after an MI and peak at 24 to 48 hours.
creatine phosphokinase (CPK)	Used to detect area of damage.
creatine kinase (CK)	Level may be 5 to 8 times normal.
creatine kinase isoenzymes	Used to indicate area of damage; CK-MB heart muscle, CK-MM skeletal muscle, and CK-BB brain.
cholesterol (kōl-lĕs′ tĕr-ŏl)	A blood test to determine the level of cholesterol in the serum. Elevated levels may indicate an increased risk of coronary heart disease. Any level greater than 200 mg/dL is considered too high for good heart health.
electrophysiology (ē-lĕk″ trō-fĭz″ ĭ-ŏl′ ō-jē)	A cardiac procedure that maps the electrical activity of the heart from within the heart itself.
Holter monitor (hōlt ər mŏn′ ĭ-tər)	A method of recording a patient's ECG for 24 hours. The device is portable and small enough to be worn by the patient during normal activity.

TEST	DESCRIPTION
lactic dehydrogenase (LDH) (lăk′ tĭk dē-hĭ-drŏj′ ĕ-nās)	Increased 6 to 12 hours after cardiac injury.
stress test (strĕs tĕst)	A method of evaluating cardiovascular fitness. The ECG is monitored while the patient is subjected to increasing levels of work. A treadmill or ergometer is used for this test.
triglycerides (trī-glĭs′ ĕr-īds)	A blood test to determine the level of triglycerides in the serum. Elevated levels (greater than 200 mg/dL) may indicate an increased risk of coronary heart disease and diabetes mellitus.
ultrasonography (ŭl-tră-sŏn-ŏg′ ră-fē)	A test used to visualize an organ or tissue by using high-frequency sound waves. It may be used as a screening test or as a diagnostic tool to determine abnormalities of the aorta, arteries and veins, and the heart.
ultrafast CT scan	Has begun to be used in the past few years to diagnose heart disease. Ultrafast CT can take multiple images of the heart within the time of a single heartbeat, thus providing much more detail about the heart's function and structures, while also greatly decreasing the amount of time required for a study. Ultrafast CT can detect very small amounts of calcium within the heart and the coronary arteries. This calcium has been shown to indicate that lesions which may eventually block off one or more coronary arteries and cause chest pain or even a heart attack are in the beginning stages of formation. Thus, ultrafast CT scanning is being used by many physicians as a means to diagnose early coronary artery disease in certain people, especially persons who have no symptoms of the disease.

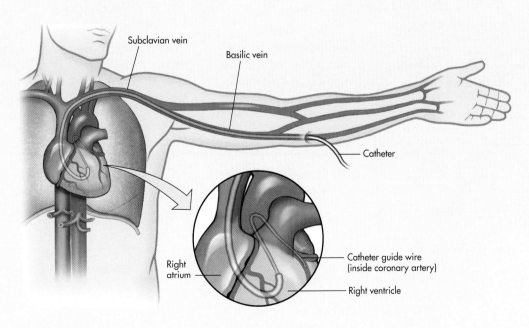

FIGURE 7–31

Cardiac catheterization.

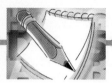

ABBREVIATIONS

ABBREVIATION	MEANING	ABBREVIATION	MEANING
ACG	angiocardiography	Hgb	hemoglobin
AI	aortic insufficiency	H&L	heart and lungs
AMI	acute myocardial infarction	IHSS	idiopathic hypertrophic subaortic stenosis
AS	aortic stenosis		
ASD	atrial septal defect	JNC	Joint National Committee
ASH	asymmetrical septal hypertrophy	LA	left atrium
		LBBB	left bundle branch block
ASHD	arteriosclerotic heart disease	LD	lactic dehydrogenase
AST	aspartate aminotransferase	LDL	low-density lipoprotein
A-V, AV	atrioventricular; arteriovenous	LEDs	light-emitting diodes
BBB	bundle branch block	LV	left ventricle
BP	blood pressure	MI	myocardial infarction
CABG	coronary artery bypass graft	MS	mitral stenosis
CAD	coronary artery disease	MVP	mitral valve prolapse
CC	cardiac catheterization	NHLBI	National Heart, Lung, and Blood Institute
CCU	coronary care unit		
CHD	coronary heart disease	NIH	National Institutes of Health
CHF	congestive heart failure	OHS	open heart surgery
CK	creatine kinase	PAT	paroxysmal atrial tachycardia
CO	cardiac output	PMI	point of maximal impulse
CPR	cardiopulmonary resuscitation	PTCA	percutaneous transluminal coronary angioplasty
CVP	central venous pressure		
DVT	deep vein thrombosis	PVC	premature ventricular contraction
ECC	extracorporeal circulation		
ECG	electrocardiogram	RA	right atrium
EKG	electrocardiogram	RV	right ventricle
FHS	fetal heart sound	S-A, SA	sinoatrial (node)
HBP	high blood pressure	SCD	sudden cardiac death
HDL	high-density lipoprotein	tPA, TPA	tissue plasminogen activator
HF	heart failure	VLDL	very-low-density lipoprotein
Hg	mercury	VSD	ventricular septal defect

STUDY AND REVIEW

Anatomy and Physiology

Write your answers to the following questions. Do not refer to the text.

1. The cardiovascular system includes:

   a. _____   b. _____

   c. _____   d. _____

2. Name the three layers of the heart.

   a. _____   b. _____

   c. _____

3. The heart weighs approximately _____ grams.

4. The _____ or upper chambers of the heart are separated by the

   _____ septum.

5. The _____ or lower chambers of the heart are separated by the

   _____ septum.

6. By listing each cardiovascular part in the proper order, trace the flow of blood through the heart, to the lungs, back to the heart, and on to the various body parts.

   a. _____   b. _____

   c. _____   d. _____

   e. _____   f. _____

   g. _____   h. _____

   i. _____   j. _____

   k. _____   l. _____

   m. _____   n. _____

7. The _____ _____ _____ controls the heartbeat.

8. The _____ _____ is called the pacemaker of the heart.

9. The _____ _____ includes the bundle of His and the peripheral fibers.

10. Name the three primary pulse points and state their locations on the body.

a. _____   located _____

b. _____   located _____

c. _____   located _____

11. Define the following terms:

a. Blood pressure _____

b. Pulse pressure _____

12. The average adult heart is about the size of a _____ and normally

beats at a pulse rate of _____ to _____ beats per minute.

13. The average adult usually has a systolic pressure between _____ and

_____ mm Hg and a diastolic pressure between _____ and

_____ mm Hg.

14. Give the purpose and function of arteries. _____

_____

15. Give the purpose and function of veins. _____

_____

Word Parts

1. In the spaces provided, write the definition of these prefixes, roots, combining forms, and suffixes. Do not refer to the listing of medical words. Leave blank those words you cannot define.

2. After completing as many as you can, refer to the medical word listings to check your work. For each word missed or left blank, write the word and its definition several times on the margins of these pages or on a separate sheet of paper.

3. To maximize the learning process, it is to your advantage to do the following exercises as directed. To refer to the word building section before completing these exercises invalidates the learning process.

PREFIXES

Give the definitions of the following prefixes:

1. a- _____   2. bi- _____

3. brady- _____   4. con- _____

5. end- _____   6. endo- _____

7. extra- _____

8. hyper- _____

9. hypo- _____

10. peri- _____

11. dys- _____

12. semi- _____

13. tachy- _____

14. tri- _____

ROOTS AND COMBINING FORMS

Give the definitions of the following roots and combining forms:

1. ang/i _____

2. angin _____

3. angi/o _____

4. anastom _____

5. aort/o _____

6. arter _____

7. arter/i _____

8. arteri/o _____

9. ather _____

10. ather/o _____

11. atri _____

12. atri/o _____

13. card _____

14. card/i _____

15. cardi/o _____

16. cyan _____

17. auscultat _____

18. dilat _____

19. electr/o _____

20. embol _____

21. glyc _____

22. hem _____

23. isch _____

24. chol/e _____

25. log _____

26. lun _____

27. man/o _____

28. mitr _____

29. my/o _____

30. circulat _____

31. oxy _____

32. phleb _____

33. phleb/o _____

34. phon/o _____

35. pulmonar _____

36. rrhythm _____

37. scler _____

38. sin/o _____

39. sphygm/o _____

40. sten _____

41. steth/o _____

42. strict _____

43. claudicat _____

44. tens _____

45. thromb _____

46. diast _____

47. vascul _____

48. vas/o _____

49. ech/o _____

50. ven/i _____

51. corpor/e _____

52. ventricul _____

53. fibrillat _____

54. hem/o _____

55. dynam _____

56. infarct _____

57. lip/o _____

58. prot/e _____

59. occlus _____

60. ox/i _____

61. palpitat _____

62. sept _____

63. syst _____

64. tel _____

65. thromb/o _____

66. sterol _____

SUFFIXES

Give the definitions of the following suffixes:

1. -ac _____

2. -al _____

3. -ar _____

4. -blast _____

5. -centesis _____

6. -ole _____

7. -cuspid _____

8. -metry _____

9. -ectasis _____

10. -ectomy _____

11. -emia _____

12. -er _____

13. -gen _____

14. -in _____

15. -graph _____

16. -graphy _____

17. -ia _____

18. -ic _____

19. -ide _____

20. -ion _____

21. -ism _____

22. -ist _____

23. -itis _____

24. -ive _____

25. -logy _____

26. -malacia _____

27. -megaly _____

28. -meter _____

29. -oma _____

30. -or _____

31. -osis _____

32. -pathy _____

33. -plasty _____

34. -puncture _____

35. -scope _____

36. -spasm _____

37. -tomy _____

38. -um _____

39. -y _____

Identifying Medical Terms

In the spaces provided, write the medical terms for the following meanings:

1. _____ A tumor of a blood vessel

2. _____ The germ cell from which blood vessels develop

3. _____ Surgical repair of a blood vessel or vessels

4. _____ A condition of narrowing of a blood vessel

5. _____ Incision into an artery

6. _____ Inflammation of an artery

7. _____ Having two points or cusps; pertaining to the mitral valve

8. _____ One who specializes in the study of the heart

9. _____ Enlargement of the heart

10. _____ Pertaining to the heart and lungs

11. _____ The process of drawing together as in the narrowing of a vessel

12. _____ A condition in which a blood clot obstructs a blood vessel

13. _____ Inflammation of a vein

14. _____ A fast heartbeat

15. _____ A widening of a blood vessel

Spelling

In the spaces provided, write the correct spelling of these misspelled terms:

1. astomosis _____

2. athrosclerosis _____

3. atriventrcular _____

4. endcarditis _____

5. extracoporal _____

6. iscemia _____

7. mycardial _____

8. oyxgen _____

9. phelebitis _____

10. palpitaiton _____

Matching

Select the appropriate lettered meaning for each word listed below.

_____ 1. cholesterol

_____ 2. claudication

_____ 3. dysrhythmia

_____ 4. diastole

_____ 5. fibrillation

_____ 6. lipoprotein

_____ 7. lubb-dupp

_____ 8. palpitation

_____ 9. percutaneous transluminal coronary angioplasty

_____ 10. systole

a. The two separate heart sounds that can be heard with the use of a stethocope
b. Quivering of muscle fiber
c. Fat and protein molecules that are bound together
d. A waxy, fat-like substance in the bloodstream of all animals
e. The process of lameness, limping
f. An abnormal, difficult, or bad rhythm
g. The relaxation phase of the heart cycle
h. The contraction phase of the heart cycle
i. Rapid throbbing or fluttering of the heart
j. The use of a balloon-tipped catheter to compress fatty plaques against an artery wall
k. The process of being closed

Abbreviations

Place the correct word, phrase, or abbreviation in the space provided.

1. acute myocardial infarction _____

2. atrioventricular _____

3. BP _____

4. CAD _____

5. cardiac catheterization _____

6. ECG, EKG _____

7. HDL _____

8. heart and lungs _____

9. MI _____

10. tPA, TPA _____

Diagnostic and Laboratory Tests

Select the best answer to each multiple choice question. Circle the letter of your choice.

1. _____ is a cardiac procedure that maps the electrical activity of the heart from within the heart itself.
   a. electrocardiogram
   b. electrocardiomyogram
   c. electrophysiology
   d. cardiac catheterization

2. Blood tests performed to determine cardiac damage in an acute myocardial infarction.
   a. cardiac enzymes
   b. cholesterol
   c. triglycerides
   d. angiogram

3. A method of recording a patient's ECG for 24 hours.
   a. stress test
   b. Holter monitor
   c. ultrasonography
   d. angiography

4. A test used to determine the size and shape of arteries and veins of organs and tissues.
   a. electrophysiology
   b. stress test
   c. angiogram
   d. cholesterol

5. The x-ray recording of a blood vessel after the injection of a radiopaque substance.
   a. angiogram
   b. angiography
   c. stress test
   d. cardiac catheterization

CASE STUDY

ANGINA PECTORIS

Read the following case study and then answer the questions that follow.

A 45-year-old male was seen by a cardiologist; the following is a synopsis of his visit.

Present History: The patient states that during a workout session he felt tightness in his chest, became short of breath, and felt very apprehensive. He states that this uncomfortable sensation went away after he stopped exercising.

Signs and Symptoms: Tightness in his chest, dyspnea, apprehension.

Diagnosis: Angina pectoris. Diagnosis was determined by a complete physical examination, an electrocardiogram, and blood enzyme studies.

Treatment: Nitroglycerin sublingual tablets 0.4 mg as needed for chest pain. The patient is instructed to seek medical attention without delay if the pain is not relieved by three tablets, taken one every 5 minutes over a 15-minute period.

Prevention: Teach the patient to avoid situations that precipitate angina attacks. Proper rest and diet, stress management, lifestyle changes, avoidance of alcohol and tobacco are recommended.

CASE STUDY QUESTIONS

1. Signs and symptoms of angina pectoris include tightness in the chest, _____ (shortness of breath), and apprehension.

2. The diagnosis of angina pectoris was determined by a complete physical examination, an _____ _____, and blood enzyme studies.

3. The medication regimen prescribed included _____ 0.4 mg as needed for chest pain.

4. If the patient follows the recommended medication regimen and it does not relieve the pain, he should _____.

MedMedia Wrap-Up

www.prenhall.com/rice

Audio Glossary
Medical Terminology Exercises & Activities
Pathology Spotlight
Terminology Translator
Animations
Videos

Additional interactive resources and activities for this chapter can be found on the Companion Website. For animations, videos, audio glossary, and review, access the accompanying CD-ROM in this book.

Objectives
Medical Terminology Exercises & Activities
Audio Glossary
Drug Updates
Medical Terminology in the News

BLOOD AND THE LYMPHATIC SYSTEM

8

OBJECTIVES

On completion of this chapter, you will be able to:

- Describe the blood.
- Describe the formed elements in blood.
- Name the four blood types.
- Describe and state the functions of the lymphatic system.
- Describe the accessory organs of the lymphatic system.
- Describe the immune system/response.
- Analyze, build, spell, and pronounce medical words.
- Describe each of the conditions presented in the Pathology Spotlights.
- Complete the Pathology Checkpoint.
- Review Drug Highlights presented in this chapter.
- Provide the description of diagnostic and laboratory tests related to blood and the lymphatic system.
- Identify and define selected abbreviations.
- Successfully complete the study and review section.

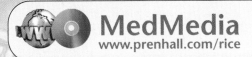

MedMedia
www.prenhall.com/rice

Additional interactive resources and activities for this chapter can be found on the Companion Website. For Terminology Translator, animations, videos, audio glossary, and review, access the accompanying CD-ROM in this book.

Anatomy and Physiology Overview

Blood and lymph are two of the body's main fluids and are circulated through two separate but interconnected vessel systems. **Blood** is circulated by the action of the heart, through the circulatory system consisting largely of arteries, veins, and capillaries. **Lymph** does not actually circulate. It is propelled in one direction, away from its source, through increasingly larger lymph vessels, to drain into large veins of the circulatory system located in the neck region. Numerous valves within the lymph vessels permit one-directional flow, opening and closing as a consequence of pressure caused by the massaging action of muscles on the vessels and the fluid they contain. The various organs and components of blood and the lymphatic system are described in this chapter.

BLOOD

Blood is a fluid consisting of formed elements and plasma, both of which are continuously produced by the body for the purpose of transporting respiratory gases (*oxygen and carbon dioxide*), chemical substances (*foods, salts, hormones*), and cells that act to protect the body from foreign substances. The blood volume within an individual depends on body weight. An individual weighing 154 lb (70 kg) has a blood volume of about 5 qt or 5 L.

Formed Elements

The formed elements in blood are the red blood cells or **erythrocytes**, **platelets** or **thrombocytes**, and white blood cells or **leukocytes**. Formed elements constitute about 45 percent of the total volume of blood and are sometimes referred to as whole blood (Table 8–1).

BLOOD AND THE LYMPHATIC SYSTEM

Organ/Structure	Primary Functions
Blood	Fluid consisting of formed elements and plasma that transport respiratory gases (oxygen and carbon dioxide), chemical substances (foods, salts, hormones), and cells that act to protect the body from foreign substances
Lymphatic System	A vessel system composed of lymphatic capillaries, lymphatic vessels, lymphatic ducts, and lymph nodes that convey lymph from the tissue to the blood. The three main functions of the lymphatic system are: 1. It transports proteins and fluids, lost by capillary seepage, back to the bloodstream 2. It protects the body against pathogens by phagocytosis and immune response 3. It serves as a pathway for the absorption of fats from the small intestines into the bloodstream
Spleen	Major site of erythrocyte destruction; serves as a reservoir for blood; acts as a filter, removing microorganisms from the blood
Tonsils	Filter bacteria and aid in the formation of white blood cells
Thymus	Essential role in the formation of antibodies and the development of the immune response in the newborn; manufactures infection-fighting T cells and helps distinguish normal T cells from those that attack the body's own tissue

TABLE 8–1 TYPES OF BLOOD CELLS AND FUNCTIONS

Blood Cell	Function
Erythrocyte (red blood cell)	Transports oxygen and carbon dioxide
Thrombocyte (platelet)	Blood clotting
Leukocyte (white blood cell)	Body's main defense against invasion of pathogens
Types of leukocytes	
Neutrophil	Protection against infection, phagocytosis
Eosinophil	Destroys parasitic organisms, plays a key role in allergic reactions
Basophil	Key role in releasing histamine and other chemicals that act on blood vessels, essential to nonspecific immune response to inflammation
Monocyte	One of the first lines of defense in the inflammatory process, phagocytosis
Lymphocyte	Provides the body with immune capacity
B lymphocyte	Identifies foreign antigens and differentiates into antibody-producing plasma cells (source for immunoglobulins–antibodies)
T lymphocyte	Essential for the specific immune response of the body

ERYTHROCYTES

Erythrocytes are doughnut-shaped cells without nuclei. They transport oxygen (most of which is bound to hemoglobin contained in the cell) and carbon dioxide. There are approximately 5 million erythrocytes per cubic millimeter, and they have a life span of 80 to 120 days. Erythrocytes are formed in the red bone marrow and are commonly called red blood cells (Fig. 8–1).

Thrombocytes

Thrombocytes are disk-shaped cells about half the size of erythrocytes. They play an important role in the clotting process by releasing *thrombokinase*, which, in the presence of calcium, reacts with *prothrombin* to form *thrombin*. There are approximately

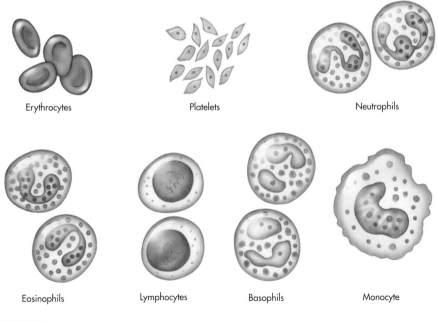

Erythrocytes   Platelets   Neutrophils

Eosinophils   Lymphocytes   Basophils   Monocyte

FIGURE 8–1

The formed elements of blood: erythrocytes, leukocytes (neutrophils, eosinophils, basophils, lymphocytes, and monocytes), and thrombocytes (platelets).

200,000 to 500,000 thrombocytes per cubic millimeter. Thrombocytes are fragments of certain giant cells called megakaryocytes, which are formed in the red bone marrow. Thrombocytes are commonly called **platelets** (Fig. 8–1).

Leukocytes

Leukocytes are sphere-shaped cells containing nuclei of varying shapes and sizes. Leukocytes are the body's main defense against the invasion of **pathogens**. At the time pathogens enter the tissue, the leukocytes leave the blood vessels through their walls and move in an amoeba-like motion to the area of infection, where they perform **phagocytosis**. There are approximately 8000 leukocytes per cubic millimeter. There are five types of leukocytes: **neutrophils**, **eosinophils**, **basophils**, **lymphocytes**, and **monocytes**.

Except for the lymphocytes, leukocytes are formed in the red bone marrow. Lymphocytes are formed in lymph nodes and other lymphoid tissue. Leukocytes are commonly called **white blood cells** (Fig. 8–1).

Blood Grouping

There are a number of human blood systems which are determined by a series of two or more genes closely linked on a single autosomal chromosome. The ABO system which was discovered in 1901 by Karl Landsteiner is of great significance in blood typing and blood transfusion. The four blood types identified in this system are types A, B, AB, and O. The differences in human blood are due to the presence or absence of certain protein molecules called antigens and antibodies. The antigens are located on the surface of the red blood cells and the antibodies are in the blood plasma. Individuals have different types and combinations of these molecules. Individuals in the A group have the A antigen on the surface of their red blood cells and anti-B antibody in the blood plasma; B group has the B antigen and the anti-A antibody; AB group has both A and B antigens and no anti-A or anti-B antibodies; and group O has neither A or B antigens and both anti-A and anti-B antibodies. Type AB blood group is known as the universal recipient and type O as the universal donor. See Table 8–2 and Figure 8–2.

Rh Factor

The presence of a substance called an **agglutinogen** in the red blood cells is responsible for what is known as the **Rh factor**. It was first discovered in the blood of the rhesus monkey from which the factor gets its name. About 85 percent of the population have the Rh factor and are called Rh positive. The other 15 percent lack the Rh factor and are designated Rh negative. There are more than 20 genetically determined blood group systems known today, but the ABO and Rh systems are the most important ones used for blood transfusions. Not all blood groups are compatible with each

TABLE 8–2 BLOOD GROUPS

Type	Antigen	Plasma Antibody	Percentage/Population
A	A	Anti-B	41
B	B	Anti-A	10
AB	Both A and B	No anti-A or anti-B	4
O	No A and B	Both anti-A and anti-B	45

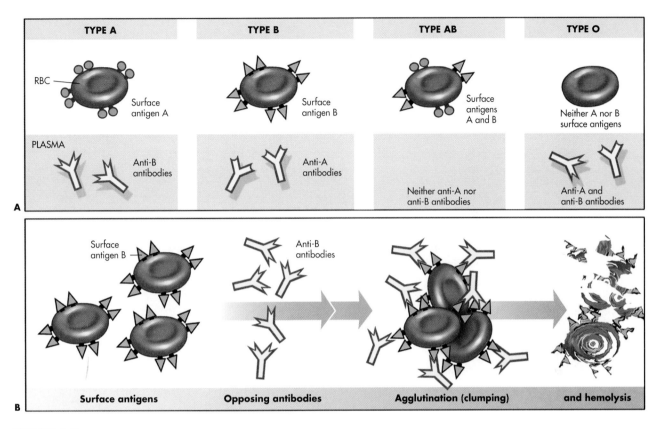

FIGURE 8–2

Blood-typing and cross-reactions: the blood type depends on the presence of surface antigens (agglutinogens) on RBC surfaces. (A) The plasma antibodies (agglutinins) that will react with foreign surface antigens. (B) In a cross-reaction, antibodies that encounter their target antigens lead to agglutination and hemolysis of the affected RBCs.

other. Mixing incompatible blood groups leads to blood clumping or agglutination, which is dangerous for individuals.

If an individual with Rh− blood receives a transfusion of Rh+ blood, it causes the formation of anti-Rh agglutinin. Subsequent transfusions of Rh+ blood may result in serious transfusion reactions (agglutination and hemolysis of red blood cells). A pregnant woman who is Rh− may become sensitized by blood of an Rh+ fetus. Sensitization can also occur if an Rh-negative woman has had a previous miscarriage, induced abortion, or ectopic pregnancy. There is also a slight chance that a woman may develop antibodies after having amniocentesis done later in pregnancy. These are all cases in which fetal blood (that might be Rh positive) could mix with maternal blood, resulting in the production of antibodies that could complicate a subsequent pregnancy. In subsequent pregnancies, if the fetus is Rh+, Rh antibodies produced in maternal blood may cross the placenta and destroy fetal cells, producing hemolytic disease of the newborn (HDN). See Figure 8–3. Today, hemolytic disease can for the most part be prevented if the Rh-negative woman has not already made antibodies against the Rh factor from an earlier pregnancy or blood transfusion. Rh immunoglobulin (Rhogam) is a product that can safely prevent sensitization of an Rh-negative mother. It suppresses her ability to respond to Rh-positive red cells. With its use, sensitization can be prevented almost all the time, although Rhogam is not helpful if the mother is already sensitized.

For a blood transfusion to be successful, ABO and Rh blood groups must be compatible between the donor and the recipient. If they are not, the red blood cells from

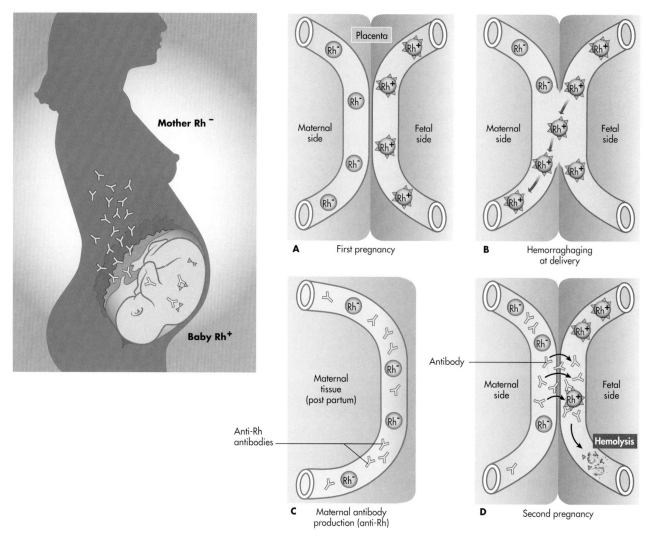

FIGURE 8–3

Rh factors and pregnancy: when an Rh-negative woman has her first Rh-positive child, fetal and maternal blood mix at delivery when the placenta breaks down. The appearance of Rh-positive blood cells in the maternal bloodstream sensitizes the mother, stimulating the production of anti-Rh antibodies. If another pregnancy occurs with an Rh-positive fetus, maternal anti-Rh antibodies can cross the placenta and attack fetal blood cells, producing hemolytic disease of the newborn (HDN).

the donated blood can clump or agglutinate and cause clogging of blood vessels and slow and/or stop the circulation of blood to various parts of the body. The agglutinated red blood cells may also hemolyze and their contents leak out in the body. The red blood cells contain hemoglobin which becomes toxic when outside the red blood cell, and this could lead to fatal consequences for the recipient.

Plasma

The fluid part of the blood is called **plasma**. It comprises about 55 percent of the total volume of blood, is clear and somewhat straw-colored, and is composed of water (91 percent) and chemical compounds (9 percent). Plasma is the medium for circulation of blood cells, it provides nutritive substances to various body structures, and it removes waste products of metabolism from body structures. There are four major plasma proteins: **albumin**, **globulin**, **fibrinogen**, and **prothrombin**.

THE LYMPHATIC SYSTEM

The **lymphatic system** is a vessel system apart from, but connected to, the circulatory system. The lymphatic system returns fluids from tissue spaces to the bloodstream. The lymphatic system is composed of *lymphatic capillaries, lymphatic vessels, lymphatic ducts,* and *lymph nodes.* The system conveys lymph from the tissues to the blood. Lymph is a clear, colorless, alkaline fluid that is about 95 percent water. The principal component of lymph is fluid from plasma that has seeped out of capillary walls into spaces among the body tissues. Lymph contains white blood cells, particularly lymphocytes. Figure

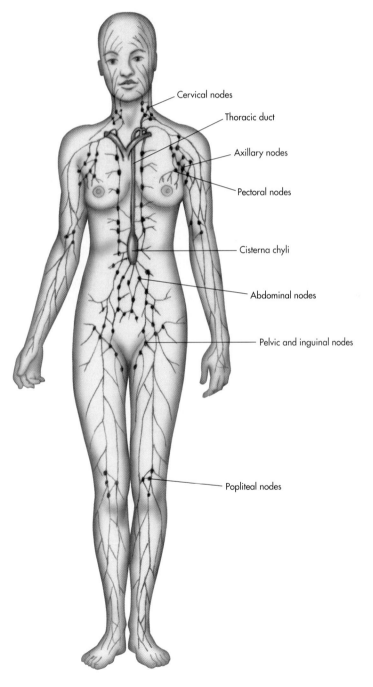

FIGURE 8–4

The lymphatic system.

8–4 shows the major lymphatics of the body. The three main functions of the lymphatic system are:

1. It transports proteins and fluids, lost by capillary seepage, back to the bloodstream.
2. It protects the body against pathogens by phagocytosis and immune response.
3. It serves as the pathway for the absorption of fats from the small intestines into the bloodstream.

ACCESSORY ORGANS

The **spleen**, the **tonsils**, and the **thymus** are not actually part of the lymphatic system; however, they are closely related to it in their functions. See Figure 8–5.

The Spleen

The **spleen** is a soft, dark red oval body lying in the upper left quadrant of the abdomen. The spleen is the major site of erythrocyte destruction. It serves as a reservoir for blood. The spleen plays an essential role in the immune response and acts as a filter, removing microorganisms from the blood.

The Tonsils

The **tonsils** are lymphoid masses located in depressions of the mucous membranes of the face and pharynx. They consist of the *palatine tonsil*, *pharyngeal tonsil* (adenoid), and the *lingual tonsil*. The tonsils filter bacteria and aid in the formation of white blood cells. See Figure 8–6.

The Thymus

The **thymus** is considered one of the endocrine glands, but because of its function and appearance, it is a part of the lymphoid system. It is located in the mediastinal cavity. The thymus plays an essential role in the formation of antibodies and the development of the immune response in the newborn. It manufactures infection-fighting **T cells** and helps distinguish normal T cells from those that attack the body's own tissue. T cells are important in the body's cellular immune response.

THE IMMUNE SYSTEM/RESPONSE

All of us live in a virtual "sea" of microorganisms, organisms so tiny that they cannot be seen with the naked eye. Many of these organisms are not harmful to humans, while others are **pathogenic**, capable of causing disease. Each day our bodies are faced with microorganisms, potentially harmful toxins in the environment, and even some of our own cells that may change into cancer. Fortunately, the average, healthy human body is equipped with natural defenses that assist the body in fighting off disease and cancer. These natural defenses are intact skin, the cleansing action of the body's secretions (such as tears, mucus), white blood cells, body chemicals (such as hormones, enzymes), and antibodies. As long as the immune system is intact and functioning properly, it can defend the body against invading foreign substances and cancer.

The **immune system** consists of the tissues, organs, and physiologic processes used by the body to identify abnormal cells, foreign substances, and foreign tissue cells that

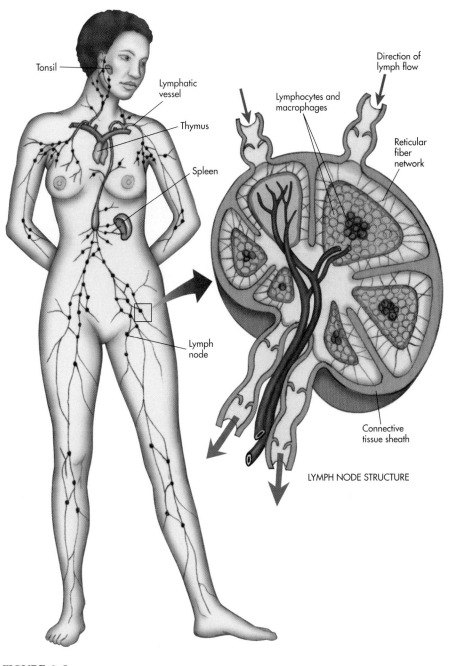

FIGURE 8–5

The tonsils, lymph nodes, thymus, spleen, and lymphatic vessels with an expanded view of a lymph node.

may have been transplanted into the body. Many of these tissues and organs are part of the lymphatic system.

THE IMMUNE RESPONSE

The **immune response** is the reaction of the body to foreign substances and the means by which it protects the body. The following is an overview of this response.

The immune response may be described as humoral immunity or antibody-mediated immunity, and cellular immunity or cell-mediated immunity.

Humoral (pertaining to body fluids or substances contained in them) **immunity** or **antibody-mediated immunity** involves the production of plasma lymphocytes (B cells)

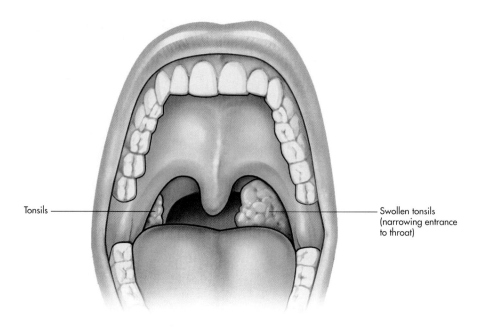

Tonsils

Swollen tonsils (narrowing entrance to throat)

FIGURE 8–6

Tonsils—normal and enlarged.

in response to antigen exposure with subsequent formation of antibodies. **Antibodies** are protein substances that are developed in response to a specific antigen. An **antigen** is a substance such as bacteria, toxins, or certain allergens that induces the formation of antibodies. Humoral immunity is a major defense against bacterial infections.

Cellular immunity or **cell-mediated immunity** involves the production of lymphocytes (T cells) that responds to any form of injury and NK (natural killer) cells that attack foreign cells, normal cells infected with viruses, and cancer cells. Cellular immunity constitutes a major defense against infections caused by viruses, fungi, and a few bacteria, such as the tubercle bacillus that causes tuberculosis. It also helps defend against the formation of tumors, especially cancer.

There are four general phases associated with the body's immune response to a foreign substance and these are:

1. The first phase is the recognition of the foreign substance or the invader (enemy).
2. Activation of the body's defenses by producing more white blood cells that are designed to seek and destroy the invader(s), especially the macrophages that eat and engulf the foreign substances and lymphocytes, B cells, and T cells (see Table 8–3), constitutes the second phase.

T cells of the helper type identify the enemy and rush to the spleen and lymph nodes, where they stimulate the production of other cells to aid in the fight of the foreign substance.

TABLE 8–3 SUMMARY OF FUNCTIONS OF LYMPHOCYTES

Type of Cell	Functions
T cells (thymus-dependent)	Cellular immunity
B cells (bone marrow-derived)	Humoral immunity
NK cells (natural killers)	Attack foreign cells, normal cells infected with viruses, and cancer cells

T cells of the natural killer (NK) type are large granular lymphocytes that also specialize in killing cells of the body that have been invaded by foreign substances and fighting cells that have turned cancerous.

The B cells reside in the spleen or lymph nodes and produce antibodies for specific antigens.

3. During the attack phase, the above defenders of the body produce antibodies and/or seek out to kill and/or remove the foreign invader. This is done by phagocytosis, where the macrophages squeeze out between the cells in the capillaries and crawl into the tissue to the site of the infection. Here they surround and eat the foreign substances that caused the infection. Other white blood cells respond to infection by producing antibodies. Antibodies are released into the bloodstream and carried to the site of the infection, where they surround and immobilize the invaders. Later, both antibody and invader may be eaten by the phagocytes.

4. In the slowdown phase, the number of defenders returns to normal, following victory over the foreign invader.

LIFE SPAN CONSIDERATIONS

■ THE CHILD

In the embryo, plasma and blood cells are formed about the 2nd week of life. At approximately the 5th week of development, blood formation occurs in the liver and later in the spleen, thymus, lymphatic system, and bone marrow. At 12 weeks the fetus is 11.5 cm (4.5 inches) from crown to head and weighs 45 g (1.6 oz). The fetal **liver** is the chief producer of red blood cells, and **bile** is secreted by the gallbladder. At 16 weeks blood vessels are visible through the now-transparent skin. Fetal circulation provides oxygenation and nutrition to the fetus and disposes of carbon dioxide and other waste products.

The **thymus gland** plays an important role in the development of the immune response in the newborn. At birth, the average weight of the thymus is 10 to 15 g. It attains a weight of 40 g at puberty, after which it begins to undergo involution, with the thymus being replaced with adipose and connective tissue.

■ THE OLDER ADULT

With advancing age, lymphatic tissue shrinks, the bone marrow becomes less productive, and the walls of peripheral vessels stiffen. There is also loss of elasticity in the peripheral vessels, which causes increases in peripheral resistance, impairs the flow of blood, and results in an increase in the workload of the left ventricle. As a result of these changes in the peripheral vascular system, the transportation of oxygen and nutrients to the tissues and the removal of wastes from the tissues are affected adversely. The transportation of oxygen may also be compromised by the decrease of **hemoglobin** of some older adults.

Immune response declines with age, limiting the body's ability to identify and fight foreign substances such as bacteria and viruses. With aging there is loss of the thymus cortex, which leads to a reduced production of T lymphocytes, including T cells, natural killer cells, and B lymphocytes. Persons at the extremes of the life span are more likely to develop immune-response problems than those in their middle years. Frequency and severity of infections are generally increased in elderly persons because of a decreased ability of the immune system to respond adequately to invading microorganisms. The incidence of **autoimmune diseases** also increases with aging, most likely due to a decreased ability of antibodies to differentiate between self and nonself. Failure of the immune response system to recognize mutant, or abnormal, cells may be the reason for the high incidence of cancer associated with increasing age.

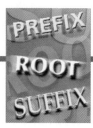

BUILDING YOUR MEDICAL VOCABULARY

This section provides the foundation for learning medical terminology. Medical words can be made up of four different types of word parts:

- Prefixes (P)
- Roots (R)
- Combining forms (CF)
- Suffixes (S)

By connecting various word parts in an organized sequence, thousands of words can be built and learned. In this text the word list is alphabetized so one can see the variety of meanings created when common prefixes and suffixes are repeatedly applied to certain word roots and/or combining forms. Words shown in pink are additional words related to the content of this chapter that are not built from word parts. These words are included to enhance your vocabulary. Note: an asterisk icon ✱ indicates words that are covered in the Pathology Spotlights section in this chapter.

MEDICAL WORD	WORD PARTS (WHEN APPLICABLE)			DEFINITION
	Part	**Type**	**Meaning**	
acquired immuno-deficiency syndrome (AIDS) (ă-kwīrd ĭm″ ū-nō dě-físh′ ěn-sē sĭn-drōm)				AIDS is a disease caused by the human immunodeficiency virus (HIV). This virus is transmitted through sexual contact, through exposure to infected blood or blood components, and perinatally from mother to infant. The HIV virus invades the T4 lymphocytes, and as the disease progresses the body's immune system becomes paralyzed. The patient becomes severely weakened, and potentially fatal infections can occur. *Pneumocystis carinii* pneumonia and Kaposi's sarcoma account for many of the deaths of AIDS patients. ✱ See Pathology Spotlight: AIDS.
agglutination (ă-gloo″ tĭ-nā′ shŭn)	agglutinat -ion	R S	clumping process	The process of clumping together, as of blood cells that are incompatible
albumin (ăl-bū′ mĭn)				One of a group of simple proteins found in blood plasma and serum
allergy (ăl′ ěr-jē)	all -ergy	R S	other work	Individual hypersensitivity to a substance that is usually harmless. ✱ See Figure 8–18 in Pathology Spotlight: Rhinitis.

MEDICAL WORD	WORD PARTS (WHEN APPLICABLE)			DEFINITION
	Part	**Type**	**Meaning**	
anaphylaxis (ăn″ ă-fĭ-lăk′ sĭs)	ana -phylaxis	P S	up protection	An unusual or exaggerated allergic reaction to foreign proteins or other substances. ✱ See Figure 8–19 in Pathology Spotlight: Anaphylaxis.
anemia (ă-nē′ mĭ-ă)	an -emia	P S	lack of blood condition	A condition of a lack of red blood cells. ✱ See Figures 8–20 and 8–21 in Pathology Spotlight: Anemia.
anisocytosis (ăn-ī″ sō-sī-tō′ sĭs)	anis/o cyt -osis	CF R S	unequal cell condition of	A condition in which the erythrocytes are unequal in size and shape
antibody (ăn′ tĭ-bŏd″ ē)	anti -body	P S	against body	A protein substance produced in the body in response to an invading foreign substance (*antigen*). ✱ See Pathology Spotlight: Antibody.
anticoagulant (ăn″ tĭ-kō-ăg′ ū-lănt)	anti coagul -ant	P R S	against clots forming	An agent that works against the formation of blood clots
antigen (ăn′ tĭ-jĕn)	anti -gen	P S	against formation, produce	An invading foreign substance that induces the formation of antibodies
autolmmune disease (aw″ tō-ĭm-mūn dĭ-zēz)				A condition in which the body's immune system becomes defective and produces antibodies against itself. Hemolytic anemia, rheumatoid arthritis, myasthenia gravis, and scleroderma are considered as autoimmune diseases.
autotransfusion (aw″ tō-trăns-fū′ zhŭn)	auto trans fus -ion	P P R S	self across to pour process	The process of reinfusing a patient's own blood. Methods used are: "harvesting" the blood 1 to 3 weeks before elective surgery; "salvaging" intraoperative blood; and collecting blood from trauma or selected surgical patients for reinfusion within 4 hours.
basocyte (bā′ sō-sīt)	bas/o -cyte	CF S	base cell	A base cell leukocyte
basophil (bā′ sō-fĭl)	bas/o -phil	CF S	base attraction	A cell that has an attraction for a base dye
blood (blŭd)				The fluid that circulates through the heart, arteries, veins, and capillaries

MEDICAL WORD	WORD PARTS (WHEN APPLICABLE)			DEFINITION
	Part	Type	Meaning	
coagulable (kō-ăg′ ū-lăb-l)	coagul -able	R S	to clot capable	Capable of forming a clot
corpuscle (kŏr′ pŭs-ĕl)				A blood cell
creatinemia (krē″ ă-tĭn-ē′ mĭ-ă)	creatin -emia	R S	flesh, creatine blood condition	A condition of excess creatine in the blood
embolus (ĕm′ bō-lŭs)				A blood clot carried in the bloodstream
eosinophil (ē″ ŏ-sĭn′ ō-fĭl)	eosin/o -phil	CF S	rose-colored attraction	A cell that stains readily with the acid stain; attraction for the rose-colored stain
erythroblast (ĕ-rĭth′ rō-blăst)	erythr/o -blast	CF S	red immature cell, germ cell	An immature red blood cell
erythrocyte (ĕ-rĭth′ rō-sīt)	erythr/o -cyte	CF S	red cell	A red blood cell
erythrocytosis (ĕ-rĭth″ rō-sī-tō′ sĭs)	erythr/o cyt -osis	CF R S	red cell condition of	An abnormal condition in which there is an increase in red blood cells
erythropoiesis (ĕ-rĭth″ rō-poy-ē′ sĭs)	erythr/o -poiesis	CF S	red formation	Formation of red blood cells
erythropoietin (ĕ-rĭth″ rō-poy′ ĕ′-tĭn)	erythr/o poiet -in	CF R S	red formation chemical	A hormone that stimulates the production of red blood cells
extravasation (ĕks-tră″ vă-sā′ shŭn)	extra vas(at) -ion	P R S	beyond vessel process	The process whereby fluids and/or medications (IVs) escape into surrounding tissue
fibrin (fī′ brĭn)	fibr -in	R S	fiber chemical	An insoluble protein formed from fibrinogen by the action of thrombin in the blood-clotting process
fibrinogen (fī-brĭn′ ō-gĕn)	fibrin/o -gen	CF S	fiber formation	A blood protein converted to fibrin by the action of thrombin in the blood-clotting process
globulin (glŏb′ ū-lĭn)	globul -in	R S	globe chemical	An albuminous protein found in body fluids and cells
granulocyte (grăn′ ū-lō-sīt″)	granul/o -cyte	CF S	little grain, granular cell	A granular leukocyte

MEDICAL WORD	WORD PARTS (WHEN APPLICABLE)			DEFINITION
	Part	**Type**	**Meaning**	
hematocrit (hē-măt′ ō-krĭt)	hemat/o -crit	CF S	blood to separate	A blood test that separates solids from plasma in the blood by centrifuging the blood sample
hematologist (hē″ mă-tŏl′ ō-jĭst)	hemat/o log -ist	CF R S	blood study of one who specializes	One who specializes in the study of the blood
hematology (hē″ mă-tŏl′ ō-jē)	hemat/o -logy	CF S	blood study of	The study of the blood
hematoma (hē″ mă-tō′ mă)	hemat -oma	R S	blood tumor	A blood tumor. See Figure 8–7.
hemochromatosis (hē″ mō-krō″ mă-tō′ sĭs)	hem/o chromat -osis	CF R S	blood color condition of	A disease condition in which iron is not metabolized properly and it accumulates in body tissues. The skin has a bronze hue, the liver becomes enlarged, and diabetes and cardiac failure may occur.
hemoglobin (hē″ mō-glō′ bĭn)	hem/o -globin	CF S	blood globe, protein	Blood protein; the iron-containing pigment of red blood cells
hemolysis (hē-mŏl′ ĭ-sĭs)	hem/o -lysis	CF S	blood destruction	Destruction of red blood cells
hemophilia (hē″ mō-fĭl′ ĭ-ă)	hem/o -philia	CF S	blood attraction	A hereditary blood disease characterized by prolonged coagulation and tendency to bleed
hemorrhage (hĕm′ ĕ-rĭj)	hem/o -rrhage	CF S	blood bursting forth	Excessive bleeding; bursting forth of blood. See Figure 8–8.
hemostasis (hē-mŏs′ tā-sĭs)	hem/o -stasis	CF S	blood control, stopping	The control or stopping of bleeding. See Figure 8–9.
heparin (hĕp′ ă-rĭn)				A substance found in the liver, lungs, and other body tissues that inhibits blood clotting
hypercalcemia (hī″ pĕr-kăl-sē′ mĭ-ă)	hyper calc -emia	P R S	excessive lime, calcium blood condition	A condition of excessive amounts of calcium in the blood
hyperglycemia (hī″ pĕr-glī-sē′ mĭ-ă)	hyper glyc -emia	P R S	excessive sweet, sugar blood condition	A condition of excessive amounts of sugar in the blood

MEDICAL WORD	WORD PARTS (WHEN APPLICABLE)			DEFINITION
	Part	Type	Meaning	
hyperlipemia (hī″ pĕr-lĭp-ē′ mĭ-ă)	hyper lip -emia	P R S	excessive fat blood condition	A condition of excessive amounts of fat in the blood
hypoglycemia (hī″ pō-glī-sē′ mĭ-ă)	hypo glyc -emia	P R S	deficient sweet, sugar blood condition	A condition of deficient amounts of sugar in the blood
immunoglobulin (Ig) (ĭm″ ū-nō-glŏb′ ū-lĭn)	immun/o globul -in	CF R S	immunity globe chemical	A blood protein capable of acting as an antibody. The five major types are IgA, IgD, IgE, IgG, and IgM.
Kaposi's sarcoma (kăp′ ō-sēz săr-kō′ mă)				A malignant neoplasm that causes violaceous vascular lesions and general lymphadenopathy; it is the most common AIDS-related tumor. See Figures 8–10 and 8–11.
leukapheresis (loo″ kă-fĕ-rē′ sĭs)	leuk/a -pheresis	CF S	white removal	Removal of white blood cells from the circulation
leukemia (loo-kē′ mē-ă)	leuk -emia	R S	white blood condition	A disease of the blood characterized by overproduction of leukocytes. The disease may be malignant, acute, or chronic. ✳ See Figure 8–22 in Pathology Spotlight: Leukemia.
leukocyte (loo′ kō-sīt)	leuk/o -cyte	CF S	white cell	A white blood cell
leukocytopenia (loo″ kō-sī″ tō-pē′ nĭ-ă)	leuk/o cyt/o -penia	CF CF S	white cell lack of	A lack of white blood cells
lymph (lĭmf)				A clear, colorless, alkaline fluid found in the lymphatic vessels
lymphadenitis (lĭm-făd″ ĕn-ī′ tĭs)	lymph aden -itis	R R S	lymph gland inflammation	Inflammation of the lymph glands
lymphadenotomy (lĭm-făd″ ĕ-nō tō-mē)	lymph aden/o -tomy	R CF S	lymph gland incision	Incision into a lymph gland
lymphangiology (lĭm-făn″ jē-ŏl′ ō-jē)	lymph angi/o -logy	R CF S	lymph vessel study of	The study of the lymphatic vessels
lymphangitis (lĭm″ făn-jī′ tĭs)	lymph ang -itis	R R S	lymph vessel inflammation	Inflammation of lymphatic vessels. See Figure 8–12.

MEDICAL WORD	WORD PARTS (WHEN APPLICABLE)			DEFINITION
	Part	Type	Meaning	
lymphedema (lĭmf-ĕ-dē′ mă)	lymph -edema	R S	lymph swelling	An abnormal accumulation of lymph in the interstitial spaces. See Figures 8–13 and 8–14.
lymphoma (lĭm-fō′ mă)	lymph -oma	R S	lymph tumor	A lymphoid neoplasm, usually malignant. See Figures 8–15 and 8–16.
lymphostasis (lĭm-fō′ stā-sĭs)	lymph/o -stasis	CF S	lymph control, stopping	The control or stopping of the flow of lymph
macrocyte (măk′ rō-sīt)	macr/o -cyte	CF S	large cell	An abnormally large erythrocyte
monocyte (mŏn′ ō-sīt)	mono -cyte	P S	one cell	The largest leukocyte, which has one nucleus
mononucleosis (mŏn″ ō-nū″ klē-ō′ sĭs)	mono nucle -osis	P R S	one kernel, nucleus condition	A condition of excessive amounts of mononuclear leukocytes in the blood
neutrophil (nū′ trō-fĭl)	neutr/o -phil	CF S	neither attraction	A leukocyte that stains with neutral dyes
opportunistic infection (ŏp″ ŏr-too-nĭs′ tĭk ĭn-fĕk′ shŭn)				A protozoal, fungal, viral, or bacterial infection that occurs when one's immune system is compromised. AIDS patients are very vulnerable and develop one or more opportunistic infections.
pancytopenia (păn″ sī-tō-pē′ nĭ-ă)	pan cyt/o -penia	P CF S	all cell lack of	A lack of the cellular elements of the blood
phagocytosis (făg″ ō-sī-tō′ sĭs)	phag/o cyt -osis	CF R S	eat, engulf cell condition of	A condition of the engulfing and eating of bacteria by the phagocytes
plasma (plăz′ mă)				The fluid part of the blood
plasmapheresis (plăz″ mă-fĕr-ē′ sĭs)	plasma -pheresis	R S	a thing formed, plasma removal	Removal of blood from the body and centrifuging it to separate the plasma from the blood
Pneumocystis carinii (nū″ mō-sĭs′ tĭs kă-rī′ nē-ī)				A protozoan that causes *Pneumocystis carinii* pneumonia (PCP)

MEDICAL WORD	WORD PARTS (WHEN APPLICABLE)			DEFINITION
	Part	Type	Meaning	
Pneumocystis carinii pneumonia (nū″ mō-sĭs′ tĭs nū-mō′ nē-ă)				An opportunistic infection that is prevalent in AIDS patients. If not treated, the mortality rate is high.
polycythemia (pŏl″ ē-sī-thē′ mĭ-ă)	poly cyth -emia	P R S	many cell blood condition	A condition of too many red blood cells
prothrombin (prō-thrŏm′ bĭn)	pro thromb -in	P R S	before clot chemical	A chemical substance that interacts with calcium salts to produce thrombin
radioimmunoassay (rā″ dē-ō-ĭm″ ū-nō-ăs′ ā)				A method of determining the concentration of protein-bound hormones in the blood plasma
reticulocyte (rĕ-tĭk′ ū-lō-sīt)	reticul/o -cyte	CF S	net cell	A red blood cell containing a network of granules
septicemia (sĕp″ tĭ-sē′ mĭ-ă)	septic -emia	R S	putrefying blood condition	A condition in which pathogenic bacteria are present in the blood
seroculture (sē′ rō-kŭl″ chūr)	ser/o -culture	CF S	whey, serum cultivation	A bacterial culture of blood serum
serum (sē′ rŭm)	ser (a) -um	R S	whey tissue	The clear, yellowish fluid that separates from the clot when blood clots
sideropenia (sĭd″ ĕr-ō-pē′ nĭ-ă)	sider/o -penia	CF S	iron lack of	Lack of iron in the blood
splenomegaly (splē″ nō-mĕg′ ă-lē)	splen/o -megaly	CF S	spleen enlargement	Enlargement of the spleen
stem cell (stĕm sĕl)				A cell in the bone marrow that gives rise to various types of blood cells
thalassemia (thăl-ă-sē′ mĭ-ă)	thalass -emia	R S	sea blood condition	Hereditary anemias occurring in populations bordering the Mediterranean Sea and in Southeast Asia
thrombectomy (thrŏm-bĕk′ tō-mē)	thromb -ectomy	R S	clot excision	Surgical excision of a blood clot
thrombin (thrŏm′ bĭn)	thromb -in	R S	clot chemical	A blood enzyme that causes clotting by forming fibrin
thrombocyte (thrŏm′ bō-sīt)	thromb/o -cyte	CF S	clot cell	A clotting cell; *a blood platelet*

MEDICAL WORD	WORD PARTS (WHEN APPLICABLE)			DEFINITION
	Part	**Type**	**Meaning**	
thromboplastin (thrŏm″ bō-plăs′ tĭn)	thromb plast -in	R R S	clot a developing chemical	An essential factor in the production of thrombin and blood clotting
thrombosis (thrŏm-bō′ sĭs)	thromb -osis	R S	clot condition of	Condition of a blood clot
thymoma (thī-mō′ mă)	thym -oma	R S	thymus tumor	A tumor of the thymus
tonsillectomy (tŏn″ sĭl-ĕk′ tō-mē)	tonsill -ectomy	R S	tonsil excision	Surgical excision of the tonsil
transfusion (trăns-fū″ zhŭn)	trans fus -ion	P R S	across to pour process	The process whereby blood is transferred from one individual to the vein of another
vasculitis (văs″ kŭ-lī′ tĭs)	vascul -itis	R S	small vessel inflammation	Inflammation of a lymph or blood vessel. See Figure 8–17.

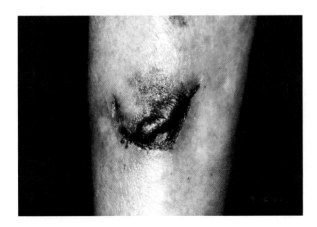

FIGURE 8–7

Traumatic hematoma. (Courtesy of Jason L. Smith, MD.)

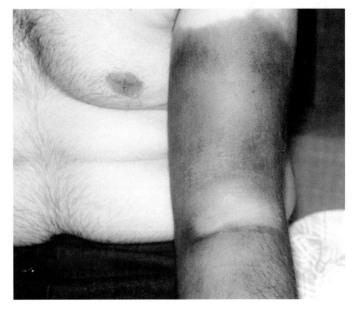

FIGURE 8–8

Hemorrhage, vein. (Courtesy of Jason L. Smith, MD.)

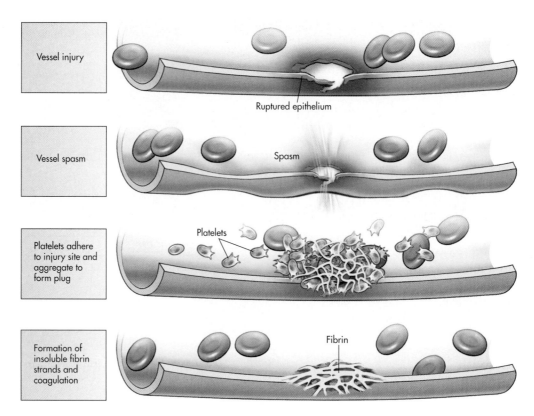

Vessel injury	Ruptured epithelium
Vessel spasm	Spasm
Platelets adhere to injury site and aggregate to form plug	Platelets
Formation of insoluble fibrin strands and coagulation	Fibrin

FIGURE 8–9

Basic steps in hemostasis.

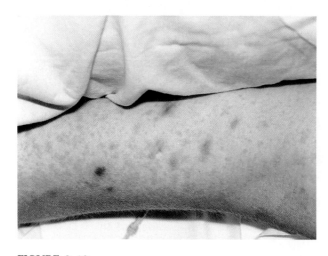

FIGURE 8–10

Kaposi's sarcoma. (Courtesy of Jason L. Smith, MD.)

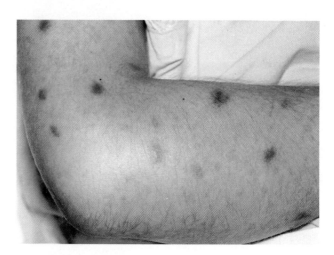

FIGURE 8–11

Kaposi's sarcoma. (Courtesy of Jason L. Smith, MD.)

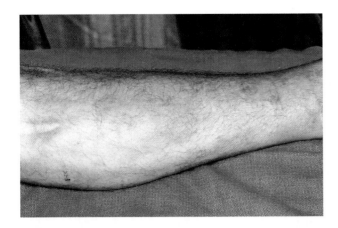

FIGURE 8–12

Lymphangitis. (Courtesy of Jason L. Smith, MD.)

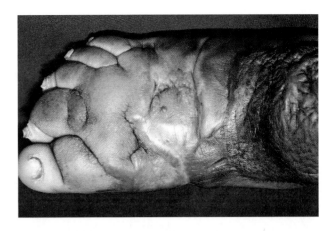

FIGURE 8–13

Congenital lymphedema. (Courtesy of Jason L. Smith, MD.)

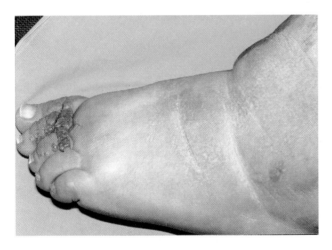

FIGURE 8–14

Chronic lymphedema. (Courtesy of Jason L. Smith, MD.)

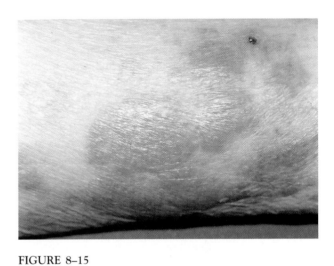

FIGURE 8–15

Lymphoma. (Courtesy of Jason L. Smith, MD.)

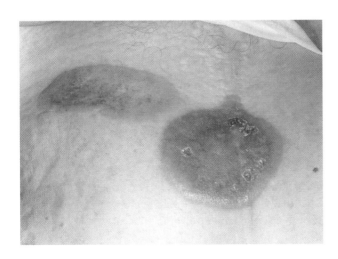

FIGURE 8–16

Cutaneous T-cell lymphoma. (Courtesy of Jason L. Smith, MD.)

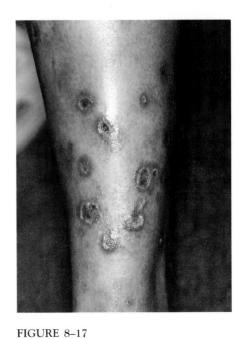

FIGURE 8–17

Vasculitis. (Courtesy of Jason L. Smith, MD.)

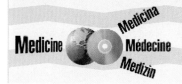

Terminology Translator

This feature, found on the accompanying CD-ROM, provides an innovative tool to translate medical words into Spanish, French, and German.

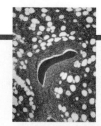

PATHOLOGY SPOTLIGHTS

Acquired Immunodeficiency Syndrome (AIDS)

AIDS is the final stage of human immunodeficiency virus (HIV) disease. AIDS is caused by the human immunodeficiency virus (HIV). The virus attacks the immune system and leaves the body vulnerable to a variety of life-threatening illnesses and cancers. Common bacteria, yeast, parasites, and viruses that ordinarily do not cause serious disease in people with healthy immune systems can cause serious or fatal illnesses in those with AIDS.

The Centers for Disease Control (CDC) defines AIDS as beginning when a person with HIV infection has a CD4 cell (also called a "T-cell", which is a type of immune cell) count below 200/mm^3. AIDS is also defined by the opportunistic infections and cancers that occur in someone with HIV infection. The statistics are sobering: AIDS is the fifth leading cause of death among persons between ages 25 and 44 in the United States. More than 47 million people worldwide have been infected with HIV since the start of the epidemic.

The symptoms of AIDS are the result of the opportunistic infections that do not normally develop in individuals with healthy immune systems. Common symptoms are flu-like and include fevers, sweats, swollen glands, chills, weakness, and weight loss. There may be no symptoms after initial infection, however. Some people with HIV infection remain without symptoms for years between the time of exposure and development of AIDS.

HIV has been found in such body fluids as saliva, tears, nervous system tissue, blood, semen, vaginal fluid, and breast milk. At this time, only blood, semen, vaginal secretions, and breast milk have been proven to transmit infection to others.

Transmission of the virus occurs in the following ways:

- Through sexual contact—including oral, vaginal, and anal sex
- Through blood, including blood transfusions (now extremely rare in the United States) or needle sharing
- From mother to child—a pregnant woman can passively transmit the virus to her fetus, or a nursing mother can transmit it to her baby

Although rare, HIV can be transmitted in other ways, including accidental needle injury, artificial insemination with donated semen, and through a donated organ.

HIV cannot be spread by casual contact such as hugging and touching, by touching dishes, doorknobs, or toilet seats previously touched by a person infected with the virus, during participation in sports, or by mosquitoes. It is not transmitted to a person who *donates* blood or organs in the United States because hospitals do not re-use syringes and sterilize all devices involved in these procedures. However, HIV can be transmitted to the person *receiving* blood or organs from an infected donor. This is the reason blood banks and organ donor programs screen donors, blood, and tissues thoroughly.

People who are at highest risk for HIV infection include homosexual or bisexual men who engage in unprotected sex, intravenous drug users who share needles, the sexual partners of those who participate in high-risk activities, infants born to mothers with HIV, and people who received blood transfusions or clotting products between 1977 and 1985 (prior to standard screening for the virus in the blood).

Although there is no cure for AIDS at this time, there are several treatments that can delay the progression of disease for many years and improve the quality of life of those who have developed symptoms.

The main form of treatment is through antiviral therapy, which suppresses the replication of the HIV virus. The newest form involves a combination of several antiretroviral agents, called highly active anti-retroviral therapy (HAART), and has been highly effective in reducing the number of HIV particles in the blood stream (as measured by a blood test called the viral load). This can help the immune system recover and improve T-cell counts.

Although HAART shows great promise, it is not a cure for HIV, and people on HAART with suppressed levels of HIV can still transmit the virus to others through sex or sharing of needles. There is good evidence that, if the levels of HIV remain suppressed and the CD4 count remains high (>200), life and quality of life can be significantly prolonged and improved. However, HIV tends to become resistant in patients who do not take their medications every day. Certain strains of HIV mutate easily and may become resistant to HAART especially quickly.

Other antiviral agents are in investigational stages and many new drugs are in the pipeline. Medications are also used to prevent opportunistic infections (such as *Pneumocystis carinii* pneumonia) and can keep AIDS patients healthier for longer periods of time. Opportunistic infections are treated as they occur.

Allergic Rhinitis

Allergic rhinitis is a collection of symptoms that typically occur in the nose and eyes after exposure to airborne particles of dust, dander, or the pollens of certain seasonal plants in people who are allergic to these substances. Symptoms include coughing, headache, sneezing, and itching nose, mouth, and eyes.

Allergies are common, and are caused by an oversensitive immune system. The immune system normally protects the body against harmful substances such as bacteria and viruses. Allergy occurs when the immune system reacts to substances (allergens) that are generally harmless and in most people do not cause an immune response. Heredity and environmental exposures may also contribute to a predisposition to allergies.

When the symptoms are caused by pollens, the allergic rhinitis is commonly known as hay fever. See Figure 8–18. This same reaction occurs with allergy to mold, animal dander, dust, and similar inhaled allergens.

When an allergen such as pollen or dust is inhaled by a person with a sensitized immune system, it triggers antibody production. See p. 275 for more information about antibodies. These antibodies bind to cells that contain histamine. When the antibodies are stimulated by pollen and dust, histamine (and other chemicals) are released. This causes itching, swelling, and mucus production. Symptoms vary in severity from person to person. Very sensitive individuals can experience hives or other rashes.

In order to diagnose allergic rhinitis, the history of the person's symptoms is important, including whether the symptoms vary according to time of day or the season, exposure to pets or other allergens, and diet.

Allergy testing may reveal the specific allergens to which the person is reacting. Skin testing is the most common method of allergy testing. This may include intradermal, scratch, patch, or other tests.

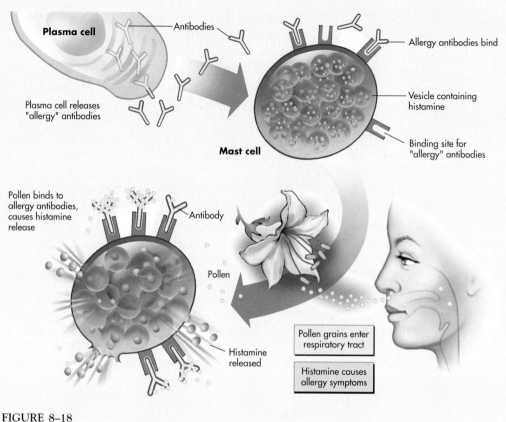

FIGURE 8–18

Allergic rhinitis.

The goal of treatment is to reduce the inflammation that causes allergy symptoms. The most effective treatment is avoidance of the allergens, or reducing exposure to allergens. Medication options include over-the-counter and prescription antihistamines, nasal corticosteroid sprays, and decongestants.

Allergy shots (immunotherapy) may be administered if the allergen cannot be avoided and if symptoms are hard to control. This includes regular injections of the allergen, given in increasing doses (each dose is slightly larger than the previous dose) that may help the body adjust to the allergen.

Anaphylaxis

Anaphylaxis is a type of allergic reaction that affects the whole body. It is a response to a substance to which a person has become very sensitive. This allergic response is sudden, severe, and involves the whole body.

During an anaphylactic allergic reaction, tissues in different parts of the body release histamine and other substances. This causes constriction of the airways, resulting in wheezing; difficulty breathing; and gastrointestinal symptoms such as abdominal pain, cramps, vomiting, and diarrhea. See Figure 8–19. Symptoms develop rapidly, often within seconds or minutes.

Shock may occur as a result of lowered blood pressure and blood volume. Hives and angioedema (hives on the lips, eyelids, throat, and/or tongue) often occur, and angioedema may be severe enough to cause obstruction of the airway. Prolonged anaphylaxis can cause heart arrhythmias.

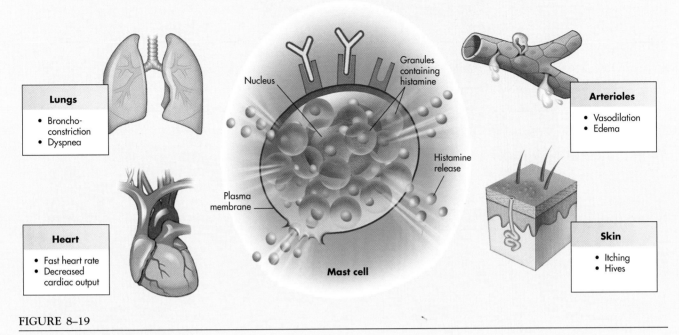

FIGURE 8–19

Symptoms of anaphylaxis.

Some drugs such as morphine, x-ray dye, and others may cause an anaphylactic-like reaction on the first exposure. Anaphylaxis can occur in response to any allergen. Common causes include insect bites/stings, food allergies, and drug allergies. Pollens and other inhaled allergens, which commonly cause allergic rhinitis, rarely cause anaphylaxis. Some people have an anaphylactic reaction with no identifiable cause.

Although anaphylaxis occurs infrequently, it is life-threatening and can occur at any time. Risks include prior history of any type of allergic reaction.

Anaphylaxis is an emergency condition that requires immediate professional medical attention. Assessment of the ABCs (airway, breathing, and circulation, per Basic Life Support protocols) should be done in all suspected anaphylactic reactions. If indicated, CPR should be initiated. People with a history of severe allergic reactions may carry an Epi-Pen or other allergy kit, and should be assisted if necessary. Paramedics or physicians may place a tube through the nose or mouth into the airway (endotracheal intubation) or conduct emergency surgery to place a tube directly into the trachea (tracheostomy).

Epinephrine (or an Epi-Pen) should be given by injection without delay. Epinephrine opens the airways and raises the blood pressure by constricting blood vessels.

If the person is in shock, treatment includes intravenous fluids and medications that support the actions of the heart and circulatory system. Antihistamines (such as diphenhydramine) and corticosteroids (such as prednisone) may be given to further reduce symptoms after lifesaving measures and epinephrine are administered.

Anemia

Anemia is a condition that is characterized by a lower than normal number of red blood cells (erythrocytes) in the blood, usually measured by a decrease in the amount of hemoglobin. See Figure 8–20. Hemoglobin is a protein, and is the red pigment in red blood cells that transports oxygen.

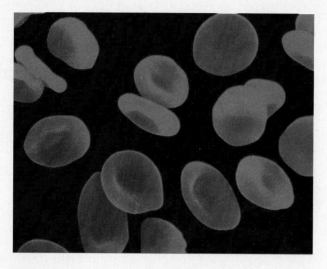

FIGURE 8–20

Normal red blood cells. (Source: Custom Medical Stock Photo, Inc.)

There are many types and causes of anemia. Some common types include sickle cell anemia (see Figure 8–21), hemolytic anemia, and pernicious anemia. Anemia can also result from nutritional deficiencies, such as B_{12}, folate, and iron.

The cause varies with the type of anemia. Potential causes include blood loss, nutritional deficits, many diseases, medication reactions, and various problems with the bone marrow.

Possible symptoms include fatigue, angina (chest pain), and shortness of breath. Anemia can be confirmed by a red blood count or hemoglobin level test. Other tests depend on the type of anemia.

Treatment is directed at the cause of the anemia, and includes blood transfusions and the medication erythropoietin.

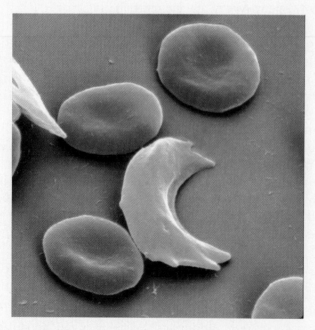

FIGURE 8–21

Iron deficiency anemia blood cells. (Source: Photo Researchers, Inc.)

TABLE 8–4 ANTIBODIES/IMMUNOGLOBULINS

Antibody	Functions
IgG	Crosses placenta to provide passive immunity for the newborn
	Opsonizing (coating) microorganisms to enhance phagocytosis
	Activates complement system (a group of proteins in the blood)
	Components of complement are labeled C1 through C9. Complement acts by directly killing organisms; by opsonizing an antigen; and by stimulating inflammation and the B-cell-mediated immune response.
IgM	Activates complement
	First antibody produced in response to bacterial and viral infections
IgA	Protects epithelial surfaces
	Activates complement
	Passed to breast-feeding newborn via the colostrum
IgE	Active in allergic reactions and some parasitic infections
	Trigger mast cells to release histamine, serotonin, kinins, slow-reacting substance of anaphylaxis, and the neutrophil factor. These mediators produce allergic skin reaction, asthma, and hay fever.
IgD	Role not clear; possibly influences B lymphocyte differentiation

Antibody

An antibody is also referred to as an immunoglobulin. It is a complex glycoprotein produced by B lymphocytes in response to the presence of an antigen. Antibodies neutralize or destroy antigens in several ways. They can initiate destruction of the antigen by activating the complement system, neutralizing toxins released by bacteria, opsonizing (coating) the antigen or forming a complex to stimulate phagocytosis, promoting antigen clumping, or preventing the antigen from adhering to host cells. See Table 8–4 for the five classes of antibodies: IgG, IgM, IgA, IgE, and IgD.

Leukemia

Leukemia is any of a group of diseases of the blood involving uncontrolled increase of white blood cells (leukocytes). Common types include chronic lymphocytic leukemia (CLL) and acute lymphocytic leukemia.

Chronic lymphocytic leukemia is a malignancy (cancer) of the white blood cells (lymphocytes) characterized by a slow, progressive increase of these cells in the blood and the bone marrow. Chronic lymphocytic leukemia (CLL) affects the B lymphocytes and causes immunosuppression, failure of the bone marrow, and invasion of malignant (cancerous) cells into organs.

Usually the symptoms develop gradually (see Figure 8–22). The incidence of CLL is about 2 per 100,000 and increases with age. 90 percent of cases are found in people over 50 years old. Many cases are detected by routine blood tests in people with no symptoms. The cause of CLL is unknown. No relationship to viruses, or exposure to radiation or carcinogenic chemicals has been determined. The disease is more common in Jewish people of Russian or Eastern European descent and is uncommon in people of Asian descent.

Acute lymphocytic leukemia (ALL) is a cancer of the lymph cells. It is characterized by large numbers of immature white blood cells that resemble lymphoblasts. These cells can be found in the blood, the bone marrow, the lymph nodes, the spleen, and other organs. This type of leukemia is responsible for 80 percent of the acute leukemias of childhood, with the peak incidence occurring between ages 3 and 7. ALL also occurs in adults, and comprises 20 percent of all adult leukemias.

In ALL, the blood cell loses its ability to mature and specialize (differentiate) its function. These malignant cells multiply rapidly and replace the normal cells. Bone marrow failure occurs

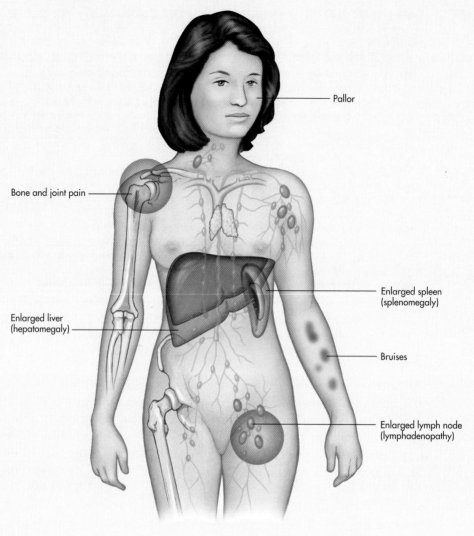

Pallor

Bone and joint pain

Enlarged spleen
(splenomegaly)

Enlarged liver
(hepatomegaly)

Bruises

Enlarged lymph node
(lymphadenopathy)

FIGURE 8–22

Signs and symptoms of leukemia.

as malignant cells replace normal bone marrow elements. The person becomes susceptible to
bleeding and infection because the normal blood cells are reduced in number.

Most cases of ALL seem to have no apparent cause. However, radiation, some toxins such
as benzene, and some chemotherapy agents are thought to contribute to this type of leukemia.
Abnormalities in chromosomes may also play a role in the development of ALL.

✔ PATHOLOGY CHECKPOINT

Following is a concise list of the pathology-related terms that you've seen in the chapter. Review this checklist to make sure that you are familiar with the meaning of each term before moving on to the next section.

Conditions and Symptoms

- ❑ acquired immunodeficiency syndrome (AIDS)
- ❑ allergy
- ❑ anaphylaxis
- ❑ anemia
- ❑ anisocytosis
- ❑ autoimmune disease
- ❑ creatinemia
- ❑ embolus
- ❑ erythrocytosis
- ❑ extravasation
- ❑ hematoma
- ❑ hemochromatosis
- ❑ hemophilia
- ❑ hemorrhage
- ❑ hypercalcemia
- ❑ hyperglycemia
- ❑ hyperlipemia
- ❑ hypoglycemia
- ❑ Kaposi's sarcoma
- ❑ leukemia
- ❑ leukocytopenia
- ❑ lymphadenitis
- ❑ lymphangitis
- ❑ lymphedema
- ❑ lymphoma
- ❑ mononucleosis
- ❑ opportunistic infection
- ❑ pancytopenia
- ❑ pneumocystis pneumonia
- ❑ polycythemia
- ❑ septicemia
- ❑ sideropenia
- ❑ splenomegaly
- ❑ thalassemia
- ❑ thrombosis
- ❑ thymoma
- ❑ tonsillectomy
- ❑ vasculitis

Diagnosis and Treatment

- ❑ anticoagulant
- ❑ autotransfusion
- ❑ hematocrit
- ❑ hemostasis
- ❑ leukapheresis
- ❑ lymphadenotomy
- ❑ lymphostasis
- ❑ plasmapheresis
- ❑ radioimmunoassay
- ❑ seroculture
- ❑ thrombectomy
- ❑ transfusion

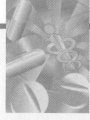

DRUG HIGHLIGHTS

Drugs that are generally used in blood and lymphatic diseases and disorders include anticoagulants, hemostatic agents, antianemic agents, epoetin alfa, and drugs used in treating megaloblastic anemias.

Anticoagulants	Used in inhibiting or preventing a blood clot formation. Hemorrhage can occur at almost any site in patients on anticoagulant therapy.
	Examples: heparin sodium, Coumadin (warfarin sodium), and Lovenox (enoxaparin).
Hemostatic Agents	Used to control bleeding and may be administered systemically or topically.
	Examples: Proplex (factor IX complement), Amicar (aminocaproic acid), vitamin K, and Surgicel (oxidized cellulose).
Antianemic Agents (irons)	Used to treat iron deficiency anemia. Oral iron preparations interfere with the absorption of oral tetracycline antibiotics. These products should not be taken within 2 hours of each other.
	Examples: Femiron (ferrous fumarate), Fergon, Fertinic (ferrous gluconate), and Feosol (ferrous sulfate).
Epoetin Alfa (EPO, Procrit)	A genetically engineered hemopoietin that stimulates the production of red blood cells. It is a recombinant version of erythropoietin and is indicated for treating anemia in patients with chronic renal failure and HIV-infected patients taking zidovudine (AZT).
Agents	Used in treating megaloblastic anemias include *Folvite (folic acid) and vitamin* B_{12} *(cyanocobalamin).*

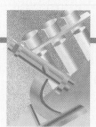

DIAGNOSTIC & LAB TESTS

TEST	DESCRIPTION
antinuclear antibodies (ANA) (ăn″ tĭ-nū′ klē-ăr ăn′ tĭ-bŏd″ ēs)	A blood test to identify antigen–antibody reactions. ANA antibodies are present in a number of autoimmune diseases.
bleeding time (blēd′ ĭng tīm)	A puncture of the ear lobe or forearm to determine the time required for blood to stop flowing. Duke method (ear lobe) 1 to 3 minutes is the normal time, and with the Ivy (forearm), 1 to 9 minutes is the normal time for the flow of blood to cease. Times greater than these may indicate thrombocytopenia, aplastic anemia, leukemia, decreased platelet count, hemophilia, and potential hemorrhage. Anticoagulant drugs delay the bleeding time.

TEST	DESCRIPTION
blood typing (ABO group and Rh factor) (blod tīp′ ĭng)	A blood test to determine an individual's blood type and Rh factor. Blood types are A, B, AB, and O. Rh factor may be negative or positive.
bone marrow aspiration (bōn măr′ ō ăs-pĭ-rā′ shŭn)	Removal of bone marrow for examination; may be performed to determine aplastic anemia, leukemia, certain cancers, and polycythemia.
complete blood count (CBC) (kom-plēt′ blod kount)	This blood test includes a hematocrit, hemoglobin, red and white blood cell count, and differential. This test is usually a part of a complete physical examination and a good indicator of hematologic system functioning.
hematocrit (Hct) (hē-măt′ ō-krĭt)	A blood test performed on whole blood to determine the percentage of red blood cells in the total blood volume.
hemoglobin (Hb, Hgb) (hē″ mō-glō′ bĭn)	A blood test to determine the amount of iron-containing pigment of the red blood cells.
immunoglobulins (Ig) (ĭm″ ŭ-nō-glŏb′ ū-lĭns)	A serum blood test to determine the presence of IgA, IgD, IgE, IgG, and/or IgM. Lymphocytes and plasma cells produce immunoglobulins in response to antigen exposure. Increased and/or decreased values may indicate certain disease conditions.
partial thromboplastin time (PTT) (păr′ shāl thrŏm″ bō-plăs′ tĭn tīm)	A test performed on blood plasma to determine how long it takes for fibrin clots to form; used to regulate heparin dosage and to detect clotting disorders.
platelet count (plāt′ lĕt kount)	A test performed on whole blood to determine the number of thrombocytes present. Increased and/or decreased amounts may indicate certain disease conditions.
prothrombin time (PT) (prō-thrŏm′ bĭn tīm)	A test performed on blood plasma to determine the time needed for oxalated plasma to clot; used to regulate anticoagulant drug therapy and to detect clotting disorders.
red blood count (RBC) (red blod kount)	A test performed on whole blood to determine the number of erythrocytes present. Increased and/or decreased amounts may indicate certain disease conditions.
sedimentation rate (ESR) (sĕd″ -ĭmĕn-tā′ shŭn rāt)	A blood test to determine the rate at which red blood cells settle in a long, narrow tube. The distance the RBCs settle in 1 hour is the rate. Higher or lower rate may indicate certain disease conditions.
viral load (vī′ ral lōd)	A blood test that measures the amount of HIV in the blood. Results can range from 50 to over one million copies per milliliter (mL) of blood. Two tests that are used to measure viral load are bDNA and PCR.
white blood count (WBC) (wīt blod kount)	A blood test to determine the number of leukocytes present. Increased level indicates infection and/or inflammation and decreased level indicates aplastic anemia, pernicious anemia, and malaria.

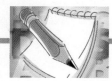

ABBREVIATIONS

ABBREVIATION	MEANING	ABBREVIATION	MEANING
ABO	blood group	HIV	human immunodeficiency virus
AHF	antihemophilic factor		
AIDS	acquired immunodeficiency syndrome	lymphs	lymphocytes
		MCH	mean corpuscular hemoglobin
ALL	acute lymphocytic leukemia	MCHC	mean corpuscular hemoglobin concentration
BAC	blood alcohol concentration		
baso	basophil	MCV	mean corpuscular volume
BSI	body systems isolation	mono	monocyte
CBC	complete blood count	PCP	*Pneumocystis carinii* pneumonia
CLL	chronic lymphocytic leukemia		
CML	chronic myelogenous leukemia	PCV	packed cell volume
diff	differential count	PMN	polymorphonuclear neutrophil
EBV	Epstein–Barr virus	poly	polymorphonuclear
ELISA	enzyme-linked immunosorbent assay	PT	prothrombin time
		PTT	partial thromboplastin time
eos, eosin	eosinophil	RBC	red blood cell (count)
ESR	erythrocyte sedimentation rate	Rh	Rhesus (factor)
Hb, Hgb, HGB	hemoglobin	RIA	radioimmunoassay
		segs	segmented (mature RBCs)
Hct, HCT	hematocrit	SRS-A	slow-reacting substances of anaphylaxis
HDN	hemolytic disease of the newborn		
		WBC	white blood cell (count)

STUDY AND REVIEW

Anatomy and Physiology

Write your answers to the following questions. Do not refer to the text.

1. Name the three formed elements of blood.

    a. _____   b. _____

    c. _____

2. State the function of erythrocytes. _____

    _____

3. There are approximately _____ million erythrocytes per cubic millimeter of blood.

4. The life span of an erythrocyte is _____.

5. State the function of leukocytes. _____

    _____

6. There are approximately _____ thousand leukocytes per cubic millimeter of blood.

7. Name the five types of leukocytes.

    a. _____   b. _____

    c. _____   d. _____

    e. _____

8. State the function of thrombocytes. _____

    _____

9. There are approximately _____ thrombocytes per cubic millimeter of
   blood.

10. Name the four blood types.

    a. _____   b. _____

    c. _____   d. _____

11. State the three main functions of the lymphatic system.

    a. _____

    b. _____

    c. _____

12. Name the three accessory organs of the lymphatic system.

    a. _____

    b. _____

    c. _____

Word Parts

1. In the spaces provided, write the definition of these prefixes, roots, combining forms, and suffixes. Do not refer to the listings of medical words. Leave blank those words you cannot define.

2. After completing as many as you can, refer to the medical word listings to check your work. For each word missed or left blank, write the word and its definition several times on the margins of these pages or on a separate sheet of paper.

3. To maximize the learning process, it is to your advantage to do the following exercises as directed. To refer to the word building section before completing these exercises invalidates the learning process.

PREFIXES

Give the definitions of the following prefixes:

1. an- _____   2. anti- _____

3. auto- _____   4. ana- _____

5. extra- _____   6. hyper- _____

7. hypo- _____   8. mono- _____

9. pan- _____   10. poly- _____

11. pro- _____   12. trans- _____

ROOTS AND COMBINING FORMS

Give the definitions of the following roots and combining forms:

1. aden _____

2. aden/o _____

3. agglutinat _____

4. all _____

5. angi/o _____

6. anis/o _____

7. bas/o _____

8. calc _____

9. chromat _____

10. fus _____

11. coagul _____

12. creatin _____

13. cyt _____

14. cyth _____

15. cyt/o _____

16. eosin/o _____

17. erythr/o _____

18. globul _____

19. granul/o _____

20. hemat _____

21. hemat/o _____

22. hem/o _____

23. leuk _____

24. leuk/o _____

25. lip _____

26. log _____

27. lymph _____

28. lymph/o _____

29. macr/o _____

30. neutr/o _____

31. nucle _____

32. phag/o _____

33. plasma _____

34. reticul/o _____

35. septic _____

36. ser/o _____

37. sider/o _____

38. fibr _____

39. splen/o _____

40. thalass _____

41. thromb _____

42. thromb/o _____

43. thym _____

44. fibrin/o _____

45. tonsill _____

46. poiet _____

47. immun/o _____

48. ang _____

49. ser (a) _____

50. plast _____

51. vas (at) _____

52. vascul _____

SUFFIXES

Give the definitions of the following suffixes:

1. -able _____

2. -ant _____

3. -blast _____

4. -body _____

5. -edema _____

6. -crit _____

7. -culture _____

8. -cyte _____

9. -ectomy _____

10. -emia _____

11. -ergy _____

12. -gen _____

13. -phylaxis _____

14. -globin _____

15. -um _____

16. -ic _____

17. -in _____

18. -ion _____

19. -ist _____

20. -itis _____

21. -logy _____

22. -lysis _____

23. -megaly _____

24. -oma _____

25. -osis _____

26. -penia _____

27. -pheresis _____

28. -phil _____

29. -philia _____

30. -poiesis _____

31. -rrhage _____

32. -stasis _____

33. -tomy _____

Identifying Medical Terms

In the spaces provided, write the medical terms for the following meanings:

1. _____ Process of clumping together, as of blood cells that are incompatible

2. _____ Individual hypersensitivity to a substance that is usually harmless

3. _____ A protein substance produced in the body in response to an invading foreign substance

4. _____ An agent that works against the formation of blood clots

5. _____ An invading foreign substance that induces the formation of antibodies

6. _____ A base cell, leukocyte

7. _____ Capable of forming a clot

8. _____ Excess of creatine in the blood

9. _____ A cell that readily stains with the acid stain

10. _____ A granular leukocyte

11. _____ One who specializes in the study of the blood

12. _____ Blood protein

13. _____ Excessive amounts of sugar in the blood

14. _____ Excessive amounts of fat in the blood

15. _____ A white blood cell

16. _____ The control or stopping of the flow of lymph

17. _____ Condition of excessive amounts of mononuclear leukocytes in the blood

18. _____ A chemical substance that interacts with calcium salts to produce thrombin

19. _____ Surgical fixation of a movable spleen

20. _____ A clotting cell; a blood platelet

Spelling

In the spaces provided, write the correct spelling of these misspelled terms:

1. allregy _____

2. cretinemia _____

3. etravasation _____

4. erythcytosis _____

5. thrombplastin _____

6. hemacrit _____

7. hemorhage _____

8. lukemia _____

9. lymphadnotomy _____

10. anphylaxis _____

Matching

Select the appropriate lettered meaning for each word listed below.

_____ 1. autotransfusion

_____ 2. erythrocyte

_____ 3. erythropoietin

_____ 4. extravasation

_____ 5. hemorrhage

_____ 6. immunoglobulin

_____ 7. hemochromatosis

_____ 8. radioimmunoassay

_____ 9. reticulocyte

_____ 10. thrombectomy

a. A method of determining the concentration of protein-bound hormones in the blood plasma
b. A disease condition in which iron is not metabolized properly and accumulates in body tissues
c. A blood protein capable of acting as an antibody
d. A red blood cell
e. A hormone that stimulates the production of red blood cells
f. Excessive bleeding
g. The process whereby fluids and/or medications escape into surrounding tissue
h. The process of reinfusing a patient's own blood
i. Surgical excision of a blood clot
j. A red blood cell containing a network of granules
k. A white blood cell

Abbreviations

Place the correct word, phrase, or abbreviation in the space provided.

1. acquired immunodeficiency syndrome _____

2. body systems isolation _____

3. CML _____

4. hemoglobin _____

5. Hct _____

6. human immunodeficiency virus _____

7. PCP _____

8. PT _____

9. RBC _____

10. radioimmunoassay _____

Diagnostic and Laboratory Tests

Select the best answer to each multiple choice question. Circle the letter of your choice.

1. A blood test to identify antigen–antibody reactions.
   a. sedimentation rate
   b. hematocrit
   c. immunoglobulins
   d. antinuclear antibodies

2. This blood test includes a hematocrit, hemoglobin, red and white blood cell count, and differential.
   a. blood typing
   b. sedimentation rate
   c. CBC
   d. Hb, Hgb

3. A blood test performed on whole blood to determine the percentage of red blood cells in the total blood volume.
   a. RBC
   b. WBC
   c. Hct
   d. PTT

4. A blood test to determine the number of leukocytes present.
   a. RBC
   b. WBC
   c. Hct
   d. PTT

5. A puncture of the ear lobe or forearm to determine the time required for blood to stop flowing.
   a. bleeding time
   b. platelet count
   c. prothrombin time
   d. PTT

CASE STUDY

ACQUIRED IMMUNODEFICIENCY SYNDROME (AIDS)

Read the following case study and then answer the questions that follow.

A 52-year-old female was seen by a physician; the following is a synopsis of her visit. *Note: More than 10% of all AIDS cases in the United States have occurred in persons age 50 or older.*

Present History: The patient states that several months after the death of her husband she became sexually involved with a younger man. She states that they didn't use condoms, as they were not concerned about pregnancy, and now she has found out that he has AIDS. She is most anxious, and states that lately she has had "night sweats," weight loss for no apparent reason, constant fatigue, diarrhea, swollen lymph nodes, and unusual confusion.

Signs and Symptoms: Night sweats, weight loss, fatigue, diarrhea, swollen lymph nodes, and unusual confusion.

Diagnosis: Acquired immunodeficiency syndrome (AIDS). Diagnosis was determined by a complete medical and social history, a physical examination, CD_4 lymphocyte count, which was 180 cells/mm^3 (normal is 600 to 1200 cells/mm^3), and laboratory evidence of immune dysfunction, identification of HIV antibodies, and signs and symptoms.

Treatment: The regimen includes treating any associated condition with proper medical intervention, and starting the patient on a combination of antiretroviral therapy of three drugs: AZT—zidovudine; 3TC—lamiudine; and a protease inhibitor, Norvir—ritonavir. Drug therapy is carefully monitored for older adults, as they may have preexisting conditions, such as cardiac disease and/or renal insufficiency, that can make them less tolerant of drugs. Clinical evaluation and laboratory monitoring every 3 to 6 months and more frequently if needed. Provide for professional assistance as needed. Information on services available for the older adult with HIV infection and AIDS may be obtained by calling the CDC's AIDS Hotline at 1-800-342-AIDS.

CASE STUDY QUESTIONS

1. Signs and symptoms of AIDS include night sweats, weight loss, fatigue, _____, swollen lymph nodes, and confusion.

2. The diagnosis of AIDS was determined by a complete physical examination, laboratory evidence of _____ dysfunction, and a CD_4 lymphocyte count of 180 cells/mm^3.

3. _____ is an antiretroviral drug that is combined with two other drugs in the treatment of AIDS.

4. Why is drug therapy carefully monitored for older adults? _____

MedMedia Wrap-Up

www.prenhall.com/rice

Additional interactive resources and activities for this chapter can be found on the Companion Website. For animation, videos, audio glossary, and review, access the accompanying CD-ROM in this book.

Audio Glossary
Medical Terminology Exercises & Activities
Pathology Spotlights
Terminology Translator
Animations
Videos

Objectives
Medical Terminology Exercises & Activities
Audio Glossary
Drug Updates
Medical Terminology in the News

THE RESPIRATORY SYSTEM

9

OBJECTIVES

On completion of this chapter, you will be able to:

- Describe the organs of the respiratory system.
- State the functions of the organs of the respiratory system.
- Define terms that are used by physiologists and respiratory specialists to describe the volume of air exchanged in breathing.
- State the vital function of respiration.
- Provide the respiratory rates for some different age groups.
- Analyze, build, spell, and pronounce medical words.
- Describe each of the conditions presented in the Pathology Spotlights.
- Complete the Pathology Checkpoint.
- Review Drug Highlights presented in this chapter.
- Provide the description of diagnostic and laboratory tests related to the respiratory system.
- Identify and define selected abbreviations.
- Successfully complete the study and review section.

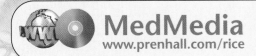

MedMedia
www.prenhall.com/rice

Additional interactive resources and activities for this chapter can be found on the Companion Website. For Terminology Translator, animations, videos, audio glossary, and review, access the accompanying CD-ROM in this book.

Anatomy and Physiology Overview

The respiratory system consists of the **nose, pharynx, larynx, trachea, bronchi,** and **lungs**. The primary function of the respiratory system is to furnish oxygen for use by individual tissue cells and to take away their gaseous waste product, carbon dioxide. See Figure 9–1. This process is accomplished through the act of *respiration*. Respiration consists of external and internal processes. **External respiration** is the process whereby the lungs are ventilated and oxygen and carbon dioxide are exchanged between the air in the lungs and the blood within capillaries of the alveoli. **Internal respiration** is the process whereby oxygen and carbon dioxide are exchanged between the blood in tissue capillaries and the cells of the body.

THE NOSE

The **nose** is the projection in the center of the face and consists of an external and internal portion. The *external portion* is a triangle of cartilage and bone that is covered with skin and lined with mucous membrane. The external entrance of the nose is known as the **nostrils** or **anterior nares**. The *internal portion* of the nose is divided into two chambers by a partition, the **septum**, separating it into a right and a left cavity. These cavities are divided into three air passages: the *superior, middle,* and *inferior conchae*. These passages lead to the pharynx and are connected by openings with the paranasal sinuses, with the ears by the eustachian tube, and with the region of the eyes by the nasolacrimal ducts.

The *palatine bones* separate the nasal cavities from the mouth cavity. When the palatine bones fail to unite during fetal development, a congenital defect known as **cleft palate** occurs. This defect may be corrected by surgery. The nose, as well as the rest of the respiratory system, is lined with mucous membrane, which is covered with *cilia*. The nasal mucosa produces about 946 mL or 1 qt of mucus per day. Four pairs of paranasal sinuses drain into the nose. These are the *frontal, maxillary, ethmoidal,* and *sphenoidal* sinuses (Fig. 9–2).

THE RESPIRATORY SYSTEM

Organ/Structure	Primary Functions
Nose	Serves as an air passageway; warms and moistens inhaled air; its cilia and mucous membrane trap dust, pollen, bacteria, and other foreign matter; contains olfactory receptors, which sort out odors; aids in phonation and the quality of voice
Pharynx	Serves as a passageway for air and for food; aids in phonation by changing its shape
Larynx	Production of vocal sounds
Trachea	Provides an open passageway for air to the lungs
Bronchi	Provide a passageway for air to and from the lungs
Lungs	Bring air into intimate contact with blood so that oxygen and carbon dioxide can be exchanged in the alveoli

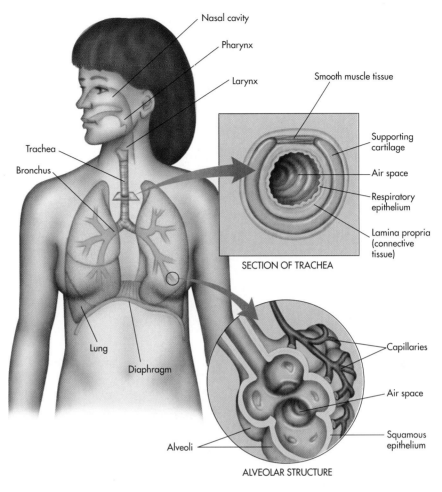

Nasal cavity

Pharynx

Larynx

Trachea

Bronchus

Lung

Diaphragm

Alveoli

Smooth muscle tissue

Supporting cartilage

Air space

Respiratory epithelium

Lamina propria (connective tissue)

SECTION OF TRACHEA

Capillaries

Air space

Squamous epithelium

ALVEOLAR STRUCTURE

FIGURE 9–1

The respiratory system: nasal cavity, pharynx, larynx, trachea, bronchus, and lung with expanded views of the trachea and alveolar structure.

Functions of the Nose

Five functions have been attributed to the nose. These functions are:

1. It serves as an air passageway.
2. It warms and moistens inhaled air.
3. Its cilia and mucous membrane trap dust, pollen, bacteria, and other foreign matter.
4. It contains olfactory receptors, which sort out odors.
5. It aids in phonation and the quality of voice.

THE PHARYNX

The **pharynx** or throat is a musculomembranous tube about 5 inches long that extends from the base of the skull, lies anterior to the cervical vertebrae, and becomes continuous with the esophagus. It is divided into three portions: the *nasopharynx* located behind the nose, the *oropharynx* located behind the mouth, and the *laryngopharynx* located behind the larynx. Seven openings are found in the pharynx: two openings from the eustachian tubes, two openings from the posterior nares into the nasopharynx,

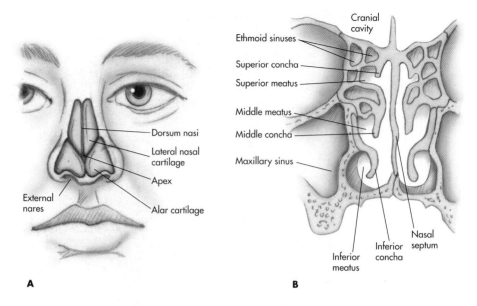

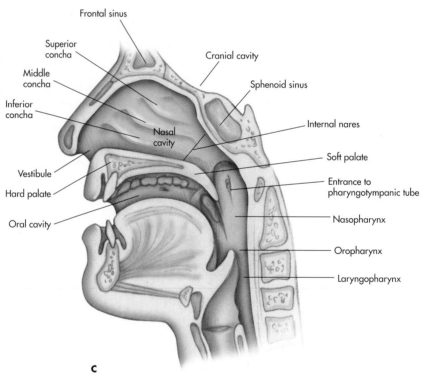

FIGURE 9–2

The nose, nasal cavity, and pharynx: (A) nasal cartilages and external structure; (B) meatuses and positions of the entrance to the ethmoid and maxillary sinuses; and (C) sagittal section of the nasal cavity and pharynx.

the fauces or opening from the mouth into the oropharynx, and the openings from the larynx and the esophagus into the laryngopharynx (Fig. 9–2). Associated with the pharynx are three pairs of lymphoid tissues, which are the **tonsils**. The nasopharynx contains the *adenoids* or *pharyngeal* tonsils. The oropharynx contains the *faucial* or *palatine* tonsils and the *lingual* tonsils. The tonsils are accessory organs of the lymphatic system and aid in filtering bacteria and other foreign substances from the circulating lymph.

Functions of the Pharynx

The following three functions are associated with the pharynx:

1. It serves as a passageway for air.
2. It serves as a passageway for food.
3. It aids in phonation by changing its shape.

THE LARYNX

The **larynx** or voicebox is a muscular, cartilaginous structure lined with mucous membrane. It is the enlarged upper end of the trachea below the root of the tongue and hyoid bone (Fig. 9–1).

Cartilage of the Larynx

The larynx is composed of nine cartilages bound together by muscles and ligaments. The three unpaired cartilages, each of which is described below, are the *thyroid*, *cricoid*, and *epiglottic*, and the three paired cartilages are the *arytenoid*, *cuneiform*, and *corniculate*.

THE THYROID CARTILAGE

The **thyroid cartilage** is the largest cartilage in the larynx and forms the structure commonly called the "*Adam's apple*." This structure is usually larger and more prominent in men than in women and contributes to the deeper male voice.

THE EPIGLOTTIC CARTILAGE

The **epiglottic cartilage** is a small cartilage attached to the superior border of the thyroid cartilage. Known as the **epiglottis**, it covers the entrance of the larynx, and during swallowing, it acts as a lid to prevent aspiration of food into the trachea. When the epiglottis fails to cover the entrance to the larynx, food or liquid intended for the esophagus may enter, causing irritation, coughing, or in extreme cases, choking.

THE CRICOID CARTILAGE

The **cricoid cartilage** is the lowermost cartilage of the larynx. It is shaped like a signet ring with the broad portion being posterior and the anterior portion forming the arch and resembling the ring's band.

The cavity of the larynx contains a pair of *ventricular folds* (false vocal cords) and a pair of vocal folds or true vocal cords. The cavity is divided into three regions: the vestibule, the ventricle, and the entrance to the glottis. The **glottis** is a narrow slit at the opening between the true vocal folds.

Function of the Larynx

The function of the larynx is the production of vocal sounds. High notes are formed by short, tense vocal cords. Low notes are produced by long, relaxed vocal cords. The nose, mouth, pharynx, and bony sinuses aid in phonation.

THE TRACHEA

The **trachea** or windpipe is a cylindrical cartilaginous tube that is the air passageway extending from the pharynx and larynx to the main bronchi. It is about 1 inch wide and $4^1/_2$ inches (11.3 cm) long. It is composed of smooth muscle that is reinforced at the front and sides by C-shaped rings of cartilage. Mucous membrane lining the trachea contains **cilia**, which sweep foreign matter out of the passageway. The function of the trachea is to provide an open passageway for air to the lungs (see Fig. 9–1).

THE BRONCHI

The **bronchi** are the two main branches of the trachea, which provide the passageway for air to the lungs. The trachea divides into the **right bronchus** and the **left bronchus**. The right bronchus is larger and extends down in a more vertical direction than the left bronchus. When a foreign body is inhaled or aspirated, it frequently lodges in the right bronchus or enters the right lung. Each bronchus enters the lung at a depression, the **hilum**. They then subdivide into the bronchial tree composed of smaller bronchi, bronchioles, and alveolar ducts. The bronchial tree terminates in the *alveoli*, which are tiny air sacs supporting a network of capillaries from pulmonary blood vessels. The function of the bronchi is to provide a passageway for air to and from the lungs (see Fig. 9–1).

THE LUNGS

The **lungs** are cone-shaped, spongy organs of respiration lying on either side of the heart within the pleural cavity of the thorax. They occupy a large portion of the thoracic cavity and are enclosed in the **pleura**, a serous membrane composed of several layers. The six layers of the pleura are the *costal, parietal, pericardiaca, phrenica, pulmonalis,* and *visceral*. The *parietal pleura* extends from the roots of the lungs and lines the walls of the thorax and the superior surface of the diaphragm. The *visceral pleura* covers the surface of the lungs and enters into and lines the interlobar fissures. The pleural cavity is a space between the parietal and visceral pleura and contains a serous fluid that lubricates and prevents friction caused by the rubbing together of the two layers. The thoracic cavity is separated from the abdominal cavity by a musculomembranous wall, the **diaphragm**. The central portion of the thoracic cavity, between the lungs, is a space called the **mediastinum**, containing the heart and other structures.

The lungs consist of elastic tissue filled with interlacing networks of tubes and sacs that carry air and with blood vessels carrying blood. The broad inferior surface of the lung is the **base**, which rests on the diaphragm, while the **apex**, or pointed upper margin, rises from 2.5 to 5 cm above the sternal end of the first rib. The lungs are divided into **lobes**, with the right lung having three lobes and the left lung having only two lobes. The left lung has an indentation, the **cardiac depression**, for the normal placement of the heart. In an average adult male, the right lung weighs approximately 625 g and the left about 570 g. In an average adult male, the total lung capacity is 3.6 to 9.4 L, whereas in an average adult female it is 2.5 to 6.9 L. The lungs contain around 300 million **alveoli**, which are the air cells where the exchange of oxygen and carbon dioxide takes place. The main function of the lungs is to bring air into intimate contact with blood so that oxygen and carbon dioxide can be exchanged in the alveoli (Fig. 9–3).

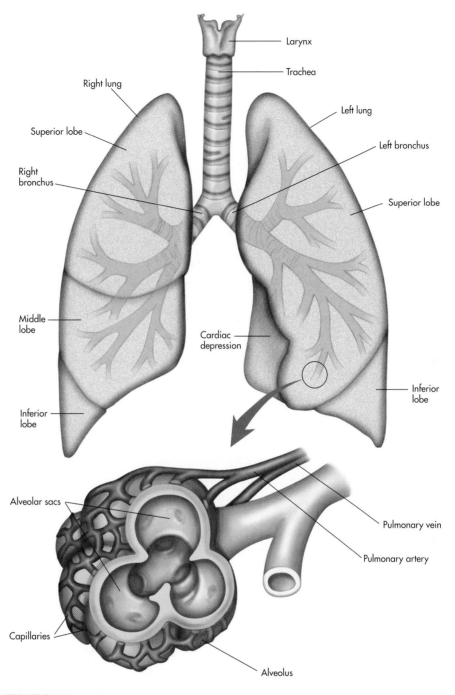

FIGURE 9–3

The larynx, trachea, bronchi, and lungs with an expanded view showing the structures of an alveolus and the pulmonary blood vessels.

RESPIRATION

Volume

The following terms are used by physiologists and respiratory specialists to describe the volume of air exchanged in breathing:

Tidal Volume. The amount of air in a single inspiration or expiration. In the average adult male, about 500 cc of air enters the respiratory tract during normal quiet breathing.

Supplemental Air. The amount of air that may be forcibly expired after a normal quiet respiration. This is also the expiratory reserve volume and measures approximately 1600 cc.

Complemental Air. The amount of air that may be forcibly inspired over and above a normal inspiration. This is known as the inspiratory reserve volume.

Residual Volume. The amount of air remaining in the lungs after maximal expiration—about 1500 cc.

Minimal Air. The small amount of air that remains in the alveoli. After death, if the thorax is opened and the lungs collapse, the minimal air pressure will allow the lungs to float.

Vital Capacity. The volume of air that can be exhaled after a maximal inspiration. This amount equals the sum of the tidal air, complemental air, and the supplemental air.

Functional Residual Capacity. The volume of air that remains in the lungs at the end of a normal expiration.

Total Lung Capacity. The maximal volume of air in the lungs after a maximal inspiration.

The Vital Function of Respiration

Temperature, pulse, respiration, and **blood pressure** are the vital signs that are essential elements for determining an individual's state of health. A deviation from normal of one or all of the vital signs denotes a state of illness. Evaluation of an individual's response to changes occurring within the body can be measured by taking his or her vital signs. Through careful analysis of these changes in the vital signs, a physician may determine a diagnosis, a prognosis, and a plan of treatment for the patient. The variations of certain vital signs signify a typical disease process and its stages of development. For example, in a patient who has pneumonia the temperature is elevated to 101° to 106°F, and pulse and respiration increase to almost twice their normal rates. When the patient's temperature falls, he or she will perspire profusely and his or her pulse and respiration will begin to return to normal rates.

The process of *respiration* is interrelated with other systems of the body. The *medulla oblongata* and the *pons* of the central nervous system regulate and control respiration. The rate, rhythm, and depth of respiration are controlled by nerve impulses from the medulla oblongata and the pons via the spinal cord and nerves to the muscles of the diaphragm, abdomen, and rib cage.

Respiratory Rates

Individuals of different ages breathe at different respiratory rates. **Respiratory rate** is regulated by the respiratory center located in the medulla oblongata. The following are respiratory rates for some different age groups:

Newborn	30 to 80 per minute
1st year	20 to 40 per minute
5th year	20 to 25 per minute
15th year	15 to 20 per minute
Adult	15 to 20 per minute

LIFE SPAN
CONSIDERATIONS

■ THE CHILD

At 12 weeks gestation the lungs of the fetus have a definite shape. At 20 weeks the fetus is able to suck its thumb and swallow amniotic fluid. The cellular structure of the **alveoli** of the lungs are complete. At 24 weeks the nostrils open, respiratory movements occur, and alveoli begin the production of **surfactant**. Surfactant is a substance in the lung that regulates the amount of surface tension of the fluid lining the alveoli. In preterm infants the lack of surfactant contributes to respiratory distress syndrome.

During fetal life gaseous exchange occurs at the placental interface. The lungs do not function until birth. The respiratory rate of the newborn is 30 to 80 per minute. During the first year it is 20 to 40 per minute and at age 5 it is 20 to 25 per minute. Around the 15th year the respiratory rate is 15 to 20, the same as the average, healthy adult rate. Diaphragmatic abdominal breathing is common in infants. Accessory muscles of respiration are not as strong in infants as in older children and adults.

Oxygen consumption and metabolic rate are higher in children than in adults. Airway diameter is smaller in children, thereby increasing the potential for airway obstruction. The mucous membranes of children are vascular and susceptible to trauma, edema, and spasm.

■ THE OLDER ADULT

With advancing age, the respiratory system is vulnerable to injuries caused by infections, environmental pollutants, and allergic reactions. Age-related changes include a decline in the protection normally provided by intact mucous barrier, a decrease in the effectiveness of the bronchial cilia, and changes in the composition of the connective tissues of the lungs and chest. Older adults rely more on the **diaphragm** for inspiration, and when lying down, breathing requires more effort. **Vital capacity** declines with age; there is a decline in the elastic recoil of the lungs and an increase in the stiffness of the chest wall. This makes it more difficult for the older adult to inspire or expire air.

In the pharynx and larynx muscle atrophy can occur, with slackening of the vocal cords and loss of elasticity of the laryngeal muscles and cartilages. These changes may cause a gravelly, softer voice with a rise in pitch, making communication more difficult, especially if there is impaired hearing.

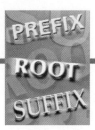

BUILDING YOUR MEDICAL VOCABULARY

This section provides the foundation for learning medical terminology. Medical words can be made up of four different types of word parts:

- Prefixes (P)
- Roots (R)
- Combining forms (CF)
- Suffixes (S)

By connecting various word parts in an organized sequence, thousands of words can be built and learned. In this text the word list is alphabetized so one can see the variety of meanings created when common prefixes and suffixes are repeatedly applied to certain word roots and/or combining forms. Words shown in pink are additional words related to the content of this chapter that are not built from word parts. These words are included to enhance your vocabulary. Note: an asterisk icon (✷) indicates words that are covered in the Pathology Spotlights section in this chapter.

MEDICAL WORD	WORD PARTS (WHEN APPLICABLE)			DEFINITION
	Part	Type	Meaning	
alveolus (ăl-vē′ ō-lŭs)	alveol	R	small, hollow air sac	Pertaining to a small air sac in the lungs
	-us	S	pertaining to	
anthracosis (ăn″ thră-kō′ sĭs)	anthrac	R	coal	Black lung; a lung condition caused by inhalation of coal dust and silica
	-osis	S	condition of	
aphasia (ă-fā′ zĭ-ă)	a	P	lack of	Absence of the ability to communicate through speech, writing, or signs because of brain dysfunction
	phas	R	speech	
	-ia	S	condition	
apnea (ăp′ -nē ă)	a	P	lack of	Temporary cessation of breathing. ✷ See Pathology Spotlight: Apnea.
	-pnea	S	breathing	
asphyxia (ăs-fĭk′ sĭ-ă)	a	P	lack of	A condition in which there is a depletion of oxygen in the blood with an increase of carbon dioxide in the blood and tissues. Symptoms include dyspnea cyanosis, and rapid pulse.
	sphyx	R	pulse	
	-ia	S	condition	
aspiration (ăs″ pĭ-rā′ shŭn)	aspirat	R	to draw in	The process of drawing in or out by suction; foreign bodies may be aspirated into the nose, throat, or lungs on inspiration
	-ion	S	process	

MEDICAL WORD	WORD PARTS (WHEN APPLICABLE)			DEFINITION
	Part	**Type**	**Meaning**	
asthma (ăz′ mă)				A disease of the bronchi characterized by wheezing, dyspnea, and a feeling of constriction in the chest. ✳ See Pathology Spotlight: Asthma.
atelectasis (ăt″ ĕ-lĕk′ tă-sĭs)	atel -ectasis	R S	imperfect dilation, expansion	A condition of imperfect dilation of the lungs; the collapse of an alveolus, a lobule, or a larger lung unit
bronchiectasis (brŏng″ kĭ-ĕk′ tă-sĭs)	bronch/i -ectasis	CF S	bronchi dilation, expansion	Chronic dilation of a bronchus or bronchi, with a secondary infection that usually involves the lower portion of a lung
bronchiolitis (brŏng″ kĭ-ō-lī′ tĭs)	bronchiol -itis	R S	bronchiole inflammation	Inflammation of the bronchioles
bronchitis (brŏng-kī′ tĭs)	bronch -itis	R S	bronchi inflammation	Inflammation of the bronchi
bronchoscope (brŏng′ kō-skōp)	bronch/o -scope	CF S	bronchi instrument	An instrument used to examine the bronchi
carbon dioxide (kăr bən dī-ŏk′ sīd)				A colorless, odorless gas used with oxygen to stimulate respiration
Cheyne-Stokes respiration (chān′ stōks′ rĕs″ pĭr-ā′ shŭn)				A rhythmic cycle of breathing with a gradual increase in respiration followed by apnea (which may last from 10 to 60 sec), then a repeat of the same cycle
cough (kawf)				Sudden, forceful expulsion of air from the lungs. It is an essential protective response that clears irritants, secretions, or foreign objects from the trachea, bronchi, and/or lungs.
croup (croop)				An acute respiratory disease characterized by obstruction of the larynx, a barking cough, dyspnea, hoarseness, and stridor
cyanosis (sī″ ăn-ō′ -sĭs)	cyan -osis	R S	dark blue condition of	A dark blue condition of the skin and mucous membrane caused by oxygen deficiency

MEDICAL WORD	WORD PARTS (WHEN APPLICABLE)			DEFINITION
	Part	Type	Meaning	
cystic fibrosis (sĭs′ tĭk fī-brō′ sĭs)	cyst -ic fibr -osis	R S R S	sac pertaining to fiber condition of	An inherited disease that affects the pancreas, respiratory system, and sweat glands. The gene responsible for this condition has been identified and persons carrying the gene can be determined through genetic testing.
diaphragmatocele (dī″ ă-frăg-măt′ ō-sēl)	dia phragmat/o -cele	P CF S	through partition hernia	A hernia of the diaphragm
dysphonia (dĭs-fō′ nĭ-ă)	dys phon -ia	P R S	difficult voice condition	A condition of difficulty in speaking
dyspnea (dĭsp-nē′ ă)	dys -pnea	P S	difficult breathing	Difficulty in breathing
emphysema (ĕm″ fĭ-sē′ mă)				A chronic pulmonary disease in which the bronchioles become obstructed with mucus
empyema (ĕm″ pī-ē′ mă)				Pus in a body cavity, especially the pleural cavity
endotracheal (ĕn″ dō-trā′ kē-ăl)	endo trach/e -al	P CF S	within trachea pertaining to	Pertaining to within the trachea
epistaxis (ĕp″ ĭ-stăk′ sĭs)	epi -staxis	P S	upon dripping	Nosebleed; usually results from traumatic or spontaneous rupture of blood vessels in the mucous membranes of the nose
eupnea (ūp-nē′ ă)	eu -pnea	P S	good, normal breathing	Good or normal breathing
exhalation (ĕks″ hə-lā′ shŭn)	ex halat -ion	P R S	out breathe process	The process of breathing out
expectoration (ĕk-spĕk″ tə′ rā′ shŭn)	ex pectorat -ion	P R S	out breast process	The process by which saliva, mucus, or phlegm is expelled from the air passages
Heimlich maneuver (hīm′ lĭk mă-nōō′ văr)				A technique for removing a foreign body (usually a bolus of food) that is blocking the trachea
hemoptysis (hē-mŏp′ tĭ-sĭs)	hem/o -ptysis	CF S	blood to spit	The spitting up of blood

MEDICAL WORD	WORD PARTS (WHEN APPLICABLE)			DEFINITION
	Part	**Type**	**Meaning**	
hyperpnea (hī″ pĕrp-nē′ ă)	hyper -pnea	P S	excessive breathing	Excessive or rapid breathing
hyperventilation (hī″ pĕr-vĕn″ tĭ-lā′ shŭn)	hyper ventilat -ion	P R S	excessive to air process	The process of excessive ventilating, thereby increasing the air in the lungs beyond the normal limit
hypoxia (hī-pŏks′ ĭ-ă)	hyp ox -ia	P R S	below, deficient oxygen condition	A condition of deficient amounts of oxygen in the inspired air
influenza (ĭn″ fl-ĕn′ ză)				An acute, contagious respiratory infection caused by a virus. Onset is usually sudden, and symptoms are fever, chills, headache, myalgia, cough, and sore throat.
inhalation (ĭn″ hă-lă′ shŭn)	in halat -ion	P R S	in breathe process	The process of breathing in
laryngeal (lăr-ĭn′ jĭ-ăl)	laryng/e -al	CF S	larynx pertaining to	Pertaining to the larynx
laryngitis (lăr″ ĭn-jī′ tĭs)	laryng -itis	R S	larynx inflammation	Inflammation of the larynx
laryngoscope (lăr-ĭn′ gō-skōp)	laryng/o -scope	CF S	larynx instrument	An instrument used to examine the larynx
Legionnaires' disease (lē jə naerz′ dĭ-zēz′)				A severe pulmonary pneumonia caused by *Legionella pneumophilia*
lobectomy (lō-bĕk′ tō-mē)	lob -ectomy	R S	lobe excision	Surgical excision of a lobe of any organ or gland, such as the lung
mesothelioma (mĕs″ ō-thē″ lĭ-ō′ mă)	mes/o thel/i -oma	CF CF S	middle nipple tumor	A malignant tumor of mesothelium (serous membrane of the pleura) caused by the inhalation of asbestos
nasopharyngitis (nā″ zō-făr′ ĭn-jī′ tĭs)	nas/o pharyng -itis	CF R S	nose pharynx inflammation	Inflammation of the nose and pharynx
olfaction (ŏl-făk′ shŭn)	olfact -ion	R S	smell process	The process of smelling
oropharynx (or″ ō-făr′ ĭnks)	or/o pharynx	CF R	mouth pharynx	The central portion of the throat that lies between the soft palate and upper portion of the epiglottis

MEDICAL WORD	WORD PARTS (WHEN APPLICABLE)			DEFINITION
	Part	Type	Meaning	
orthopnea (or″ thŏp-nē′ ă)	orth/o -pnea	CF S	straight breathing	Inability to breathe unless in an upright or straight position
palatopharyngo- plasty (păl″ ăt-ō-făr″ ĭn′ gō-plăs″ tē)	palat/o pharyng/o -plasty	CF CF S	palate pharynx surgical repair	A type of surgery that relieves snoring and sleep apnea by removing the uvula and the tonsils and reshaping the lining at the back of the throat to enlarge the air passageway
pertussis (pĕr-tŭs′ ĭs)				An acute, infectious disease caused by a bacterium *Bordetella pertussis*; it is characterized by a peculiar paroxysmal cough ending in a "crowing" or "whooping" sound; also called whooping cough
pharyngitis (făr″ ĭn-jī′ tĭs)	pharyng -itis	R S	pharynx inflammation	Inflammation of the pharynx
pleurisy (ploo′ rĭsē)				Inflammation of the pleura caused by injury, infection, or a tumor
pleuritis (ploo-rī′ tĭs)	pleur -itis	R S	pleura inflammation	Inflammation of the pleura
pleurodynia (ploo″ rō-dĭn′ ĭ-ă)	pleur/o -dynia	CF S	pleura pain	Pain in the pleura
pneumoconiosis (nū″ mō-kō″ nĭ-ō′ sĭs)	pneum/o con/i -osis	CF CF S	lung dust condition of	A condition of the lung caused by the inhalation of dust
pneumonia (nū-mō′ nĭ-ă)	pneumon -ia	R S	lung condition	Inflammation of the lung caused by bacteria, viruses, fungi, or chemical irritants. ✱ See Pathology Spotlight: Pneumonia.
pneumonitis (nū″ mō-nī′ tĭs)	pneumon -itis	R S	lung inflammation	Inflammation of the lung
pneumothorax (nū″ mō-thō′ răks)	pneum/o thorax	CF R	air chest	A collection of air in the chest cavity
polyp (pŏl′ ĭp)				A tumor with a stem; may occur where there are mucous membranes, such as the nose, ears, mouth, uterus, and intestines
pulmonectomy (pŭl″ mō-nĕk′ tō-mē)	pulmon -ectomy	R S	lung excision	Surgical excision of the lung or a part of a lung

MEDICAL WORD	WORD PARTS (WHEN APPLICABLE)			DEFINITION
	Part	Type	Meaning	
pyothorax (pī″ ō-thō′ răks)	py/o thorax	CF R	pus chest	Pus in the chest cavity
rale (rahl)				An abnormal sound heard on auscultation of the chest; a crackling, rattling, or bubbling sound
respirator (rĕs′ pĭ-rā″ tor)	respirat -or	R S	breathing a doer	A type of machine used for prolonged artificial respiration
respiratory distress syndrome (rĕs′ pĭ-ră-tō″ rē dĭs-trĕs′ sĭn′ drōm) **(hyaline membrane disease)**				A condition that may occur in a premature infant in which the lungs are not matured to the point of manufacturing lecithin, a pulmonary surfactant. This results in collapse of the alveoli, which leads to cyanosis and hypoxia.
rhinoplasty (rī′ nō-plăs″ tē)	rhin/o -plasty	CF S	nose surgical repair	Surgical repair of the nose
rhinorrhea (rī″ nō-rē′ ă)	rhin/o -rrhea	CF S	nose flow, discharge	Discharge from the nose
rhinovirus (rī″ nō-vī′ rŭs)	rhin/o vir -us	CF R S	nose virus pertaining to	One of a subgroup of viruses that causes the common cold (coryza) in humans
rhonchus (rŏng′ kŭs)	rhonch -us	R S	snore pertaining to	A rale or rattling sound in the throat or bronchial tubes caused by a partial obstruction
sarcoidosis (sar″ koyd-ō′ sĭs)	sarc -oid -osis	R S S	flesh resemble condition of	A chronic granulomatous condition that may involve almost any organ system of the body. The lungs are usually involved and this causes dyspnea on exertion
severe acute respiratory syndrome (SARS) (si-vir′ ă-kūt′ rĕs′ pĭ-ră-tō″ -rē sin′ drōm)				A contagious respiratory infection that was first described in February, 2003. SARS is a serious form of pneumonia, resulting in acute respiratory distress and sometimes death.
sinusitis (sī″ nūs-ī′ tĭs)	sinus -itis	R S	a curve, hollow inflammation	Inflammation of a sinus
spirometer (spī-rŏm′ ĕt-ĕr)	spir/o -meter	CF S	breath instrument to measure	An instrument used to measure the volume of respired air

MEDICAL WORD	WORD PARTS (WHEN APPLICABLE)			DEFINITION
	Part	Type	Meaning	
sputum (spū′ tŭm)				Substance coughed up from the lungs; may be watery, thick, purulent, clear, or bloody and may contain microorganisms
stridor (strī′ dōr)				A high-pitched sound caused by obstruction of the air passageway
tachypnea (tăk″ ĭp-nē′ ă)	tachy -pnea	P S	fast breathing	Fast breathing
thoracocentesis (thō″ răk-ō-sĕn-tē′ sĭs)	thorac/o -centesis	CF S	chest surgical puncture	Surgical puncture of the chest for removal of fluid
thoracoplasty (thō′ ră-kō-plăs″ tē)	thorac/o -plasty	CF S	chest surgical repair	Surgical repair of the chest
thoracotomy (thō″ răk- ŏt′ ō-mē)	thorac/o -tomy	CF S	chest incision	Incision of the chest
tonsillectomy (tŏn″ sĭl-ĕk′ tō-mē)	tonsil -ectomy	R S	almond, tonsil excision	Surgical excision of the tonsils
tonsillitis (tŏn″ sĭl-ī′ tĭs)	tonsil -itis	R S	almond, tonsil inflammation	Inflammation of the tonsils
tracheal (trā′ kē-ăl)	trach/e -al	CF S	trachea pertaining to	Pertaining to the trachea
trachealgia (trā″ kē-ăl′ jĭ-ă)	trach/e -algia	CF S	trachea pain	Pain in the trachea
tracheolaryngotomy (trā″ kē-ō-lăr″ ĭn-gŏt′ ō-mē)	trache/o laryng/o -tomy	CF CF S	trachea larynx incision	Incision into the larynx and trachea
tracheostomy (trā″ kē-ŏs′ tō-mē)	trache/o -stomy	CF S	trachea new opening	New opening into the trachea
tuberculosis (tū-bĕr″ kū-lō′ sĭs)	tubercul -osis	R S	a little swelling condition of	An infectious disease caused by the tubercle bacillus, *Mycobacterium tuberculosis*. ✱ See Pathology Spotlight: Tuberculosis.
wheeze (hwēz)				A whistling sound caused by obstruction of the air passageway

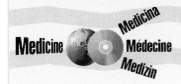
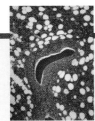

PATHOLOGY SPOTLIGHTS

Apnea

Apnea is defined as a temporary cessation of breathing. Sleep apnea is cessation of breathing during sleep. The disruption of sleep patterns due to an obstruction of airways affects about 18 million Americans. To be so classified, the apnea must last for at least 10 seconds and occur 30 or more times during a 7-hour period of sleep. This definition may not apply to older adults, in whom periods of sleep apnea are increased. Sleep apnea is classified according to the mechanisms involved.

- Obstructive apnea is caused by obstruction to the upper airway. This condition generally occurs in middle-aged men who are obese and have a history of excessive daytime sleepiness. It is associated with loud snorting, snoring, and gasping sounds.

- Central apnea is marked by absence of respiratory muscle activity. A person with this type of apnea may exhibit excessive daytime sleepiness, but the snorting and gasping sounds during sleep are absent.

Sleep deprivation can make a person tired, sluggish, irritable, prone to accidents, and less productive. Although the amount of sleep needed is different for every person, adults need at least 7 hours of sleep in a 24-hour period, children under the age of 10 need 11 to 13 hours of sleep, and teenagers need 10 to 12 hours of sleep.

Asthma

Asthma is an inflammatory disease of the bronchi characterized by wheezing, dyspnea, and a feeling of constriction in the chest. Inflammation of the airways causes airflow into and out of the lungs to be restricted. During an asthma attack, the muscles of the bronchial tree constrict and the lining of the air passages swells, reducing airflow and producing the characteristic wheezing sound. See Figure 9–4.

Most people with asthma experience periodic wheezing attacks as well as symptom-free periods. Specific symptoms can vary. Some asthmatics have chronic shortness of breath with episodes of increased shortness of breath. Other asthmatics may have cough as their predominant symptom. The duration of asthma attacks varies, from minutes to days. The attack can become dangerous if the airflow becomes severely restricted.

In asthma-prone individuals, symptoms can be triggered by inhaled allergens, such as pet dander, dust mites, cockroach allergens, molds, or pollens. A variety of other situations can also trigger symptoms, including respiratory infections, exercise, cold air, tobacco smoke and other pollutants, stress, and food or drug allergies. Aspirin and other non-steroidal anti-inflammatory drugs (NSAIDs) provoke asthma in some patients.

Asthma occurs in 3 to 5 percent of adults and 7 to 10 percent of children. Most people with asthma develop it before age 30, and half develop it before age 10. Asthma symptoms can decrease over time, especially in children. Many people with asthma have an individual and/or

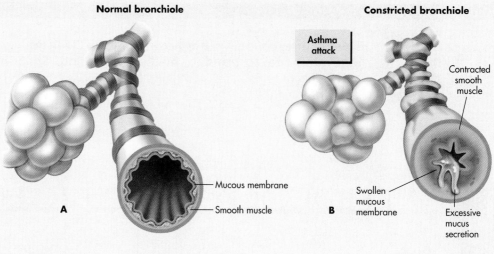

Normal bronchiole

Constricted bronchiole

Asthma attack

Contracted smooth muscle

Mucous membrane

Smooth muscle

A

B

Swollen mucous membrane

Excessive mucus secretion

FIGURE 9–4

Changes in bronchioles during an asthma attack: (A) normal bronchiole; and (B) in asthma attack.

family history of allergies, such as hay fever (allergic rhinitis) or eczema. Others have no history of allergies or evidence of allergic problems.

The goal of treatment is to avoid known allergens and respiratory irritants and control symptoms and airway inflammation through medication. Two basic types of medication are used to treat asthma. The first type, long-term control medications such as inhaled glucocorticoids, are used on a regular basis to prevent attacks (not for treatment during an attack). The second type, quick relief (rescue) medications such as short-acting bronchodilators, are used to relieve symptoms during an attack.

Allergens can sometimes be identified by noting which substances cause an allergic reaction. Allergy testing may also be helpful in identifying allergens in patients with persistent asthma.

Pneumonia

Pneumonia is an inflammation of the lung (or lungs) caused by many different organisms such as bacteria, viruses, fungi, and chemical irritants. Bacterial pneumonias tend to be the most serious. In adults, bacteria are the most common cause of pneumonia, and of these *Streptococcus pneumoniae* (pneumococcus) is the most common. In some people, particularly the elderly and those who are debilitated, pneumonia may follow influenza.

Pneumonia affects 3–4 million people each year in the United States. Symptoms include a cough with greenish mucus or pus-like sputum, chills, fever, fatigue, chest pain, and muscle aches. Initial diagnosis is made through auscultation of the chest with a stethoscope. In patients with pneumonia, rales and other abnormal breathing sounds may be heard. Tests that are used to confirm the diagnosis include a chest x-ray (Fig. 9–5) and a sputum culture.

Treatment of pneumonia is determined by the organism that caused it. If the cause is bacterial, the infection is treated with antibiotics. However, if the pneumonia is caused by a virus, antibiotics will not be effective. Supportive therapy includes oxygen and respiratory treatments to remove secretions, if needed.

Tuberculosis

Tuberculosis (TB) is a contagious disease caused by the bacillus *Mycobacterium tuberculosis*. This bacillus is carried in airborne particles, known as droplets. An infected person releases large and small droplets through talking, coughing, sneezing, laughing, or singing. The large droplets set-

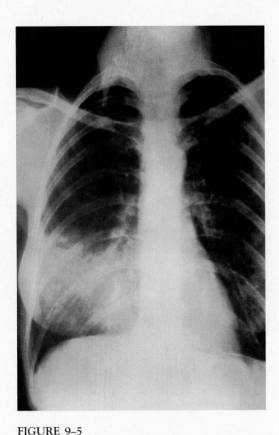

FIGURE 9–5

Lobar pneumonia. (Source: Photo Researchers, Inc.)

tle, while the small droplets remain suspended in the air and can be inhaled by a susceptible person. Virtually anyone who comes in contact with an infected person is at risk of contracting TB.

Symptoms of TB depend on where in the body the TB bacteria are growing. The disease is characterized by the development of granulomas (granular tumors) in the infected tissues. TB bacteria usually grow in the lungs and symptoms include a chronic cough, hemoptysis, and in the early stages, scanty, whitish or grayish-yellow frothy sputum. Other symptoms are fatigue, low-grade fever, night sweats, weakness, chills, anorexia, and weight loss.

Diagnosis includes examination of the lungs by stethoscope (auscultation), which can reveal rales or crackles. Enlarged or tender lymph nodes may be present in the neck or other areas. Fluid may be detectable around a lung (pleural effusion). Tests to confirm diagnosis often include a chest x-ray, sputum cultures, a tuberculin skin test, and bronchoscopy. Rarely, biopsy of the affected tissue (typically lungs, pleura, or lymph nodes) is required.

Treatment of TB requires long-term drug therapy (9 to 12 months), often using a regimen that includes a combination of antituberculosis agents. The primary drug regimen for active tuberculosis combines the drugs *rifampin*, *isoniazid*, and *ethambutol HCl*. Diet and rest are also important aspects of the treatment regimen.

Multidrug-resistant tuberculosis (MDR TB) occurs when the TB bacteria become resistant to two or more of the drugs that are used to treat tuberculosis. Appropriate measures must be instituted promptly to treat and prevent the spread of MDR TB.

Infants, the elderly, and individuals who are immunocompromised (for example, those with AIDS, those undergoing chemotherapy, or transplant recipients taking antirejection medications) are at higher risk for developing tuberculosis.

TB is still a major cause of death worldwide, killing 2 million people each year. An estimated 10 million people in the United States are infected with the TB bacterium. At the present time TB occurs primarily among AIDS patients, the homeless, drug abusers, prison inmates, and immigrants.

✓ PATHOLOGY CHECKPOINT

Following is a concise list of the pathology-related terms that you've seen in the chapter. Review this checklist to make sure that you are familiar with the meaning of each term before moving on to the next section.

Conditions and Symptoms

- ❏ anthracosis
- ❏ aphasia
- ❏ apnea
- ❏ asphyxia
- ❏ asthma
- ❏ atelectasis
- ❏ bronchiectasis
- ❏ bronchiolitis
- ❏ bronchitis
- ❏ Cheyne-Stokes respiration
- ❏ cough
- ❏ croup
- ❏ cyanosis
- ❏ cystic fibrosis
- ❏ diaphragmatocele
- ❏ dysphonia
- ❏ dyspnea
- ❏ emphysema
- ❏ empyema
- ❏ epistaxis
- ❏ eupnea
- ❏ hemoptysis
- ❏ hyperpnea
- ❏ hyperventilation

- ❏ hypoxia
- ❏ influenza
- ❏ laryngitis
- ❏ Legionnaires' disease
- ❏ mesothelioma
- ❏ nasopharyngitis
- ❏ orthopnea
- ❏ pertussis
- ❏ pharyngitis
- ❏ pleurisy
- ❏ pleuritis
- ❏ pleurodynia
- ❏ pneumoconiosis
- ❏ pneumonia
- ❏ pneumonitis
- ❏ pneumothorax
- ❏ polyp
- ❏ pyothorax
- ❏ rale
- ❏ respiratory distress syndrome (hyaline membrane disease)
- ❏ rhinorrhea
- ❏ rhonchus
- ❏ sarcoidosis
- ❏ severe acute respiratory syndrome (SARS)

- ❏ sinusitis
- ❏ sputum
- ❏ stridor
- ❏ tachypnea
- ❏ tonsillitis
- ❏ trachealgia
- ❏ tuberculosis
- ❏ wheeze

Diagnosis and Treatment

- ❏ bronchoscope
- ❏ laryngoscope
- ❏ lobectomy
- ❏ palatopharyngoplasty
- ❏ pulmonectomy
- ❏ respirator
- ❏ rhinoplasty
- ❏ spirometer
- ❏ thoracocentesis
- ❏ thoracoplasty
- ❏ thoracotomy
- ❏ tonsillectomy
- ❏ tracheolaryngotomy
- ❏ tracheostomy

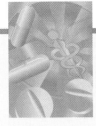

DRUG HIGHLIGHTS

Drugs that are generally used in respiratory system diseases and disorders include antihistamines, decongestants, antitussives, expectorants, mucolytics, bronchodilators, inhalational glucocorticoids, and antituberculosis agents. See Figure 9–6.

Antihistamines

Act to counter the effects of histamine by blocking histamine 1 (H_1) receptors. They are used in the treatment of allergy symptoms, for preventing or controlling motion sickness, and in combination with cold remedies to decrease mucus secretion and produce bedtime sedation.

Examples: Benadryl (diphenhydramine HCl), Dimetane (brompheniramine maleate), Allegra (fexofenadine), Claritin (loratadine), and Zyrtec (cetirizine).

Decongestants

Act to constrict dilated arterioles in the nasal mucosa. These agents are used for the temporary relief of nasal congestion associated with the common cold, hay fever, other upper respiratory allergies, and sinusitis.

Examples: Sudafed (pseudoephedrine HCl), Coricidin (phenylephrine HCl), Sinutab Long-Lasting Sinus Spray (xylometazoline HCl), and Afrin (oxymetazoline HCl).

Antitussives
Non-narcotic agents

May be classified as non-narcotic and narcotic.
Anesthetize the stretch receptors located in the respiratory passages, lungs, and pleura by dampening their activity and thereby reducing the cough reflex at its source.

Examples: Tessalon (benzonatate), Benylin (diphenhydramine HCl), and dextromethorphan hydrobromide.

Narcotic agents

Depress the cough center that is located in the medulla, thereby raising its threshold for incoming cough impulse.

Examples: codeine and Codimal (hydrocodone bitartrate).

Expectorants

Promote and facilitate the removal of mucus from the lower respiratory tract.

Examples: Robitussin (guaifenesin) and SSKI (saturated solution of potassium iodide).

Mucolytics

Break chemical bonds in mucus, thereby lowering its thickness.

Example: Mucomyst (acetylcysteine).

Bronchodilators

Are used to improve pulmonary airflow.

Examples: Adrenalin (epinephrine), Proventil (albuterol), ephedrine sulfate, aminophylline, and Theo-24 (theophylline).

Inhalational Glucocorticoids

Used in the treatment of bronchial asthma, and in seasonal or perennial allergic conditions when other forms of treatment are not effective.

Examples: Beclovent (beclomethasone dipropionate), Azmacort (triamcinolone acetonide), Flovent (fluticasone), and Aerobid (flunisolide).

Antituberculosis Agents

Used in the long-term treatment of tuberculosis (9 months to 1 year). They are often used in *combination of two or more drugs and the primary drug regimen for active tuberculosis combines the drugs Myambutol (ethambutol HCl); INH, Nydrazid (isoniazid); and Rifadin, Rimactane (rifampin).*

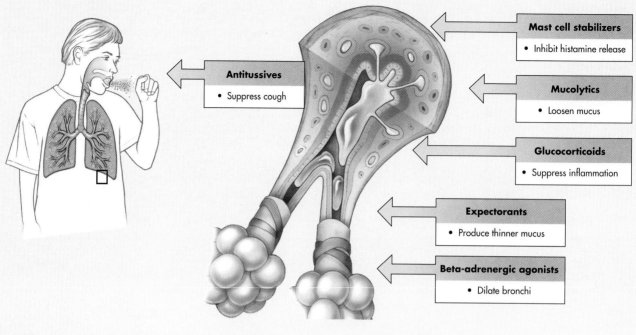

FIGURE 9–6

Drugs used to treat respiratory disorders.

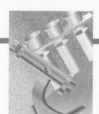

DIAGNOSTIC & LAB TESTS

TEST	DESCRIPTION
acid-fast bacilli (AFB) (ăs ĭd-făst″ bă-sĭl′ ī)	A test performed on sputum to detect the presence of *Mycobacterium tuberculosis*, an acid-fast bacilli. Positive results indicate tuberculosis.
antistreptolysin O (ASO) (ăn″ tĭ-strĕp-tŏl′ ĭ-sĭn)	A test performed on blood serum to detect the presence of streptolysin enzyme O, which is secreted by beta-hemolytic streptococcus. Positive results indicate streptococcal infection.
arterial blood gases (ABGs) (ăr-tē′ rē-ăl blod găs′ ĕs)	A series of tests performed on arterial blood to establish acid–base balance. Important in determining respiratory acidosis and/or alkalosis, metabolic acidosis and/or alkalosis.
bronchoscopy (brŏng-kŏs′ kō-pē)	Visual examination of the larynx, trachea, and bronchi via a flexible bronchoscope. With the use of biopsy forceps, tissues and secretions can be removed for further analysis.
culture, sputum (kŭl tūr, spū tŭm)	Examination of the sputum to determine the presence of microorganisms. Abnormal results may indicate tuberculosis, bronchitis, pneumonia, bronchiectasis, and other infectious respiratory diseases.
culture, throat (kŭl′ tūr, thrōt)	A test done to identify the presence of microorganisms in the throat, especially beta-hemolytic streptococci.

TEST	DESCRIPTION
laryngoscopy (lăr″ ĭn-gŏs′ kō-pē)	Visual examination of the larynx via a laryngoscope.
nasopharyngography (nā″ zō-făr-ĭn-ŏg′ ră-fē)	X-ray examination of the nasopharynx.
pulmonary function test (pŭl′ mō-nĕ-rē fŭng′ shŭn test)	A series of tests performed to determine the diffusion of oxygen and carbon dioxide across the cell membrane in the lungs. Tests included are: tidal volume (TV), vital capacity (VC), expiratory reserve volume (ERV), inspiratory capacity (IC), residual volume (RV), forced inspiratory volume (FIV), functional residual capacity (FRC), maximal voluntary ventilation (MVV), total lung capacity (TLC), and flow volume loop (F-V loop). Abnormal results may indicate various respiratory diseases and conditions.
rhinoscopy (rī-nŏs′ kō-pē)	Visual examination of the nasal passages.

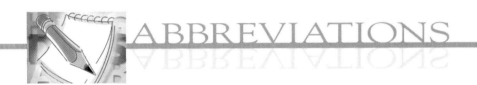

ABBREVIATIONS

ABBREVIATION	MEANING	ABBREVIATION	MEANING
ABGs	arterial blood gases	MBC	maximal breathing capacity
AFB	acid-fast bacilli	MV	minute volume
ARD	acute respiratory disease	MVV	maximal voluntary ventilation
ARDS	adult respiratory distress syndrome	O_2	oxygen
CF	cystic fibrosis	PE	pulmonary embolism
CO_2	carbon dioxide	PEEP	positive end-expiratory pressure
COLD	chronic obstructive lung disease	PND	postnasal drip, paroxysmal nocturnal dyspnea
COPD	chronic obstructive pulmonary disease	PPD	purified protein derivative
CXR	chest x-ray	R	respiration
ENT	ear, nose, and throat	RD	respiratory disease
ERV	expiratory reserve volume	RDS	respiratory distress syndrome
ET	endotracheal	SARS	severe acute respiratory syndrome
FEF	forced expiratory flow	SIDS	sudden infant death syndrome
FEV	forced expiratory volume	SOB	shortness of breath
HBOT	hyperbaric oxygen therapy	T & A	tonsillectomy and adenoidectomy
HMD	hyaline membrane disease	TB	tuberculosis
IPPB	intermittent positive-pressure breathing	TLC	total lung capacity
IRDS	infant respiratory distress syndrome	TV	tidal volume
		URI	upper respiratory infection
IRV	inspiratory reserve volume	VC	vital capacity

STUDY AND REVIEW

Anatomy and Physiology

Write your answers to the following questions. Do not refer to the text.

1. List the organs of the respiratory system.

   a. _____   b. _____

   c. _____   d. _____

   e. _____   f. _____

2. State the primary function of the respiratory system. _____

   _____

3. Define external respiration. _____

4. Define internal respiration. _____

5. List the five functions of the nose.

   a. _____

   b. _____

   c. _____

   d. _____

   e. _____

6. Name the three divisions of the pharynx.

   a. _____   b. _____

   c. _____

7. List the three functions of the pharynx.

   a. _____

   b. _____

   c. _____

8. State the function of the epiglottis. _____

9. Define glottis. _____

10. State the function of the larynx. _____

11. State the function of the trachea. _____

12. The trachea divides into the _____ _____ and

    the _____ _____.

13. State the function of the bronchi. _____

14. Give a brief description of the lungs. _____

    _____

15. Define pleura. _____

16. The thoracic cavity is separated from the abdominal cavity by a musculomem-

    branous wall commonly known as the _____.

17. The central portion of the thoracic cavity, between the lungs, is a space called

    the _____.

18. The right lung has _____ lobes and the left lung has _____ lobes.

19. The air cells of the lungs are the _____.

20. State the main function of the lungs. _____

    _____.

21. The vital signs, which are essential elements for determining an individual's state

    of health, are _____, _____, _____, and _____.

22. Define the following terms:

    a. Tidal volume _____

    b. Residual volume _____

    c. Vital capacity _____

23. The _____ _____ and the _____ of the central nervous
    system regulate and control respiration.

24. The respiratory rate for a newborn is _____ to _____ breaths per
    minute.

25. The respiratory rate for an adult is _____ to _____ breaths per
    minute.

Word Parts

1. In the spaces provided, write the definition of these prefixes, roots, combining forms, and suffixes. Do not refer to the listings of medical words. Leave blank those words you cannot define.

2. After completing as many as you can, refer to the medical word listings to check your work. For each word missed or left blank, write the word and its definition several times on the margins of these pages or on a separate sheet of paper.

3. To maximize the learning process, it is to your advantage to do the following exercises as directed. To refer to the word building section before completing these exercises invalidates the learning process.

PREFIXES

Give the definitions of the following prefixes:

1. a- _____

2. epi- _____

3. dia- _____

4. dys- _____

5. endo- _____

6. eu- _____

7. ex- _____

8. hyp- _____

9. hyper- _____

10. in- _____

11. tachy- _____

ROOTS AND COMBINING FORMS

Give the definitions of the following roots and combining forms:

1. aspirat _____

2. alveol _____

3. anthrac _____

4. atel _____

5. bronch _____

6. bronch/i _____

7. bronchiol _____

8. bronch/o _____

9. con/i _____

10. cyan _____

11. halat _____

12. hem/o _____

13. laryng _____

14. larynge _____

15. laryng/o _____

16. lob _____

17. cyst _____

18. fibr _____

19. nas/o _____

20. orth/o _____

21. mes/o _____

22. tubercul _____

23. palat/o _____

24. pectorat _____

25. pharyng _____

26. pharyng/o _____

27. thel/i _____

28. phragmat/o _____

29. phas _____

30. pleur _____

31. pleura _____

32. pleur/o _____

33. pneum/o _____

34. pneumon _____

35. pulm/o _____

36. pulmon _____

37. py/o _____

38. rhin/o _____

39. sinus _____

40. spir/o _____

41. respirat _____

42. thorac/o _____

43. ventilat _____

44. tonsill _____

45. trach/e _____

46. trache/o _____

47. rhonch _____

48. sarc _____

SUFFIXES

Give the definitions of the following suffixes:

1. -al _____

2. -algia _____

3. -cele _____

4. -centesis _____

5. -dynia _____

6. -ectasis _____

7. -ectomy _____

8. -ic _____

9. -ia _____

10. -ion _____

11. -itis _____

12. -meter _____

13. -osis _____

14. -oma _____

15. -staxis _____

16. -plasty _____

17. -or _____

18. -pnea _____

19. -ptysis _____

20. -rrhea _____

21. -scope _____

22. -stomy _____

23. -tomy _____

24. -us _____

Identifying Medical Terms

In the spaces provided, write the medical terms for the following meanings:

1. _____ Pertaining to a small air sac in the lungs

2. _____ Dilation of the bronchi

3. _____ Inflammation of the bronchi

4. _____ Difficulty in speaking

5. _____ Good or normal breathing

6. _____ The spitting up of blood

7. _____ The process of breathing in

8. _____ Inflammation of the larynx

9. _____ A collection of air in the chest cavity

10. _____ Surgical repair of the nose

11. _____ Discharge from the nose

12. _____ Inflammation of a sinus

Spelling

In the spaces provided, write the correct spelling of these misspelled words.

1. bronchscope _____

2. diaphramatcele _____

3. expectorion _____

4. laryngal _____

5. orthpnea _____

6. peluritis _____

7. pulmnectomy _____

8. rhoncus _____

9. trachypnea _____

10. trachal _____

Matching

Select the appropriate lettered meaning for each word listed below.

_____ 1. cough

_____ 2. cystic fibrosis

_____ 3. influenza

_____ 4. inhalation

_____ 5. olfaction

_____ 6. pleurodynia

_____ 7. rhinovirus

_____ 8. sputum

_____ 9. tachypnea

_____10. thoracocentesis

a. Substance coughed up from the lungs
b. Pain in the pleura
c. The process of smelling
d. One of a subgroup of viruses that causes the common cold in humans
e. Fast breathing
f. The process of breathing in
g. Surgical puncture of the chest for removal of fluid
h. Sudden, forceful expulsion of air from the lungs
i. An inherited disease that affects the pancreas, respiratory system, and sweat glands
j. Slow breathing
k. An acute, contagious respiratory infection caused by a virus

Abbreviations

Place the correct word, phrase, or abbreviation in the space provided.

1. acid-fast bacilli _____

2. CF _____

3. Chest x-ray _____

4. chronic obstructive lung disease _____

5. ET _____

6. PND _____

7. respiration _____

8. SIDS _____

9. shortness of breath _____

10. TB _____

Diagnostic and Laboratory Tests

Select the best answer to each multiple choice question. Circle the letter of your choice.

1. A test performed on sputum to detect the presence of *Mycobacterium tuberculosis*.
   a. antistreptolysin O
   b. acid-fast bacilli
   c. pulmonary function test
   d. bronchoscopy

2. The visual examination of the nasal passages.
   a. bronchoscopy
   b. laryngoscopy
   c. rhinoscopy
   d. nasopharyngography

3. _____ is/are important in determining respiratory acidosis and/or alkalosis, metabolic acidosis and/or alkalosis.
   a. Acid-fast bacilli
   b. Antistreptolysin O
   c. Arterial blood gases
   d. Pulmonary function test

4. A series of tests to determine the diffusion of oxygen and carbon dioxide across the cell membrane in the lungs.
   a. acid-fast bacilli
   b. antistreptolysin O
   c. arterial blood gases
   d. pulmonary function test

5. The visual examination of the larynx, trachea, and bronchi via a flexible scope.
   a. bronchoscopy
   b. laryngoscopy
   c. nasopharyngography
   d. rhinoscopy

CASE STUDY

Please read the following case study and then answer the questions that follow.

A 28-year-old male was seen by a physician and the following is a synopsis of the visit.

Present History: The patient states that he has had a persistent cough for the past 3 weeks, is very tired, has lost 8 lb recently, doesn't have an appetite, and wakes up in the middle of the night soaked in sweat.

Signs and Symptoms: Chronic cough, fatigue, night sweats, weakness, anorexia, and weight loss.

Diagnosis: Pulmonary tuberculosis. The diagnosis was determined by a physical examination, a sputum culture that was positive for *Mycobacterium tuberculosis*, a positive PPD (purified protein derivative) test, and a chest x-ray that revealed lesions in the upper right lobe.

Treatment: The physician ordered a regimen of diet, rest, and a combination of three antituberculosis agents: *isoniazid*, *rifampin*, and *ethambutol*. The medication is to be taken as ordered for 9 months. A follow-up visit was scheduled for 2 weeks.

Prevention: Avoid exposure to *Mycobacterium tuberculosis* bacillus. The Centers for Disease Control and Prevention has published a booklet on *Guidelines for Preventing the Transmission of Tuberculosis in Health-Care Settings*. The following are specific actions to reduce the risk of tuberculosis transmission:

- Screening patients for active TB and TB infection
- Providing rapid diagnostic services
- Prescribing an appropriate curative and preventive therapy
- Maintaining physical measures to reduce microbial contamination of the air
- Providing isolation rooms for persons with, or suspected of having, infectious TB
- Screening health-care-facility personnel for TB infection
- Promptly investigating and controlling outbreaks

CASE STUDY QUESTIONS

1. Signs and symptoms of pulmonary tuberculosis include a chronic cough, fatigue, night sweats, weakness, _____, and weight loss.

2. The diagnosis was determined by a physical examination, a positive PPD test, and a positive sputum culture for _____ _____ bacillus.

3. Treatment included diet, rest, and a medication regimen of three antituberculosis agents: _____, rifampin, and ethambutol.

4. What does the abbreviation PPD mean? _____

 MedMedia Wrap-Up
www.prenhall.com/rice

Additional interactive resources and activities for this chapter can be found on the Companion Website. For animations, videos, audio glossary, and review, access the accompanying CD-ROM in this book.

 Audio Glossary
Medical Terminology Exercises & Activities
Pathology Spotlight
Terminology Translator
Animations
Videos

Objectives
Medical Terminology Exercises & Activities
Audio Glossary
Drug Updates
Medical Terminology in the News

THE URINARY SYSTEM 10

OBJECTIVES

On completion of this chapter, you will be able to:

- Describe the organs of the urinary system.
- State the vital function of the urinary system.
- Describe the formation of urine.
- Describe urinalysis.
- Identify the normal constituents of urine.
- Identify abnormal constituents of urine.
- Analyze, build, spell, and pronounce medical words.
- Describe each of the conditions presented in the Pathology Spotlights.
- Complete the Pathology Checkpoint.
- Review Drug Highlights presented in this chapter.
- Provide the description of diagnostic and laboratory tests related to the urinary system.
- Identify and define selected abbreviations.
- Successfully complete the study and review section.

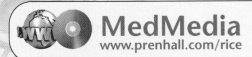

MedMedia
www.prenhall.com/rice

Additional interactive resources and activities for this chapter can be found on the Companion Website. For Terminology Translator, animations, videos, audio glossary, and review, access the accompanying CD-ROM in this book.

Anatomy and Physiology Overview

The urinary system consists of two **kidneys,** two **ureters,** one **bladder,** and one **urethra** (Fig. 10–1). It may be referred to as the excretory system, genitourinary system, or urogenital system. The vital function of the urinary system is extraction of certain wastes from the bloodstream, conversion of these materials to urine, transport of the urine from the kidneys via the ureters to the bladder, and elimination of it at appropriate intervals via the urethra. Through this vital function, homeostasis of body fluids is maintained. See Figure 10–2.

THE KIDNEYS

The **kidneys** are purplish-brown, bean-shaped organs located at the back of the abdominal cavity (*retroperitoneal area*). They lie, one on each side of the spinal column, just above the waistline, against the muscles of the back. Each kidney is surrounded by three capsules; the **true capsule,** the **perirenal fat,** and the **renal fascia.** The true capsule is a smooth, fibrous connective membrane that is loosely adherent to the surface of the kidney. The perirenal fat is the adipose capsule that embeds each kidney in fatty tissue. The renal fascia is a sheath of fibrous tissue that helps to anchor the kidney to the surrounding structures and helps to maintain its normal position.

External Structure

Each kidney has a *concave* border and a *convex* border. The center of the concave border opens into a notch called the **hilum.** The renal artery and vein, nerves, and lymphatic vessels enter and leave through the hilum. The ureter enters the kidney through the hilum into a sac-like collecting portion called the *renal pelvis*.

Internal Structure

When a cross section is made through the kidney, two distinct areas are seen comprising its anterior: the **cortex,** which is the outer layer, and the **medulla** or inner portion. The cortex contains the arteries, veins, convoluted tubules, and glomerular capsules. The medulla contains the renal pyramids, cone-like masses with papillae projecting into calyces of the pelvis.

THE URINARY SYSTEM

Organ/Structure	Primary Functions
Kidneys	Produce urine and help regulate body fluids
Ureters	Transport urine from the kidneys to the bladder
Urinary Bladder	Serves as a reservoir for urine
Urethra	Conveys urine to the outside of the body; in the male conveys both urine and semen

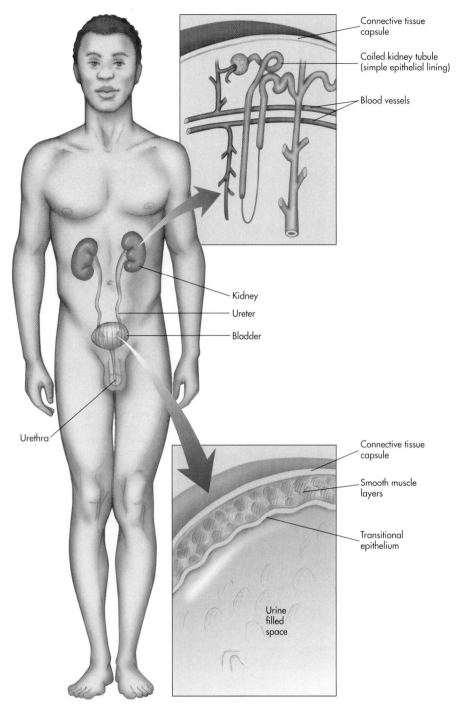

FIGURE 10–1

The urinary system: kidneys, ureters, bladder, and urethra with expanded view of a nephron and the urine-filled space within a bladder.

Microscopic Anatomy

Microscopic examination of the kidney reveals about 1 million **nephrons**, which are the structural and functional units of the organ. Each nephron consists of a **renal corpuscle** and **tubule**. The renal corpuscle or malpighian body consists of a glomerulus and Bowman's capsule. Extending from each **Bowman's capsule** is a tubule consisting of the proximal convoluted portion, the loop of Henle, and a distal convoluted portion that opens into a collecting tubule.

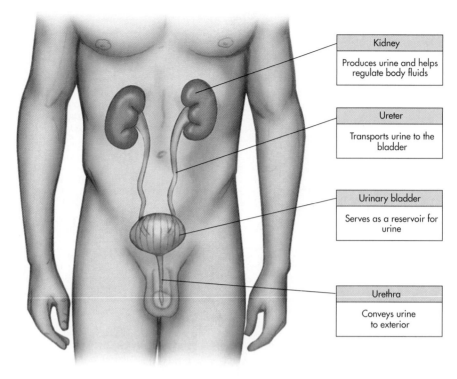

FIGURE 10–2

The organs of the urinary system with major functions.

The Nephron

The vital function of the **nephron** is to remove the waste products of metabolism from the blood plasma. These waste products are urea, uric acid, and creatinine, plus any excess sodium, chloride, and potassium ions and ketone bodies. The nephron plays a vital role in the maintenance of normal fluid balance in the body by allowing for reabsorption of water and some electrolytes back into the blood. Approximately 1000 to 1200 mL of blood pass through the kidney per minute. At a rate of 1000 mL of blood per minute about 1.5 million mL pass through the kidney in each 24-hour day (Fig. 10–3).

THE URETERS

There are two **ureters**, one for each kidney. They are narrow, muscular tubes that transport urine from the kidneys to the bladder. They are from 28 to 34 cm long and vary in diameter from 1 mm to 1 cm. The walls of the ureters consist of three layers: an inner coat of mucous membrane, a middle coat of smooth muscle, and an outer coat of fibrous tissue.

THE URINARY BLADDER

The **urinary bladder** is the muscular, membranous sac that serves as a reservoir for urine. It is located in the anterior portion of the pelvic cavity and consists of a lower portion, the **neck**, which is continuous with the urethra, and an upper portion, the

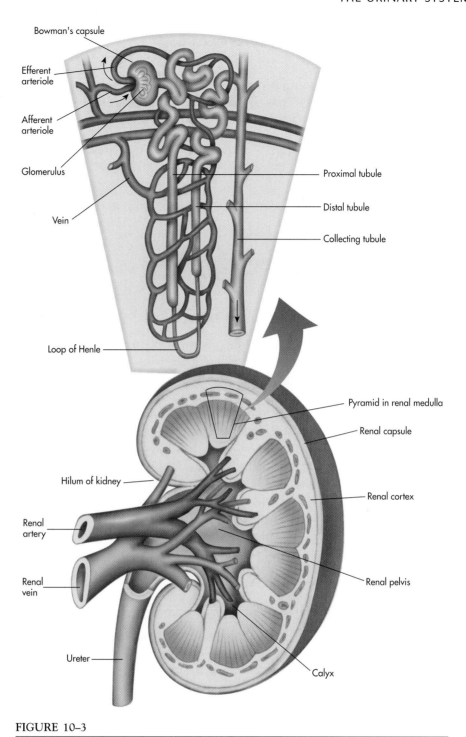

Bowman's capsule

Efferent
arteriole

Afferent
arteriole

Glomerulus

Vein

Proximal tubule

Distal tubule

Collecting tubule

Loop of Henle

Pyramid in renal medulla

Renal capsule

Hilum of kidney

Renal cortex

Renal
artery

Renal
vein

Renal pelvis

Ureter

Calyx

FIGURE 10–3

The kidney with an expanded view of a nephron.

apex, which is connected with the umbilicus by the median umbilical ligament. The **trigone** is a small triangular area near the base of the bladder. The wall of the bladder consists of four layers: an inner layer of epithelium, a muscular coat of smooth muscle, an outer layer comprised of longitudinal muscle (*detrusor urinae*), and a fibrous layer. An empty bladder feels firm as the muscular wall becomes thick. As the bladder fills with urine, the muscular wall becomes thinner and it distends according to the amount of urine present.

THE URETHRA

The **urethra** is the musculomembranous tube extending from the bladder to the outside of the body. The external urinary opening is the **urinary meatus**. The male urethra is approximately 20 cm long and is divided into three sections: *prostatic, membranous,* and *penile.* It conveys both urine and semen. The female urethra is approximately 3 cm long. The urinary meatus is situated between the clitoris and the opening of the vagina. The female urethra conveys only urine.

URINE

The Formation of Urine

Urine is formed by the process of *filtration* and *reabsorption* in the nephron. Blood enters the nephron via the afferent arteriole. As it passes through the glomerulus, water and dissolved substances are filtered through the glomerular membrane and collect in the Bowman's capsule. The glomerular filtrate passes through the proximal tubule, into the loop of Henle, into the distal tubule, and then into the collecting tubule. Water and some selected substances are reabsorbed into the capillaries surrounding the tubules. Substances such as uric acid and hydrogen ions, through the process of secretion, may be added to the fluid now known as urine. Urine consists of 95% water and 5% solid substances. It is secreted by the kidneys and transported by the ureters to the bladder, where it is stored before being discharged from the body via the urethra. An average normal adult feels the need to void when the bladder contains around 300 to 350 mL of urine. An average of 1000 to 1500 mL of urine is voided daily. Normal urine is clear, is yellow to amber in color, and has a faintly aromatic odor, a specific gravity of 1.003 to 1.030, and a slightly acid pH.

Urinalysis

Urinalysis is a laboratory procedure that may involve the physical, chemical, and microscopic examination of urine. A freshly voided urine specimen will provide for more accurate test results as certain changes may occur in urine that is left standing. If the urinalysis cannot be performed on the specimen within 1 hour of the time voided, it should be refrigerated, with the time of collection written on the label of the container. Urine should be collected in a clean, dry container. A disposable container is preferred. When a bacteriologic culture is to be done on urine, the specimen is collected by **catheterization**.

Urinalysis is a valuable diagnostic tool, as abnormal conditions or diseases may be quickly and easily detected because of the fact that the physical and chemical constituents of normal urine are constant. See Table 10–1.

TABLE 10–1 NORMAL AND ABNORMAL CONSTITUENTS OF URINE

Constituent	Normal	Abnormal/Significance
Color	Yellow to amber	Red or reddish — presence of hemoglobin Orange — due to pyridum or santonin Greenish-brown or black — caused by bile pigments. *The color of urine darkens upon standing.*
Appearance	Clear	Milky — fat globules, pus, bacteria Smoky — blood cells Hazy — refrigeration
Reaction	Acid, between 5.0 to 7.0 pH, with an average of 6.0	High acidity — diabetic acidosis, fever, diarrhea, dehydration Alkaline (pH of 8-14) — chronic cystitis, urinary tract infection, renal failure
Specific Gravity	Between 1.003 and 1.030	Low (1.001 to 1.002) — diabetes insipidus High (over 1.030) — diabetes mellitus, hepatic disease, congestive heart failure
Odor	Faintly aromatic	Fruity sweet — acetone, associated with diabetes mellitus Unpleasant — decomposition of drugs, foods, alcohol
Quantity	Around 1000 to 1500 mL per day	High — diabetes mellitus, diabetes insipidus, nervousness, diuretics, excessive intake Low — acute neprhritis, heart disease, diarrhea, vomiting None — uremia, renal failure
Protein	Negative	Positive — renal disease, pyelonephritis
Glucose	Negative	Positive — diabetes mellitus, pain, excitement, liver damage
Ketones	Negative	Positive — uncontrolled diabetes mellitus, high-protein, low-carbohydrate diet
Bilirubin	Negative	Positive — liver disease, biliary obstruction, congestive heart failure
Blood	Negative	Positive — renal disease or disorders, trauma
Nitrites	Negative	Positive — bacteriuria
Urobilinogen	0.1 to 1.0	Absent — biliary obstruction Reduced — antibiotic therapy Increased — early warning of hepatic or hemolytic disease

LIFE SPAN
CONSIDERATIONS

■ THE CHILD

Soon after implantation, the embryonic mass differentiates into three distinct layers of cells: the **ectoderm**, **mesoderm**, and **endoderm**. The urinary and reproductive organs originate from the mesoderm. At 10 weeks urine forms and enters the bladder. At about the third month of gestation, the fetal kidneys begin to secrete urine. The amount increases gradually as the fetus matures. The newborn's kidneys are immature and lack the ability to concentrate urine. Glomerular filtration and absorption are relatively low until the child is 1 or 2 years of age. In the child the kidneys are more susceptible to trauma, because they usually do not have as much fat padding as in the adult. Infants are more prone to fluid volume changes, excess, and/or dehydration.

Urinary tract infections (UTIs) are common in children. The microorganisms *Escherichia coli*, *Klebsiella*, and *Proteus* cause most urinary tract infections seen in children. The signs and symptoms of urinary tract infection are age related. See Table 10–2.

■ THE OLDER ADULT

With advancing age, the **kidneys** may lose mass as blood vessels degenerate. The loss of glomerular capillaries causes a decrease in glomerular filtration and the kidneys lose their ability to conserve water and sodium. Additionally, the tubules of the aging kidneys diminish in their capacity for conserving base and ridding the body of excess hydrogen ions. Because the renal system helps to regulate acid–base balance, fluid and electrolyte imbalances may occur quickly in the older adult. Additional changes noted in the urinary system of the older adult are loss of muscle tone in the **ureters**, **bladder**, and **urethra**. The bladder capacity may be reduced by half and the older adult may have to make frequent trips to the bathroom. **Urge incontinence** (or the inability to retain urine voluntarily) is a concern for older adults.

During the fourth decade the kidneys begin to decrease in size and function. By the eighth decade the kidneys have generally shrunk 30% and have lost a proportionate amount of function. If stressed, kidneys respond more slowly to changes in one's internal environment. Some causes of stressful situations that may cause the kidneys to respond more slowly and contribute to fluid and electrolyte imbalance are:

- Vomiting and diarrhea
- Surgery
- Diuretics
- Decreased fluid intake
- Fever
- Renal damage from medications

TABLE 10–2 SIGNS AND SYMPTOMS OF URINARY TRACT INFECTION IN CHILDREN

Infants	Fever, loss of weight, nausea, vomiting, increased urination, foul-smelling urine, persistent diaper rash, failure to thrive
Older Child	Increased urination (frequency), pain during urination, abdominal pain, hematuria, fever, chills, bedwetting in a "trained" child

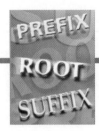

BUILDING YOUR MEDICAL VOCABULARY

This section provides the foundation for learning medical terminology. Medical words can be made up of four different types of word parts:

- Prefixes (P)
- Roots (R)
- Combining forms (CF)
- Suffixes (S)

By connecting various word parts in an organized sequence, thousands of words can be built and learned. In this text the word list is alphabetized so one can see the variety of meanings created when common prefixes and suffixes are repeatedly applied to certain word roots and/or combining forms. Words shown in pink are additional words related to the content of this chapter that are not built from word parts. These words are included to enhance your vocabulary. Note: an asterisk icon (✱) indicates words that are covered in the pathology spotlights section in this chapter.

MEDICAL WORD	WORD PARTS (WHEN APPLICABLE)			DEFINITION
	Part	Type	Meaning	
albuminuria (ăl-bū″ mĭn-oo′ rĭ-ă)	albumin -uria	R S	protein urine	Presence of serum protein in the urine
antidiuretic (ăn″ tĭ-dī″ ū-rĕt′ ĭk)	anti di(a) uret -ic	P P R S	against through urine pertaining to	Pertaining to a medication that decreases urine secretion
anuria (ăn-ū′ rĭ-ă)	an -uria	P S	without urine	Without the formation of urine
bacteriuria (băk-tē″ rĭ-ū′ rĭ-ă)	bacter/i -uria	CF S	bacteria urine	Presence of bacteria in the urine
calciuria (kăl″ sĭ-ū′ rĭ-ă)	calc/i -uria	CF S	calcium urine	Presence of calcium in the urine
calculus (kăl′ kū-lŭs)				A pebble; any abnormal concretion (stone); plural: calculi
catheter (kăth′ ĕ-tĕr)				A tube of elastic, elastic web, rubber, glass, metal, or plastic that is inserted into a body cavity to remove fluid or to inject fluid
cystectomy (sĭs-tĕk′ tō-mē)	cyst -ectomy	R S	bladder excision	Surgical excision of the bladder or part of the bladder
cystitis (sĭs-tī′ tĭs)	cyst -itis	R S	bladder inflammation	Inflammation of the bladder. ✱ See Pathology Spotlight: Cystitis.
cystocele (sĭs′ tō-sēl)	cyst/o -cele	CF S	bladder hernia	Hernia of the bladder that protrudes into the vagina
cystodynia (sĭs″ tō-dĭn′ ĭ-ă)	cyst/o -dynia	CF S	bladder pain	Pain in the bladder
cystogram (sĭs′ tō-grăm)	cyst/o -gram	CF S	bladder a mark, record	An x-ray record of the bladder
cystolithectomy (sĭs″ tō-lĭ-thĕk′ tō-mē)	cyst/o -lith -ectomy	CF S S	bladder stone excision	Surgical excision of a stone from the bladder
cystoscope (sĭst′ ō-skōp)	cyst/o -scope	CF S	bladder instrument	An instrument used for examination of the bladder
dialysis (dī-ăl′ ĭ-sĭs)	dia -lysis	P S	through destruction, to separate	A procedure to separate waste material from the blood and to maintain fluid, electrolyte, and acid–base balance in impaired kidney function or in the absence of the kidney

MEDICAL WORD	WORD PARTS (WHEN APPLICABLE)			DEFINITION
	Part	Type	Meaning	
diuresis (dī″ ū-rē′ sĭs)	di(a) ure -sis	P R S	through urinate condition	A condition of increased or excessive flow of urine
dysuria (dĭs-ū′ rĭ-ă)	dys -uria	P S	difficult, painful urine	Difficult or painful urination
edema (ĕ-dē′ mă)				An abnormal condition in which the body tissues contain an accumulation of fluid
enuresis (ĕn″ ū-rē′ sĭs)	en ure -sis	P R S	within urinate condition of	A condition of involuntary emission of urine; *bedwetting*
excretory (ĕks′ krə-tō-rē)	excret -ory	R S	sifted out like, resemble	Pertaining to the elimination of waste products from the body
extracorporeal shock-wave lithotriptor (ĕks″ tră-kor-por′ ē-ăl lĭth′ ō-trip″ tor)	extra corpor/e -al	P CF S	outside of body pertaining to	A device used to crush kidney stones *(renal calculi)*. The patient is sedated and immersed in a water bath while shock waves pound the stones until they crumble into small pieces. These pieces are flushed out with urine.
glomerular (glō-mĕr′ ū-lăr)	glomerul -ar	R S	glomerulus, little ball pertaining to	Pertaining to the glomerulus
glomerulitis (glō-mĕr″ ū-lī′ tĭs)	glomerul -itis	R S	glomerulus, little ball inflammation	Inflammation of the renal glomeruli
glomerulonephritis (glō-mĕr″ ū-lō-nĕ-frī′ tĭs)	glomerul/o nephr -itis	CF R S	glomerulus, little ball kidney inflammation	Inflammation of the kidney involving primarily the glomeruli
glycosuria (glī″ kō-soo′ rĭ-ă)	glycos -uria	R S	sweet, sugar urine	Presence of glucose in the urine
hematuria (hē″ mă-tū′ rĭ-ă)	hemat -uria	R S	blood urine	Presence of blood in the urine
hemodialysis (hē″ mō-dī-ăl′ ĭ-sĭs)	hem/o dia -lysis	CF P S	blood through to separate	The use of an artificial kidney to separate waste from the blood. The blood is circulated through tubes made of semipermeable membranes, and these tubes are continually bathed by solutions that remove waste.

MEDICAL WORD	WORD PARTS (WHEN APPLICABLE)			DEFINITION
	Part	**Type**	**Meaning**	
hydronephrosis (hī″ drō-něf-rō′ sǐs)	hydro nephr -osis	P R S	water kidney condition of	A condition in which urine collects in the renal pelvis because of an obstructed outflow. See Figure 10–4.
hypercalciuria (hī″ pěr-kǎl sǐ-ū′ rǐ-ǎ)	hyper calci -uria	P R S	excessive calcium urine	An excessive amount of calcium in the urine
incontinence (ǐn-kən′ tǐn-əns)	in continence	P R	not to hold	The inability to hold urine
interstitial cystitis (ǐn″ ter-stǐsh′ al sǐs-tī′ tǐs)				A chronically irritable and painful inflammation of the bladder wall
ketonuria (kě″ tō-nū′ rǐ-ǎ)	keton -uria	R S	ketone urine	Presence of ketones in the urine
lithotripsy (lǐth′ ō trǐp″ sē)	lith/o -tripsy	CF S	stone crushing	The crushing of a kidney stone. ✱ See Figure 10–5 in Pathology Spotlight: Kidney Stones.
meatotomy (mē″ ǎ-tǒt′ ō-mē)	meat/o -tomy	CF S	passage incision	Incision of the urinary meatus to enlarge the opening
meatus (mē-ā′ tǔs)				An opening or passage; the external opening of the urethra
micturition (mǐk′ tū-rǐ′ shǔn)	micturit -ion	R S	to urinate process	The process of urination
nephrectomy (ně-frěk′ tō-mē)	nephr -ectomy	R S	kidney excision	Surgical excision of a kidney
nephritis (něf-rī′ tǐs)	nephr -itis	R S	kidney inflammation	Inflammation of the kidney
nephrocystitis (něf″ rō-sǐs′ tī′ tǐs)	nephr/o cyst -itis	CF R S	kidney bladder inflammation	Inflammation of the bladder and the kidney
nephrolith (něf′ rō-lǐth)	nephr/o -lith	CF S	kidney stone, calculus	Kidney stone, calculus. ✱ See Pathology Spotlight: Kidney Stones.
nephrology (ně-frǒl′ ō-jē)	nephr/o -logy	CF S	kidney study of	The study of the kidney
nephroma (ně-frō′ mǎ)	nephr -oma	R S	kidney tumor	Kidney tumor
nephron (něf′ rǒn)				The structural and functional unit of the kidney

MEDICAL WORD	WORD PARTS (WHEN APPLICABLE)			DEFINITION
	Part	Type	Meaning	
nephropathy (nĕ-frŏp′ ă-thē)	nephr/o -pathy	CF S	kidney disease	Disease of the kidney
nephrosclerosis (nĕf″ rō-sklē-rō′ sĭs)	nephr/o scler -osis	CF R S	kidney hardening condition of	A condition of hardening of the kidney
nocturia (nŏk-tū′ rĭ-ă)	noct -uria	R S	night urine	Excessive urination during the night
oliguria (ŏl-ĭg-ū′ rĭ-ă)	olig -uria	P S	scanty urine	Scanty urination
percutaneous **ultrasonic** **lithotripsy** (pĕr″ kū-tā′ nē-ŭs) ŭl-tră-sŏn′ ĭk lĭth′ ō-trĭp″ sē)	per cutan/e -ous ultra son -ic lith/o -tripsy	P CF S P R S CF S	through skin pertaining to beyond sound pertaining to stone crushing	The crushing of a kidney stone by using ultrasound. This is an invasive surgical procedure performed by using a nephroscope or fluoroscopy.
peritoneal dialysis (pĕr″ ĭ-tō-nē′ ăl dī-ăl′ ĭ-sĭs)	periton/e -al dia -lysis	CF S P S	peritoneum pertaining to through to separate	Separation of waste from the blood by using a peritoneal catheter and dialysis. Fluid is introduced into the peritoneal cavity, and wastes from the blood pass into this fluid. The fluid and waste are then removed from the body. Types of peritoneal dialysis are IPD—intermittent—and CAPD—continuous ambulatory.
periurethral (pĕr″ ĭ-ū-rē′ thrăl)	peri urethr -al	P R S	around urethra pertaining to	Pertaining to around the urethra
polyuria (pŏl″ ē-ū′ rĭ-ă)	poly -uria	P S	excessive urine	Excessive urination
pyelocystitis (pī″ ĕ-lō-sĭs-tī′ tĭs)	pyel/o cyst -itis	CF R S	renal pelvis bladder inflammation	Inflammation of the bladder and renal pelvis
pyelolithotomy (pī″ ĕ-lō-lĭth-ŏt′ ō-mē)	pyel/o lith/o -tomy	CF CF S	renal pelvis stone incision	Surgical incision into the renal pelvis for removal of a stone
pyelonephritis (pī″ ĕ-lō-nĕ-frī′ tĭs)	pyel/o nephr -itis	CF R S	renal pelvis kidney inflammation	Inflammation of the kidney and renal pelvis. ✱ See pathology Spotlight: Pyelonephritis.

MEDICAL WORD	WORD PARTS (WHEN APPLICABLE)			DEFINITION
	Part	Type	Meaning	
pyuria (pī-ū′ rǐ-ǎ)	py -uria	R S	pus urine	Pus in the urine
renal (rē′ nǎl)	ren -al	R S	kidney pertaining to	Pertaining to the kidney
renal colic (rē′ nǎl kŏl′ ǐk)				An acute pain that occurs in the kidney area and is caused by blockage during the passage of a stone
renal failure (rē′ nǎl fāl′ yǔr)				Cessation of proper functioning of the kidney. ✳ See Pathology Spotlight: Renal Failure.
renal transplant (rē′ nǎl trăns′ plǎnt)				Surgical procedure to implant a donor kidney to a recipient
renin (rěn′ ǐn)				An enzyme produced by the kidney
residual urine (rē-zǐd′ ǔ-ǎl ū′ rǐn)				Urine that is left in the bladder after urination
sediment (sěd′ ǐ-měnt)				The substance that settles at the bottom of a liquid; a precipitate
specific gravity (spě-sǐf′ ǐk grăv′ ǐ-tē)				The weight of a substance compared with an equal amount of water. Urine has a specific gravity of 1.003 to 1.030.
specimen (spěs′ ǐ-měn)				A sample of tissue, blood, urine, or other material intended to show the nature of the whole
sterile (stěr′ ǐl)				A state of being free from living microorganisms; asepsis
stricture (strik′ chǔr)	strict -ure	R S	to draw, to bind process	An abnormal narrowing of a duct or passage such as the esophagus, ureter, or urethra
trigonitis (trǐg″ ō-nī′ tǐs)	trigon -itis	R S	trigone inflammation	Inflammation of the trigone of the bladder
urea (ū-rē′ ǎ)				The chief nitrogenous constituent of urine
uremia (ū-rē′ mǐ-ǎ)	ur -emia	R S	urine blood condition	A condition of excess urea and other nitrogenous waste in the blood

MEDICAL WORD	WORD PARTS (WHEN APPLICABLE)			DEFINITION
	Part	**Type**	**Meaning**	
ureterocolostomy (ū-rē″ tĕr-ō-kō-lŏs′ tō-mē)	ureter/o col/o -stomy	CF CF S	ureter colon new opening	Surgical implantation of the ureter into the colon
ureteropathy (ū-rē″ tĕr-ŏp′ ă-thē)	ureter/o -pathy	CF S	ureter disease	Disease of the ureter
ureteroplasty (ū-rē′ tĕr-ō-plăs″ tē)	ureter/o -plasty	CF S	ureter surgical repair	Surgical repair of the ureter
urethralgia (ū-rē-thrăl′ jĭ-ă)	urethr -algia	R S	urethra pain	Pain in the urethra
urethral stricture (ū-rē′ thrăl strĭk′ chŭr)	urethr -al strict -ure	R S R S	urethra pertaining to to draw, to bind process	A narrowing or constriction of the urethra
urethroperineal (ū-rē″ thrō-pĕr″ ĭ nē′ ăl)	urethr/o perine -al	CF R S	urethra perineum pertaining to	Pertaining to the urethra and perineum
urgency (ŭr-jĕn′ sē)				The sudden need to void, urinate
uric acid (ū′ rĭk ăs′ ĭd)				An end product of purine metabolism; a common component of urinary and renal stones
urinal (ū′ rĭn-ăl)	urin -al	R S	urine pertaining to	A container, toilet, or bathroom fixture into which one urinates
urinalysis (ū′ rĭ-năl′ i-sĭs)	urin a -lysis	R P S	urine apart destruction, to separate	Analysis of the urine; a separating of the urine for examination to determine the presence of abnormal elements
urination (ū″ rĭ-nā′ shŭn)	urinat -ion	R S	urine process	The process of voiding urine
urine (ū′ rĭn)				A waste product of fluid and dissolved substances secreted by the kidneys, stored in the bladder, and excreted through the urethra
urinometer (ū″ rĭ-nŏm′ ĕ-tĕr)	urin/o -meter	CF S	urine instrument to measure	An instrument used to measure the specific gravity of urine
urobilin (ū″ rō-bī′ lĭn)	ur/o bil -in	CF R S	urine bile chemical	A brown pigment formed by the oxidation of urobilinogen; may be formed in the urine after exposure to air

MEDICAL WORD	WORD PARTS (WHEN APPLICABLE)			DEFINITION
	Part	**Type**	**Meaning**	
urochrome (ū′ rō-krōm)				The pigment that gives urine the normal yellow color
urologist (ū-rŏl′ ō-jĭst)	ur/o log -ist	CF R S	urine study of one who specializes	One who specializes in the study of the urinary system
urology (ū-rŏl′ ō-jē)	ur/o -logy	CF S	urine study of	The study of the urinary system
void (voyd)				To empty the bladder

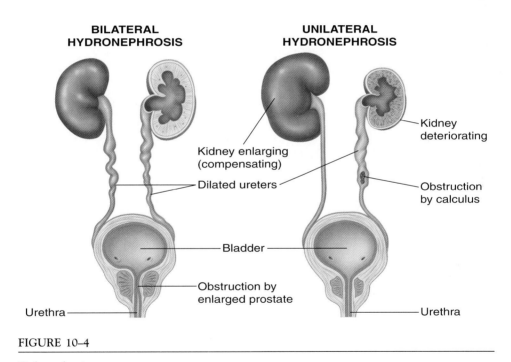

BILATERAL HYDRONEPHROSIS

UNILATERAL HYDRONEPHROSIS

Kidney enlarging (compensating)

Dilated ureters

Bladder

Obstruction by enlarged prostate

Urethra

Kidney deteriorating

Obstruction by calculus

Urethra

FIGURE 10–4

Hydronephrosis.

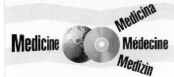

Terminology Translator

This feature, found on the accompanying CD-ROM, provides an innovative tool to translate medical words into Spanish, French, and German.

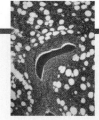

PATHOLOGY SPOTLIGHTS

Cystitis

Cystitis is an inflammation of the bladder, usually occurring secondary to ascending urinary tract infections. Associated organs such as the kidney, prostate (male), and urethra may also be involved. Cystitis may be acute or chronic.

Cystitis occurs when the lower urinary tract (urethra and bladder) is infected by bacteria and becomes irritated and inflamed. More than 85 percent of cases of cystitis are caused by *Escherichia coli*, a bacterium found in the lower gastrointestinal tract.

It is very common and occurs in more than 6 million Americans a year. The condition frequently affects sexually active women ages 20 to 50, but may also occur in those who are not sexually active or in young girls. During sexual activity, bacteria can be introduced into the bladder through the urethra. Once bacteria enter the bladder, they normally are removed through urination. When bacteria multiply faster than they are removed by urination, infection results.

Older adults are also at high risk for developing cystitis (see Table 10–3). Females are more prone to cystitis because of their shorter urethra (bacteria do not have to travel as far to enter the bladder) and because of the short distance between the opening of the urethra and the anus. Cystitis in men is usually secondary to some other type of infection such as epididymitis, prostatitis, gonorrhea, syphilis, and/or kidney stones.

The most common symptom is frequent, painful urination. Other symptoms include a burning sensation during urination, chills, and fever. With chronic cystitis, pyuria may be the only symptom.

Interstitial cystitis (IC) is a painful inflammation of the bladder wall. Approximately 450,000 people suffer from this condition, of whom 90 percent are women. Symptoms can vary from mild to severe. The cause is unknown, and IC does not respond to antibiotic therapy.

See Table 10–3 for prevalence of urinary tract infections according to age and sex.

Kidney Stones

Kidney stones (**nephroliths**) are deposits of mineral salts, called calculi, in the kidney. These stones can pass into the ureter, irritate kidney tissue, and block urine flow. Kidney stones occur when the urine has a high level of minerals that form stones. Most kidney stones are made from calcium. Minerals such as uric acid and oxalate may also form stones.

Kidney stones are one of the most common and painful disorders of the urinary tract. An estimated 10 percent of people in the United States will have a kidney stone at some point in their lives. Men tend to be affected more frequently than women. A person with a family his-

TABLE 10–3 THE PREVALENCE OF URINARY TRACT INFECTION ACCORDING TO AGE AND SEX

Age Group	Prevalence	Male:Female Ratio
Pre-school	2 to 3%	1:10
School age	1 to 2%	1:30
Reproductive years	25%	1:50
Elderly (65 to 70)	20%	1:10

tory of kidney stones may be more likely to develop stones. Urinary tract infections, kidney disorders, and metabolic disorders such as hyperparathyroidism are also linked to stone formation.

In more than half of patients, the cause is hypercalciuria. In this inherited condition, calcium is absorbed from food in excess and is lost into the urine. This high level of calcium in the urine causes crystals of calcium oxalate or calcium phosphate to form in the kidneys or urinary tract.

Most kidney stones pass out of the body without any intervention by a physician. Stones that cause lasting symptoms or other complications may be treated by various techniques, most of which do not involve major surgery. Some of these techniques include **extracorporeal shock-wave lithotripsy** (see Figure 10–5) and **percutaneous ultrasonic lithotripsy**.

Usually, the first symptom of a kidney stone is extreme pain. The pain often begins suddenly when a stone moves in the urinary tract, causing irritation or blockage. The person feels a sharp, cramping pain in the back and side in the area of the kidney or in the lower abdomen. Nausea and vomiting may occur. If the stone is too large to pass easily, pain continues and blood may appear in the urine.

People with a history of kidney stones should drink enough fluid to produce at least two liters, or about two quarts, of urine each day. People prone to forming calcium oxalate stones may be instructed by their physician to cut back on certain foods. This is especially true if their urine contains an excess of oxalate.

Food and drinks that contain oxalate:

- Beets
- Chocolate
- Coffee
- Cola
- Nuts
- Rhubarb
- Spinach

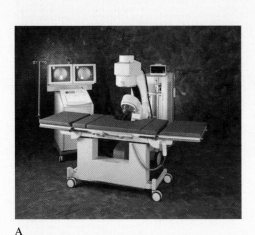

A

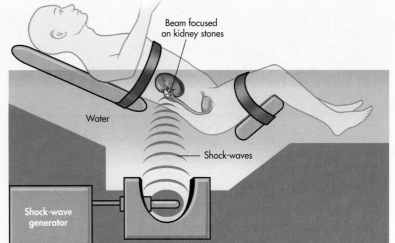

B

FIGURE 10–5

(A) The Dornier Compact Delta® lithotripsy system. Acoustic shock waves generated by the shock-wave generator travel through soft tissue to shatter the renal stone into fragments, which are then eliminated in the urine. (B) An illustration of water immersion lithotripsy procedure. ([A] Source: Courtesy of Dornier Medical Products, Inc.)

- Strawberries
- Tea
- Wheat bran

Pyelonephritis

Pyelonephritis is an infection of the kidney and renal pelvis. It may come on suddenly (acute) or it may be a long-term problem (chronic).

Pyelonephritis is usually caused by bacteria entering the kidneys from the bladder. *Escherichia coli* is a bacterium that is normally found in the large intestine. It causes about 90 percent of kidney infections. These infections usually spread from the genital area through the ureters to the bladder. In a healthy urinary tract, the infection is prevented from going to the kidneys by the flow of urine, which washes organisms out. When bacteria enter the normally sterile urinary tract, they can cause pyelonephritis.

Other possible causes of infection include the use of a catheter to drain urine from the bladder, use of a **cystoscope** to examine the bladder and urethra, and conditions such as prostate enlargement and kidney stones that prevent the efficient flow of urine from the bladder.

Symptoms include back, side, and groin pain; urgent, frequent urination; pain or burning during urination; fever; nausea and vomiting; and pus and blood in the urine.

Diagnosis is made with a urine test to identify bacteria and formations of white blood cells. If an infection cannot be easily cured, x-rays might be done to look for abnormalities in the kidneys, ureters, and bladder. A kidney infection is treated with an appropriate antibiotic, and abnormalities may need to be surgically treated.

An untreated or recurrent kidney infection can lead to chronic pyelonephritis, scarring of the kidneys, and permanent kidney damage.

Renal Failure

There are two types of renal (kidney) failure: acute and chronic.

Acute renal failure occurs when the filtering function of the kidneys changes so that the kidneys are not able to maintain healthy body function. The following conditions can lead to acute renal failure:

- A blockage of urine flow out of the kidneys and into the bladder
- Exposure to certain drugs and/or toxic substances
- Significant loss of blood or sudden drop in blood flow to the kidneys

People who have preexisting kidney disease or damage are at higher risk for acute renal failure.

At first, there are no specific signs or symptoms of acute renal failure. But as the disease progresses, many people have decreased urine output. As a result, fluid builds up in the body tissues and organs. Some common symptoms of acute renal failure include irregular heartbeats (arrhythmias), excess fluid in the abdomen (ascites), and swelling of the extremities (edema).

In *chronic* renal failure, there is a gradual and progressive loss of kidney function. It most often results from any disease that causes gradual loss of kidney function. It can range from mild dysfunction to severe kidney failure. Chronic renal failure usually occurs over a number of years as the internal structures of the kidney are slowly damaged. In the early stages, there may be no symptoms. In fact, progression may be so gradual that symptoms do not occur until kidney function is less than one-tenth of normal.

Chronic renal failure affects more than 2 out of 1,000 people in the United States. Diabetes and hypertension are the two most common causes and account for approximately two-thirds of the cases of chronic renal failure.

The goal of treatment of acute and chronic renal failure is to identify and treat any reversible causes of the kidney failure (e.g., use of kidney-toxic medications). Treatment also focuses on preventing excess accumulation of fluids and wastes, while allowing the kidneys to heal and gradually resume their normal function. Hospitalization is required for treatment and monitoring. Antibiotics may be used to treat or prevent infection. Diuretics may be used to remove fluid from the kidney.

In some cases, **dialysis** may be necessary. Dialysis is a method of removing toxic substances (impurities or wastes) from the blood when the kidneys are unable to do so. In addition to being used for patients who have renal failure, it may also be used to quickly remove drugs or poisons in acute situations.

Some patients may require a renal transplant, which is a surgical procedure to implant a healthy kidney into a patient with kidney disease or kidney failure. The kidney transplant may be taken from a living donor or from a recently deceased donor. Kidney transplants are the second most common transplant operation in the United States. There are over 9,000 kidney transplants performed each year.

✓PATHOLOGY CHECKPOINT

Following is a concise list of the pathology-related terms that you've seen in the chapter. Review this checklist to make sure that you are familiar with the meaning of each term before moving on to the next section.

Conditions and Symptoms

- ❑ albuminuria
- ❑ anuria
- ❑ bacteriuria
- ❑ calciuria
- ❑ calculus
- ❑ cystitis
- ❑ cystocele
- ❑ cystodynia
- ❑ diuresis
- ❑ dysuria
- ❑ edema
- ❑ enuresis
- ❑ glomerulitis
- ❑ glomerulonephritis
- ❑ glycosuria
- ❑ hematuria
- ❑ hydronephrosis
- ❑ hypercalciuria
- ❑ incontinence
- ❑ interstitial cystitis
- ❑ ketonuria
- ❑ micturition
- ❑ nephritis
- ❑ nephrocystitis

- ❑ nephrolith
- ❑ nephroma
- ❑ nephropathy
- ❑ nephrosclerosis
- ❑ nocturia
- ❑ oliguria
- ❑ polyuria
- ❑ pyelocystitis
- ❑ pyelonephritis
- ❑ pyuria
- ❑ renal colic
- ❑ renal failure
- ❑ residual urine
- ❑ stricture
- ❑ trigonitis
- ❑ uremia
- ❑ ureteropathy
- ❑ urethralgia
- ❑ urethral stricture
- ❑ urgency
- ❑ uric acid

Diagnosis and Treatment

- ❑ antidiuretic
- ❑ catheter

- ❑ cystectomy
- ❑ cystogram
- ❑ cystolithectomy
- ❑ cystoscope
- ❑ dialysis
- ❑ extracorporeal shock-wave lithotriptor
- ❑ hemodialysis
- ❑ lithotripsy
- ❑ meatotomy
- ❑ nephrectomy
- ❑ percutaneous ultrasonic lithotripsy
- ❑ peritoneal dialysis
- ❑ pyelolithotomy
- ❑ renal transplant
- ❑ specific gravity
- ❑ specimen
- ❑ ureterocolostomy
- ❑ urinometer
- ❑ ureteroplasty
- ❑ urinalysis

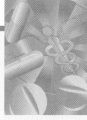

DRUG HIGHLIGHTS

Drugs that are generally used for urinary system diseases and disorders include diuretics, urinary tract antibacterials and antiseptics, and other drugs.

Diuretics	Decrease reabsorption of sodium chloride by the kidneys, thereby increasing the amount of salt and water excreted in the urine. This action reduces the amount of fluid retained in the body and prevents edema. Diuretics are classified according to site and mechanism of action.
Thiazide	Appear to act by inhibiting sodium and chloride reabsorption in the early portion of the distal tubule.
	Examples: Diuril (chlorothiazide), HydroDiuril (hydrochlorothiazide), and Lozol (indapamide).
Loop	Act by inhibiting the reabsorption of sodium and chloride in the ascending loop of Henle.
	Examples: Bumex (bumetanide) and Lasix (furosemide).
Potassium-sparing	Act by inhibiting the exchange of sodium for potassium in the distal tubule. They inhibit potassium excretion.
	Examples: Aldactone (spironolactone) and Dyrenium (triamterene).
Osmotic	Are capable of being filtered by the glomerulus, but have a limited capability of being reabsorbed into the bloodstream.
	Example: Osmitrol (mannitol).
Carbonic anhydrase inhibitor	Act to increase the excretion of bicarbonate ion, which carries out sodium, water, and potassium.
	Example: Diamox (acetazolamide).
Urinary Tract Antibacterials	Sulfonamides are generally the drugs of choice for treating acute, uncomplicated urinary tract infections, especially those caused by *Escherichia coli* and *Proteus mirabilis* bacterial strains. They exert a bacteriostatic effect against a wide range of gram-positive and gram-negative microorganisms.
	Examples: Gantrisin (sulfisoxazole), Gantanol (sulfamethoxazole), Microsulfon (sulfadiazine), and Bactrim and Septra, which are mixtures of trimethoprim and sulfamethoxazole.
Urinary Tract Antiseptics	May inhibit the growth of microorganisms by bactericidal, bacteriostatic, anti-infective, and/or antibacterial action.
	Examples: NegGram (nalidixic acid), Furadanton and Macrodantin (nitrofurantoin), Mandelamine and Hiprex (methenamine), and Cipro (ciprofloxacin HCl).
Other Drugs	Disorders of the lower urinary tract may be treated with drugs that either stimulate or inhibit smooth muscle activity, thereby improving urinary bladder functions. These functions are the storage of urine and its subsequent excretion from the body.
	Examples: Cystospaz-M and Levsin (hyoscyamine sulfate), Urispas (flavoxate HCl), and Urecholine (bethanechol chloride).
Rimso-50 (dimethyl sulfoxide)	Used in the treatment of interstitial cystitis.

Pyridium (phenazopyridine HCl)	Analgesic, anesthetic action on the urinary tract mucosa. This medication causes the urine to turn an orange color.
Urispas (flavoxate HCl)	Reduces dysuria, nocturia, and urinary frequency.
Tofranil (imipramine HCl)	Treatment of nocturnal enuresis in children.
Ditropan XL (oxybutynin chloride)	Relaxes the muscles in the bladder, thereby decreasing the occurrence of wetting accidents.
Detrol (tolterodine tartrate)	Helps control involuntary contractions of the bladder muscle.

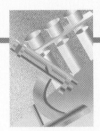

DIAGNOSTIC & LAB TESTS

TEST	DESCRIPTION
blood urea nitrogen (BUN) (blod ū-rē′ ă nǐ′ trō-jěn)	A blood test to determine the amount of urea that is excreted by the kidneys. Abnormal results indicate urinary tract disease.
creatinine (krē′ ă-tǐn ēn)	A blood test to determine the amount of creatinine present. Abnormal results indicate kidney disease.
creatinine clearance (krē′ ă-tǐn ēn klir′ ăns)	A urine test to determine the glomerular filtration rate (GFR). Abnormal results indicate kidney disease.
culture, urine (kūl′ tūr, ū′ rǐn)	A urine test to determine the presence of microorganisms. Abnormal results indicate urinary tract infection.
cystoscopy (sǐs-tǒs′ kə-pě)	Visual examination of the bladder and urethra via a lighted cystoscope. Abnormal results may indicate the presence of renal calculi, a tumor, prostatic hyperplasia, and/or bleeding.
intravenous pyelography (pyelogram) (ǐn-tră-vē′ nǔs pǐ″ ě-lǒg′ ră-fē)	A test to visualize the kidneys, ureters, and bladder. A radiopaque substance is intravenously injected, and x-rays are taken. Abnormal results may indicate renal calculi, kidney or bladder tumors, and kidney disease.
kidney, ureter, bladder (KUB) (kǐd′ nē, ū′ rě-těr, blăd′ děr)	A flat-plate x-ray is taken of the abdomen to indicate the size and position of the kidneys, ureters, and bladder.
renal biopsy (rē′ năl bī′ ǒp-sē)	The removal of tissue from the kidney. Abnormal results may indicate kidney cancer, kidney transplant rejection, and glomerulonephritis.
ultrasonography, kidneys (ŭl-tră-sǒn-ǒg′ ră-fē, kǐd′ nēs)	The use of high-frequency sound waves to visualize the kidneys. The sound waves (echoes) are recorded on an oscilloscope and film. Abnormal results may indicate kidney tumors, cysts, abscess, and kidney disease.

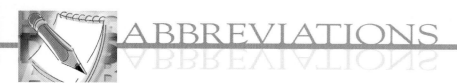

ABBREVIATIONS

ABBREVIATION	MEANING	ABBREVIATION	MEANING
ADH	antidiuretic hormone	HCO_3	bicarbonate
A/G	albumin/globulin ratio	HD	hemodialysis
AGN	acute glomerulonephritis	H_2O	water
ATN	acute tubular necrosis	I & O	intake and output
BUN	blood urea nitrogen	IPD	intermittent peritoneal dialysis
CAPD	continuous ambulatory peritoneal dialysis	IVP	intravenous pyelogram
		IVU	intravenous urogram
CC	clean catch	K	potassium
CGN	chronic glomerulonephritis	KUB	kidney, ureter, bladder
Cl	chlorine	LPF	low-power field
CMG	cystometrogram	Na	sodium
CRF	chronic renal failure	PD	peritoneal dialysis
C & S	culture and sensitivity	pH	hydrogen ion concentration
cysto	cystoscopic examination	PKU	phenylketonuria
ECF	extracellular fluid	PUL	percutaneous ultrasonic lithotripsy
ECSL	extracorporeal shockwave lithotriptor		
		RP	retrograde pyelogram
ESRD	end-stage renal disease	UA	urinalysis
ESWL	extracorporeal shockwave lithotripsy	UTI	urinary tract infection
		VCU,	voiding cystourethrogram
GFR	glomerular filtration rate	VCUG	
GU	genitourinary		

STUDY AND REVIEW

Anatomy and Physiology

Write your answers to the following questions. Do not refer to the text.

1. List the organs of the urinary system.

   a. _____   b. _____

   c. _____   d. _____

2. State the vital function of the urinary system. _____

   _____

3. Name the three capsules that surround each kidney.

   a. _____   b. _____

   c. _____

4. Define hilum. _____

5. Define renal pelvis. _____

6. The cortex of the kidney contains the _____, _____,

   _____ _____, and _____ _____.

7. The medulla is the _____ portion of the kidney.

8. Define nephron. _____

9. Each nephron consists of a _____ _____ and a

   _____.

10. The malpighian corpuscle consists of _____ and _____

    _____.

11. State the vital function of the nephron. _____

    _____

12. Urine is formed by the process of _____ and _____ in the
    nephron.

13. Urine consists of _____ percent water and _____ percent
    solid substances.

14. An average of _____ to _____ mL of urine is voided daily.

15. Describe the ureters and state their function. _____

    _____

16. Describe the urinary bladder and state its function. _____

    _____

17. Define trigone. _____

18. State the function of the male urethra. _____

19. State the function of the female urethra. _____

20. The external urinary opening is the _____ _____.

21. Define urinalysis. _____

    _____

22. Give the normal constituents for the physical examination of urine.

    a. Color _____   b. Appearance _____

    c. Reaction _____   d. Specific gravity _____

    e. Odor _____   f. Quantity _____

23. Name the three types of epithelial cells that may be found in urine.

    a. _____   b. _____

    c. _____

24. A urine that has a fruity, sweet odor may indicate _____

    _____.

25. Under chemical examination, the presence of protein in urine is an important

    sign of _____

    _____.

Word Parts

1. In the spaces provided, write the definition of these prefixes, roots, combining forms, and suffixes. Do not refer to the listings of medical words. Leave blank those words you cannot define.

2. After completing as many as you can, refer to the medical word listings to check your work. For each word missed or left blank, write the word and its definition several times on the margins of these pages or on a separate sheet of paper.

3. To maximize the learning process, it is to your advantage to do the following exercises as directed. To refer to the word building section before completing these exercises invalidates the learning process.

PREFIXES

Give the definitions of the following prefixes:

1. an- _____

2. anti- _____

3. di(a)- _____

4. dia- _____

5. dys- _____

6. en- _____

7. hydro- _____

8. extra- _____

9. in- _____

10. olig- _____

11. per- _____

12. ultra- _____

13. poly- _____

ROOTS AND COMBINING FORMS

Give the definitions of the following roots and combining forms:

1. excret _____

2. albumin _____

3. bacter/i _____

4. bil _____

5. calc/i _____

6. col/o _____

7. continence _____

8. cyst _____

9. corpor/e _____

10. cyst/o _____

11. cutan/e _____

12. glomerul _____

13. glomerul/o _____

14. glycos _____

15. hemat _____

16. keton _____

17. lith/o _____

18. log _____

19. hem/o _____

20. meat/o _____

21. micturit _____

22. nephr _____

23. nephr/o _____

24. noct _____

25. periton/e _____

26. perine _____

27. son _____

28. strict _____

29. py _____

30. pyel/o _____

31. ren _____

32. scler _____

33. trigon _____

34. ur _____

35. ure _____

36. uret _____

37. ureter/o _____

38. urethr _____

39. urethr/o _____

40. urin _____

41. urinat _____

42. urino _____

43. ur/o _____

SUFFIXES

Give the definitions of the following suffixes:

1. -al _____

2. -algia _____

3. -ar _____

4. -cele _____

5. -dynia _____

6. -ory _____

7. -ous _____

8. -ectomy _____

9. -emia _____

10. -gram _____

11. -ic _____

12. -in _____

13. -ion _____

14. -ist _____

15. -itis _____

16. -lith _____

17. -logy _____

18. -lysis _____

19. -tripsy _____

20. -ure _____

21. -meter _____

22. -oma _____

23. -osis _____

24. -pathy _____

25. -plasty _____

26. -scope _____

27. -sis _____

28. -stomy _____

29. -tomy _____

30. -uria _____

Identifying Medical Terms

In the spaces provided, write the medical terms for the following meanings:

1. _____ Pertaining to a medication that decreases urine secretion

2. _____ Surgical excision of the bladder or part of the bladder

3. _____ Inflammation of the bladder

4. _____ Difficult or painful urination

5. _____ Inflammation of the renal glomeruli

6. _____ An excessive amount of calcium in the urine

7. _____ The process of urinating

8. _____ Kidney stone

9. _____ Pertaining to around the urethra

10. _____ Pus in the urine

11. _____ Disease of the ureter

12. _____ Pain in the urethra

13. _____ One who specializes in the study of the urinary system

Spelling

In the spaces provided, write the correct spelling of these misspelled words:

1. excreteory _____

2. euresis _____

3. glycouria _____

4. hemauria _____

5. incontence _____

6. nephrcysitis _____

7. nocuria _____

8. ueteroplasty _____

9. urinalsis _____

10. urbilin _____

Matching

Select the appropriate lettered meaning for each word listed below.

_____ 1. lithotriptor

_____ 2. hemodialysis

_____ 3. lithotripsy

_____ 4. peritoneal dialysis

_____ 5. renal colic

_____ 6. urethral stricture

_____ 7. urgency

_____ 8. urination

_____ 9. urochrome

_____ 10. urinometer

a. An acute pain that occurs in the kidney area and is caused by blockage during the passage of a stone

b. The crushing of a kidney stone

c. The process of voiding urine

d. A device used to crush kidney stones

e. The use of an artificial kidney to separate waste from the blood

f. Separation of waste from the blood by using a peritoneal catheter and dialysis

g. A narrowing or constriction of the urethra

h. Pigment that gives urine its normal yellow color

i. An instrument used to measure the specific gravity of urine

j. The sudden need to void, urinate

k. Analysis of the urine

Abbreviations

Place the correct word, phrase, or abbreviation in the space provided.

1. antidiuretic hormone _____

2. BUN _____

3. chronic renal failure _____

4. cysto _____

5. GU _____

6. HD _____

7. intravenous pyelogram _____

8. PD _____

9. pH _____

10. urinalysis _____

Diagnostic and Laboratory Tests

Select the best answer to each multiple choice question. Circle the letter of your choice.

1. A urine test to determine the glomerular filtration rate.
   a. BUN
   b. creatinine
   c. creatinine clearance
   d. KUB

2. A urine test to determine the presence of microorganisms.
   a. BUN
   b. creatinine
   c. urine culture
   d. KUB

3. A test to visualize the kidneys, ureters, and bladder.
   a. cystoscopy
   b. intravenous pyelography
   c. KUB
   d. renal biopsy

4. The use of high-frequency sound waves to visualize the kidneys.
   a. retrograde pyelography
   b. intravenous pyelography
   c. ultrasonography
   d. cystoscopy

5. A flat-plate x-ray of the abdomen to indicate the size and position of the kidneys, ureters, and bladder.
   a. cystoscopy
   b. KUB
   c. BUN
   d. retrograde pyelography

CASE STUDY   ACUTE CYSTITIS

Read the following case study and then answer the questions that follow.

A 21-year-old female was seen by a physician and the following is a synopsis of the visit.

Present History: The patient states that she goes to the bathroom a lot and that it "burns" and "hurts." She also has chills and fever.

Signs and Symptoms: Frequency, burning sensation and pain during urination, chills, and fever.

Diagnosis: Acute cystitis. The diagnosis was determined by a history of the symptoms, a complete urinalysis (physical, chemical, and microscopic) that revealed red blood cells, white blood cells, and bacteria.

Treatment: The physician ordered a sulfonamide, Pyridium, and provided her with written Guidelines to Help Avoid Cystitis (female).

Prevention: In the United States, approximately 10 million people seek treatment for urinary tract infection each year, with cystitis being the most common. Cystitis is most often caused by an ascending infection from the urethra and it is more common in the female because of the short length of the urethra, which promotes the transmission of bacteria from the skin and genitals to the internal bladder. The most common type of bacteria that causes cystitis in females is *Escherichia coli* (*E. coli*), the colon bacillus.

Guidelines to Help Avoid Cystitis (Female)

- Drink 8 glasses or more of water/day.
- Females should wipe themselves from front to back after a bowel movement to avoid contaminating the urinary meatus.
- Have sexual partner wear a condom.
- Do not use vaginal deodorants, bubble baths, colored toilet paper, and other substances that could cause irritation to the urinary meatus.
- Wear cotton underclothes and keep the genital area dry.

CASE STUDY QUESTIONS

1. Signs and symptoms of cystitis include frequency, burning ——————— and pain during urination, chills, and fever.
2. The diagnosis was determined by a history of the symptoms, a complete ——————— that revealed red blood cells, white blood cells, and bacteria.
3. Treatment included a ———————, Pyridium, and written Guidelines to Help Avoid Cystitis.
4. Why is cystitis more common in the female than in the male?
5. What type of bacteria generally causes cystitis in the female?
6. After a bowel movement, why is it important for the female to wipe herself from front to back?

MedMedia Wrap-Up
www.prenhall.com/rice

Additional interactive resources and activities for this chapter can be found on the Companion Website. For animations, videos, audio glossary, and review, access the accompanying CD-ROM in this book.

Audio Glossary
Medical Terminology Exercises & Activities
Pathology Spotlight
Terminology Translator
Animations
Videos

Objectives
Medical Terminology Exercises & Activities
Audio Glossary
Drug Updates
Medical Terminology in the News

THE ENDOCRINE SYSTEM 11

OUTLINE

OBJECTIVES

On completion of this chapter, you will be able to:

- Describe the primary glands of the endocrine system.
- State the primary functions of the endocrine glands.
- Describe the secondary glands of the endocrine system.
- State the vital function of the endocrine system.
- Identify and state the functions of the various hormones secreted by the endocrine glands.
- Analyze, build, spell, and pronounce medical words.
- Describe each of the conditions presented in the Pathology Spotlights.
- Complete the Pathology Checkpoint.
- Review Drug Highlights presented in this chapter.
- Provide the description of diagnostic and laboratory tests related to the endocrine system.
- Identify and define selected abbreviations.
- Successfully complete the study and review section.

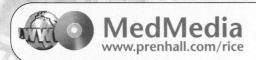

MedMedia
www.prenhall.com/rice

Additional interactive resources and activities for this chapter can be found on the Companion Website. For Terminology Translator, animations, videos, audio glossary, and review, access the accompanying CD-ROM in this book.

Anatomy and Physiology Overview

The endocrine system is made up of glands and the hormones they secrete. Although the endocrine glands are the body's main hormone producers, some other organs such as the brain, heart, lungs, liver, skin, thymus, and the placenta during pregnancy and the gastrointestinal mucosa produce and release hormones. The primary glands of the endocrine system are the pituitary, pineal, thyroid, parathyroid, islets of Langerhans, adrenals, ovaries in the female, and testes in the male. See Table 11–1.

The vital function of the endocrine system involves the production and regulation of chemical substances called hormones. A hormone is a chemical transmitter that is released in small amounts and transported via the bloodstream to a target organ or other cells. The word hormone is derived from the Greek language and means "to excite" or "to urge on." As the body's chemical messengers, hormones transfer information and instructions from one set of cells to another. They regulate growth, development, mood, tissue function, metabolism, and sexual function in the male and female.

Many pathological conditions are caused by or associated with hyposecretion or hypersecretion of specific hormones of the endocrine system. Too much or too little of any hormone can be harmful to the body. Controlling the production of or replacing specific hormones can treat many hormonal disorders and/or conditions.

The endocrine system and the nervous system work closely together to help maintain homeostasis. The hypothalamus, a collection of specialized cells that are located in the lower central part of the brain, is the primary link between the endocrine and nervous system. Nerve cells in the hypothalamus control the pituitary gland by producing chemicals that either stimulate or suppress hormone secretions from the pituitary.

THE ENDOCRINE SYSTEM

Gland	Primary Functions
Pituitary (Hypophysis)	Master gland; regulatory effects on other endocrine glands
Anterior lobe	Influences growth and sexual development, thyroid function, adrenocortical function; regulates skin pigmentation
Posterior lobe	Stimulates the reabsorption of water and elevates blood pressure; stimulates the release of milk and the uterus to contract during labor, delivery, and parturition
Pineal	Helps regulate the release of gonadotropin and controls body pigmentation
Thyroid	Vital role in metabolism and regulates the body's metabolic processes, influences bone and calcium metabolism, helps maintain plasma calcium homeostasis
Parathyroid	Maintenance of a normal serum calcium level, plays a role in the metabolism of phosphorus
Pancreas (Islets of Langerhans)	Regulates blood glucose levels and plays a vital role in metabolism of carbohydrates, proteins, and fats
Adrenals (Suprarenals)	
Adrenal cortex	Regulates carbohydrate metabolism, anti-inflammatory effect; helps body cope during stress; regulates electrolyte and water balance; promotes development of male characteristics
Adrenal medulla	Synthesizes, secretes, and stores catecholamines (dopamine, epinephrine, norepinephrine)
Ovaries	Promote growth, development, and maintenance of female sex organs
Testes	Promote growth, development, and maintenance of male sex organs

TABLE 11–1 SUMMARY OF THE ENDOCRINE GLANDS, HORMONES, AND HORMONAL FUNCTIONS

Endocrine Glands	Hormones	Hormonal Functions
Pituitary Gland		
Anterior lobe	Growth hormone (GH)	Growth and development of bones, muscles, and other organs
	Adrenocorticotropin hormone (ACTH)	Growth and development of the adrenal cortex
	Thyroid-stimulating hormone (TSH)	Growth and development of the thyroid gland
	Follicle-stimulating hormone (FSH)	Stimulates the growth of ovarian follicles in the female and sperm in the male
	Luteinizing hormone (LH)	Stimulates the development of the corpus luteum in the female and the production of testosterone in the male
	Prolactin hormone (PRL)	Stimulates the mammary glands to produce milk after childbirth
	Melanocyte-stimulating hormone (MSH)	Regulates skin pigmentation and promotes the deposit of melanin in the skin after exposure to sunlight
Posterior lobe	Antidiuretic hormone (ADH)	Stimulates the reabsorption of water by the renal tubules and has a pressor effect that elevates the blood pressure
	Oxytocin	Acts on the mammary glands to stimulate the release of milk and stimulates the uterus to contract during labor, delivery, and parturition
Pineal Gland	Melatonin	Helps regulate the release of gonadotropin and influences the body's internal clock
	Serotonin	Neurotransmitter, vasoconstrictor, and smooth muscle stimulant; acts to inhibit gastric secretion
Thyroid Gland	Thyroxine	Maintenance and regulation of the basal metabolic rate (BMR)
	Triiodothyronine	Influences the basal metabolic rate
	Calcitonin	Influences calcium metabolism
Parathyroid Glands	Parathormone hormone (PTH)	Plays a role in maintenance of a normal serum calcium level and in the metabolism of phosphorus
Islets of Langerhans	Glucagon	Facilitates the breakdown of glycogen to glucose
	Insulin	Plays a role in maintenance of normal blood sugar
	Somatostatin	Suppresses the release of glucagon and insulin
Adrenal Glands		
Cortex	Cortisol	Principal steroid hormone. Regulates carbohydrate, protein, and fat metabolism; gluconeogenesis; increases blood sugar level; anti-inflammatory effect; helps body cope during times of stress.
	Corticosterone	Steroid hormone. Essential for normal use of carbohydrates, the absorption of glucose, and gluconeogenesis. Also influences potassium and sodium metabolism.
	Aldosterone	Principal mineralocorticoid. Essential in regulating electrolyte and water balance.
	Testosterone	Development of male secondary sex characteristics
	Androsterone	Development of male secondary sex characteristics
Medulla	Dopamine	Dilates systemic arteries, elevates systolic blood pressure, increases cardiac output, increases urinary output
	Epinephrine (adrenaline)	Vasoconstrictor, vasopressor, cardiac stimulant, antispasmodic, and sympathomimetic
	Norepinephrine	Vasoconstrictor, vasopressor, and neurotransmitter
Ovaries	Estrogens (estradiol, estrone, and estriol)	Female sex hormones. Essential for the growth, development, and maintenance of female sex organs and secondary sex characteristics. Promotes the development of the mammary glands, and plays a vital role in a woman's emotional well-being and sexual drive.
	Progesterone	Prepares the uterus for pregnancy
Testes	Testosterone	Essential for normal growth and development of the male accessory sex organs. Plays a vital role in the erection process of the penis and, thus, is necessary for the reproductive act, copulation.
Thymus Gland	Thymosin	Promotes the maturation process of T lymphocytes
	Thymopoietin	Influences the production of lymphocyte precursors and aids in their process of becoming T lymphocytes
Gastrointestinal Mucosa	Gastrin	Stimulates gastric acid secretion
	Secretin	Stimulates pancreatic juice, bile, and intestinal secretion
	Pancreozymin	Stimulates the pancreas to produce pancreatic juice
	Cholecystokinin	Contraction and emptying of the gallbladder
	Enterogastrone	Regulates gastric secretions

The hypothalamus synthesizes and secretes releasing hormones such as thyrotropin-releasing hormone (TRH) and gonadotropin-releasing hormone (GnRH) and releasing factors such as corticotropin-releasing factor (CRF), growth hormone-releasing factor (GHRF), prolactin-releasing factor (PRF), and melanocyte-stimulating hormone-releasing factor (MRF). The hypothalamus also synthesizes and secretes release-inhibiting hormones such as growth hormone release-inhibiting hormone. It also produces release-inhibiting factors such as prolactin release-inhibiting factor (PIF) and melanocyte-stimulating hormone release-inhibiting factor (MIF). The hypothalamus also exerts direct nervous control over the anterior pituitary and the adrenal medulla and controls the secretion of the hormones epinephrine and norepinephrine.

THE PITUITARY GLAND (HYPOPHYSIS)

The **pituitary gland** is a small gray gland located at the base of the brain. It lies or rests in a shallow depression of the sphenoid bone known as the *sella turcica*. It is attached by the infundibulum stalk to the hypothalamus. The pituitary is approximately 1 cm in diameter and weighs approximately 0.6 g. It is divided into the anterior lobe or adenohypophysis and the posterior lobe or neurohypophysis. The pituitary is called the **master gland** of the body because of its regulatory effects on the other endocrine glands (see Fig. 11–1).

The Anterior Lobe

The **adenohypophysis** or anterior lobe secretes several hormones that are essential for the growth and development of bones, muscles, other organs, sex glands, the thyroid gland, and the adrenal cortex. The hormones secreted by the anterior lobe and their functions are described below and shown in Figure 11–2.

GROWTH HORMONE (GH)

Growth hormone, also called somatotropin hormone (STH), is essential for the growth and development of bones, muscles, and other organs. It also enhances protein synthesis, decreases the use of glucose, and promotes fat destruction (lipolysis). Hyposecretion of this hormone may result in **dwarfism** and **Simmonds' disease**. Hypersecretion of the hormone may result in **gigantism** during early life and **acromegaly** in adults.

ADRENOCORTICOTROPIN (ACTH)

Adrenocorticotropin is essential for growth and development of the middle and inner zones of the adrenal cortex. The adrenal cortex secretes the glucocorticoids cortisol and corticosterone.

THYROID-STIMULATING HORMONE (TSH)

Thyroid-stimulating hormone is essential for the growth and development of the thyroid gland. It stimulates the production of thyroxine and triiodothyronine. It also influences the body's metabolic processes and plays an important role in metabolism.

FOLLICLE-STIMULATING HORMONE (FSH)

Follicle-stimulating hormone is a gonadotropic hormone that is essential in stimulating the growth of ovarian follicles in the female and the production of sperm in the male.

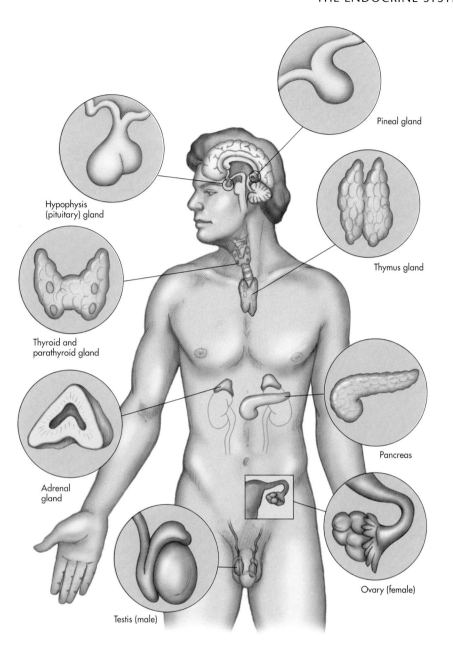

FIGURE 11–1

The primary glands of the endocrine system.

LUTEINIZING HORMONE (LH)

Luteinizing hormone is a gonadotropic hormone that is essential in the maturation process of the ovarian follicles and stimulates the development of the corpus luteum in the female and the production of testosterone in the male.

PROLACTIN (PRL)

Prolactin is also known as *lactogenic hormone* (LTH). It is a gonadotropic hormone that stimulates the mammary glands to produce milk after childbirth.

MELANOCYTE-STIMULATING HORMONE (MSH)

Melanocyte-stimulating hormone regulates skin pigmentation and promotes the deposit of melanin in the skin after exposure to sunlight.

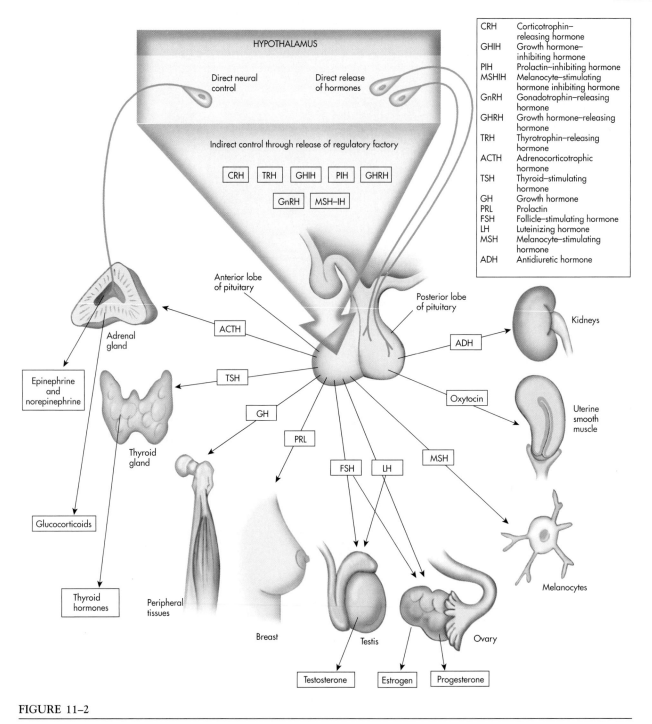

FIGURE 11–2

The pituitary hormones and their target cells, tissues, and/or organs.

The Posterior Lobe

The *neurohypophysis* or posterior lobe secretes two known hormones: antidiuretic hormone and oxytocin (see Fig. 11–2). The following is a description of the functions of these hormones.

ANTIDIURETIC HORMONE (ADH)

Antidiuretic hormone is also known as *vasopressin* (VP). It stimulates the reabsorption of water by the renal tubules and has a pressor effect that elevates blood pressure. Hyposecretion of this hormone may result in **diabetes insipidus.**

OXYTOCIN

Oxytocin acts on the mammary glands to stimulate the release of milk and stimulates the uterus to contract during labor, delivery, and parturition.

THE PINEAL GLAND (BODY)

The **pineal gland** is a small, pine cone–shaped gland located near the posterior end of the corpus callosum. It is less than 1 cm in diameter and weighs approximately 0.1 g (see Fig. 11–1). The pineal gland secretes **melatonin** and **serotonin**. Melatonin is a hormone that may be released at night to help regulate the release of gonadotropin. Serotonin is a hormone that is a neurotransmitter, vasoconstrictor, and smooth muscle stimulant and acts to inhibit gastric secretion.

THE THYROID GLAND

The **thyroid gland** is a large, bilobed gland located in the neck. It is anterior to the trachea and just below the thyroid cartilage. The thyroid is approximately 5 cm long and 3 cm wide and weighs approximately 30 g (see Fig. 11–1 and Fig. 11–3). It plays a vital role in metabolism and regulates the body's metabolic processes. The hormones described below are stored and secreted by the thyroid gland.

THYROXINE (T_4)

Thyroxine is essential for the maintenance and regulation of the *basal metabolic rate* (BMR). It contains four iodine atoms, which are attached to its nucleus. Thyroxine influences growth and development, both physical and mental, and the metabolism of

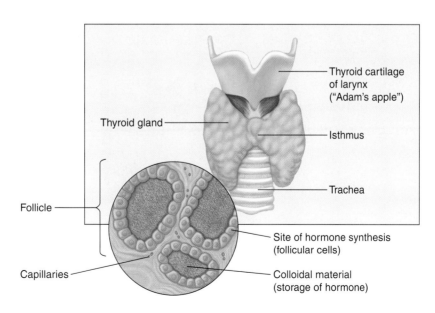

FIGURE 11–3

The thyroid gland. (Source: Pearson Education/PH College.)

fats, proteins, carbohydrates, water, vitamins, and minerals. It can be synthetically produced or extracted from animal thyroid glands in crystalline form to be used in the treatment of thyroid dysfunction, especially cretinism, myxedema, and Hashimoto's disease.

TRIIODOTHYRONINE (T_3)

Triiodothyronine is an effective thyroid hormone that contains three iodine atoms. It influences the basal metabolic rate and is more biologically active than thyroxine.

CALCITONIN

Also known as thyrocalcitonin, *calcitonin* is a thyroid hormone that influences bone and calcium metabolism. It helps maintain plasma calcium homeostasis.

Hyposecretion of the thyroid hormones T_3 and T_4 results in **cretinism** during infancy, **myxedema** during adulthood, and **Hashimoto's disease**, which is a chronic thyroid disease. Hypersecretion of the thyroid hormones T_3 and T_4 results in **hyperthyroidism**, which is also called **thyrotoxicosis**, and **Graves' disease, exophthalmic goiter, toxic goiter,** or **Basedow's disease.** Simple or endemic goiter is an enlargement of the thyroid gland caused by a deficiency of iodine in the diet.

THE PARATHYROID GLANDS

The **parathyroid glands** are small, yellowish-brown bodies occurring as two pairs and located on the dorsal surface and lower aspect of the thyroid gland. Each parathyroid gland is approximately 6 mm in diameter and weighs approximately 0.033 g (Fig. 11–1 and Fig. 11–4). The hormone secreted by the parathyroids is *parathormone* (PTH). This hormone is essential for the maintenance of a normal serum calcium level. It also plays a role in the metabolism of phosphorus. Hyposecretion of PTH may result in **hypoparathyroidism,** which may result in **tetany** (see Fig. 11–5). Hypersecretion of PTH may result in **hyperparathyroidism,** which may result in **osteoporosis, kidney stones,** and **hypercalcemia.**

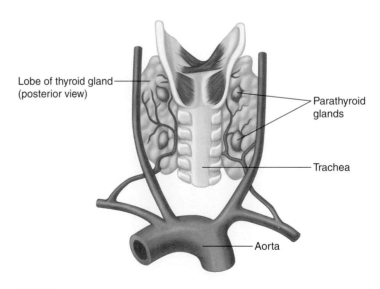

FIGURE 11–4

Parathyroid glands. (Source: Pearson Education/PH College.)

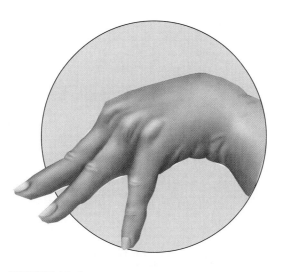

FIGURE 11–5

Tetany of the hand in hypoparathyroidism. (Source:
Pearson Education/PH College.)

THE PANCREAS (THE ISLETS OF LANGERHANS)

The **islets of Langerhans** are small clusters of cells located within the pancreas (see Fig.
11–1 and Fig. 11–6). They are composed of three major types of cells: **alpha**, **beta**, and
delta. The alpha cells secrete the hormone glucagon (see Fig. 11–7), which facilitates
the breakdown of glycogen to glucose, thereby elevating blood sugar. The beta cells
secrete the hormone insulin (see Fig. 11–7), which is essential for the maintenance of
normal blood sugar (70–110 mg/100 mL of blood). Insulin is essential to life. It
promotes the use of glucose in cells, thereby lowering the blood glucose level, and
plays a vital role in carbohydrate, protein, and fat metabolism. Insulin can be synthetically produced in various types and was first discovered and used successfully by

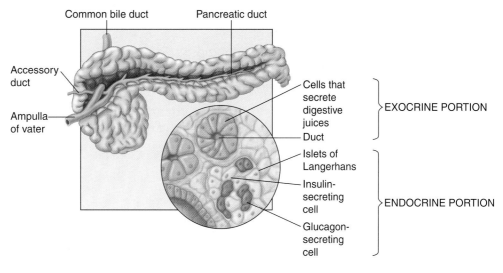

FIGURE 11–6

The pancreas—an endocrine and exocrine gland. (Source: Pearson Education/PH College.)

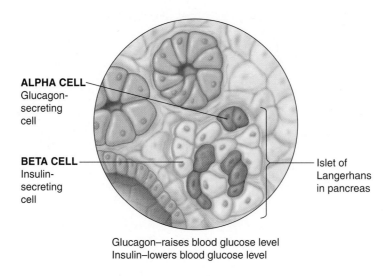

ALPHA CELL
Glucagon-
secreting
cell

BETA CELL
Insulin-
secreting
cell

Islet of
Langerhans
in pancreas

Glucagon–raises blood glucose level
Insulin–lowers blood glucose level

FIGURE 11–7

Islets of Langerhans.

Sir F. G. Banting. Hyposecretion or inadequate use of insulin may result in **diabetes mellitus**. Hypersecretion of insulin may result in **hyperinsulinism**. The delta cells secrete a hormone, *somatostatin*, that suppresses the release of glucagon and insulin.

THE ADRENAL GLANDS (SUPRARENALS)

The **adrenal glands** are two small, triangular-shaped glands located on top of each kidney. Each gland weighs about 5 g and consists of an outer portion or cortex and an inner portion called the *medulla* (Fig. 11–1 and Fig. 11–8).

The Adrenal Cortex

The *cortex* is essential to life as it secretes a group of hormones, the glucocorticoids, the mineralocorticoids, and the androgens. These hormones and their effects on the body are described below.

THE GLUCOCORTICOIDS

The two glucocorticoid hormones are *cortisol* and *corticosterone*.

Cortisol.   *Cortisol* (hydrocortisone) is the principal steroid hormone secreted by the cortex. The following are some of the known influences and functions of this hormone:

- It regulates carbohydrate, protein, and fat metabolism.
- It stimulates output of glucose from the liver (gluconeogenesis).
- It increases the blood sugar level.
- It regulates other physiologic body processes.
- It promotes the transport of amino acids into extracellular tissue, thereby making them available for energy.
- It influences the effectiveness of catecholamines such as dopamine, epinephrine, and norepinephrine.

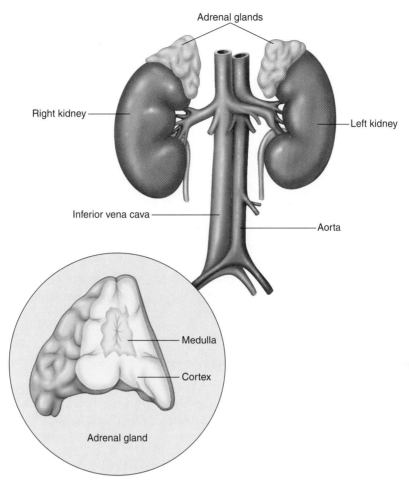

Adrenal glands

Right kidney

Left kidney

Inferior vena cava

Aorta

Medulla

Cortex

Adrenal gland

FIGURE 11–8

The adrenal glands.

- It has an anti-inflammatory effect.
- It helps the body cope during times of stress.

Hyposecretion of this hormone may result in **Addison's disease.** Hypersecretion of cortisol may result in **Cushing's disease.**

Corticosterone.   *Corticosterone* is a steroid hormone secreted by the adrenal cortex. It is essential for the normal use of carbohydrates, the absorption of glucose, and the process known as **gluconeogenesis.** It also influences potassium and sodium metabolism.

THE MINERALOCORTICOIDS

Aldosterone is the principal *mineralocorticoid* secreted by the adrenal cortex. It is essential in regulating electrolyte and water balance by promoting sodium and chloride retention and potassium excretion. Hyposecretion of this hormone may result in a **reduced plasma volume.** Hypersecretion of this hormone may result in a condition known as **primary aldosteronism.**

THE ANDROGENS

Androgen refers to a substance or hormone that promotes the development of male characteristics. The two main androgen hormones are *testosterone* and *androsterone*. These hormones are essential for the development of the male secondary sex characteristics.

The Adrenal Medulla

The *medulla* synthesizes, secretes, and stores catecholamines, specifically, dopamine, epinephrine, and norepinephrine. A discussion of these substances and their effects on the body follows.

Dopamine

Dopamine acts to dilate systemic arteries, elevates systolic blood pressure, increases cardiac output, and increases urinary output. It is used in the treatment of shock and is a neurotransmitter in the nervous system.

EPINEPHRINE

Epinephrine (Adrenalin, adrenaline) acts as a vasoconstrictor, vasopressor, cardiac stimulant, antispasmodic, and sympathomimetic. Its main function is to assist in the regulation of the sympathetic branch of the autonomic nervous system. It can be synthetically produced and may be administered parenterally *(by an injection)*, topically *(on a local area of the skin)*, or by inhalation *(by nose or mouth)*. The following are some of the known influences and functions of this hormone:

- It elevates the systolic blood pressure.
- It increases the heart rate and cardiac output.
- It increases glycogenolysis, thereby hastening the release of glucose from the liver. This action elevates the blood sugar level and provides the body with a spurt of energy; referred to as the "fight-or-flight" syndrome.
- It dilates the bronchial tubes and relaxes air passageways.
- It dilates the pupils so that one can see more clearly.

NOREPINEPHRINE

Norepinephrine (noradrenaline) acts as a vasoconstrictor, vasopressor, and neurotransmitter. It elevates systolic and diastolic blood pressure, increases the heart rate and cardiac output, and increases glycogenolysis.

THE OVARIES

The **ovaries** produce *estrogens (estradiol, estrone,* and *estriol)* and *progesterone.* Estrogen is the female sex hormone secreted by the graafian follicles of the ovaries. Progesterone is a steroid hormone secreted by the corpus luteum. These hormones are essential for promoting the growth, development, and maintenance of secondary female sex organs and characteristics. They also prepare the uterus for pregnancy, promote development of the mammary glands, and play a vital role in a woman's emotional well-being and her sexual drive (see Fig. 11–1).

THE TESTES

The **testes** produce the male sex hormone *testosterone,* which is essential for normal growth and development of the male accessory sex organs. Testosterone plays a vital role in the erection process of the penis and, thus, is necessary for the reproductive act, copulation (see Fig. 11–1).

THE PLACENTA

During pregnancy the **placenta,** a spongy structure joining mother and child, serves as an endocrine gland. It produces chorionic gonadotropin hormone, estrogen, and progesterone.

THE GASTROINTESTINAL MUCOSA

The **mucosa** of the pyloric area of the stomach secretes the hormone *gastrin*, which stimulates gastric acid secretion. Gastrin also affects the gallbladder, pancreas, and small intestine secretory activities.

The mucosa of the duodenum and jejunum secretes the hormone *secretin*, which stimulates pancreatic juice, bile, and intestinal secretion. The mucosa of the duodenum also secretes *pancreozymin-cholecystokinin*, which stimulates the pancreas. *Enterogastrone*, a hormone that regulates gastric secretions, is also secreted by the duodenal mucosa.

THE THYMUS

The **thymus** is a bilobed body located in the mediastinal cavity in front of and above the heart (Fig. 11–9). It is composed of lymphoid tissue and is a part of the lymphatic system. It is a ductless gland-like body and secretes the hormones *thymosin* and *thymopoietin*. Thymosin promotes the maturation process of T lymphocytes (thymus-dependent). Thymopoietin is a hormone that influences the production of lymphocyte precursors and aids in their process of becoming T lymphocytes.

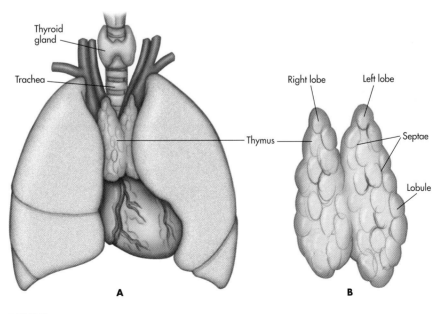

FIGURE 11–9

The thymus gland. (A) Appearance and position; (B) with anatomic structures.

LIFE SPAN
CONSIDERATIONS

■ THE CHILD

Most of the structures and glands of the endocrine system develop during the first 3 months of pregnancy. The endocrine system of the newborn is supplemented by hormones that cross the placental barrier. Both male and female newborns may have swelling of the breast and genitalia from maternal hormones.

Either excessively high or insufficient production of growth hormone (GH) by the anterior lobe of the pituitary gland can cause abnormal growth patterns. Excessive production of GH can cause **gigantism**. Insufficient production of GH can cause **dwarfism**.

Diabetes mellitus is the most common endocrine system disorder of childhood. The rate of occurrence is highest among 5–7-year-olds and 11–13-year-olds. The classic symptoms of diabetes mellitus—**polyuria** (frequent urination), **polydipsia** (excessive thirst), and **polyphagia** (extreme hunger)—appear more rapidly in children. Other symptoms seen during childhood are weakness, loss of weight, lethargy, anorexia, irritability, dry skin, vaginal yeast infections in the female child and/or recurrent infections, and abdominal cramps. The management of diabetes mellitus during childhood is very difficult, because diet, exercise, and medication have to be adjusted and regulated according to the various stages of growth and development of the child.

■ THE OLDER ADULT

With aging, **hormonal changes** vary with each individual. Generally the number of tissue receptors decreases, thus diminishing the body's response to hormones. This is especially the case with older adults who develop Type 2 **diabetes mellitus.** In this condition sufficient insulin is produced, but because the number of cell receptors is reduced, glucose does not enter the cells.

An older adult may not be diagnosed with diabetes until he or she goes in for a regular eye exam and the ophthalmologist discovers a problem and/or one goes in for a physical examination and the blood test indicates an elevated blood glucose level. There are multiple risk factors associated with the older adult and the development of diabetes; these are:

- Age-related decreased insulin production
- Age-related insulin resistance
- Heredity
- Decreased physical activity
- Multiple diseases
- Polypharmacy
- Obesity
- New stressors in life

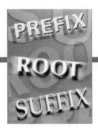

BUILDING YOUR MEDICAL VOCABULARY

This section provides the foundation for learning medical terminology. Medical words can be made up of four different types of word parts:

- Prefixes (P)
- Roots (R)
- Combining forms (CF)
- Suffixes (S)

By connecting various word parts in an organized sequence, thousands of words can be built and learned. In this text the word list is alphabetized so one can see the variety of meanings created when common prefixes and suffixes are repeatedly applied to certain word roots and/or combining forms. Words shown in pink are additional words related to the content of this chapter that are not built from word parts. These words are included to enhance your vocabulary. Note: an asterisk icon (✱) indicates words that are covered in the Pathology Spotlights section in this chapter.

MEDICAL WORD	WORD PARTS (WHEN APPLICABLE)			DEFINITION
	Part	**Type**	**Meaning**	
acidosis (ăs″ ĭ-dō′ sĭs)	acid -osis	R S	acid condition of	A condition of excessive acidity of body fluids
acromegaly (ăk″ rō-mĕg′ ă-lē)	acr/o -megaly	CF S	extremity enlargement, large	A chronic disease marked by enlargement of the extremities caused by excessive growth hormone
Addison's disease (ăd′ ĭ-sŭns dĭ-zēz)				Results from a deficiency in the secretion of adrenocortical hormones. Also called hypo-adrenocorticism. ✱ See Pathology Spotlight: Addison's Disease.
adenectomy (ăd″ ĕn-ĕk′ tō-mē)	aden -ectomy	R S	gland excision	Surgical excision of a gland
adenoma (ăd″ ĕ-nō′ mă)	aden -oma	R S	gland tumor	A tumor of a gland
adenosis (ăd″ ĕ-nō′ sĭs)	aden -osis	R S	gland condition of	Any disease condition of a gland
adrenal (ăd-rē′ năl)	ad ren -al	P R S	toward kidney pertaining to	Pertaining to toward the kidney
adrenalectomy (ăd-rē″ năl-ĕk′ tō-mē)	ad ren -al -ectomy	P R S S	toward kidney pertaining to excision	Surgical excision of the adrenal gland
adrenopathy (ăd″ rĕn-ŏp′ ă-thē)	ad ren/o -pathy	P CF S	toward kidney disease	Any disease of the adrenal gland
aldosterone (ăl-dŏs′ tĕr-ōn)				A mineralocorticoid hormone secreted by the adrenal cortex that helps regulate metabolism of sodium, chloride, and potassium
androgen (ăn′ drō-jĕn)	andr/o -gen	CF S	man formation, produce	Hormones that produce or stimulate the development of male characteristics. The two major androgens are testosterone and androsterone.

MEDICAL WORD	WORD PARTS (WHEN APPLICABLE)			DEFINITION
	Part	**Type**	**Meaning**	
catecholamines (kăt″ ĕ-kōl′ ăm-ēns)				Biochemical substances, epinephrine, norepinephrine, and dopamine
cortisone (kŏr′ tĭ-sōn)	cortis -one	R S	cortex hormone	A glucocorticoid hormone that is isolated from the adrenal cortex; *used as an anti-inflammatory agent*
cretinism (krē′ tĭn-ĭzm)	cretin -ism	R S	cretin condition of	A congenital deficiency in secretion of the thyroid hormones T_3 and T_4
Cushing's disease (koosh′ ĭngs dĭ-zēz)				Results from hypersecretion of cortisol. Symptoms include fatigue, muscular weakness, and changes in body appearance. Prolonged administration of large doses of ACTH can cause Cushing's syndrome. A "buffalo hump" and a "moon face" are characteristic signs of this condition.
diabetes (dī″ ă-bē′ tēz)	dia -betes	P S	through to go	A disease characterized by excessive discharge of urine. ✳ See Pathology Spotlight: Diabetes Mellitus.
dopamine (dō′ pă-mēn)				An intermediate substance in the synthesis of norepinephrine; used in the treatment of shock as it acts to elevate blood pressure and increase urinary output
dwarfism (dwar′ fizm)	dwarf -ism	R S	small condition of	A condition of being abnormally small
endocrine (ĕn′ dō-krĭn)	endo crine	P R	within to secrete	A ductless gland that produces an internal secretion
endocrinologist (ĕn″ dō-krĭn-ŏl′ ō-gĭst)	endo crin/o log -ist	P CF R S	within to secrete study of one who specializes	One who specializes in the study of the endocrine glands
endocrinology (ĕn″ dō-krĭn-ŏl′ ō-jē)	endo crin/o -logy	P CF S	within to secrete study of	The study of the endocrine glands
epinephrine (ĕp″ ĭ-nĕf′ rĭn)	epi nephr -ine	P R S	upon kidney pertaining to	A hormone produced by the adrenal medulla; used as a vasoconstrictor, as a cardiac stimulant, to relax bronchospasm, and to relieve allergic symptoms; *also called adrenaline, Adrenalin*

MEDICAL WORD	WORD PARTS (WHEN APPLICABLE)			DEFINITION
	Part	Type	Meaning	
estrogen (ĕs' trō-jĕn)	estr/o -gen	CF S	mad desire formation, produce	Hormones produced by the ovaries, including estradiol, estrone, and estriol; female sex hormones important in the development of secondary sex characteristics and regulation of the menstrual cycle
euthyroid (ū-thī' royd)	eu thyr -oid	P R S	good, normal thyroid, shield resemble	Normal activity of the thyroid gland
exocrine (ĕks' ō-krĭn)	exo crine	P R	out, away from to secrete	External secretion of a gland
exophthalmic (ĕks" ŏf-thăl' mĭk)	ex ophthalm -ic	P R S	out, away from eye pertaining to	Pertaining to an abnormal protrusion of the eye
galactorrhea (gă-lăk" tō-rĭ' ă)	galact/o -rrhea	CF S	milk flow, discharge	Excessive secretion of milk after cessation of nursing
gigantism (ji' găn-tĭzm)	gigant -ism	R S	giant condition of	A condition of being abnormally large
glandular (glăn' dū-lăr)	glandul -ar	R S	little acorn pertaining to	Pertaining to a gland
glucocorticoid (glū" kō-kŏrt' ĭ-koyd)	gluc/o cortic -oid	CF R S	sweet, sugar cortex resemble	A general classification of the adrenal cortical hormones
hirsutism (hŭr' sūt-ĭzm)	hirsut -ism	R S	hairy condition of	An abnormal condition characterized by excessive growth of hair, especially in women. See Figure 11–10.
hormone (hor' mōn)				A chemical substance produced by the endocrine glands
hydrocortisone (hĭ" drō-kŏr' tĭ-sōn)	hydro cortis -one	R R S	water cortex hormone	A glucocorticoid hormone produced by the adrenal cortex; *used as an anti-inflammatory agent*
hypergonadism (hĭ" pĕr-gō' năd-ĭzm)	hyper gonad -ism	P R S	excessive seed condition of	A condition of excessive secretion of the sex glands
hyperinsulinism (hĭ" pĕr-ĭn' sū-lĭn-ĭzm)	hyper insulin -ism	P R S	excessive insulin condition of	A condition of excessive amounts of insulin in the blood

MEDICAL WORD	WORD PARTS (WHEN APPLICABLE)			DEFINITION
	Part	Type	Meaning	
hyperkalemia (hī″ pĕr-kă-lē′ mĭ-ă)	hyper kal -emia	P R S	excessive potassium (K) blood condition	A condition of excessive amounts of potassium in the blood
hyperthyroidism (hī″ pĕr-thī′ royd-ĭzm)	hyper thyr -oid -ism	P R S S	excessive thyroid, shield resemble condition of	A condition caused by excessive secretion of the thyroid gland. ✳ See Pathology Spotlight: Hyperthyroidism.
hypogonadism (hī″ pō-gō′ năd-ĭzm)	hypo gonad -ism	P R S	deficient seed condition of	A condition caused by deficient internal secretion of the gonads
hypoparathyroidism (hī″ pō-păr″ ă-thī′ royd-ĭzm)	hypo para thyr -oid -ism	P P R S S	deficient beside thyroid, shield resemble condition of	Deficient internal secretion of the parathyroid glands
hypophysis (hī-pŏf′ ĭ-sĭs)	hypo -physis	P S	deficient, under growth	Any undergrowth; the pituitary body
hypothyroidism (hī″ pō-thī′ royd-ĭzm)	hypo thyr -oid -ism	P R S S	deficient thyroid, shield resemble condition of	Deficient secretion of the thyroid gland. ✳ See Pathology Spotlight: Hypothyroidism.
insulin (in′ sū-lĭn)	insul -in	R S	insulin, island chemical	A hormone produced by the beta cells of the islets of Langerhans of the pancreas; essential for the metabolism of carbohydrates and fats; *used in the management of diabetes mellitus*
insulinogenic (ĭn″ sū-lĭn″ ō-jĕn′ ĭk)	insulin/o -genic	CF S	insulin, island formation produce	The formation or production of insulin
iodine (ī′ ō-dīn)				A trace mineral that aids in the development and functioning of the thyroid gland
lethargic (lĕ-thar′ jĭk)	letharg -ic	R S	drowsiness pertaining to	Pertaining to drowsiness, sluggish
myxedema (mĭks″ ĕ-dē′ mă)	myx -edema	R S	mucus swelling	A condition of mucus swelling resulting from hypofunction of the thyroid gland. See Figure 11–11.
norepinephrine (nŏr-ĕp″ ĭ-nĕf′ rĭn)	nor epi nephr -ine	P P R S	not upon kidney pertaining to	A hormone produced by the adrenal medulla; used as a vasoconstrictor of peripheral blood vessels in acute hypotensive states

MEDICAL WORD	WORD PARTS (WHEN APPLICABLE)			DEFINITION
	Part	**Type**	**Meaning**	
oxytocin (ŏk″ sĭ-tō′ sĭn)				A hormone produced by the pituitary gland that stimulates uterine contraction during childbirth and stimulates the release of milk during nursing
pancreatic (păn″ krē-ăt′ ĭk)	pan creat -ic	P R S	all flesh pertaining to	Pertaining to the pancreas
parathyroid (păr″ ă-thī′ royd)	para thyr -oid	P R S	beside thyroid, shield resemble	An endocrine gland located beside the thyroid gland
pineal (pĭn′ ē-ăl)	pine -al	R S	pine cone pertaining to	An endocrine gland that is shaped like a small pine cone
pituitarism (pĭt-ū′ ĭ-tă-rĭzm)	pituitar -ism	R S	phlegm condition	Any condition of the pituitary gland
pituitary (pĭ-tū′ ĭ-tăr″ ē)	pituitar -y	R S	phlegm pertaining to	Pertaining to phlegm; the pituitary body or gland, the hypophysis
progeria (prō-jē′ rĭ-ă)	pro ger -ia	P R S	before old age condition	A condition of premature old age occurring in childhood
progesterone (prō-jĕs′ tĕr-ōn)	pro gester -one	P R S	before to bear hormone	A hormone produced by the corpus luteum of the ovary, the adrenal cortex, or the placenta; released during the second half of the menstrual cycle
somatotropin (sō-măt′ ō-trō″ pĭn)	somat/o trop -in	CF R S	body turn chemical	Growth-stimulating hormone produced by the anterior lobe of the pituitary gland
steroids (stĕr′ oydz)	ster -oid	R S	solid resemble	A group of chemical substances that includes hormones, vitamins, sterols, cardiac glycosides, and certain drugs
testosterone (tĕs-tŏs′ tĕr-ōn)	test/o ster -one	CF R S	testicle solid hormone	A hormone produced by the testes; male sex hormone important in the development of secondary sex characteristics and masculinization
thymectomy (thī-mĕk′ tō-mē)	thym -ectomy	R S	thymus excision	Surgical excision of the thymus gland
thymitis (thī-mī′ tĭs)	thym -itis	R S	thymus inflammation	Inflammation of the thymus gland
thyroid (thī′ royd)	thyr -oid	R S	thyroid, shield resemble	Resembling a shield; one of the endocrine glands

MEDICAL WORD	WORD PARTS (WHEN APPLICABLE)			DEFINITION
	Part	**Type**	**Meaning**	
thyroidectomy (thī″ royd-ĕk′ tō-mē)	thyr -oid -ectomy	R S S	thyroid, shield resemble excision	Surgical excision of the thyroid gland
thyroiditis (thī″ royd′ ī′ tĭs)	thyr -oid -itis	R S S	thyroid, shield resemble inflammation	Inflammation of the thyroid gland
thyrotoxicosis (thī″ rō-tŏks″ ĭ-kō′ sĭs)	thyr/o toxic -osis	CF R S	thyroid, shield poison condition of	A poisonous condition of the thyroid gland caused by hyperactivity
thyroxine (thī-rŏks′ ēn)	thyro -ine	R S	thyroid, shield pertaining to	A hormone produced by the thyroid gland; important in growth and development and regulation of the body's metabolic rate and metabolism of carbohydrates, fats, and proteins
vasopressin (văs″ ō-prĕs′ ĭn)	vas/o press -in	CF R S	vessel to press chemical	A hormone produced by the hypothalamus and stored in the posterior lobe of the pituitary gland; also called antidiuretic hormone, ADH
virilism (vĭr′ ĭl-ĭzm)	viril -ism	R S	masculine condition of	The condition of masculinity developed in a woman

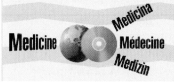

Terminology Translator

This feature, found on the accompanying CD-ROM, provides an innovative tool to translate medical words into Spanish, French, and German.

Medicine Medicina Médecine Medizin

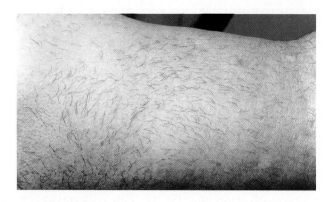

FIGURE 11–10

Hirsutism. (Courtesy of Jason L. Smith, MD.)

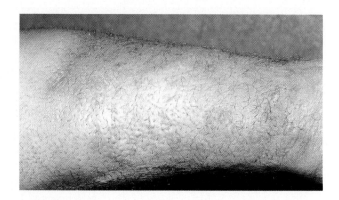

FIGURE 11–11

Pretibial myxedema. (Courtesy of Jason L. Smith, MD.)

PATHOLOGY SPOTLIGHTS

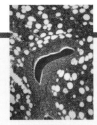

PATHOLOGY SPOTLIGHTS

Addison's Disease

Addison's disease occurs when the cortex of the adrenal gland is damaged and there is a deficiency in the production of the adrenocortical hormones. The most common cause of this condition is the result of the body attacking itself (autoimmune disease). For unknown reasons, the immune system views the adrenal cortex as a foreign body, something to attack and destroy. Other causes of Addison's disease include infections of the adrenal glands, spread of cancer to the glands or hemorrhage into the glands.

Addison's disease is named for the 19th century English physician, Thomas Addison, who identified and described the condition. It can occur at any age, including infancy, and is equally prevalent among males and females. It is a rare disease occurring about 1 in 100,000 Americans.

The signs and symptoms of Addison's disease may include:

- Weight loss
- Anorexia
- Weakness and lethargy
- Increased pigmentation of the skin and mucous membranes
- Low blood sugar (hypoglycemia)
- Joint and muscle aches
- Persistent fever
- Nausea, vomiting, diarrhea, abdominal discomfort

The signs and symptoms usually develop slowly over several months, but they may appear suddenly. In acute adrenal failure (addisonian crisis), the signs and symptoms include dehydration, shock and loss of consciousness. This condition is life-threatening and requires immediate medical care. Prescribed adrenocortical steroids along with intravenous fluids and sodium are administered to the patient.

The diagnosis of Addison's disease is determined by blood and urine tests which measure the amount of corticosteroid hormones present. With Addison's, the level of the hormones is very low.

When Addison's disease is diagnosed early, treatment generally consists of replacement of the adrenocortical hormones and supplemental sodium. Both the patient and family are taught the importance of lifelong replacement therapy and the proper technique of how to give an intramuscular injection of hydrocortisone. The patient is advised to wear or carry a medical identification at all times.

Diabetes Mellitus

Diabetes mellitus is a complex disorder of metabolism. It is a disease in which the body does not produce or properly use insulin. Insulin is a hormone that is needed to convert sugar, starches and other food into energy needed for daily life.

According to the American Diabetes Association (ADA) approximately 17 million people in the United States, or 6.2 percent of the population, have diabetes. While an estimated 11.1 million have been diagnosed, unfortunately, 5.9 million people are unaware that they have the disease.

There are three major types of diabetes: Type 1, Type 2, and gestational diabetes. Type 1 diabetes used to be known as insulin-dependent diabetes mellitus, IDDM, or juvenile-onset diabetes. It results from the body's failure to produce insulin, the hormone that "unlocks" the cells of the body, allowing glucose to enter and fuel them. So an individual with this type of diabetes will need to take insulin injections each day for the rest of his or her life. It is estimated that 5–10 percent of Americans who are diagnosed with diabetes have Type 1 diabetes.

Type 2 diabetes used to be known as noninsulin-dependent diabetes mellitus, NIDDM, or adult-onset diabetes. It results from insulin resistance combined with relative insulin deficiency. This is by far the most common type of diabetes. Approximately 90–95 percent of Americans (16 million) have Type 2 diabetes. Someone with Type 2 diabetes might make healthy or even high levels of insulin, but obesity makes the body resistant to its effect. Type 2 diabetes used to be rare in children. But with the increase in obesity in children, doctors are now finding that as many as 1 out of each 20 children who have diabetes has Type 2 diabetes. Of these children, 85 percent are obese. Obesity is the main cause of Type 2 diabetes in both adults and children. A recent study showed a 33 percent increase in the number of Americans with Type 2 diabetes over the past 8 years. The increase was 70 percent in people ages 30 to 39 years old and was linked to a sharp rise in obesity in this group.

It may be possible to prevent Type 2 diabetes. Even modest lifestyle changes can help prevent the onset of Type 2 diabetes. The key is to eat a healthy diet, exercise 30 minutes a day at least 5 days a week and maintain a proper body weight for age and body type.

Gestational diabetes or pregnancy-induced diabetes develops in a pregnant woman. In most cases, this type of diabetes goes away after the woman's child is born. It affects about 4 percent of all pregnant women, about 135,000 cases in the United States each year.

Prediabetes is a condition that occurs when a person's blood glucose levels are higher than normal but not high enough for a diagnosis of Type 2 diabetes. It is estimated that at least 16 million Americans have prediabetes, in addition to the 17 million with diabetes. Without lifestyle changes, most people who have prediabetes will progress to Type 2 diabetes within 10 years.

Are you at risk for diabetes? Do you have any, some, or many of the signs and symptoms of diabetes? See Table 11–2 for the warning signs and symptoms of diabetes mellitus.

Hypothyroidism

Hypothyroidism is a condition in which the thyroid gland does not produce adequate amounts of thyroid hormone. Approximately 6 to 7 million Americans, mainly women older than age 40, have an underactive thyroid. Because hypothyroidism usually develops slowly, only about half of all cases are diagnosed early.

Symptoms may be subtle, and may occur early in the course of hypothyroidism. These may include fatigue, decreased concentration, intolerance to cold environments, constipation, loss of appetite, muscle cramping and stiffness, and weight gain. Some individuals may notice hair loss, dry skin, or nail changes.

TABLE 11–2 WARNING SIGNS AND SYMPTOMS OF DIABETES MELLITUS

Type 1	*Type 2*
Frequent urination (**polyuria**)	Any Type 1 symptom
Excessive thirst (**polydipsia**)	Tingling or numbing in the feet
Extreme hunger (**polyphagia**)	Frequent vaginal or skin infection
Unusual weight loss	
Increased fatigue	
Blurred vision	
Irritability	

Untreated hypothyroidism can lead to a number of health problems. Constant stimulation of the thyroid to release more hormones may cause the gland to become larger, a condition known as a goiter. Hashimoto's thyroiditis, an autoimmune inflammation of the thyroid, is one of the most common causes of a goiter. Hypothyroidism may also be associated with an increased risk of heart disease, primarily because of high levels of low-density lipoprotein (LDL) cholesterol—the bad cholesterol—can occur in people with an underactive thyroid. Hypothyroidism can also lead to an enlarged heart.

Other complications of this condition include depression, decreased sexual desire, and slowed mental functioning. **Myxedema** is a rare, life-threatening condition that is the result of long-term, undiagnosed hypothyroidism. It symptoms include intense cold intolerance and drowsiness followed by profound lethargy and unconsciousness. A myxedema coma may be triggered by sedatives, infection or other stress on the body. One should seek immediate emergency medical treatment if there are symptoms of myxedema.

Standard treatment for an underactive thyroid involves daily use of the synthetic thyroid hormone levothyroxine (Levothroid, Synthroid). The oral medication restores adequate hormone levels and soon after starting treatment, changes such as feeling less fatigued, weight loss, and gradual lowering of cholesterol levels will be noted. Treatment with levothyroxine is usually lifelong. To determine the right dosage of medication, the physician will check the level of TSH after 2 to 3 months of therapy.

Hyperthyroidism

Hyperthyroidism is a disorder that is caused by elevated levels of thyroid hormone. The symptoms of hyperthyroidism are caused by high levels of thyroid hormone. Symptoms can include: nervousness, palpitations, tremors, sweating, increased activity in the intestinal tract, changes in menstruation, and weight loss. Some people find it more difficult to tolerate heat. Some feel anxious or restless. Changes in fingernails and hair may be noticed. The heart may beat irregularly, or even become enlarged.

Sometimes an uncommon condition called Graves' ophthalmopathy may affect the eyes. In this disorder, the eyeball protrudes beyond its normal protective orbit when tissues and muscles behind the eye swell, pushing the eyeball forward.

Graves' disease, the most common cause of hyperthyroidism, is an autoimmnue disease in which antibodies produced by the immune system stimulate the thyroid to produce too much thyroxine. Other forms of hyperthyroidism may be caused by **thyroiditis,** or inflammation of the thyroid gland. Certain benign or malignant tumors can also produce too much thyroid hormone.

Some of the most serious complications of hyperthyroidism involve the heart. These include a rapid heart rate, atrial fibrillation and congestive heart failure. Untreated hyperthyroidism can also lead to weak, brittle bones (osteoporosis). People with Graves' ophthalmopathy develop eye problems, including bulging, red or swollen eyes, sensitivity to light and blurring or double vision. In rare cases, Graves' disease also affects the skin, causing redness and swelling on the shins and feet. A person who has hyperthyroidism is at risk of thyrotoxic crisis, a sudden intensification of the symptoms, leading to a fever, a rapid pulse and even delirium. If this occurs, one should seek immediate medical care.

Hyperthyroidism is usually treated with antithyroid medications, radioactive iodine (which destroys the thyroid and thus stops the excess production of hormones), or surgery (thyroidectomy). If the thyroid must be removed and/or destroyed, replacement thyroid hormones (levothyroxine) must be taken for the rest of the person's life. If the parathyroid glands are also removed, the patient will need medication to keep the blood calcium levels normal.

✔ PATHOLOGY CHECKPOINT

Following is a concise list of the pathology-related terms that you've seen in the chapter. Review this checklist to make sure that you are familiar with the meaning of each term before moving on to the next section.

Conditions and Symptoms

- ❏ acidosis
- ❏ acromegaly
- ❏ Addison's disease
- ❏ adenoma
- ❏ adenosis
- ❏ adrenopathy
- ❏ cretinism
- ❏ Cushing's disease
- ❏ diabetes
- ❏ dwarfism
- ❏ exophthalmic
- ❏ galactorrhea
- ❏ gigantism
- ❏ hirsutism
- ❏ hypergonadism
- ❏ hyperinsulinism
- ❏ hyperkalemia
- ❏ hyperthyroidism

- ❏ hypogonadism
- ❏ hypoparathyroidism
- ❏ hypothyroidism
- ❏ lethargic
- ❏ myxedema
- ❏ pituitarism
- ❏ progeria
- ❏ thymitis
- ❏ thyroiditis
- ❏ thyrotoxicosis
- ❏ virilism

Diagnosis and Treatment

- ❏ adenectomy
- ❏ adrenalectomy
- ❏ aldosterone
- ❏ androgen
- ❏ catecholamines
- ❏ cortisone

- ❏ dopamine
- ❏ epinephrine
- ❏ estrogen
- ❏ glucocorticoid
- ❏ hormone
- ❏ hydrocortisone
- ❏ insulin
- ❏ iodine
- ❏ norepinephrine
- ❏ oxytocin
- ❏ progesterone
- ❏ somatotropin
- ❏ steroids
- ❏ testosterone
- ❏ thymectomy
- ❏ thyroidectomy
- ❏ thyroxine
- ❏ vasopressin

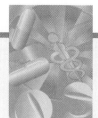

DRUG HIGHLIGHTS

Drugs that are generally used for endocrine system diseases and disorders include thyroid hormones, antithyroid hormones, insulin, and oral hypoglycemic agents.

Thyroid Hormones   Increase metabolic rate, cardiac output, oxygen consumption, body temperature, respiratory rate, blood volume, and carbohydrate, fat, and protein metabolism, and influence growth and development at cellular level. Thyroid hormones are used as supplements or replacement therapy in hypothyroidism, myxedema, and cretinism.

Examples: Levothroid and Synthroid (levothyroxine sodium), Cytomel (liothyronine sodium), Thyrolar (liotrix), and thyroid, USP.

Antithyroid Hormones	Inhibit the synthesis of thyroid hormones by decreasing iodine use in manufacture of thyroglobin and iodothyronine. They do not inactivate or inhibit thyroxine or triiodothyronine. They are used in the treatment of hyperthyroidism.

Example: Tapazole (methimazole), potassium iodide solution, Lugol's solution (strong iodine solution), and PTU (propylthiouracil).

Insulin Stimulates carbohydrate metabolism by increasing the movement of glucose and other monosaccharides into cells. It also influences fat and carbohydrate metabolism in the liver and adipose cells. It decreases blood sugar, phosphate, and potassium, and increases blood pyruvate and lactate. *Insulin* is used in the treatment of insulin-dependent diabetes mellitus (Type 1), non-insulin-dependent diabetes mellitus (Type 2) when other regimens are not effective, and to treat ketoacidosis.

Insulin Preparations Insulin is given by subcutaneous injection and is available in rapid-acting, intermediate-acting, and long-acting preparations.

Rapid-acting *Examples: Regular, Novolin R, Velosulin, and Humalog.*

Onset of Action ½ hour   Appearance—clear

Intermediate-acting *Examples: NPH, Novolin N, Humulin N, Lente Insulin, and Novolin L.*

Onset of Action 1–1½ hours   Appearance—cloudy

Long-acting *Examples: Ultralente and Humulin U.*

Onset of Action 3–5 hours   Appearance—cloudy

Oral Hypoglycemic Agents Are agents of the sulfonylurea class and are used to stimulate insulin secretion from pancreatic cells in non-insulin-dependent diabetics with some pancreatic function.

Examples: Diabinese (chlorpropamide), Glucotrol (glipizide), DiaBeta and Micronase (glyburide), Tolinase (tolazamide), and Orinase (tolbutamide).

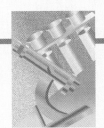

DIAGNOSTIC & LAB TESTS

TEST	DESCRIPTION
catecholamines (kăt″ ě-kōl′ ă-mēns)	A test performed on urine to determine the amount of epinephrine and norepinephrine present. These adrenal hormones increase in times of stress.
corticotropin, corticotropin-releasing factor (CRF) (kor″ tĭ-kō-trō′ pin)	A test performed on blood plasma to determine the amount of corticotropin present. Increased levels may indicate stress, adrenal cortical hypofunction, and/or pituitary tumors. Decreased levels may indicate adrenal neoplasms and/or Cushing's syndrome.
fasting blood sugar (FBS) (făs-tĭng blŭd shoog′ ar)	A test performed on blood to determine the level of sugar in the bloodstream. Increased levels may indicate diabetes mellitus, diabetic acidosis, and many other conditions. Decreased levels may indicate hypoglycemia, hyperinsulinism, and many other conditions.

TEST	DESCRIPTION
glucose tolerance test (GTT) (gloo′ kōs tŏl′ ĕr-ăns test)	A blood sugar test performed at specified intervals after the patient has been given a certain amount of glucose. Blood samples are drawn, and the blood glucose level of each sample is determined. It is more accurate than other blood sugar tests, and it is used to diagnose diabetes mellitus.
17-hydroxycorticosteroids (17-OHCS) (hī-drŏk″ sē-kor tĭ-kō-stĕr′ oyd)	A test performed on urine to identify adrenocorticosteroid hormones. It is used to determine adrenal cortical function.
17-ketosteroids (17-KS) (kē″ tō-stĕr′ oyd)	A test performed on urine to determine the amount of 17-KS present. 17-KS is the end product of androgens and is secreted from the adrenal glands and testes. It is used in the diagnosing of adrenal tumors.
protein-bound iodine (PBI) (prō′ tēn bound ī′ ō-dīn)	A test performed on serum to indicate the amount of iodine that is attached to serum protein. It may be used to indicate thyroid function.
radioactive iodine uptake (RAIU) (rā″ dē-ō-ăk′ tīv ī′ ō-dīn ŭp′ tāk)	A test to measure the ability of the thyroid gland to concentrate ingested iodine. Increased level may indicate hyperthyroidism, cirrhosis, and/or thyroiditis. Decreased level may indicate hypothyroidism.
radioimmunoassay (rā″ dē-ō-ĭmŭ″ -nō-ăs′ ā)	A standard assay method that is used for the measurement of minute quantities of specific antibodies and/or antigens. It may be used for clinical laboratory measurements of hormones, therapeutic drug monitoring, and substance abuse screening.
thyroid scan (thī′ royd skăn)	A test to detect tumors of the thyroid gland. The patient is given radioactive iodine 131, which localizes in the thyroid gland, and the gland is then visualized with a scanner device.
thyroxine (T_4) (thī-rōks′ ĭn)	A test performed on blood serum to determine the amount of thyroxine present. Increased levels may indicate hyperthyroidism. Decreased levels may indicate hypothyroidism.
triiodothyronine uptake (T_3) (trī″ ī-ō″ dō-thī′ rō-nĭn ŭp′ tāk)	A test performed on blood serum to determine the amount of triiodothyronine present. Increased levels may indicate thyrotoxicosis, toxic adenoma, and/or Hashimoto's struma. Decreased levels may indicate starvation, severe infection, and severe trauma.
total calcium (tōt′ l kăl′ sē-ŭm)	A test performed on blood serum to determine the amount of calcium present. Increased levels may indicate hyperparathyroidism. Decreased levels may indicate hypoparathyroidism.
ultrasonography (ŭl-tră-sŏn-ŏg′ ră-fē)	The use of high-frequency sound waves to visualize the structure being studied. May be used to visualize the pancreas, thyroid, and any other gland. It is used as a screening test or as a diagnostic tool.

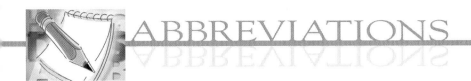

ABBREVIATIONS

ABBREVIATION	MEANING	ABBREVIATION	MEANING
ACTH	adrenocorticotropic hormone	MSH	melanocyte-stimulating hormone
ADA	American Diabetes Association	NIDDM	non-insulin-dependent diabetes mellitus
ADH	antidiuretic hormone	PBI	protein bound iodine
BG, bG	blood glucose	PIF	prolactin release-inhibiting factor
BMR	basal metabolic rate		
CRF	corticotropin-releasing factor	PRF	prolactin-releasing factor
DI	diabetes insipidus	PTH	parathormone
DM	diabetes mellitus	RAIU	radioactive iodine uptake
FBS	fasting blood sugar	RIA	radioimmunoassay
FSH	follicle-stimulating hormone	SMBG	self-monitoring of blood glucose
GH	growth hormone		
GnRF	gonadotropin-releasing factor	STH	somatotropin hormone
GTT	glucose tolerance test	T_3	triiodothyronine
IDDM	insulin-dependent diabetes mellitus	T_3RU	triiodothyronine resin uptake
		T_4	thyroxine
K	potassium	TFS	thyroid function studies
LH	luteinizing hormone	TSH	thyroid-stimulating hormone
LTH	lactogenic hormone	VMA	vanillylmandelic acid
MIF	melanocyte-stimulating hormone release-inhibiting factor	VP	vasopressin

STUDY AND REVIEW

Anatomy and Physiology

Write your answers to the following questions. Do not refer to the text.

1. Name the primary glands of the endocrine system.

   a. _____

   b. _____

   c. _____

   d. _____

   e. _____

   f. _____

   g. _____

   h. _____

2. Name the secondary glands of the endocrine system.

   a. _____

   b. _____

   c. _____

3. State the vital function of the endocrine system. _____

   _____

4. Define hormone. _____

5. State the vital role of the hypothalamus in regulating endocrine functions.

   _____

   _____

   _____

6. Why is the pituitary gland known as the master gland of the body? _____

   _____

7. Name the hormones secreted by the adenohypophysis.

   a. _____

   b. _____

   c. _____

   d. _____

   e. _____

   f. _____

   g. _____

8. Name the hormones secreted by the neurohypophysis.

   a. _____   b. _____

9. The pineal gland secretes the hormones _____ and _____.

10. State the vital role of the thyroid gland. _____

   _____

11. Name the hormones stored and secreted by the thyroid gland.

   a. _____   b. _____

   c. _____

12. Parathormone is essential for the maintenance of a normal level of

   _____ and also plays a role in the metabolism of _____.

13. Insulin is essential for the maintenance of a normal level of _____.

14. The adrenal cortex secretes a group of hormones known as the

   _____, the _____, and the _____.

15. Name four functions of cortisol.

   a. _____   b. _____

   c. _____   d. _____

16. Name four functions of corticosterone.

   a. _____   b. _____

   c. _____   d. _____

17. _____ is the principal mineralocorticoid secreted by the adrenal cortex.

18. Define androgen. _____

   _____

19. Name the three main catecholamines synthesized, secreted, and stored by the
    adrenal medulla.

   a. _____   b. _____

   c. _____

20. Name three functions of the hormone epinephrine.

   _____

   _____

   _____

21. The ovaries produce the hormones _____ and _____.

22. The testes produce the hormone _____.

23. Name the two hormones secreted by the thymus.

    a. _____   b. _____

24. Name the four hormones secreted by the gastrointestinal mucosa.

    a. _____   b. _____

    c. _____   d. _____

Word Parts

1. In the spaces provided, write the definitions of these prefixes, roots, combining forms, and suffixes. Do not refer to the listings of medical words. Leave blank those words you cannot define.

2. After completing as many as you can, refer to the medical word listings to check your work. For each word missed or left blank, write the word and its definition several times on the margins of these pages or on a separate sheet of paper.

3. To maximize the learning process, it is to your advantage to do the following exercises as directed. To refer to the word building section before completing these exercises invalidates the learning process.

PREFIXES

Give the definitions of the following prefixes:

1. ad- _____   2. dia- _____

3. endo- _____   4. eu- _____

5. ex- _____   6. exo- _____

7. hyper- _____   8. hypo- _____

9. pan- _____   10. para- _____

11. pro- _____   12. epi- _____

13. hydro- _____

ROOTS AND COMBINING FORMS

Give the definitions of the following roots and combining forms:

1. acid _____

2. acr/o _____

3. aden _____

4. aden/o _____

5. cortic _____

6. creat _____

7. cretin _____

8. andr/o _____

9. crine _____

10. crin/o _____

11. dwarf _____

12. galact/o _____

13. ger _____

14. gigant _____

15. glandul _____

16. gluc/o _____

17. gonad _____

18. hirsut _____

19. insul _____

20. cortis _____

21. insulin/o _____

22. kal _____

23. letharg _____

24. log _____

25. myx _____

26. ophthalm _____

27. pine _____

28. nephr _____

29. pituitar _____

30. ren _____

31. ren/o _____

32. estr/o _____

33. thym _____

34. gester _____

35. thyr _____

36. thyr/o _____

37. toxic _____

38. trop _____

39. viril _____

40. somat/o _____

41. test/o _____

42. ster _____

43. thyrox _____

44. vas/o _____

45. press _____

SUFFIXES

Give the definitions of the following suffixes:

1. -al _____

2. -gen _____

3. -ar _____

4. -betes _____

5. -ectomy _____

6. -edema _____

7. -emia _____

8. -genic _____

9. -ia _____

10. -ic _____

11. -ism _____

12. -ist _____

13. -itis _____

14. -logy _____

15. -one _____

16. -megaly _____

17. -oid _____

18. -oma _____

19. -osis _____

20. -pathy _____

21. -ine _____

22. -physis _____

23. -in _____

24. -rrhea _____

25. -y _____

Identifying Medical Terms

In the spaces provided, write the medical terms for the following meanings:

1. _____ Any disease condition of a gland

2. _____ A congenital deficiency in secretion of the thyroid hormone

3. _____ A disease characterized by excessive discharge of urine

4. _____ The study of the endocrine system

5. _____ Normal activity of the thyroid gland

6. _____ External secretion of a gland

7. _____ A condition of being abnormally large

8. _____ A general classification of the adrenal cortex hormones

9. _____ An excessive amount of potassium in the blood

10. _____ Deficient internal secretion of the gonads

11. _____ Pertaining to drowsiness; sluggishness

12. _____ Inflammation of the thymus

Spelling

In the spaces provided, write the correct spelling of these misspelled words:

1. catcholamines _____
2. crtinism _____
3. exopthalmic _____
4. hypthyoidism _____
5. myexdema _____
6. pinael _____
7. pitutary _____
8. thyoid _____
9. oxytoin _____
10. virlism _____

Matching

Select the appropriate lettered meaning for each word listed below.

_____ 1. aldosterone
_____ 2. androgen
_____ 3. catecholamines
_____ 4. cortisone
_____ 5. dopamine
_____ 6. epinephrine
_____ 7. insulin
_____ 8. iodine
_____ 9. thyroxine
_____ 10. vasopressin

a. Also called antidiuretic hormone, ADH
b. Biochemical substances, epinephrine, norepinephrine, and dopamine
c. A hormone essential for the metabolism of carbohydrates and fats
d. A hormone produced by the thyroid gland
e. The principal mineralocorticoid secreted by the adrenal cortex
f. Hormones that produce or stimulate the development of male characteristics
g. A glucocorticoid hormone used as an anti-inflammatory agent
h. An intermediate substance in the synthesis of norepinephrine
i. Also called adrenaline, Adrenalin
j. A trace mineral that aids in the development and functioning of the thyroid gland
k. A hormone produced by the testes

Abbreviations

Place the correct word, phrase, or abbreviation in the space provided.

1. basal metabolic rate _____
2. diabetes mellitus _____
3. FBS _____

4. GTT _____

5. protein bound iodine _____

6. PTH _____

7. RIA _____

8. somatotropin hormone _____

9. TFS _____

10. VP _____

Diagnostic and Laboratory Tests

Select the best answer to each multiple choice question. Circle the letter of your choice.

1. A test performed on urine to determine the amount of epinephrine and norepinephrine present.
   a. catecholamines
   b. corticotropin
   c. protein bound iodine
   d. total calcium

2. Increased levels may indicate diabetes mellitus, diabetes acidosis, and many other conditions.
   a. protein bound iodine
   b. total calcium
   c. fasting blood sugar
   d. thyroid scan

3. A test used to detect tumors of the thyroid gland.
   a. thyroxine
   b. total calcium
   c. thyroid scan
   d. protein-bound iodine

4. A blood sugar test performed at specific intervals after the patient has been given a certain amount of glucose.
   a. fasting blood sugar
   b. glucose tolerance test
   c. protein bound iodine
   d. corticotropin

5. A test used in the diagnosing of adrenal tumors.
   a. 17-HCS
   b. 17-OHCS
   c. 17-KS
   d. 17-HDL

CASE STUDY

DIABETES MELLITUS TYPE 1

Read the following case study and then answer the questions that follow.

A 20-year-old female was seen by a physician and the following is a synopsis of the visit.

Present History: The patient states that she has been very thirsty and hungry and urinating a lot. She says that diabetes runs in her family, and she is concerned that she may be developing the disease.

Signs and Symptoms: Polydipsia, polyphagia, polyuria.

Diagnosis: Diabetes mellitus Type 1. The diagnosis was determined by the characteristic symptoms, family history, a blood glucose test, and a glucose tolerance test.

Treatment: The management of diabetes mellitus Type 1 is based on trying to normalize insulin activity and blood glucose levels to reduce the development of complications of the disease. The patient was instructed in insulin therapy, diet therapy, an exercise program, and lifestyle modifications. The patient was taught how to properly administer insulin, with dosage based on her blood glucose test performed before breakfast, lunch, and dinner. A follow-up visit was scheduled for 2 weeks with instructions to call if there were any questions or problems.

CASE STUDY QUESTIONS

1. Signs and symptoms of diabetes mellitus Type 1 include _____, polyphagia, and polyuria.
2. The diagnosis was determined by the characteristic symptoms, family history, a blood glucose test, and a _____ tolerance test.
3. Treatment for diabetes mellitus Type 1 includes insulin therapy, _____ therapy, an exercise program, and lifestyle changes.
4. The medical word for excessive thirst is _____.
5. The medical word for frequent urination is _____.
6. The medical word for extreme hunger is _____.

MedMedia Wrap-Up
www.prenhall.com/rice

Additional interactive resources and activities for this chapter can be found on the Companion Website. For animations, videos, audio glossary, and review, access the accompanying CD-ROM in this book.

Audio Glossary
Medical Terminology Exercises & Activities
Pathology Spotlight
Terminology Translator
Animations
Videos

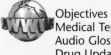

Objectives
Medical Terminology Exercises & Activities
Audio Glossary
Drug Updates
Medical Terminology in the News

THE NERVOUS SYSTEM 12

OBJECTIVES

On completion of this chapter, you will be able to:

- Describe the tissues of the nervous system.
- Describe nerve fibers, nerves, and tracts.
- Describe the transmission of nerve impulses.
- Describe the central nervous system.
- Describe the peripheral nervous system.
- Describe the autonomic nervous system.
- Analyze, build, spell, and pronounce medical words.
- Describe each of the conditions presented in the Pathology Spotlights.
- Complete the Pathology Checkpoint.
- Review Drug Highlights presented in this chapter.
- Provide the description of diagnostic and laboratory tests related to the nervous system.
- Identify and define selected abbreviations.
- Successfully complete the study and review section.

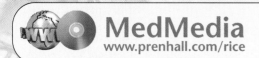

MedMedia
www.prenhall.com/rice

Additional interactive resources and activities for this chapter can be found on the Companion Website. For Terminology Translator, animations, videos, audio glossary, and review, access the accompanying CD-ROM in this book.

Anatomy and Physiology Overview

The nervous system is usually described as having two interconnected divisions: the CNS or **central nervous system** and the PNS or **peripheral nervous system**. The CNS includes the brain and spinal cord. It is enclosed by the bones of the skull and spinal column. The PNS consists of the network of nerves and neural tissues branching throughout the body from 12 pairs of cranial nerves and 31 pairs of spinal nerves. See Figure 12–1. A general description of the nervous system and its functions is provided in this overview.

TISSUES OF THE NERVOUS SYSTEM

There are two principal tissue types in the nervous system. These tissues are made up of **neurons** or nerve cells and their supporting tissues, collectively called **neuroglia**. Neurons are the structural and functional units of the nervous system. These cells are specialized conductors of impulses that enable the body to interact with its internal and external environments. There are several types of neurons, three of which are described for you.

Motor Neurons

Motor neurons cause contractions in muscles and secretions from glands and organs. They also act to inhibit the actions of glands and organs, thereby controlling most of the body's functions. Motor neurons may be described as being **efferent** processes, as they transmit impulses away from the neural cell body to the muscles or organs to be

THE NERVOUS SYSTEM

Organ/Structure	Primary Functions
Neurons (nerve cells)	Structural and functional units of the nervous system. Specialized conductors of impulses that enable the body to interact with its internal and external environments
Neuroglia	Supporting tissue
Nerve Fibers and Tracts	Conduct impulses from one location to another
Central Nervous System	Receives impulses from throughout the body, processes the information, and responds with an appropriate action
Brain	Governs sensory perception, emotions, consciousness, memory, and voluntary movements
Spinal cord	Conduct sensory impulses to the brain; conduct motor impulses from the brain to body parts, and serves as a reflex center for impulses entering and leaving the spinal cord without involvement of the brain
Peripheral Nervous System	Links the central nervous system with other parts of the body
Cranial nerves (12 pairs)	Provide sensory input and motor control, or a combination of these
Spinal nerves (31 pairs)	Carry impulses to the spinal cord and to muscles, organs, and glands
Autonomic Nervous System	Controls involuntary bodily functions such as sweating and arterial blood pressure

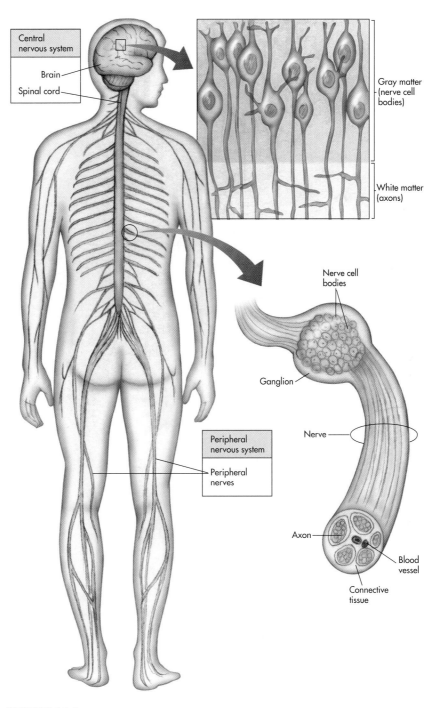

FIGURE 12–1

The nervous system is described as having two interconnected divisions: the central nervous system (CNS) consisting of the brain and spinal cord, and the peripheral nervous system (PNS) consisting of peripheral nerves.

innervated. Motor neurons consist of a nucleated cell body with protoplasmic processes extending away from it in several directions. These processes are known as the **axon** and **dendrites**. Most axons are long and are covered with a fatty substance, the myelin sheath, that acts as an insulator and increases the transmission velocity of the nerve fiber it surrounds. Axons may be as long as several feet and reach from the cell body to the area to be activated. Dendrites resemble the branches of a tree, are short, or unsheathed, and transmit impulses to the cell body. Neurons usually have several dendrites and only one axon (Fig. 12–2).

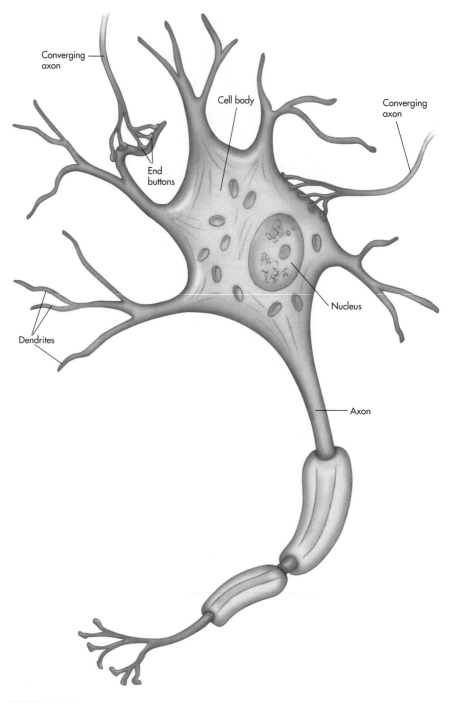

FIGURE 12–2

A neuron (nerve cell) with two converging axons.

Sensory Neurons

Sensory neurons differ in structure from motor neurons because they do not have true dendrites. The processes transmitting sensory information to the cell bodies of these neurons are called peripheral processes, are sheathed, and resemble axons. They are attached to sensory receptors and transmit impulses to the central nervous system (CNS). In turn, the CNS may stimulate motor neurons in response to this sensory information. Sensory neurons are sometimes referred to as **afferent nerves**, as they carry impulses to the cell body and the central nervous system.

Interneurons

Interneurons are sometimes called *central* or *associative neurons* and are located entirely within the central nervous system. They function to mediate impulses between sensory and motor neurons.

NERVE FIBERS, NERVES, AND TRACTS

The terms *nerve fiber*, *nerve*, and *tract* are used to describe neuronal processes conducting impulses from one location to another. Each term is defined.

Nerve Fiber

A single elongated process, usually a long axon or a peripheral process from a sensory neuron, is called a **nerve fiber**. Each peripheral nerve fiber is wrapped by a protective membrane called a **sheath**. There are two types of sheaths, *myelinated (thick)* and *unmyelinated (thin)*, formed by accessory cells. Some nerve fibers have only the unmyelinated sheath or neurilemma composed of *Schwann cells*. Myelinated fibers have an inner sheath of myelin, a thick fatty substance, and an outer sheath, the **neurilemma**. Nerve fibers of the central nervous system (*within the brain and spinal cord*) do not contain Schwann cells, which are necessary for the regeneration of a damaged nerve fiber. Therefore, damage to fibers of the CNS is permanent, whereas damage to a peripheral nerve may be reversible.

Nerve

A **nerve** is a bundle of nerve fibers, located outside the brain and spinal cord, that connects to various parts of the body. Nerves are usually described as being **afferent** (*conducting to the CNS*) or **efferent** (*conducting to muscles, organs, and glands*). Some nerves contain a mixture of afferent and efferent fibers and are called **mixed nerves**. Nerves are also referred to as sensory (**afferent**) and motor (**efferent**).

Tracts

Groups of nerve fibers within the central nervous system are sometimes referred to as **tracts** when they have the same origin, function, and termination. The spinal cord contains afferent sensory tracts ascending to the brain and efferent motor tracts descending from the brain. The brain itself contains numerous tracts, the largest of which is the *corpus callosum* joining the left and right hemispheres.

TRANSMISSION OF NERVE IMPULSES

Stimulation of a nerve occurs at a *receptor*. Sensory receptors are of different types, ranging from the simplest, which are free nerve endings for pain, to the most complex, as in the retina of the eye for vision. Receptors are generally specialized to specific types of stimulation such as heat, cold, light, pressure, or pain and react by initiating a chemical change or impulse. The transmission of an impulse by a nerve fiber is based on the

all-or-none principle. This means that no transmission occurs until the stimulus reaches a set minimum strength, which may vary with different receptors. Once the minimum stimulus or threshold is reached, a maximum impulse is produced. A stimulation that is stronger than the minimum needed does not produce a larger impulse. Impulses travel from receptors, through dendrites or peripheral processes, to the neural cell bodies and on to an axon that terminates in several specialized knob-like branch endings. At this point, called a **synapse**, the impulse is transmitted, with the help of certain chemical agents, across a space separating the axon's end knobs from the dendrites of the next neuron or from a motor end plate attached to a muscle. This space is called a **synaptic cleft**, and the chemical agents released are called **neurotransmitters**. They are discharged into the synaptic cleft and alter the permeability of the postsynaptic membrane in which the cleft is located. This alternation may have an excitatory effect or, in some cases, an inhibitory effect, depending on the chemical reaction that occurs when the neurotransmitter crosses the synaptic cleft.

THE CENTRAL NERVOUS SYSTEM (CNS)

Consisting of the brain and spinal cord, the **central nervous system** receives impulses from throughout the body, processes the information, and responds with an appropriate action. This activity may be at the conscious or unconscious level, depending on the source of the sensory stimulus. Both the brain and spinal cord can be divided into **gray** and **white matter**. The gray matter consists of unsheathed cell bodies and true dendrites. The white matter is composed of myelinated nerve fibers. In the spinal cord, the arrangement of white and gray matter results in an H-shaped core of gray cell bodies surrounded by tracts of nerve fibers interconnected to the brain. The reverse is generally true of the brain where the surface layer or cortex is gray matter and most of the internal structures are white matter.

The Brain

The nervous tissue of the **brain** consists of millions of nerve cells and fibers. It is the largest mass of nervous tissue in the body, weighing about 1380 g in the male and 1250 g in the female. When fully developed, the brain fills the cranial cavity and is enclosed by three membranes known collectively as the **meninges**. From the outside in, these are the *dura mater, arachnoid,* and *pia mater.* The major substructures or divisions of the brain are the *cerebrum, diencephalon, midbrain, cerebellum, pons, medulla oblongata,* and the *reticular formation* (Fig. 12–3).

THE CEREBRUM

Representing seven-eighths of the brain's total weight, the **cerebrum** contains nerve centers that govern all sensory and motor activity, including sensory perception, emotions, consciousness, memory, and voluntary movements. See Table 12–1. It is divided by the longitudinal fissure into two cerebral hemispheres, the right and left, that are joined by large fiber tracts (*the corpus callosum*) that allow information to pass from one hemisphere to the other. The surface or *cortex* of each hemisphere is arranged in folds creating bulges and shallow furrows. Each bulge is called a **gyrus** or **convolution**. A furrow is known as a **sulcus**. This surface is composed of gray, unmyelinated cell bodies and is known as the **cerebral cortex**. The cortex has been divided into lobes as a means of identifying certain locations. These lobes correspond to the overlying bones of the skull and are the *frontal lobe, parietal lobe, temporal lobe,* and *occipital lobe.*

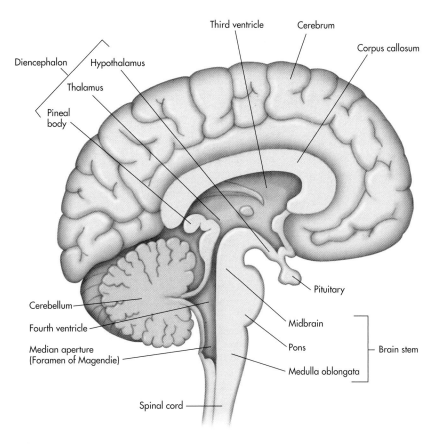

Third ventricle

Cerebrum

Corpus callosum

Diencephalon

Hypothalamus

Thalamus

Pineal body

Pituitary

Cerebellum

Fourth ventricle

Median aperture (Foramen of Magendie)

Midbrain

Pons

Brain stem

Medulla oblongata

Spinal cord

FIGURE 12–3

The major divisions of the brain.

Another reference system for locating areas of the cerebral cortex is by way of **fissures** and **sulci**. As noted earlier, the cerebrum is divided by a deep longitudinal fissure. Each hemisphere, thus created, contains **six major sulci**. The two most often used as reference points are the lateral and central sulci. The lateral sulcus lies below the frontal and parietal lobes and forms the upper border of the temporal lobe. The central sulcus runs from the longitudinal fissure to the lateral sulcus and separates the frontal lobe from the parietal lobe. The occipital lobe is the lower rear part of the cerebrum beneath the parietal lobe and posterior to the temporal lobe (Fig. 12–4).

Electrical stimulation of the various areas of the cortex during neurosurgery has identified specialized cell activity within the different lobes. The **frontal lobe** has been identified as the brain's major motor area. The **parietal lobe** contains centers for sensory input from all parts of the body and is known as the somesthetic area. Temperature, pressure, touch, and an awareness of muscle control are some of the sensory activities centered in this area. The **temporal lobe** contains centers for auditory and language input, and the **occipital lobe** is considered to be the primary sensory area for vision.

Throughout the cortex are areas known to integrate and store information. These memory or association areas comprise more than three-fourths of the cerebral cortex. Below the cortex are masses of nerve fibers, the white matter, that interconnect areas within the brain and lead to the spinal cord. Four paired masses of gray matter, the **dorsal ganglia**, have been found embedded within the white fibers. The dorsal ganglia function in the control of motor activity and an injury or a disease in this area can result in a loss of motor control.

TABLE 12–1 MAJOR DIVISIONS OF THE BRAIN AND THEIR FUNCTIONS

Brain Area	Functions
Cerebrum	Governs all sensory and motor activity; sensory perception, emotions, consciousness, memory, and voluntary movements.
Diencephalon	
Thalamus	Relay center for all sensory impulses (except olfactory) being transmitted to the sensory areas of the cortex. Also relays motor impulses from the cerebellum and the basal ganglia to motor areas of the cortex. Thought to be involved with emotions and arousal mechanisms.
Hypothalamus	Principal regulator of autonomic nervous activity that is associated with behavior and expression. It also produces neurosecretions for the control of water balance, sugar and fat metabolism, regulation of body temperature, sleep-cycle control, appetite, and sexual arousal. Additionally, the hypothalamus produces hormones for the posterior pituitary gland.
Midbrain	Two-way conduction pathway; relay center for visual and auditory impulses. Contains afferent and efferent pathways connecting major motor areas of the forebrain and hindbrain, thereby serving as a two-way conduction pathway. Also found in the midbrain are four small masses of gray cells known collectively as the corpora quadrigemina. The upper two, called the superior colliculi, are associated with visual reflexes. The lower two, or inferior colliculi, are involved with the sense of hearing.
The Hindbrain	
Cerebellum	Coordination of voluntary movement.
Pons	Links the cerebellum and medulla to higher cortical areas; two-way conduction pathway between areas of the brain and other areas of the body; influences respiration.
Medulla oblongata	Cardiac, respiratory, and vasomotor control center. Regulation and control of breathing, swallowing, coughing, sneezing, and vomiting. Also regulates arterial blood pressure, thereby exerting control over the circulation of blood.
Reticular formation	Exerts control over or influences wakefulness, sleep, and certain reflex activities of the spinal nerves.

THE DIENCEPHALON

The word **diencephalon** means "second portion of the brain" and refers to the thalamus and hypothalamus.

The Thalamus. The **thalamus** is the largest of the two divisions of the diencephalon and is actually two large masses of gray cell bodies joined by a third or intermediate mass. The thalamus serves as a relay center for all sensory impulses (*except olfactory*) being transmitted to the sensory areas of the cortex. Besides its sensory function, the thalamus also relays motor impulses from the cerebellum and the basal ganglia to motor areas of the cortex. Some impulses related to emotional behavior are also passed from the hypothalamus, through the thalamus, to the cerebral cortex. See Table 12–1.

The Hypothalamus. The **hypothalamus** lies beneath the thalamus and is a principal regulator of autonomic nervous activity that is associated with behavior and emotional expression. It also produces neurosecretions for the control of water balance, sugar and fat metabolism, regulation of body temperature, and other metabolic activities. Additionally, the hypothalamus produces hormones for the posterior pituitary gland and exerts control over secretions from both the anterior and posterior pituitary. See Table 12–1. The pituitary gland is attached to the hypothalamus by a narrow stalk, the *infundibulum*.

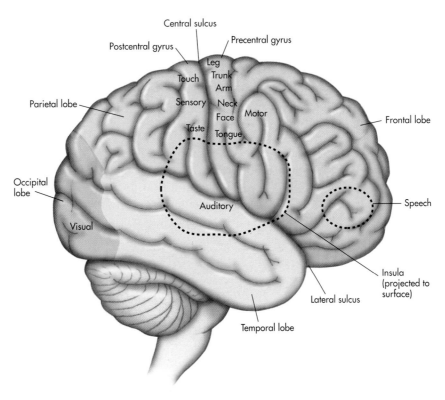

FIGURE 12–4

The brain, its lobes, and principal sulci. The location of certain sensory and motor areas are shown.

THE MIDBRAIN

Located between the forebrain, which has just been described, and the hindbrain, the **midbrain** contains a number of large afferent and efferent pathways connecting major motor areas of the fore- and hindbrain. Also found in the midbrain are four small masses of gray cells known collectively as the **corpora quadrigemina**. The upper two, called the **superior colliculi**, are associated with visual reflexes such as the tracking movements of the eyes. The lower two, or **inferior colliculi**, are involved with the sense of hearing. See Table 12–1.

THE HINDBRAIN

The **hindbrain** consists of the cerebellum, the pons, the medulla oblongata, and the recticular formation.

The Cerebellum.   The largest part of the hindbrain is the **cerebellum**. It occupies a space in the back of the skull, inferior to the cerebrum and dorsal to the pons and medulla oblongata. The cerebellum is oval in shape and divided into lobes by deep fissures. The surface of the cerebellum has a cortex of gray cell bodies, and its interior contains nerve fibers, white matter, connecting it to every part of the central nervous system. The cerebellum plays an important part in the coordination of voluntary movement. See Table 12–1.

The Pons.   The **pons** is a broad band of white matter located anterior to the cerebellum and between the midbrain and the medulla oblongata. The pons contains fiber tracts linking the cerebellum and medulla to higher cortical areas. See Table 12–1.

The Medulla Oblongata. That part of the brain stem that connects the pons and the rest of the brain to the spinal cord is called the **medulla oblongata**. All the afferent and efferent tracts from the spinal cord either pass through or terminate in the medulla oblongata. The medulla also contains nerve centers instrumental to the regulation and control of breathing, swallowing, coughing, sneezing, and vomiting. Other centers in the medulla regulate arterial blood pressure, thereby exerting control over the circulation of blood. See Table 12–1.

The Reticular Formation. The **reticular formation** is a diffuse network, consisting of small groups of cell bodies and their processes, located in the area of the brain stem. The reticular formation exerts control over or influences wakefulness, sleep, and certain reflex activities of the spinal nerves. See Table 12–1.

The Spinal Cord

As previously mentioned, the **spinal cord** has an H-shaped gray area of cell bodies encircled by an outer region of white matter. The white matter consists of nerve tracts and fibers providing sensory input to the brain and conducting motor impulses from the brain to spinal neurons. Other fibers connect nerve cells within the spinal cord with other areas of the cord. The spinal cord is about 44 cm long and extends down the vertebral canal from the medulla to terminate near the junction of the first and second lumbar vertebrae. The functions of the spinal cord are to conduct sensory impulses to the brain, to conduct motor impulses from the brain, and to serve as a reflex center for impulses entering and leaving the spinal cord without involvement of the brain (Fig. 12–5).

The Cerebrospinal Fluid

The brain and spinal cord are surrounded by **cerebrospinal fluid**. This colorless fluid is produced by the *choroid plexuses* within the *ventricles* of the brain. There are four cavities or ventricles within the brain that are interconnected and are continuous with a small central canal that extends through the length of the spinal cord. Cerebrospinal fluid circulates through the ventricles, the central canal, and the subarachnoid space. This is a thin space between the arachnoid membrane and the pia mater, which is the membrane covering the surface of the brain and spinal cord. Cerebrospinal fluid is removed from circulation by the **arachnoid villi**, which are small projections of the arachnoid membrane that penetrate the tough outer membrane, the dura mater. The arachnoid villi allow the fluid to drain into the superior sagittal sinus. The normal adult will have between 120 and 150 mL of cerebrospinal fluid in circulation. The fluid serves to cushion the brain and cord from shocks that might cause injury. It also helps to support the brain by allowing it to float within the supporting liquid. It also contains neurotransmitters such as monoamines, acetylcholine, and neuropeptides.

THE PERIPHERAL NERVOUS SYSTEM (PNS)

The network of nerves branching throughout the body from the brain and spinal cord is known as the **peripheral nervous system**. There are 12 pairs of cranial nerves that attach to the brain and 31 pairs of spinal nerves connected to the spinal cord.

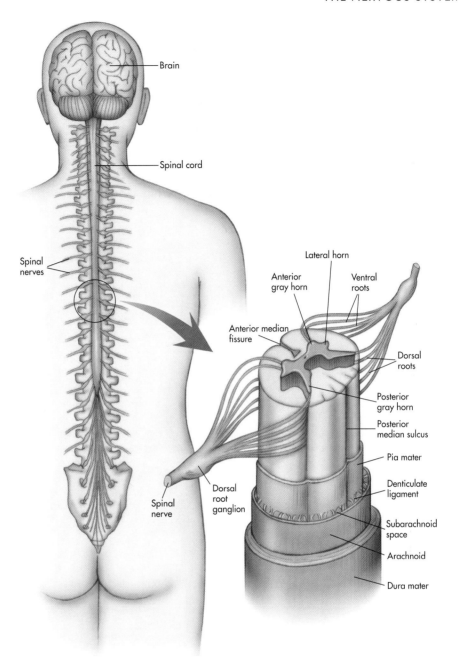

FIGURE 12–5

The brain, spinal cord, and spinal nerves. An expanded view of a spinal nerve is shown.

The Cranial Nerves

The nerves described below attach to the brain and provide sensory input, motor control, or a combination of these functions. They are arranged symmetrically, 12 to each side of the brain, and generally are named for the area or function they serve (Fig. 12–6 and Table 12–2).

THE OLFACTORY NERVE (I)

The **olfactory nerve** provides sensory input only and carries impulses for smell to the brain. The cell bodies of these nerve fibers are located in the nasal mucous membrane and serve as receptors for the sense of smell.

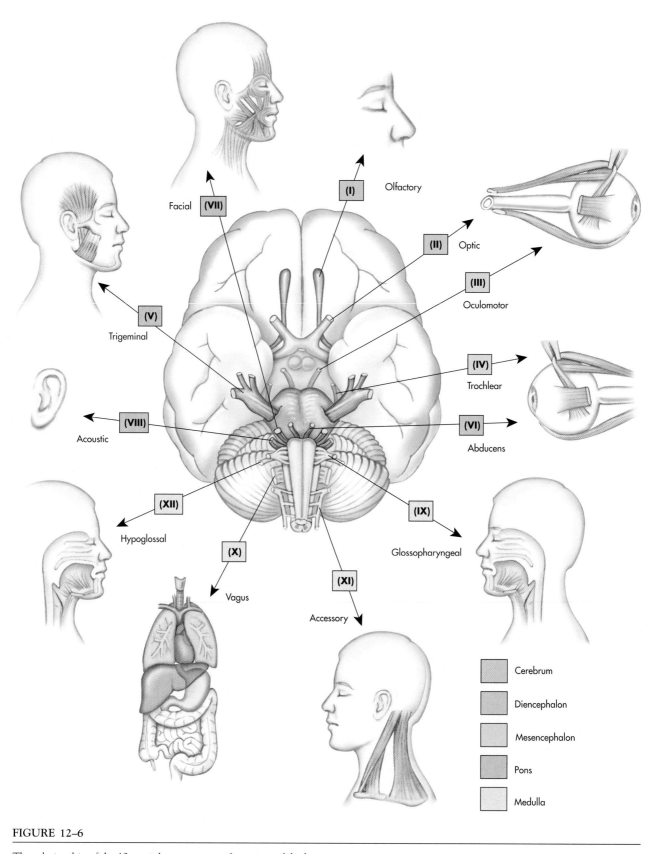

FIGURE 12–6

The relationship of the 12 cranial nerves to specific regions of the brain.

TABLE 12–2 CRANIAL NERVES AND FUNCTIONS

Nerve/Number	Function
Olfactory (I)	Sense of smell
Optic (II)	Vision
Oculomotor (III)	Motor impulses to four of the six external muscles of the eye and to the muscle that raises the eyelid
Trochlear (IV)	Motor impulses to control the superior oblique muscle of the eyeball
Trigeminal (V)	Provide sensory input from the face, nose, mouth, forehead, and top of the head; motor fibers to the muscles of the jaw (chewing)
Abducens (VI)	Conducts motor impulses to the lateral rectus muscle of the eyeball
Facial (VII)	Controls the muscles of the face and scalp; controls the lacrimal glands of the eye and the submandibular and sublingual salivary glands; input from the tongue for the sense of taste
Acoustic (VIII)	Input for hearing and equilibrium
Glossopharyngeal (IX)	General sense of taste; swallowing; control secretion of saliva
Vagus (X)	Controls muscles of the pharynx and larynx and of the thoracic and abdominal organs; swallowing, voice production, slowing of heartbeat, acceleration of peristalsis
Accessory (XI)	Control of the trapezius and sternocleidomastoid muscles, permitting movement of the head and shoulders
Hypoglossal (XII)	Control of the tongue; tongue movements

THE OPTIC NERVE (II)

The **optic nerve** provides sensory input only and carries impulses for vision to the brain. The rods and cones of the eyes are receptors and transmit images through the cells of the retina to processes that form the optic nerve. The optic nerves from each eye unite after entering the cranial cavity to form the optic chiasm from which tracts, carrying images from both eyes, connect to the brain.

THE OCULOMOTOR NERVE (III)

The **oculomotor nerve** conducts motor impulses to four of the six external muscles of the eye and to the muscle that raises the eyelid. The cell bodies of motor nerves are located in the brain.

THE TROCHLEAR NERVE (IV)

The **trochlear nerve** conducts motor impulses to control the superior oblique muscle of the eyeball.

THE TRIGEMINAL NERVE (V)

The **trigeminal nerve** has both sensory and motor fibers. Its fibers form three sensory divisions, the ophthalmic, maxillary, and mandibular. These fibers provide sensory input from the face, nose, mouth, forehead, and top of the head. The mandibular division also contains motor fibers to the muscles of the jaw.

THE ABDUCENS NERVE (VI)

The **abducens nerve** conducts motor impulses to the lateral rectus muscle of the eyeball.

THE FACIAL NERVE (VII)

The **facial nerve** has both sensory and motor fibers. Its motor fibers control the muscles of the face and scalp, thereby providing for facial expression. It also provides efferent fibers to control the lacrimal glands of the eyes as well as the submandibular and sublingual salivary glands. Sensory fibers of the facial nerve provide input from the forward two thirds of the tongue for the sense of taste.

THE ACOUSTIC NERVE (VIII)

Sometimes called the vestibulocochlear or auditory nerve, the **acoustic nerve** provides sensory input for hearing and equilibrium. Fibers of the cochlear division connect with receptors in the cochlea of the ear for hearing. Fibers of the vestibular division connect to receptors in the semicircular canals and vestibule located in the ear for the sense of equilibrium.

THE GLOSSOPHARYNGEAL NERVE (IX)

The **glossopharyngeal nerve** has both sensory and motor fibers. The sensory fibers provide for the general sense of taste and attach to the back of the tongue and pharynx. Motor fibers innervate the stylopharyngeus muscle and are important to the act of the swallowing. Other efferent fibers control the secretion of saliva from the parotid gland.

THE VAGUS NERVE (X)

The **vagus nerve** contains both sensory and motor fibers and is the longest of the cranial nerves. The motor fibers control muscles of the pharynx and larynx. The sensory fibers provide input from the autonomic control of most of the organs in the thoracic and abdominal cavities.

THE ACCESSORY NERVE (XI)

The **accessory nerve** conducts motor impulses for the control of the trapezius and sternocleidomastoid muscles, permitting movement of the head and shoulders.

THE HYPOGLOSSAL NERVE (XII)

The **hypoglossal nerve** conducts motor impulses for control of the muscles of the tongue.

The Spinal Nerves

There are 31 pairs of **spinal nerves** distributed along the length of the spinal cord and emerging from the vertebral canal on either side through the intervertebral foramina. At the point of attachment, each nerve is divided into *two roots* (see Fig. 12–5). The **dorsal** or **sensory root** is composed of afferent fibers carrying impulses to the cord, and the **ventral root** contains motor fibers carrying efferent impulses to muscles and organs. The cell bodies of the motor fibers lie in the gray matter of the spinal cord. The cell bodies for the sensory fibers are clustered just outside the spinal cord in small enlargements on each dorsal root. These enlargements are called the **spinal ganglia**. Named for the region of the vertebral column from which they exit, there are 8 pairs of **cervical spinal nerves**, 12 pairs of **thoracic spinal nerves**, 5 pairs of **lumbar spinal nerves**, 5 pairs of **sacral spinal nerves**, and 1 pair of **coccygeal spinal nerves**. A short distance from the cord, the fibers of the two roots unite to form a spinal nerve. Having formed a single nerve composed of afferent and efferent fibers, each spinal nerve then branches into several smaller nerves. The two primary branches from each spinal nerve are the **dorsal** and **ventral rami**. The dorsal rami (*branches*) carry motor and sensory fibers to the muscles and skin of the back and serve an area from the back of the head to the coccyx. The ventral rami, serving a much larger area, carry both motor and sensory fibers to the muscles and organs of the body, including the arms, legs, hands, and feet. The following describes the origin and purpose of the ventral branches of the 31 pairs of spinal nerves.

The ventral fibers from the first four cervical nerves form a network of interlaced nerve fibers called a **plexus**, which gives rise to peripheral nerves. Located in the neck, the **cervical plexus** innervates the muscles and skin of the neck and back of the head. The phrenic nerve, serving the diaphragm, also arises from the cervical plexus. Ventral fibers of cervical nerves 4 through 8 and the first thoracic nerve interlace to form the **brachial plexus**. Located in the area of the shoulder, the peripheral nerves from the brachial plexus innervate the shoulder, arm, forearm, wrist, and hand. The ventral rami of thoracic nerves 1 through 12 form the intercostal (*between the ribs*) nerves and the subcostal (*below the ribs*) nerves. Fibers of these nerves serve the muscles and skin of the thorax and upper abdomen. Ventral fibers of the first three and most of the fourth lumbar nerves interlace to form the **lumbar plexus**. Peripheral nerves from the lumbar plexus serve the muscles of the thigh and leg and the skin of the hip, scrotum, thigh, and leg. The ventral rami of the fourth and fifth lumbar together with those of the five sacral nerves interlace to form the **sacral plexus**. Peripheral nerves from the sacral plexus innervate the skin and muscles of the leg, foot, and external genitalia. Part of the fifth sacral and the entire coccygeal nerve are of limited importance and innervate the coccygeus muscle and the skin over the coccyx.

THE AUTONOMIC NERVOUS SYSTEM (ANS)

Actually a part of the peripheral nervous system, the **autonomic nervous system** controls involuntary bodily functions such as sweating, secretions of glands, arterial blood pressure, smooth muscle tissue, and the heart. The autonomic nervous system is primarily composed of efferent fibers from certain cranial and spinal nerves and can be functionally divided into two divisions, the **sympathetic** and **parasympathetic**. These two divisions counteract each other's activity to keep the body in a state of homeostasis.

The Sympathetic Division

Branches from the ventral roots of the 12 thoracic and the first 3 lumbar spinal nerves form the first part of the **sympathetic division**. The cell bodies of these nerve fibers are located in the *gray matter* of the spinal cord. Just outside the spinal cord, axons of these nerve cells leave the spinal nerves and enter almost immediately into masses of nerve cell bodies, the **sympathetic ganglia**, which form a chain that runs next to the vertebral column. This chain of about 23 ganglia runs from the base of the head to the coccyx and is known as the **sympathetic trunk**. Within the ganglia of the sympathetic trunk, fibers from the spinal nerves synapse with ganglionic nerve cell bodies. These ganglionic neurons produce long axons that reach to the parts of the body to be innervated. This arrangement, characteristic of autonomic nerves, creates a two-neuron chain as opposed to single-neuron control of regular motor nerves (Fig. 12–7).

Because of the arrangement whereby *sympathetic fibers* from spinal nerves synapse with many cell bodies in the sympathetic ganglia, they tend to produce widespread innervation when activated. This condition has been described as preparing the individual for "fight or flight." On the other hand, fibers from the *parasympathetic division* have only the two-neuron chain and do not interact with as many cell bodies; therefore, their transmissions result in localized responses.

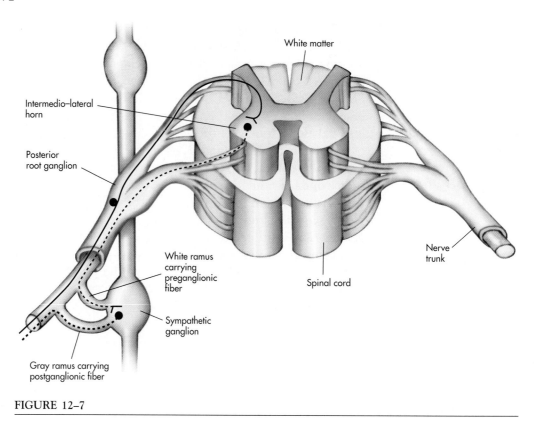

White matter

Intermedio–lateral
horn

Posterior
root ganglion

White ramus
carrying
preganglionic
fiber

Spinal cord

Nerve
trunk

Sympathetic
ganglion

Gray ramus carrying
postganglionic fiber

FIGURE 12–7

The origin of sympathetic neurons of the autonomic nervous system.

The Parasympathetic Division

Very long fibers branching from cranial nerves 3, 7, 9, and 10 along with long fibers of sacral nerves 2, 3, and 4 form the first stage of the **parasympathetic division**. Cell bodies for these long fibers are located in the brain and spinal cord. These long fibers extend to ganglia located close by the organs to be innervated. Fibers of **cranial** and **sacral nerves** synapse with ganglionic cell bodies, which then conduct impulses over short axons to the gland, smooth muscle tissue, or organ to be innervated. Fibers from the cranial nerves serve the iris and ciliary muscles of the eye, lacrimal glands, and salivary glands through four ganglia located in the head. Cranial nerve fibers extend via the vagus nerve to ganglia serving the thoracic, abdominal, and pelvic viscera. The fibers of the sacral spinal nerves form the pelvic nerve, which branches to synapse with small ganglia near or within the organs to be innervated. The cell bodies of these ganglia serve the lower colon, rectum, bladder, and reproductive organs. The **hypothalamus** is instrumental in the control of parasympathetic and sympathetic activity and is discussed elsewhere in this chapter and in Chapter 11, The Endocrine System.

LIFE SPAN
CONSIDERATIONS

■ THE CHILD

Neural tube development occurs about the third to fourth week of embryonic life. This development becomes the **central nervous system**. At 6 weeks a developing baby's brain waves are measurable. At 28 weeks the fetal nervous system begins some regulatory functions. At 32 weeks the fetal nervous system is continuing to mature, so that rhythmic respirations and regulation of body temperature are possible if delivery of the fetus occurs at this time. Brain and nerve cell growth are most rapid from birth until about 4 years of age.

A baby's **brain** has three main structural parts: the **cerebrum**, the **cerebellum**, and the **brain stem**. The cerebrum serves as a control center as it receives, processes, and acts on information. The cerebellum helps coordinate muscle activities and maintains posture and balance. The brain stem maintains vital body functions, such as breathing, heartbeat, blood pressure, digestion, and swallowing. While an infant's brain resembles an adult's, there is one area that is relatively unrefined. In an infant, the right and left hemispheres of the brain have not yet developed their own specific tasks. By the time a child is 3 years old, the two sides of the brain are well on their way to becoming specialized in different tasks.

While a baby is still in the womb, the brain is forging connections in the cerebellum, and the kicks and twitches that the fetus delivers to the mother are proof of this. At about four to six weeks of life, motor function is the main connection taking place in the brain. The initial movements characteristics of an infant soon give way to the repetition of smoother, deliberate ones as the brain's motor cortex process new signals and strengthens connections. Over the next 12 months, a baby's brain focuses first on gross-motor skills, such as holding up the head, rolling over, pushing up to a seated position, crawling, using the pincer grasp to pick up food. Between 2 and 4 years, the child will learn to run and kick a ball.

■ THE OLDER ADULT

With aging, the number of nerve cells decrease, and there is a reduction in brain mass. Loss may occur in different areas of the brain and to varying degrees. In many older adults there is very little change in function, because a person has more nerve cells than needed. There are decreasing levels of **neurotransmitters** or chemicals communicating in synapses between nerve cells. This generally affects short-term memory, motor coordination and control. The older adult has slower response time and decreased reflexes. Loss of cells in the brainstem changes sleep patterns. The older adult generally does not sleep as long or as well as a younger person. As one ages, the learning of new information and skills continues.

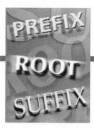

BUILDING YOUR MEDICAL VOCABULARY

This section provides the foundation for learning medical terminology. Medical words can be made up of four different types of word parts:

- Prefixes (P)
- Roots (R)
- Combining forms (CF)
- Suffixes (S)

By connecting various word parts in an organized sequence, thousands of words can be built and learned. In this text the word list is alphabetized so one can see the variety of meanings created when common prefixes and suffixes are repeatedly applied to certain word roots and/or combining forms. Words shown in pink are additional words related to the content of this chapter that are not built from word parts. These words are included to enhance your vocabulary. Note: an asterisk icon (✶) indicates words that are covered in the Pathology Spotlights section in this chapter.

MEDICAL WORD	WORD PARTS (WHEN APPLICABLE)			DEFINITION
	Part	Type	Meaning	
acetylcholine (ACh) (ăs″ ĕ-tĭl-kō′ lēn)				A cholinergic neurotransmitter that occurs in various tissues and organs of the body. It is thought to play an important role in the transmission of nerve impulses at synapses and myoneural junctions.
acrophobia (ăk″ rō-fō′ bĭ-ă)	acr/o -phobia	CF S	extremity fear	An abnormal fear of high places
agoraphobia (ăg″ ō-ră-fō′ bĭ ă)	agor/a -phobia	CF S	marketplace fear	Abnormal fear of being alone in public places; an anxiety syndrome and panic disorder
akathesia (ăk″ ă-thĕ′ zĭ ă)				The inability to remain still, motor restlessness, and anxiety
akinesia (ă″ kĭ-nē′ zĭ-ă)	a -kinesia	P S	lack of motion	A loss or lack of the power of voluntary motion
Alzheimer's disease (ahlts′ hĭ-merz dĭ-zēz′)				A severe form of senile dementia that may be due to some defect in the neurotransmitter system. There is cortical destruction that causes variable degrees of confusion, memory loss, and other cognitive defects. ✶ See Pathology Spotlight: Alzheimer's Disease.

MEDICAL WORD	WORD PARTS (WHEN APPLICABLE)			DEFINITION
	Part	Type	Meaning	
amnesia (ăm-nē′ zĭ-ă)	a mnes -ia	P R S	lack of memory condition	A condition in which there is a loss or lack of memory
amyotrophic lateral sclerosis (ALS) (ă-mī″ ō-trŏf′ ĭk lăt′ ĕr-ăl sklĕ-rō′ sĭs)	a my/o -troph (y) -ic later -al scler -osis	P CF S S R S R S	not muscle development pertaining to side pertaining to hardening condition of	Muscular weakness, atrophy, with spasticity caused by degeneration of motor neurons of the spinal cord, medulla, and cortex; *also called Lou Gehrig's disease*
analgesia (ăn″ ăl-jē′ zĭ-ă)	an -algesia	P S	lack of pain	A lack of the sense of pain
anencephaly (ăn″ ĕn-sĕf′ ăl-ē)	an encephal -y	P R S	lack of brain condition	A congenital condition in which there is a lack of development of the brain
anesthesia (ăn″ ĕs-thē′ zĭ-ă)	an -esthesia	P S	lack of feeling	A loss or lack of the sense of feeling
anesthesiologist (ăn″ ĕs-thē″ zĭ-ŏl′ ō-jĭst)	an esthesi/o log -ist	P CF R S	lack of feeling study of one who specializes	A physician who specializes in the science of anesthesia
aphagia (ă-fā′ jĭ-ă)	a -phagia	P S	lack of to eat	A loss or lack of the ability to eat or swallow
aphasia (ă-fā′ zĭ-ă)	a -phasia	P S	lack of to speak	A loss or lack of the ability to speak
apoplexy (ăp′ ō-plĕk″ sē)				A sudden loss of consciousness caused by an embolus, a thrombus, or rupture of an artery in the brain; *also called a stroke, CVA (cerebrovascular accident) or "brain attack."* ✱ See Figures 12–14 and 12–15, in Pathology Spotlight: Stroke.
apraxia (ă-prăks′ ĭ-ă)	a -praxia	P S	lack of action	A loss or lack of the ability to use objects properly
asthenia (ăs-thē′ nĭ-ă)	a -sthenia	P S	lack of strength	A loss or lack of strength
astrocyte (ăs′ trō-sīt)	astro -cyte	P S	star-shaped cell	A star-shaped neuroglial cell with many branching processes

MEDICAL WORD	WORD PARTS (WHEN APPLICABLE)			DEFINITION
	Part	Type	Meaning	
astrocytoma (ăs″ trō-sī-tō′ mă)	astro cyt -oma	P R S	star-shaped cell tumor	A tumor composed of astrocytes
ataxia (ă-tăks′ ĭ-ă)	a -taxia	P S	lack of order	A loss or lack of muscular coordination
atelomyelia (ăt″ ĕ-lō-mī-ē′ lĭ-ă)	atel/o myel -ia	CF R S	imperfect spinal cord condition	A condition of imperfect development of the spinal cord
autism (ŏ′ tĭzm)	aut -ism	R S	self condition of	A mental disorder in which the individual is self-absorbed, inaccessible, and unable to relate to others and has language disturbances. A syndrome usually beginning in infancy and becoming apparent in the first or second year of life.
bradykinesia (brăd″ ĭ-kĭ-nē′ sĭ-ă)	brady -kinesia	P S	slow motion	An abnormal slowness of motion
cephalalgia (sĕf″ ă-lăl′ jĭ-ă)	cephal -algia	R S	head pain	Head pain; *headache*
cerebellar (sĕr″ ĕ-bĕl′ ăr)	cerebell -ar	R S	little brain pertaining to	Pertaining to the cerebellum
cerebellospinal (sĕr″ ĕ-bĕl″ ō-spī′ năl)	cerebell/o spin -al	CF R S	little brain a thorn, spine pertaining to	Pertaining to the cerebellum and spinal cord
cerebrospinal (sĕr″ ĕ-brō-spī′ năl)	cerebr/o spin -al	CF R S	cerebrum a thorn, spine pertaining to	Pertaining to the cerebrum and the spinal cord
chorea (kō-rē′ ă)				A condition of rapid, jerky involuntary muscular movements of the limbs or face
coma (kō′ mă)				An unconscious state or stupor from which the patient cannot be aroused
concussion (brain) (kŏn-kŭsh′ ŭn)	concuss -ion	R S	shaken violently process	A loss of consciousness, temporary or prolonged, caused by a blow to the head
craniectomy (krā″ nĭ-ĕk′ tō-mē)	cran/i -ectomy	CF S	skull excision	Surgical excision of a portion of the skull
craniotomy (krā″ nĭ-ŏt′ ō-mē)	crani/o -tomy	CF S	skull incision	Surgical incision of the skull

MEDICAL WORD	WORD PARTS (WHEN APPLICABLE)			DEFINITION
	Part	Type	Meaning	
deep brain stimulation (dēp brān stĭm′ ū-lā′ shŭn)				A technique used to stop uncontrollable movements in Parkinson's disease. Electrodes are implanted in the thalamus or globus pallidus of the brain and connected to a pacemaker-like device, which the patient can switch on or off as symptoms dictate.
delirium (dē-lĭr′ ĭ-ŭm)				A state of mental confusion marked by illusions, hallucinations, excitement, restlessness, delusions, and speech incoherence
dementia (dē-měn′ shē-ă)	de ment -ia	P R S	down mind condition of	Refers to a group of symptoms marked by memory loss and other cognitive functions
diskectomy (dĭs-kěk′ tō-mē)	disk -ectomy	R S	a disk excision	Surgical excision of an intervertebral disk
dyslexia (dĭs-lěks′ ĭ-ă)	dys -lexia	P S	difficult diction	A condition in which an individual has difficulty in comprehending written language
dysphasia (dĭs-fā′ zĭ-ă)	dys -phasia	P S	difficult speak	Impairment of speech caused by a brain lesion
egocentric (ē″ gō-sěn′ trĭk)	eg/o centr -ic	CF R S	I, self center pertaining to	Pertaining to being self-centered
electroencephalo-graph (ē-lěk″ trō-ěn-sěf′ ă-lō-grăf)	electr/o encephal/o -graph	CF CF S	electricity brain to write	An instrument used to record the electrical activity of the brain
electromyography (ē-lěk″ trō-mī-ŏg′ ră-fē)	electr/o my/o -graphy	CF CF S	electricity muscle recording	The recording of the contraction of a skeletal muscle as a result of electrical stimulation; used in diagnosing disorders of nerves supplying muscles
encephalitis (ěn-sěf″ ă-lī′ tĭs)	encephal -itis	R S	brain inflammation	Inflammation of the brain. ✱ See Pathology Spotlight: Encephalitis.
encephalomalacia (ěn-sěf″ ă-lō-mă-lā′ sĭ-ă)	encephal/o -malacia	CF S	brain softening	A softening of the brain
endorphins (ěn-dor′ fĭns)				Chemical substances produced in the brain that act as natural analgesics *(opiates)*

MEDICAL WORD	WORD PARTS (WHEN APPLICABLE)			DEFINITION
	Part	**Type**	**Meaning**	
epidural (ĕp″ ĭ-dū′ răl)	epi dur -al	P R S	upon dura, hard pertaining to	Pertaining to situated upon the dura mater
epiduroscopy (ep″ ĭ-du-ros′ kō-pē)	epi dur/o -scopy	P CF S	upon dura, hard to view, examine	A minimally invasive form of surgery that introduces medication via an endoscope into the epidural space. It is used for back pain relief when all other conservative treatments have failed.
epilepsy (ĕp′ ĭ-lĕp″ sē)	epi -lepsy	P S	upon seizure	A disorder of cerebral function resulting from abnormal electrical activity or malfunctioning of the chemical substances of the brain. ✱ See Pathology Spotlight: Epilepsy.
ganglionectomy (gang″ lĭ-ō-nĕk′ tō-mē)	ganglion -ectomy	R S	knot excision	Surgical excision of a ganglion (a mass of nerve tissue outside the brain and spinal cord)
glioma (glī-ō′ mă)	gli -oma	R S	glue tumor	A tumor composed of neuroglial tissue
hemiparesis (hĕm″ ĭ-păr′ ĕ-sĭs)	hemi -paresis	P S	half weakness	Slight paralysis that affects one side of the body
hemiplegia (hĕm″ ĭ-plē′ jĭ-ă)	hemi -plegia	P S	half stroke, paralysis	Paralysis that affects one half of the body
herpes zoster (hĕr′ pēz zŏs′ tĕr)				An acute viral disease characterized by painful vesicular eruptions along the segment of the spinal or cranial nerves; *also called shingles*. See Figures 12–8 and 12–9.
hydrocephalus (hī″ drō-sĕf′ ă-lŭs)	hydro cephal -us	P R S	water head pertaining to	Pertaining to an increased amount of cerebrospinal fluid within the brain. See Figure 12–10.
hyperesthesia (hī″ pĕr-ĕs-thē′ zĭ-ă)	hyper -esthesia	P S	excessive feeling	Excessive feelings of sensory stimuli, such as pain, touch, or sound
hyperkinesis (hī″ pĕr-kĭn-ē′ sĭs)	hyper -kinesis	P S	excessive motion	Excessive muscular movement and motion; inability to be still; *also known as hyperactivity*
hypnosis (hĭp-nō′ sĭs)	hypn -osis	R S	sleep condition of	An artificially induced condition of sleep

MEDICAL WORD	WORD PARTS (WHEN APPLICABLE)			DEFINITION
	Part	**Type**	**Meaning**	
intracranial (ĭn″ trăh-krā′ nĕ-ăl)	intra	P	within	Pertaining to within the skull
	crani	R	skull	
	-al	S	pertaining to	
laminectomy (lăm″ ĭ-nĕk′ tō-mē)	lamin	R	thin plate	Surgical excision of a vertebral posterior arch
	-ectomy	S	excision	
lobotomy (lō-bŏt′ ō-mē)	lob/o	CF	lobe	Surgical incision into the prefrontal or frontal lobe of the brain
	-tomy	S	incision	
meningioma (mĕn-ĭn″ jĭ-ō′ mă)	mening/i	CF	membrane	A tumor of the meninges that originates in the arachnoidal tissue
	-oma	S	tumor	
meningitis (mĕn″ ĭn-jī′ tĭs)	mening	R	membrane	Inflammation of the meninges of the spinal cord or brain. ✱ See Pathology Spotlight: Meningitis.
	-itis	S	inflammation	
meningocele (mĕn-ĭn-gō-sēl)	mening/o	CF	membrane	Congenital herniation of the skull or spinal column in which the meninges protrude through an opening. See Figure 12–11.
	-cele	S	hernia	
meningomyelocele (mĕn-ĭn″ gō-mī-ĕl′ ō-sēl)	mening/o	CF	membrane	Congenital herniation of the spinal cord and meninges through a defect in the vertebral column. See Figure 12–11.
	myel/o	CF	spinal cord	
	-cele	S	hernia	
microcephalus (mī″ krō-sĕf′ ă-lŭs)	micro	P	small	Pertaining to an individual with a very small head
	cephal	R	head	
	-us	S	pertaining to	
multiple sclerosis (mŭl′ tĭ-pl sklē′ -rō′ sĭs)	scler	R	hardening	A chronic disease of the central nervous system marked by damage to the myelin sheath. Plaques occur in the brain and spinal cord causing tremor, weakness, incoordination, paresthesia, and disturbances in vision and speech. ✱ See Pathology Spotlight: Multiple Sclerosis.
	-osis	S	condition of	
myelitis (mī″ ĕ-lī′ tĭs)	myel	R	spinal cord	Inflammation of the spinal cord
	-itis	S	inflammation	
myelography (mī″ ĕ-lŏg′ ră-fē)	myel/o	CF	spinal cord	An x-ray recording of the spinal cord after injection of a radiopaque medium into the spinal canal
	-graphy	S	recording	
narcolepsy (nar′ kō-lĕp″ sē)	narc/o	CF	numbness	A chronic condition in which there are recurrent attacks of uncontrollable drowsiness and sleep
	-lepsy	S	seizure	
neuralgia (nū-răl′ jĭ-ă)	neur	R	nerve	Pain in a nerve or nerves
	-algia	S	pain	

MEDICAL WORD	WORD PARTS (WHEN APPLICABLE)			DEFINITION
	Part	**Type**	**Meaning**	
neurasthenia (nū″ răs-thē′ nĭ-ă)	neur -asthenia	R S	nerve weakness	Nervous weakness, exhaustion, prostration common after depressed states
neurectomy (nū-rĕk′ tō-mē)	neur -ectomy	R S	nerve excision	Surgical excision of a nerve
neurilemma (nū′ rĭ-lĕm″ mă)	neur/i -lemma	CF S	nerve a sheath, husk, rind	A thin membranous sheath that envelops a nerve fiber; *also called sheath of Schwann or neurolemma*
neuritis (nū-rī′ tĭs)	neur -itis	R S	nerve inflammation	Inflammation of a nerve
neuroblast (nū′ rō-blăst)	neur/o -blast	CF S	nerve germ cell	The germ cell from which nervous tissue is formed
neuroblastoma (nū″ rō-blăs-tō′ mă)	neur/o -blast -oma	CF S S	nerve germ cell tumor	A malignant tumor composed chiefly of neuroblast; occurs mostly in infants and children
neurocyte (nū′ rō-sīt)	neur/o -cyte	CF S	nerve cell	A nerve cell, a neuron
neurofibroma (nū″ rō-fī-brō′ mă)	neur/o fibr -oma	CF R S	nerve fiber tumor	A fibrous connective tissue tumor, especially involving the Schwann cells of a nerve. See Figure 12–12.
neuroglia (nū-rŏg′ lĭ-ă)	neur/o -glia	CF S	nerve glue	The supporting elements of the nervous system (*astrocytes, oligodendrocytes, and macroglia*)
neuroleptic (nū rō-lĕp′ tĭk)	neur/o lept -ic	CF R S	nerve seizure pertaining to	Medicine that produces psychomotor slowing, emotional quieting, and extrapyramidal effects; also called antipsychotic
neurologist (nū-rŏl′ ō-jĭst)	neur/o log -ist	CF R S	nerve study of one who specializes	One who specializes in the study of the nervous system
neurology (nū-rŏl′ ō-jē)	neur/o -logy	CF S	nerve study of	The study of the nervous system
neuroma (nū-rō′ mă)	neur -oma	R S	nerve tumor	A tumor of nerve cells and nerve fibers
neuropathy (nū-rŏp′ ă-thē)	neur/o -pathy	CF S	nerve disease	Any nerve disease
neurosis (nū-rō′ sĭs)	neur -osis	R S	nerve condition of	An emotional condition or disorder

MEDICAL WORD	WORD PARTS (WHEN APPLICABLE)			DEFINITION
	Part	**Type**	**Meaning**	
neurotransmitter (nū″ rō-trăns′ mĭt-ĕr)				Substances within neurons and the cerebrospinal fluid that allow nerve cells to communicate with one another
oligodendroglioma (ŏl″ ĭ-gō-dĕn″ drō-glĭ-ō′ mă)	oligo dendr/o gli -oma	P CF R S	little tree glue tumor	A malignant tumor derived and composed of oligodendroglia
pallidotomy (păl″ ĭ-dŏt-ō-mē)	pallid/o -tomy	CF S	globus pallidus incision	Surgical destruction of the globus pallidus of the brain done to treat involuntary movements or muscular rigidity in Parkinson's disease
palsy (pawl′ zē)				A loss of sensation or an impairment of motor function; *also called paralysis.* There are many types of palsy. See Figure 12–13.
papilledema (păp″ ĭl-ĕ-dē′ mă)	papill -edema	R S	papilla swelling	Swelling of the optical disk, usually caused by increased intracranial pressure; *also called choked disk*
paranoia (păr″ ă-noy′ ă)	para -noia	P S	beside mind	A mental disorder
paraplegia (păr″ ă-plē′ jĭ-ă)	para -plegia	P S	beside stroke, paralysis	Paralysis of both legs and, in some cases, the lower portion of the body
paresis (păr′ ē-sĭs)				A slight, partial, or incomplete paralysis
paresthesia (păr″ ĕs-thē′ zĭ-ă)	par -esthesia	P S	beside feeling	An abnormal sensation, feeling of numbness, prickling, or tingling
Parkinson's disease (păr′ kĭn-sŭnz dĭ-zēz′)				A chronic disease of the nervous system. It is characterized by a loss of equilibrium and by salivation, frustration, nausea, dryness of the mouth, and muscular tremors; *also called paralysis agitans, shaking palsy.* ✱ See Pathology Spotlight: Parkinson's Disease.
paroxysm (păr′ ok-sĭzm)				A sudden recurrence of the symptoms of a disease, an exacerbation; *also means a spasm or seizure*

MEDICAL WORD	WORD PARTS (WHEN APPLICABLE)			DEFINITION
	Part	**Type**	**Meaning**	
pheochromocytoma (fē-ō-krō″ mō-sī-tō′ mă)	phe/o chrom/o cyt -oma	CF CF R S	dusky color cell tumor	A chromaffin cell tumor of the adrenal medulla or of the sympathetic nervous system
phobia (fō′ bē-ă)				A morbid and persistent fear of a specific object, activity, or situation that results in a compelling desire to avoid the feared stimulus. **Examples: claustrophobia** (fear of enclosed places), **acrophobia** (fear of heights), **photophobia** (fear of light), **arachnophobia** (fear of spiders), **nyctophobia** (fear of darkness/night), and **hematophobia** or **hemophobia** (fear of blood/bleeding).
poliomyelitis (pōl″ ĭ-ō-mī″ ĕl-ī′ tĭs)	poli/o myel -itis	CF R S	gray spinal cord inflammation	Inflammation of the gray matter of the spinal cord
polyneuritis (pŏl″ ē nū-rī′ tĭs)	poly neur -itis	P R S	many nerve inflammation	Inflammation of many nerves
psychiatrist (sī-kī′ ă-trĭst)				A physician who specializes in the study, treatment, and prevention of mental disorders
psychoanalysis (sī″ kō-ă-năl′ĭ-sĭs)				A method of obtaining a detailed account of past and present mental and emotional experiences and repressions
psychologist (sī-kŏl′ ō-jĭst)	psych/o log -ist	CF R S	mind study of one who specializes	One who specializes in the study of the mind
psychology (sī-kŏl′ ō-jē)	psych/o -logy	CF S	mind study of	The study of the mind
psychopath (sī′ kō-păth)				An individual with a psychopathic personality
psychosis (sī-kō′ sĭs)	psych -osis	R S	mind condition of	An abnormal condition of the mind
psychosomatic (sī″ kō-sō-măt′ ĭk)	psych/o somat -ic	CF R S	mind body pertaining to	Pertaining to the interrelationship of the mind and the body

MEDICAL WORD	WORD PARTS (WHEN APPLICABLE)			DEFINITION
	Part	Type	Meaning	
psychotropic (sī′ kō-trŏp″ ĭk)				A drug that affects psychic function, behavior, or experience
pyromania (pī″ rō-mā′ nĭ-ă)	pyro -mania	P S	fire madness	A madness for fire
quadriplegia (kwŏd″ rĭ plē′ jĭ-ă)	quadri -plegia	P S	four stroke, paralysis	Paralysis of all four extremities
receptor (rē-sĕp′ tōr)				A sensory nerve ending that receives and relays responses to stimuli
Reye's syndrome (rīz sĭn′ drōm)				An acute disease that causes edema of the brain and increased intracranial pressure, hypoglycemia, and fatty infiltration of the liver and other vital organs. Occurs in children and has a relation to aspirin administration. May be viral in origin.
sciatica (sī-ăt′ ĭ-kă)				Severe pain along the course of the sciatic nerve
sleep (slēp)				A state of rest for the body and mind. There are two distinct types: REM for rapid eye movement, sometimes called dream sleep, and NREM for no rapid eye movement.
somnambulism (sŏm-năm′ bū-lĭzm)	somn ambul -ism	R R S	sleep to walk condition of	A condition of sleepwalking
spondylosyndesis (spŏn″ dĭ-lō-sĭn′ dĕ-sĭs)	spondyl/o syn -desis	CF P S	vertebra together binding	A surgical procedure to bind vertebra after removal of a herniated disk; *also called spinal fusion*
subdural (sŭb-dū′ răl)	sub dur -al	P R S	below dura, hard pertaining to	Pertaining to below the dura mater
sympathectomy (sĭm″ pă-thĕk′ tō-mē)	sympath -ectomy	R S	sympathy excision	Surgical excision of a portion of the sympathetic nervous system
syncope (sĭn′ kŭ-pē)	syn -cope	P S	together strike	A temporary loss of consciousness caused by a lack of blood supply to the brain; *also called fainting*
tactile (tăk′ tĭl)				Pertaining to the sense of touch

MEDICAL WORD	WORD PARTS (WHEN APPLICABLE)			DEFINITION
	Part	Type	Meaning	
Tay-Sachs disease (tā săks′ dĭ-zēz′)				An inherited disease that predominantly affects Jewish children of Ashkenazi origin. It is a progressive disease marked by degeneration of brain tissue.
transcutaneous electrical nerve stimulations (TENS) (trăns-kū-tā′ nē-ŭs nerv stĭm′ ŭ-lā′ shŭn)				The use of mild electrical stimulation to interfere with the transmission of painful stimuli. It has proved useful in relieving pain in some patients.
vagotomy (vā-gŏt′ ō-mē)	vag/o	CF	vagus, wandering	Surgical incision of the vagus nerve
	-tomy	S	incision	
ventriculometry (vĕn-trĭk″ ū-lōm′ ĕtrē)	ventricul/o	CF	little belly	Measurement of intracranial pressure
	-metry	S	measurement	

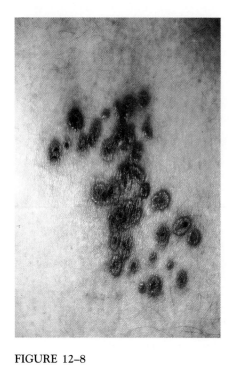

FIGURE 12–8

Herpes zoster. (Courtesy of Jason L. Smith, MD.)

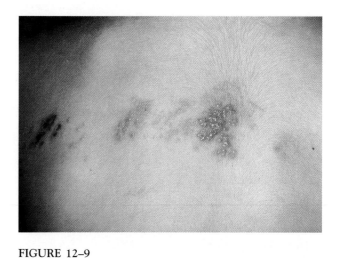

FIGURE 12–9

Herpes zoster. (Courtesy of Jason L. Smith, MD.)

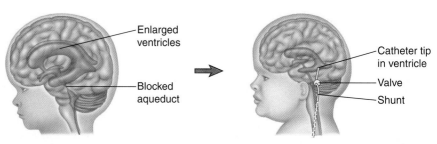

FIGURE 12–10

Hydrocephalus. (Source: Pearson Education/PH College.)

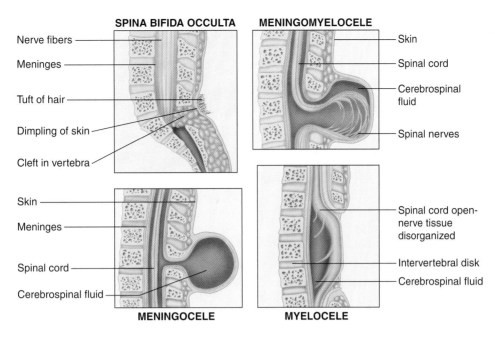

SPINA BIFIDA OCCULTA

Nerve fibers

Meninges

Tuft of hair

Dimpling of skin

Cleft in vertebra

MENINGOMYELOCELE

Skin

Spinal cord

Cerebrospinal fluid

Spinal nerves

Skin

Meninges

Spinal cord

Cerebrospinal fluid

MENINGOCELE

Spinal cord open-nerve tissue disorganized

Intervertebral disk

Cerebrospinal fluid

MYELOCELE

FIGURE 12–11

Forms of spina bifida. (Source: Pearson Education/PH College.)

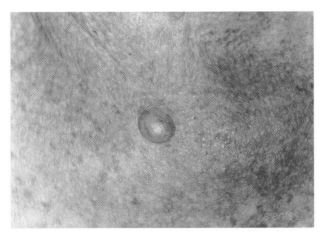

FIGURE 12–12

Neurofibroma. (Courtesy of Jason L. Smith, MD.)

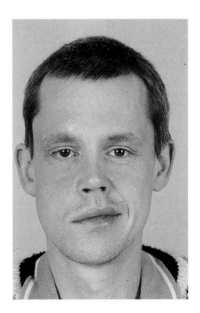

FIGURE 12–13

This man with Bell's palsy shows typical drooping of the one side of the face. (Courtesy of Phototake, Inc.)

Terminology Translator

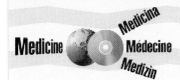

This feature, found on the accompanying CD-ROM, provides an innovative tool to translate medical words into Spanish, French, and German.

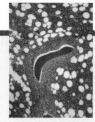

PATHOLOGY SPOTLIGHTS

PATHOLOGY SPOTLIGHTS

Alzheimer's Disease

Alzheimer's disease (AD) is a progressive, degenerative disease of the brain that is characterized by loss of memory and other cognitive functions. It is the most common cause of dementia among people aged 65 or older.

This disease is named after Dr. Alois Alzheimer, a German physician. In 1906 he noticed changes in the brain tissue of a woman who had died of an unusual mental illness. He found abnormal clumps (now called amyloid plaques) and tangled bundles of fibers (now called neurofibrillary tangles). Today, these plaques and tangles in the brain are considered signs of Alzheimer's disease.

AD seriously affects a person's ability to carry out daily activities. It involves the parts of the brain that control thought, memory, and language. Scientists estimate that up to 4 million Americans suffer from this disease. Alzheimer's usually begins after age 60, and risk goes up with age. It is important to note, however, that AD is not a normal part of aging.

Alzheimer's begins slowly. At first, the only symptom may be mild forgetfulness. In this stage, people may have trouble remembering recent events, activities, or the names of familiar people or things. They may not be able to solve simple math problems. Such difficulties may be a bother, but usually they are not serious enough to cause alarm.

However, as the disease goes on, symptoms are more easily noticed and become serious enough to cause people with AD or their family members to seek medical help. For example, people in the middle stages of Alzheimer's may forget how to do simple tasks, like brushing their teeth or combing their hair. They can no longer think clearly. They begin to have problems speaking, understanding, reading, or writing. Later on, people with this disease may become anxious or aggressive, or wander away from home. Eventually, patients need total care.

Although scientists are learning more every day, the cause is still not known, and there is no cure. There probably is not one single cause, but several factors that affect each person differently. Age is the most important known risk factor for Alzheimer's. The number of people with the disease doubles every 5 years beyond age 65.

Family history is another risk factor. Scientists believe that genetics may play a role in many Alzheimer's cases. Also, the role of diet, environment, and viruses is being studied to learn what role they might play in the development of this disease.

No treatment can stop Alzheimer's disease. However, for some people in the early and middle stages of the disease, the drugs tacrine (Cognex), donepezil (Aricept), rivastigmine (Exelon), or galantamine (Reminyl) may help prevent some symptoms from becoming worse for a limited time. Also, some medicines may help control behavioral symptoms of AD such as sleeplessness, agitation, wandering, anxiety, and depression. Treating these symptoms often makes patients more comfortable and makes their care easier for caregivers.

Developing new treatments for Alzheimer's is an active area of research. Scientists are testing a number of drugs to see if they prevent or slow the disease, or help reduce symptoms. There is evidence that inflammation in the brain may contribute to Alzheimer's damage. Some scientists believe that drugs such as nonsteroidal anti-inflammatory drugs (NSAIDs) might help slow the progression of the disease, although recent studies of two of these drugs, rofecoxib (Vioxx) and naproxen (Aleve), have shown that they did not delay the progression of Alzheimer's in people who already have the disease. Scientists are now testing other NSAIDs to find out if they can slow the onset of the disease.

Encephalitis and Meningitis

Encephalitis is an inflammation of the brain. There are many types of encephalitis, many of which are caused by viral infection. Symptoms include sudden fever, headache, vomiting, photophobia (abnormal visual sensitivity to light), stiff neck and back, confusion, drowsiness, clumsiness, unsteady gait, and irritability. Symptoms that require emergency treatment include loss of consciousness, poor responsiveness, seizures, muscle weakness, sudden severe dementia, memory loss, withdrawal from social interaction, and impaired judgement. In the United States, encephalitis affects approximately 1,500 people per year. The elderly and infants are more vulnerable and may have a more severe course of the disease.

Antiviral medications may be prescribed for herpes encephalitis or other severe viral infections. Antibiotics may be prescribed for bacterial infections. Anticonvulsants are used to prevent or treat seizures. Corticosteroids are used to reduce brain swelling and inflammation. Sedatives may be needed for irritability or restlessness. Over-the-counter medications may be used for fever and headache. Individuals with encephalitis or bacterial meningitis are usually hospitalized for treatment.

The prognosis for encephalitis varies. Some cases are mild, short and relatively benign and patients have full recovery. Other cases are severe, and permanent impairment or death is possible. The acute phase of encephalitis may last for 1 to 2 weeks, with gradual or sudden resolution of fever and neurological symptoms. Neurological symptoms may require many months before full recovery.

Meningitis is an infection of the membranes (called meninges) that surround the brain and spinal cord. Symptoms, which may appear suddenly, often include high fever, severe and persistent headache, stiff neck, nausea, and vomiting. Changes in behavior such as confusion, sleepiness, and difficulty waking up are extremely important symptoms and may require emergency treatment. In infants symptoms of meningitis may include irritability or tiredness, poor feeding and fever. Meningitis may be caused by many different viruses and bacteria. Viral meningitis cases are usually self-limited to 10 days or less. Some types of meningitis can be deadly if not treated promptly. Anyone experiencing symptoms of meningitis or encephalitis should see a doctor immediately.

With early diagnosis and prompt treatment, most patients recover from meningitis. However, in some cases, the disease progresses so rapidly that death occurs during the first 48 hours, despite early treatment.

Epilepsy

Epilepsy is a brain disorder involving repeated seizures of any type. Seizures are episodes of disturbed brain function that cause changes in attention and/or behavior. They are caused by abnormal electrical excitation in the brain.

In epilepsy, clusters of nerve cells, or neurons, in the brain sometimes signal abnormally. The normal pattern of neuronal activity becomes disturbed, causing strange sensations, emotions, and behavior or sometimes convulsions, muscle spasms, and loss of consciousness. Epilepsy is a disorder with many possible causes. Anything that disturbs the normal pattern of neuron activity—from illness to brain damage to abnormal brain development—can lead to seizures. Epilepsy may develop because of an abnormality in brain wiring, an imbalance of nerve signaling chemicals called neurotransmitters, or some combination of these factors. In other cases, injury to the brain (e.g., stroke or head injury) causes brain tissue to be abnormally excitable. In some people, an inherited abnormality affects nerve cells in the brain, which leads to seizures. In some cases, no cause at all can be identified.

Seizure disorders affect about 0.5 percent of the population. Approximately 1.5 to 5.0 percent of the population may have a seizure in their lifetime. Epilepsy can affect people of any age. Having a seizure does not necessarily mean that a person has epilepsy. Only when a person has had two or more seizures is he or she considered to have epilepsy. EEGs and brain scans are common diagnostic tests for epilepsy.

For about 80 percent of those diagnosed with epilepsy, seizures can be controlled with modern medicines and surgical techniques. Some antiepileptic drugs can interfere with the effectiveness of oral contraceptives.

Multiple Sclerosis

Multiple sclerosis (MS) is a chronic, potentially debilitating disease that affects the brain and spinal cord (central nervous system). The illness is probably an autoimmune disease, which means the immune system responds as if part of the body is a foreign substance.

In MS, the body directs antibodies and white blood cells against proteins in the myelin sheath surrounding nerves in the brain and spinal cord. This causes inflammation and injury to the sheath and ultimately to the nerves. The result may be multiple areas of scarring. The damage slows or blocks muscle coordination, visual sensation and other nerve signals.

The disease varies in severity, ranging from a mild illness to one that results in permanent disability. Treatments can modify the course of the disease and relieve symptoms. Symptoms vary because the location and extent of each attack varies. There is usually a stepwise progression of the disorder, with episodes that last days, weeks, or months alternating with times of reduced or no symptoms (remission). Recurrence (relapse) is common although non-stop progression without periods of remission may also occur.

Symptoms include weakness, paralysis, and/or tremor of one or more extremities; muscle spasticity (uncontrollable spasm of muscle groups); numbness, decreased or abnormal sensation (in any area); tingling; urinary hesitancy, urgency, and/or frequency. Symptoms may vary with each attack. They may last days to months, then reduce or disappear, then recur periodically. With each recurrence, the symptoms are as different as new areas affected. Fever can trigger or worsen attacks, as can hot baths, sun exposure, and stress.

An estimated 400,000 Americans have MS. It generally first occurs in people between the ages of 20 and 50. The disease is twice as common in women as in men.

The exact cause of the inflammation associated with MS is unknown. Geographic studies indicate there may be an environmental factor involved and it is more likely to occur in northern Europe, the northern United States, southern Australia, and New Zealand than in other areas. There seems to be a genetic link to the disease, with some families more likely to be affected than others. Certain genetic markers are more common in people with MS than in the general population.

Symptoms of multiple sclerosis may mimic many other neurologic disorders. Diagnosis is made by ruling out other conditions. A history of at least two attacks separated by a period of reduced or no symptoms may indicate one pattern of attack/remission seen in MS (known as relapsing remitting pattern). If there are observable decreases in any functions of the central nervous system (such as abnormal reflexes), the diagnosis of MS may be suspected.

Tests that indicate or confirm multiple sclerosis include:

- Head MRI scan that shows scarring or a new lesion
- Spine MRI scan that shows scarring or a new lesion
- Lumbar puncture (spinal tap)

There is no known cure for multiple sclerosis at this time. However, there are promising therapies that may decrease exacerbations and delay progression of the disease. Treatment is aimed at controlling symptoms and maintaining function to give the maximum quality of life.

Physical therapy, speech therapy, occupational therapy, and support groups may be useful. A planned exercise program early in the course of the disorder can help with maintaining muscle tone. A healthy lifestyle is encouraged, including good general nutrition. Adequate rest and relaxation can help maintain energy levels. Patients should avoid fatigue, stress, temperature extremes, and illness to reduce factors that may trigger an MS attack.

Parkinson's Disease

Parkinson's disease is a progressive disorder caused by degeneration of nerve cells in the part of the brain that controls movement. This degeneration creates a shortage of the brain signaling chemical (neurotransmitter) known as dopamine, causing the movement impairments that characterize the disease.

Often, the first symptom of Parkinson's disease is tremor (trembling or shaking) of a limb, especially when the body is at rest. The tremor often begins on one side of the body, frequently in one hand. Other common symptoms include slow movement (**bradykinesia**), an inability to move (**akinesia**), rigid limbs, a shuffling gait, and a stooped posture. People with Parkinson's disease often show reduced facial expressions and speak in a soft voice. The disease may also cause depression, personality changes, dementia, sleep disturbances, speech impairments, or sexual difficulties. The severity of Parkinson's symptoms tends to worsen over time.

An estimated 1.5 million Americans have Parkinson's disease and 50,000 new cases are reported annually. The disorder appears to be slightly more common in men than women. The average age of onset is about 60. Both prevalence and incidence increase with advancing age; the rates are very low in people under 40 and rise among people in their 70s and 80s.

Although there are many theories about the cause of Parkinson's disease, none has ever been proved. Researchers have reported families with apparently inherited Parkinson's for more than a century. However, until recently, the prevailing theory held that one or more environmental factors caused the disease. Recent studies of twins and families with Parkinson's have suggested that some people have an inherited susceptibility to the disease that may be influenced by environmental factors. The strong familial inheritance of the chromosome 4 gene is the first evidence that a gene alteration alone may lead to Parkinson's disease in some people.

Parkinson's disease is usually diagnosed by a neurologist who can evaluate symptoms and their severity. Test, such as a brain scan, can help a physician decide if a patient has true Parkinson's disease or some other disorder that resembles it.

There is no cure for Parkinson's disease. Many patients are only mildly affected and need no treatment for several years after the initial diagnosis. When symptoms grow severe, physicians generally prescribe medications that are used for palliative relief of the symptoms. Drug therapy involves an attempt to replenish dopamine levels and/or inhibit the effects of the neurotransmitter acetylcholine. Surgical interventions that may be used to stop uncontrollable movements include pallidotomy and deep brain stimulation (brain implant).

The FDA has approved the brain implant device, called the Activa Parkinson's Control System, for use in both sides of the brain to help reduce some of the symptoms of advanced Parkinson's that cannot be adequately controlled with medication. This system consists of electrodes that are implanted into the brain and connected by leads (wires) under the skin to a pulse generator implanted in the abdomen or chest. The pulse generator sends a constant stream of tiny electrical pulses to the brain, blocking tremors. When the device is implanted in both sides of the brain, two separate systems are used. To turn the stimulator on and off, the patient holds a magnet over the pulse generator. The generator must be replaced every three to five years, the life of the battery.

Stroke

A **stroke**, which is also called a cerebrovascular accident (CVA), apoplexy or "brain attack," is the death of brain tissue that occurs when the brain does not get enough blood and oxygen. If the flow of blood in an artery supplying the brain is interrrupted for longer than a few seconds, brain cells can die, causing permanent damage. The interruption can be caused by either bleeding or blood clots in the brain. See Figure 12–14.

Stroke is the third leading cause of death in the United States and many other countries, and the leading cause of disability in adults. The risk doubles with each decade after age 35. Stroke occurs in men more often than women.

A very common cause of stroke is atherosclerosis. Fatty deposits and blood platelets collect on the wall of the arteries, forming plaques. Over time, the plaques slowly begin to block the flow of blood. The plaque itself may block the artery enough to cause a stroke.

In some cases, the plaque causes the blood to flow abnormally, which leads to a blood clot. A clot can stay at the site of narrowing and prevent blood flow to all of the smaller arteries it supplies. (This type of clot, which doesn't travel, is called a **thrombus**.) In other cases, the clot

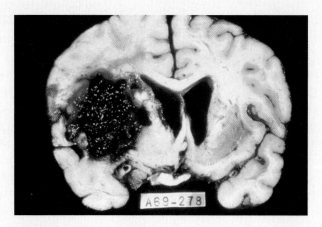

FIGURE 12–14

Cross-section of brain showing cerebrovascular accident. (Source: Pearson Education/PH College.)

can travel and wedge into a smaller vessel. (A clot that travels is called an **embolism,** as shown in Figure 12–15.)

Strokes caused by embolism are most commonly caused by heart disorders. An embolism may originate in the aortic arch, especially where there is atherosclerotic plaque. A clot can form elsewhere in the body for any number of reasons, and then travel to the brain, causing a stroke. Arrhythmias of the heart, such as atrial fibrillation, can be associated with this type of stroke and may contribute to clot formation.

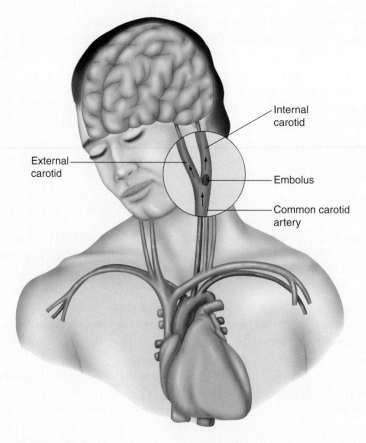

FIGURE 12–15

Embolus traveling to the brain. (Source: Pearson Education/PH College.)

Other causes of embolic stroke include endocarditis (an infection of the heart valves) or use of a mechanical heart valve. A clot can form on the valve and break off and travel to the brain.

A second major cause of stroke is bleeding in the brain (hemorrhagic stroke). This can occur when small blood vessels in the brain become weak and burst. Some people have defects in the blood vessels of the brain that makes this more likely. The flow of blood after the break damages brain cells. This kind of stroke can also occur if a clot caused by atherosclerosis or other conditions blocks a vessel, which then breaks and damages surrounding tissue.

Following are the warning signs of stroke:

- Sudden numbness or weakness of face, arm, or leg, especially on one side of the body
- Sudden confusion; trouble speaking or understanding
- Sudden trouble seeing in one or both eyes
- Sudden trouble walking, dizziness, loss of balance or coordination
- Sudden, severe headache with no known cause

✔ PATHOLOGY CHECKPOINT

Following is a concise list of the pathology-related terms that you've seen in the chapter. Review this checklist to make sure that you are familiar with the meaning of each term before moving on to the next section.

Conditions and Symptoms

- acrophobia
- agoraphobia
- akathesia
- akinesia
- Alzheimer's disease
- amnesia
- amyotrophic lateral sclerosis (ALS)
- anencephaly
- aphagia
- aphasia
- apoplexy
- apraxia
- asthenia
- astrocytoma
- ataxia
- atelomyelia
- autism
- bradykinesia

- cephalalgia
- chorea
- coma
- concussion (brain)
- delirium
- dementia
- dyslexia
- dysphasia
- egocentric
- encephalitis
- encephalomalacia
- epilepsy
- glioma
- hemiparesis
- hemiplegia
- herpes zoster
- hydrocephalus
- hyperesthesia
- hyperkinesis
- meningioma

- meningitis
- meningocele
- meningomyelocele
- microcephalus
- multiple sclerosis (MS)
- myelitis
- narcolepsy
- neuralgia
- neurasthenia
- neuritis
- neuroblastoma
- neurofibroma
- neuroma
- neuropathy
- neurosis
- oligodendroglioma
- palsy
- papilledema
- paranoia
- paraplegia

❏ paresis
❏ paresthesia
❏ Parkinson's disease
❏ paroxysm
❏ pheochromocytoma
❏ phobia
❏ poliomyelitis
❏ polyneuritis
❏ psychopath
❏ psychosis
❏ psychosomatic
❏ pyromania
❏ quadriplegia
❏ Reye's syndrome
❏ sciatica

❏ somnambulism
❏ spondylosyndesis
❏ syncope
❏ Tay-Sachs disease

Diagnosis and Treatment

❏ analgesia
❏ anesthesia
❏ craniectomy
❏ craniotomy
❏ deep brain stimulation
❏ diskectomy
❏ electroencephalograph
❏ electromyography
❏ epiduroscopy

❏ gangionectomy
❏ hypnosis
❏ laminectomy
❏ lobotomy
❏ myelography
❏ neurectomy
❏ neuroleptic
❏ pallidotomy
❏ psychoanalysis
❏ psychotropic
❏ sympathectomy
❏ transcutaneous electrical nerve stimulations (TENS)
❏ vagotomy
❏ ventriculometry

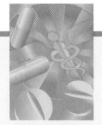

DRUG HIGHLIGHTS

Drugs that are generally used for nervous system diseases and disorders include analgesics, analgesic-antipyretics, sedatives and hypnotics, antiparkinsonism drugs, anticonvulsants, and anesthetics.

Analgesics	Inhibit ascending pain pathways in the central nervous system. They increase pain threshold and alter pain perception.
Narcotic	*Examples: codeine phosphate, codeine sulfate, Dilaudid (hydromorphone HCl), Demerol (meperidine HCl), Darvon-N (propoxyphene napsylate), morphine sulfate, and Talwin (pentazocine HCl).*
Non-narcotic	*Examples: Stadol (butorphanol tartrate) and Nubain (nalbuphine HCl).*
Analgesics–Antipyretics	Act to relieve pain (analgesic effect) and reduce fever (antipyretic effect).
	Examples: Tylenol (acetaminophen); Bayer aspirin; Advil, Motrin, Nuprin (ibuprofen); and Naprosyn (naproxen).
Sedatives and Hypnotics	Depress the central nervous system by interfering with the transmission of nerve impulses. Depending upon the dosage, barbiturates, benzodiazepines, and certain other drugs can produce either a sedative or a hypnotic effect. When used as a sedative, the dosage is designed to produce a calming effect without causing sleep. Used as a hypnotic, the dosage is sufficient to cause sleep.
Barbiturates	*Examples: Nembutal (pentobarbital), Seconal (secobarbital), and Luminal (phenobarbital).*
Non-barbiturates	*Examples: Aquachloral (chloral hydrate), Dalmane (flurazepam HCl), Restoril (temazepam), Halcion (triazolam), and Ativan (lorazepam).*

Antiparkinsonism Drugs   Are used for palliative relief from such major symptoms as bradykinesia, rigidity, tremor, and disorder of equilibrium and posture. Therapy involves an attempt to replenish dopamine levels and/or inhibit the effects of the neurotransmitter acetylcholine.

Examples: Symmetrel (amantadine HCl), Dopar (levodopa), Artane (trihexyphenidyl HCl), Cogentin (benztropine mesylate), Requip (ropinirole), Tasmar (tolcapone), and Stalevo (carbidopa, levodopa, and entacapone).

Anticonvulsants   Inhibit the spread of seizure activity in the motor cortex.

Examples: Dilantin (phenytoin), Depakene (valproic acid), Tegretol (carbamazepine), Klonopin (clonazepam), and Mysoline (primidone).

Cholinesterase Inhibitors   Increase the brain's levels of acetylcholine, which helps to restore communication between brain cells. These medications may be used to improve global functioning (including activities of daily living, behavior, and cognition) in some patients with Alzheimer's disease.

Examples: Cognex (tacrine), Aricept (donepezil hydrochloride), and Exelon (rivastigmine tartrate).

Anesthetics   Interfere with the conduction of nerve impulses and are used to produce loss of sensation, muscle relaxation, and/or complete loss of consciousness. Block nerve transmission in the area to which they are applied.

Local   Block nerve transmission in the area to which they are applied.

Examples: Novocain (procaine HCl), Xylocaine (lidocaine HCl), Marcaine (bupivacaine HCl), Dyclone (dyclonine HCl), and Pontocaine (tetracaine HCl).

General   Affect the central nervous system and produce either partial or complete loss of consciousness. They also produce analgesia, skeletal muscle relaxation, and reduction of reflex activity.

Examples: Pentothal (thiopental sodium), Fluothane (halothane), Penthrane (methoxyflurane), and nitrous oxide.

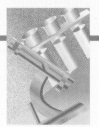

DIAGNOSTIC & LAB TESTS

TEST	DESCRIPTION
cerebral angiography (sĕr′ ĕ-brăl ăn jĭ-ŏg′ ră-fē)	The process of making an x-ray record of the cerebral arterial system. A radiopaque substance is injected into an artery of the arm or neck, and x-ray films of the head are taken. Cerebral aneurysms, tumors, or ruptured blood vessels may be visualized.
cerebrospinal fluid (CSF) analysis (sĕr ĕ-brŏ-spī′ năl floo′ ĭd ă-năl′ ĭ-sĭs)	Examination of spinal fluid for color, pressure, pH, and the level of protein, glucose, and leukocytes. Abnormal results may indicate hemorrhage, a tumor, and various disease processes.

TEST	DESCRIPTION
computed tomography (CT) (kŏm-pū′ tĕd tō-mŏg″ ră-fē)	A diagnostic procedure used to study the structure of the brain. Computerized three-dimensional x-ray images allow the radiologist to differentiate between intracranial tumors, cysts, edema, and hemorrhage.
echoencephalography (ĕk ō-ĕn-sĕf′ ă-lŏg′ ră-fē)	The process of using ultrasound to determine the presence of a centrally located mass in the brain.
electroencephalography (EEG) (ē-lĕk-trō-ĕn-sĕf′ ă-lŏg′ ră-fē)	The process of determining the electrical activity of the brain via an electroencephalograph. Abnormal results may indicate epilepsy, brain tumor, infection, abscess, hemorrhage, and/or coma. Also, brain "death" may be determined by an EEG.
lumbar puncture (lŭm′ băr pŭnk′ chūr)	Insertion of a needle into the lumbar subarachnoid space for removal of spinal fluid. The fluid is examined for color, pressure, and the level of protein, chloride, glucose, and leukocytes. See Figure 12–16.
myelogram (mī′ ĕ-lō-grăm)	The x-ray of the spinal canal after the injection of a radiopaque dye. Useful in diagnosing spinal lesions, cysts, herniated disks, tumors, and nerve root damage.
neurologic examination (nū″ -rō-lŏj′ ĭk ĕks-ăm ĭ-nā′ shŭn)	Assessment of a patient's vision, hearing, sense of taste, smell, touch and pain, position, temperature, gait, muscle strength, coordination, and reflex action. Used to determine a patient's neurologic status.

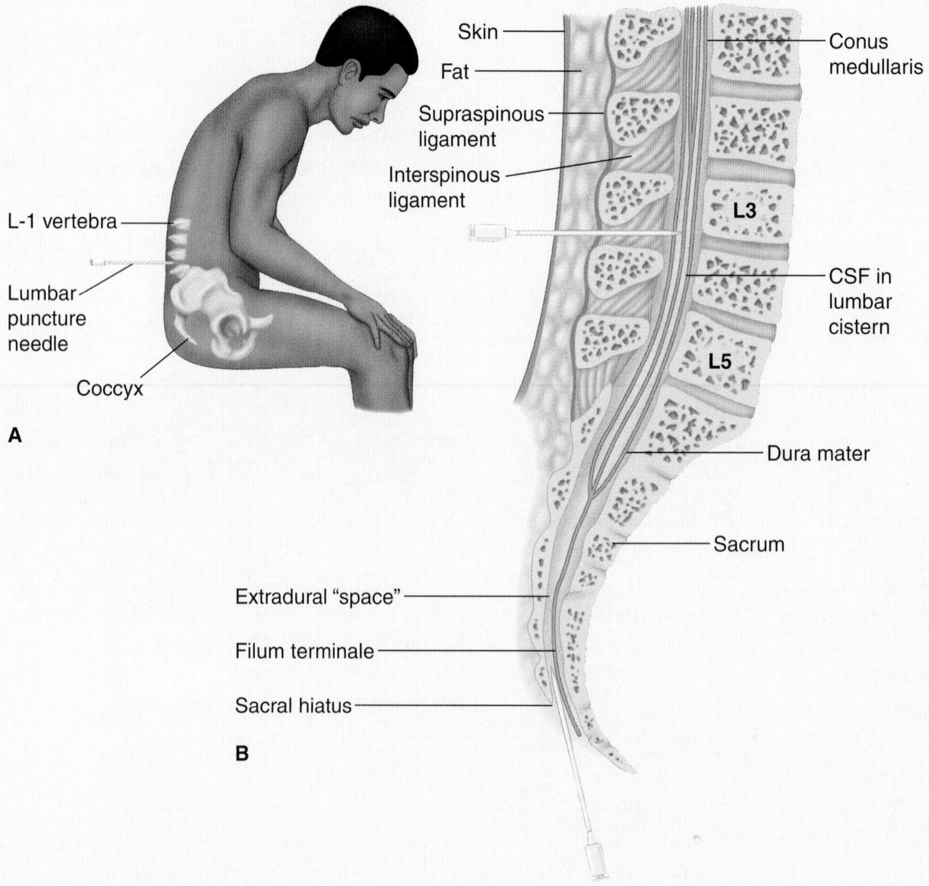

FIGURE 12–16

(A) Shows lumbar puncture, also known as spinal tap. (B) Section of the vertebral column showing the spinal cord and membranes. A lumbar puncture needle is shown at L3–4 and in the sacral hiatus. (Source: Pearson Education/PH College.)

TEST	DESCRIPTION
positron emission tomography (PET) (pŏz′ ĭ-trŏn ē-mĭsh′ ŭn tō-mŏg ră-fē)	A computer-based nuclear imaging procedure that can produce three-dimensional pictures of actual organ functioning. Useful in locating a brain lesion, in identifying blood flow and oxygen metabolism in stroke patients, in showing metabolic changes in Alzheimer's disease, and in studying biochemical changes associated with mental illness.
ultrasonography, brain (ŭl-tră-sŏn-ŏg′ ră-fē, brān)	The use of high-frequency sound waves to record echoes on an oscilloscope and film. Used as screening test or diagnostic tool.

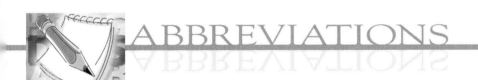

ABBREVIATIONS

ABBREVIATION	MEANING	ABBREVIATION	MEANING
ACh	acetylcholine	HDS	herniated disk syndrome
AD	Alzheimer's disease	HNP	herniated nucleus pulposus
ADHD	attention-deficit hyperactivity disorder	ICP	intracranial pressure
		IVC	intraventricular catheter
ALS	amyotrophic lateral sclerosis	LP	lumbar puncture
ANS	autonomic nervous system	MR	mental retardation
CBS	chronic brain syndrome	MS	multiple sclerosis
CNS	central nervous system	NCV	nerve conduction velocity
CP	cerebral palsy	OCD	obsessive-compulsive disorder
CSF	cerebrospinal fluid	PET	positron emission tomography
CT	computerized tomography	PNS	peripheral nervous system
CVA	cerebrovascular accident	SAD	seasonal affective disorder
DBS	deep brain stimulation	TENS	transcutaneous electrical
DCS	dorsal cord stimulation		nerve stimulation
ECT	electroconvulsive therapy	TIAs	transient ischemic attacks
EEG	electroencephalogram	TNS	transcutaneous nerve
GPi	globus pallidus		stimulation

STUDY AND REVIEW

Anatomy and Physiology

Write your answers to the following questions. Do not refer to the text.

1. Name the two interconnected divisions of the nervous system.

   a. _____   b. _____

2. _____ are the structural and functional units of the nervous system.

3. State the three actions of motor neurons.

   a. _____

   b. _____

   c. _____

4. Describe an axon._____

5. Describe a dendrite. _____

6. State an action of sensory nerves._____

   _____

7. _____ function to mediate impulses between sensory and motor neurons.

8. Define the following terms:

   a. Nerve fiber _____

   b. Nerve _____

   c. Tracts _____

9. The central nervous system consists of the _____ and the

   _____ _____.

10. State three functions of the central nervous system.

    a. _____   b. _____

    c. _____

11. Name the three meninges enclosing the brain.

    a. _____   b. _____   c. _____

12. Name the seven major divisions of the brain.

    a. _____   b. _____

    c. _____   d. _____

    e. _____   f. _____

    g. _____

13. The _____ _____ has been identified as the brain's major motor area.

14. The parietal lobe is also known as the _____ _____.

15. The temporal lobe contains centers for _____ and

    _____ input.

16. The occipital lobe is the primary area for _____.

17. State the functions of the thalamus.

    a. _____   b. _____

18. State three functions of the hypothalamus.

    a. _____   b. _____

    c. _____

19. The cerebellum plays an important part in the _____ of

    _____ .

20. State five functions of the medulla oblongata.

    a. _____   b. _____

    c. _____   d. _____

    e. _____

21. State the three functions of the spinal cord.

    a. _____   b. _____

    c. _____

22. The normal adult will have between _____ and _____ mL of cerebrospinal fluid in circulation.

23. Name the 12 pairs of cranial nerves.

a. _____ b. _____ c. _____

d. _____ e. _____ f. _____

g. _____ h. _____ i. _____

j. _____ k. _____ l. _____

24. Name the four plexuses that are formed from the spinal nerves.

a. _____ b. _____

c. _____ d. _____

25. State four functions of the autonomic nervous system.

a. _____ b. _____

c. _____ d. _____

26. Name the two divisions of the autonomic nervous system.

a. _____ b. _____

Word Parts

1. In the spaces provided, write the definitions of these prefixes, roots, combining forms, and suffixes. Do not refer to the listings of medical words. Leave blank those words you cannot define.

2. After completing as many as you can, refer to the medical word listings to check your work. For each word missed or left blank, write the word and its definition several times on the margins of these pages or on a separate sheet of paper.

3. To maximize the learning process, it is to your advantage to do the following exercises as directed. To refer to the word building section before completing these exercises invalidates the learning process.

PREFIXES

Give the definitions of the following prefixes:

1. a- _____

2. an- _____

3. astro- _____

4. brady- _____

5. de- _____

6. dys- _____

7. epi- _____

8. hemi- _____

9. hydro- _____

10. hyper- _____

11. intra- _____

12. micro- _____

13. oligo- _____

14. par- _____

15. para- _____

16. poly- _____

17. pyro- _____

18. quadri- _____

19. sub- _____

20. syn- _____

ROOTS AND COMBINING FORMS

Give the definitions of the following roots and combining forms:

1. acr/o _____

2. ambul _____

3. agor/a _____

4. dur/o _____

5. atel/o _____

6. centr _____

7. cephal _____

8. later _____

9. cerebell _____

10. cerebell/o _____

11. cerebr/o _____

12. chrom/o _____

13. aut _____

14. concuss _____

15. cran/i _____

16. crani/o _____

17. cyt _____

18. dendr/o _____

19. disk _____

20. dur _____

21. eg/o _____

22. electr/o _____

23. encephal _____

24. encephal/o _____

25. esthesi/o _____

26. narc/o _____

27. ganglion _____

28. gli _____

29. lept _____

30. hypn _____

31. pallid/o _____

32. lamin _____

33. lob/o _____

34. log _____

35. mening _____

36. mening/i _____

37. mening/o _____

38. ment _____

39. mnes _____

40. myel _____

41. myel/o _____

42. my/o _____

43. neur _____

44. neur/i _____

45. neur/o _____

46. papill _____

47. phe/o _____

48. poli/o _____

49. psych _____

50. psych/o _____

51. scler _____

52. spin _____

53. spondyl/o _____

54. somat _____

55. somn _____

56. sympath _____

57. vag/o _____

58. ventricul/o _____

SUFFIXES

Give the definitions of the following suffixes:

1. -al _____

2. -algesia _____

3. -algia _____

4. -ar _____

5. -asthenia _____

6. -blast _____

7. -cele _____

8. -cyte _____

9. -desis _____

10. -ectomy _____

11. -edema _____

12. -esthesia _____

13. -glia _____

14. -gram _____

15. -graph _____

16. -graphy _____

17. -ia _____

18. -ic _____

19. -ion _____

20. -ism _____

21. -ist _____

22. -itis _____

23. -kinesia _____

24. -kinesis _____

25. -lepsy _____

26. -lemma _____

27. -lexia _____

28. -logy _____

29. -cope _____

30. -malacia _____

31. -mania _____

32. -troph(y) _____

33. -metry _____

34. -scopy _____

35. -noia _____

36. -oma _____

37. -osis _____

38. -paresis _____

39. -pathy _____

40. -phagia _____

41. -phasia _____

42. -phobia _____

43. -praxia _____

44. -sthenia _____

45. -taxia _____

46. -tomy _____

47. -us _____

48. -y _____

Identifying Medical Terms

In the spaces provided, write the medical terms for the following meanings:

1. _____ A condition in which there is a loss or lack of memory

2. _____ A lack of the sense of pain

3. _____ A loss or lack of the ability to eat or swallow

4. _____ A loss or lack of muscular coordination

5. _____ Head pain; headache

6. _____ Pertaining to the cerebellum

7. _____ Surgical excision of a portion of the skull

8. _____ A condition in which an individual has difficulty in comprehending written language

9. _____ Inflammation of the brain

10. _____ Pertaining to situated on the dura mater

11. _____ Paralysis that affects one side of the body

12. _____ Inflammation of the meninges of the spinal cord or brain

13. _____ Pain in a nerve or nerves

14. _____ Inflammation of a nerve

15. _____ A nerve cell, a neuron

16. _____ The study of the nervous system

17. _____ A tumor of nerve cells and nerve fibers

18. _____ An emotional condition or disorder

19. _____ Inflammation of many nerves

20. _____ The study of the mind

21. _____ Surgical incision of the vagus nerve

22. _____ Measurement of intracranial pressure

Spelling

In the spaces provided, write the correct spelling of these misspelled words.

1. anestesia _____

2. atelomylia _____

3. cerebospinal _____

4. cranitomy _____

5. epilepisy _____

6. meningoma _____

7. meningmyelcele _____

8. neurpathy _____

9. polomyelitis _____

10. ventriulometry _____

Matching

Select the appropriate lettered meaning for each word listed below.

_____ 1. acetylcholine

_____ 2. Alzheimer's disease

_____ 3. apoplexy

_____ 4. endorphins

_____ 5. epilepsy

_____ 6. palsy

_____ 7. percutaneous diskectomy

_____ 8. epiduroscopy

_____ 9. dementia

_____ 10. sciatica

a. A group of symptoms marked by memory loss and other cognitive functions

b. Chemical substances produced in the brain that act as natural analgesics

c. A stroke

d. A severe form of senile dementia

e. A disorder of cerebral function resulting from abnormal electrical activity or malfunctioning of the chemical substances of the brain

f. Used for back pain relief

g. A cholinergic neurotransmitter that occurs in various tissues and organs of the body

h. A loss of sensation or an impairment of motor function

i. Severe pain along the course of the sciatic nerve

j. A surgical procedure that can be done on an outpatient basis for slipped disk

k. An anxiety syndrome and panic disorder

Abbreviations

Place the correct word, phrase, or abbreviation in the space provided.

1. Alzheimer's disease _____

2. amyotrophic lateral sclerosis _____

3. CNS _____

4. CP _____

5. computerized tomography _____

6. herniated disk syndrome _____

7. ICP _____

8. LP _____

9. MS _____

10. positron emission tomography _____

Diagnostic and Laboratory Tests

Select the best answer to each multiple choice question. Circle the letter of your choice.

1. A diagnostic procedure used to study the structure of the brain.
   a. computed tomography
   b. echoencephalography
   c. electroencephalography
   d. myelogram

2. The process of using ultrasound to determine the presence of a centrally located mass in the brain.
   a. computed tomography
   b. echoencephalography
   c. electroencephalography
   d. myelogram

3. The x-ray of the spinal canal after the injection of a radiopaque dye.
   a. cerebral angiography
   b. computed tomography
   c. myelogram
   d. ultrasonography

4. A computer-based nuclear imaging procedure that can produce three-dimensional pictures of actual organ functioning.
   a. electroencephalography
   b. myelogram
   c. ultrasonography
   d. positron emission tomography

5. The use of high-frequency sound waves to record echoes on an oscilloscope and film.
   a. electroencephalography
   b. myelogram
   c. ultrasonography
   d. positron emission tomography

CASE STUDY   ALZHEIMER'S DISEASE

Read the following case study and then answer the questions that follow.

A 68-year-old female was seen by a physician and the following is a synopsis of the visit.

Present History: The husband states that he is very concerned about his wife. He has noticed that she has become confused and forgets where she puts things, and even puts things in the wrong place. Last Monday she put the iron in the freezer. The patient had very little to say about herself.

Signs and Symptoms: Confusion, memory loss, and inappropriate placing of iron in the freezer.

Diagnosis: Alzheimer's. The diagnosis was determined by a complete physical examination, a medical history, neuropsychological testing, an electroencephalogram (EEG), and a computerized tomography (CT) scan.

Treatment: The primary symptoms of Alzheimer's disease include memory loss, disorientation, confusion, and problems with reasoning and thinking. These symptoms worsen as brain cells die and the connections between cells are lost. Although current drugs cannot alter the progressive loss of cells, they may help minimize or stabilize symptoms. These medications may also delay the need for nursing home care.

There are four drugs approved by the U.S. Food and Drug Administration for the treatment of Alzheimer's disease:

- Cognex (*tacrine*)
- Aricept (*donepezil*)
- Exelon (*rivastigmine*)
- Reminyl (*galantamine*)

These four medications are in a class of drugs known as cholinesterase inhibitors. They are designed to prevent the breakdown of acetylcholine, a chemical messenger in the brain that is important for memory and other thinking skills. The drug works to keep levels of the chemical messenger high, even while the cells that produce the messenger continue to become damaged or die. About half of the people who take cholinesterase inhibitors experience a modest improvement in cognitive symptoms. Management of a patient with Alzheimer's involves support and assistance to the patient and her family. For more information you may call the Alzheimer's Association at 1–800–272–3900.

Prevention: There is no known prevention.

Ten Warning Signs of Alzheimer's Disease: The Alzheimer's Association believes that it is critical for people with dementia and their families to receive information, care, and support as early as possible. To help family members and health care professionals recognize warning signs of Alzheimer's disease, the Association has developed a checklist of common symptoms.

1. **Memory loss.** One of the most common early signs of dementia is forgetting recently learned information. While it's normal to forget appointments, names, or telephone numbers, those with dementia will forget such things more often and not remember them later.

2. **Difficulty performing familiar tasks.** People with dementia often find it hard to complete everyday tasks that are so familiar we usually do not think about how to do them. A person with Alzheimer's may not know the steps for preparing a meal,

using a household appliance, or participating in a lifelong hobby.

3. **Problems with language.** Everyone has trouble finding the right word sometimes, but a person with Alzheimer's disease often forgets simple words or substitutes unusual words, making his or her speech or writing hard to understand. If a person with Alzheimer's is unable to find his or her toothbrush, for example, the individual may ask for "that thing for my mouth."

4. **Disorientation to time and place.** It's normal to forget the day of the week or where you're going. But people with Alzheimer's disease can become lost on their own street, forget where they are and how they got there, and not know how to get back home.

5. **Poor or decreased judgment.** No one has perfect judgment all of the time. Those with Alzheimer's may dress without regard to the weather, wearing several shirts or blouses on a warm day or very little clothing in cold weather. Individuals with dementia often show poor judgment about money, giving away large amounts of money to telemarketers or paying for home repairs or products they don't need.

6. **Problems with abstract thinking.** Balancing a checkbook may be hard when the task is more complicated than usual. Someone with Alzheimer's disease could forget completely what the numbers are and what needs to be done with them.

7. **Misplacing things.** Anyone can temporarily misplace a wallet or key. A person with Alzheimer's disease may put things in unusual places: an iron in the freezer or a wristwatch in the sugar bowl.

8. **Changes in mood or behavior.** Everyone can become sad or moody from time to time. Someone with Alzheimer's disease can show rapid mood swings—from calm to tears to anger—for no apparent reason.

9. **Changes in personality.** People's personalities ordinarily change somewhat with age. But a person with Alzheimer's disease can change a lot, becoming extremely confused, suspicious, fearful, or dependent on a family member.

10. **Loss of initiative.** It's normal to tire of housework, business activities, or social obligations at times. The person with Alzheimer's disease may become very passive, sitting in front of the television for hours, sleeping more than usual, or not wanting to do usual activities.

If you recognize any warning signs in yourself or a loved one, the Alzheimer's Association recommends consulting a physician. Early diagnosis of Alzheimer's disease or other disorders causing dementia is an important step in getting appropriate treatment, care, and support services.

CASE STUDY QUESTIONS

1. Signs and symptoms of Alzheimer's disease include confusion, _____ loss, and the inappropriate placing of an object.

2. The diagnosis was determined by a complete physical examination, a medical history, neuro-psychological testing, an _____, and a computerized tomography scan.

3. Management of Alzheimer's involves support and _____.

4. As the disease progresses, why do the symptoms of Alzheimer's disease worsen?

5. The four drugs approved for the treatment of Alzheimer's disease are classified as cholinesterase inhibitors. What are these drugs designed to do?

6. Why is it important to be familiar with the ten warning signs of Alzheimer's disease?

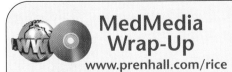 **MedMedia Wrap-Up**
www.prenhall.com/rice

Additional interactive resources and activities for this chapter can be found on the Companion Website. For animation, videos, audio glossary, and review, access the accompanying CD-ROM in this book.

Audio Glossary
Medical Terminology Exercises & Activities
Pathology Spotlight
Terminology Translator
Animations
Videos

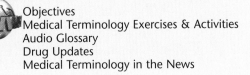
Objectives
Medical Terminology Exercises & Activities
Audio Glossary
Drug Updates
Medical Terminology in the News

SPECIAL SENSES: THE EAR 13

OUTLINE

OBJECTIVES

On completion of this chapter, you will be able to:

- Describe the anatomical structures of the ear.
- Describe the external ear.
- Describe the middle ear.
- Describe the inner ear.
- Analyze, build, spell, and pronounce medical words.
- Describe each of the conditions presented in the Pathology Spotlights.
- Complete the Pathology Checkpoint.
- Review Drug Highlights presented in this chapter.
- Provide the description of diagnostic and laboratory tests related to the ear.
- Identify and define selected abbreviations.
- Successfully complete the study and review section.

MedMedia
www.prenhall.com/rice

Additional interactive resources and activities for this chapter can be found on the Companion Website. For Terminology Translator, animations, videos, audio glossary, and review, access the accompanying CD-ROM in this book.

Anatomy and Physiology Overview

The **ear** is the site of **hearing** and **equilibrium**. It contains specially designed anatomical structures that receive sound vibrations, are sensitive to the force of gravity, and react to the movements of the head. These anatomical structures are connected to sensory areas of the brain by specialized fibers from the eighth cranial nerve. The ear is generally described as having three distinct divisions: the **external ear**, the **middle ear**, and the **inner ear**. The following is a listing of the major components of the ear and some of their functions.

THE EXTERNAL EAR

The **external ear** is the appendage on the side of the head consisting of the *auricle* or *pinna*, the *external acoustic meatus* or *auditory canal*, and the *tympanic membrane* or *eardrum*. The auricle collects sound waves that then pass through the auditory canal to vibrate the tympanic membrane that separates the external ear from the middle ear. The auditory canal is an S-shaped tubular structure about 2.5 cm long. Numerous glands line the canal and secrete **cerumen** or **earwax** to lubricate and protect the ear (Fig. 13–1).

SPECIAL SENSES: THE EAR

Organ/Structure	*Primary Functions*
The External Ear	
Auricle (pinna)	Collects and directs sound waves into the auditory canal and then into the tympanic membrane
Auditory canal (external acoustic meatus)	Numerous glands line the canal and secrete earwax to lubricate and protect the ear
Tympanic membrane (eardrum)	Separates the external ear from the middle ear
The Middle Ear	
Contains the ossicles: malleus, incus, and stapes; has five openings, and is lined with mucous membrane	Transmits sound vibrations
	Equalizes external/internal air pressure on the tympanic membrane
	Exerts control over potentially damaging or disruptive loud sounds
The Inner Ear	
Cochlea	Contains the organ of Corti, the organ of hearing
Vestibule	Contains the utricle and saccule, membranous pouches containing perilymph. The utricle communicates with the semicircular canals and contains hair cell sensory receptors connected to fibers from the eighth cranial nerve. These hair cells react to the force of gravity and movement and are a part of the sense of equilibrium.
The semicircular canals	Contains nerve endings in the form of hair cells that note changes in the position of the head and reports such movement to the brain through fibers leading to the eighth cranial nerve.

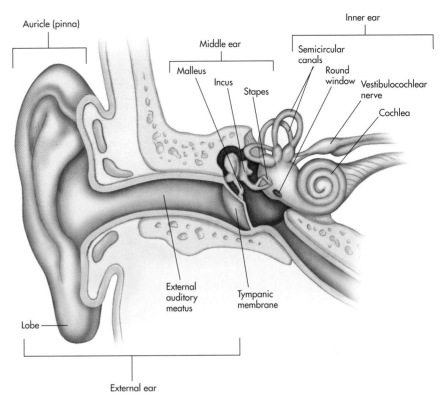

FIGURE 13–1

The ear and its anatomic structures.

THE MIDDLE EAR

Beyond the tympanic membrane is a tiny cavity in the temporal bone of the skull. This cavity contains three small bones or **ossicles** instrumental to the hearing process. These ossicles are the **malleus, incus**, and **stapes**. Sometimes referred to as the **hammer, anvil, and stirrup** because of their shapes, these bones mechanically transmit sound vibrations from the tympanic membrane, to which the malleus is attached, through the incus to the stapes, which attaches to a thin membrane covering a small opening, the oval window, that marks the beginning of the inner ear. During transmission, tympanic vibrations may be amplified as much as 22 times their original force.

The cavity of the middle ear has five openings, one covered by the tympanic membrane, another to the auditory or eustachian tube, a third to the mastoid cells, and two openings to the inner ear, the oval and round windows (Fig. 13–1). The cavity is lined by mucous membrane that is continuous with that found in the mastoid air cells, the eustachian tube, and the throat. The spread of infection from the throat along this membrane to the middle ear is called otitis media. The continued spread of infection to the mastoid air cells is called mastoiditis.

Three functions have been attributed to the middle ear:

- It transmits sound vibrations.
- It equalizes external/internal air pressure on the tympanic membrane.
- It exerts control over potentially damaging or disruptive loud sounds through reflex contractions of the stapedius and tensor tympani muscles, which are attached to the stapes and the malleus, respectively.

THE INNER EAR

The **inner ear** consists of a membranous labyrinth or maze located within a bony labyrinth. These structures are called **labyrinths** because of their complicated shapes. The bony labyrinth, located in the temporal bone, consists of the *cochlea, vestibule,* and *three semicircular canals.* Within the bony labyrinth, but separated from it by a fluid called **perilymph,** is the membranous labyrinth. It has much the same shape as the bony labyrinth and has three distinct divisions: the *cochlear duct* inside the cochlea, the *semicircular ducts* within the semicircular canals, and two sac-like structures, the **utricle** and **saccule,** located in the vestibule. Nerve endings in the form of hair cells located in various parts of the inner ear serve as receptors for the senses of *hearing* and *equilibrium.*

The Cochlea

The **cochlea** is a spiral-shaped bony structure containing the cochlear duct and so named because it resembles a snail shell. The spiral cavity of the bony cochlea is partitioned into three tube-like channels that run the entire length of the spiral. Two membranes form these tube-like areas. The *basilar membrane* forms the lower channel or *scala tympani,* and the *vestibular membrane (Reissner's membrane)* forms the upper channel, which is called the *scala vestibuli.* Between the two scala is a space, the *cochlear duct,* formed by the vestibular membrane on top and the basilar membrane as a floor. Located on the basilar membrane is the **organ of Corti** containing hair cell sensory receptors for the sense of hearing. A pale fluid, **perilymph,** fills the scala vestibuli and scala tympani. A different fluid, **endolymph,** fills the cochlear duct (Fig. 13–2).

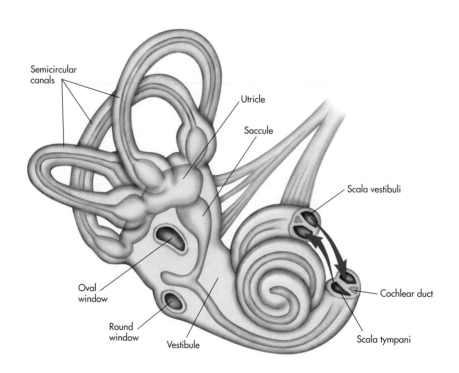

FIGURE 13–2

The cochlea.

THE HEARING PROCESS IN THE INNER EAR

The scala vestibuli and scala tympani open to the middle ear through the oval and round windows, respectively. The stapes fits into the round window and causes vibration of the perilymph, which, in turn, vibrates the basilar membrane and endolymph of the cochlear duct, thereby exciting the nerve endings contained on the **organ of Corti**. These nerve endings transmit the sounds, via the *eighth cranial nerve*, to the auditory areas of the brain. The sound waves, having excited the fluid of the cochlear duct, then pass on to the perilymph of the scala tympani and are dissipated against the membrane covering the round window.

The Vestibule

The **vestibule** is a bony structure located between the cochlea and the three semicircular canals. The bony vestibule contains the **utricle** and **saccule**, membranous pouches containing perilymph. The utricle communicates with the semicircular canals and contains hair cell sensory receptors connected to fibers from the eighth cranial nerve. These hair cells react to the forces of gravity and movement and are a part of the sense of *equilibrium*.

The Semicircular Canals

Located at right angles to each other, there are the superior, posterior, and inferior **semicircular canals**. Within the bony canals are the membranous semicircular ducts containing endolymph. At the base of each canal is an enlargement called an **ampulla** containing nerve endings in the form of hair cells. Changes in the position of the head causes the fluid in the canals to move against these sensory receptors, which, in turn, report such movement to the brain through fibers leading to the eighth cranial nerve. *Dizziness* and motion sickness are associated with rapid or erratic movement and the resulting sensory sensation in these areas.

LIFE SPAN
CONSIDERATIONS

■ THE CHILD

At 36 weeks the identifying characteristics of the fetus are soft ear lobes, few creases on the soles of the foot, ample vernix caseosa, and diminishing lanugo. At 40 weeks there are firm **ear lobes**. In newborns the wall of the ear canal is pliable because of underdeveloped cartilage and bone. The **eustachian tube** in infants is shorter and straighter than in older children and adults.

Babies respond to "mother-ese" and "parent-ese," whose melodic sounds actually provide a tutorial in the sounds that make up language. It is recommended that parents sing and talk to even the youngest infants, because verbal stimulation is crucial to how well a child develops thinking and language skills later.

According to Dr. William Staso, an expert in neurologic development, different kinds of stimulation should be emphasized at different ages.

First Month	A low level of stimulation reduces stress and increases the infant's wakefulness and alertness.
1 to 3 Months	The brain starts to discriminate among acoustic patterns of language, like intonation and pitch.
3 to 5 Months	Infants rely primarily on vision to acquire information about the world.

6 to 7 Months	Infants become alert to relationships such as cause and effect, the location of objects, and the function of objects.
7 to 8 Months	The brain is oriented to make association between sound and some meaningful activity or object.
9 to 12 Months	Learning adds up to a new level of awareness of the environment and increased interest in exploration; sensory and motor skills coordinate in a more mature fashion.

■ THE OLDER ADULT

With aging, changes occur in the **external, middle,** and **inner ear**. The skin of the **auricle** may become dry and wrinkled. Production of **cerumen** declines and it is drier. There is also dryness of the external canal, which causes itching. Hairs in the external canal become coarser and longer, especially in males. The eardrum thickens and the bony joints in the middle ear degenerate.

Changes in the inner ear affect sensitivity to sound, understanding of speech, and balance. Degenerative changes include atrophy of the cochlea, the cochlear nerve cells, and the organ of Corti. These changes lead to the hearing loss, **presbycusis**, that is common in the older adult. Noisy surroundings make it difficult for older adults to discriminate between sounds, thereby impairing communication and socialization.

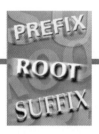

BUILDING YOUR MEDICAL VOCABULARY

This section provides the foundation for learning medical terminology. Medical words can be made up of four different types of word parts:

- Prefixes (P)
- Roots (R)
- Combining forms (CF)
- Suffixes (S)

By connecting various word parts in an organized sequence, thousands of words can be built and learned. In this text the word list is alphabetized so one can see the variety of meanings created when common prefixes and suffixes are repeatedly applied to certain word roots and/or combining forms. Words shown in pink are additional words related to the content of this chapter that are not built from word parts. These words are included to enhance your vocabulary. Note: an asterisk icon (✱) indicates words that are covered in the Pathology section in this chapter.

MEDICAL WORD	WORD PARTS (WHEN APPLICABLE)			DEFINITION
	Part	**Type**	**Meaning**	
acoustic (ă-koos′ tĭk)	acoust	R	hearing	Pertaining to the sense of hearing
	-ic	S	pertaining to	
audiogram (ŏ′ dĭ-ō-grăm″)	audi/o	CF	to hear	A record of hearing by audiometry
	-gram	S	a mark, record	

MEDICAL WORD	WORD PARTS (WHEN APPLICABLE)			DEFINITION
	Part	Type	Meaning	
audiologist (ŏ″ dĭ-ŏl′ ō-jĭst)	audi/o log -ist	CF R S	to hear study of one who specializes	One who specializes in disorders of hearing
audiology (ŏ″ dĭ-ŏl′ ō-jĭ)	audi/o -logy	CF S	to hear study of	The study of hearing disorders. ✱ See Pathology Spotlight: Audiology.
audiometer (ŏ dĭ-ŏm′ ĕ-tĕr)	audi/o -meter	CF S	to hear instrument to measure	An instrument used to measure hearing
audiometry (ŏ″ dĭ-ŏm′ ĕ-trē)	audi/o -metry	CF S	to hear measurement	Measurement of the hearing sense
audiphone (ŏ′ dĭ-fōn)	aud/i phone	CF R	to hear voice	An instrument that conveys sound to the auditory nerve through teeth or bone
auditory (ŏ′ dĭ-tō″ rē)	auditor -y	R S	hearing pertaining to	Pertaining to the sense of hearing
aural (ŏ′ răl)	aur -al	R S	the ear pertaining to	Pertaining to the ear
auricle (ŏ′ rĭ-kl)	aur/i -cle	CF S	ear small	The external portion of the ear, known as the flap of the ear; *the pinna* (pin′ na)
binaural (bīn-aw′ răl)	bin (bis) aur -al	P R S	twice ear pertaining to	Pertaining to both ears
cerumen (sē-roo′ mĕn)				Earwax, the yellowish substance secreted by the glands in the canal of the external ear
cholesteatoma (kō″ lē-stē″ ă-tō′ mă)	chol/e steat -oma	CF R S	gall or bile fat tumor	A tumor-like mass filled with epithelial cells and cholesterol
cochlea (kŏk′ lē-ă)				A portion of the inner ear shaped like a snail shell; contains the organ of hearing referred to as the organ of Corti
deafness (dĕf′ nĕs)				Complete or partial loss of the ability to hear
ear (ēr)				Organ of hearing and equilibrium

MEDICAL WORD	WORD PARTS (when applicable)			DEFINITION
	Part	**Type**	**Meaning**	
electrococh-leography (ē-lĕk″ trō-kŏk″ lē-ŏg′ ră-fē)	electr/o cochle/o -graphy	CF CF S	electricity land snail recording	A recording of the electrical activity produced when the cochlea is stimulated
endaural (ĕn′ dŏ″ ral)	end aur -al	P R S	within ear pertaining to	Pertaining to within the ear
endolymph (ĕn′ dō-lĭmf)	endo -lymph	P S	within serum, clear fluid	The clear fluid contained within the labyrinth of the ear
equilibrium (ē″ kwĭ-lĭb′ rē-ŭm)	equ/i libr/i -um	CF CF S	equal balance tissue	A state of balance. In the inner ear, the semicircular canals are the site of the organs of balance.
eustachian tube (yoo-stā′ shən tūb)				A narrow tube between the middle ear and the throat that serves to equalize pressure on both sides of the eardrum
fenestration (fĕn″ ĕs-trā′ shŭn)	fenestrat -ion	R S	window process	Surgical operation in which a new opening is made in the labyrinth of the inner ear for restoration of hearing
incus (ing′ kŭs)				The anvil, the middle of the three ossicles
labyrinth (lăb′ ĭ-rĭnth)				The inner ear; *made up of the vestibule, cochlea, and semicircular canals*
labyrinthectomy (lăb″ ĭ-rĭn-thĕk′ tō-mē)	labyrinth -ectomy	R S	maze excision	Surgical excision of the labyrinth
labyrinthitis (lăb″ ĭ-rĭn-thĭ′ tĭs)	labyrinth -itis	R S	maze inflammation	Inflammation of the labyrinth
labyrinthotomy (lăb″ ĭ-rĭn-thŏt′ ō-mē)	labyrinth/o -tomy	CF S	maze incision	Incision of the labyrinth
malleus (măl′ ē-ŭs)				The hammer, the largest of the three ossicles
mastoidalgia (măs″ toyd-ăl′ jĭ-ă)	mast oid -algia	R S S	breast form pain	Pain in the mastoid
mastoiditis (măs″ toyd-ī′ tĭs)	mast -oid -itis	R S S	breast form inflammation	Inflammation of the mastoid

MEDICAL WORD	WORD PARTS (WHEN APPLICABLE)			DEFINITION
	Part	**Type**	**Meaning**	
Ménière's disease (mān″ ē-ārz)				A disease of the inner ear *(labyrinth)* that presents a group of symptoms that recur. In acute attacks, bedrest is recommended. Vertigo and dizziness are the classic symptoms, and the patient experiences nausea, tinnitus, and a sensation of fullness or pressure in the ears. Deafness can occur. ✱ See Pathology Spotlight: Ménière's Disease.
monaural (mŏn-aw′ răl)	mon(o) aur -al	P R S	one ear pertaining to	Pertaining to one ear
myringectomy (mĭr-ĭn-jĕk′ tō-mē)	myring -ectomy	R S	drum membrane excision	Surgical excision of the tympanic membrane
myringoplasty (mĭr-ĭn′ gō-plăst″ ē)	myring/o -plasty	CF S	drum membrane surgical repair	Surgical repair of the tympanic membrane
myringoscope (mĭr-ĭn′ gō-skōp)	myring/o -scope	CF S	drum membrane instrument	An instrument used to examine the eardrum
myringotome (mĭ-rĭn′ gō-tō)	myring/o -tome	CF S	drum membrane instrument to cut	An instrument used for cutting the eardrum
myringotomy (mĭr-ĭn-gŏt′ ō-mē)	myring/o -tomy	CF S	drum membrane incision	Surgical incision of the tympanic membrane. It is used to remove unwanted fluids from the ear
ossicle (ŏs′ ĭ-kl)				Small bone. Any one of the three bones of the middle ear: the malleus, the incus, or the stapes
otic (ō′ tĭk)	ot -ic	R S	ear pertaining to	Pertaining to the ear
otitis (ō-tī′ tĭs)	ot -itis	R S	ear inflammation	Inflammation of the ear. ✱ See Pathology Spotlight: Otitis Media.
otitis media (ō-tī′ tĕs mē′ dē-ă)	ot -itis med -ia	R S R S	ear inflammation middle condition of	Inflammation of the middle ear. ✱ See Pathology Spotlight: Otitis Media.
otodynia (ō″ tō-dĭn′ ĭ-ă)	ot/o -dynia	CF S	ear pain	Pain in the ear, earache

MEDICAL WORD	WORD PARTS (WHEN APPLICABLE)			DEFINITION
	Part	**Type**	**Meaning**	
otolaryngologist (ō″ tō-lar″ ĭn-gŏl″ ō-jĭst)	ot/o laryng/o log -ist	CF CF R S	ear larynx study of one who specializes	One who specializes in the study of the ear and larynx
otolaryngology (ō″ tō-lar″ ĭn-gŏl′ ō-jē)	ot/o laryng/o -logy	CF CF S	ear larynx study of	The study of the ear and larynx
otolith (ō′ tō-lĭth)	ot/o -lith	CF S	ear stone	Ear stone
otomycosis (ō″ tō-mī-kō′ sĭs)	ot/o myc -osis	CF R S	ear fungus condition of	A fungus condition of the ear
otoneurology (ō″ tō-nū-rŏl′ ō-jē)	ot/o neur/o -logy	CF CF S	ear nerve study of	The study of ear conditions with nerve complications
otopharyngeal (ō″ tō-far-ĭn′ jē-āl)	ot/o pharyng/e -al	CF CF S	ear pharynx pertaining to	Pertaining to the ear and pharynx
otoplasty (ō′ tō-plăs″ tē)	ot/o -plasty	CF S	ear surgical repair	Surgical repair of the ear
otopyorrhea (ō″ tō-pī″ ō-rē′ ă)	ot/o py/o -rrhea	CF CF S	ear pus flow	Flow of pus from the ear
otorhinolaryngology (ō″ tō-rī″ nō-lăr″ ĭn-gŏl′ ō-jē)	ot/o rhin/o laryng/o -logy	CF CF CF S	ear nose larynx study of	The study of the ear, nose, and larynx
otosclerosis (ō″ tō-sklē-rō′ sĭs)	ot/o scler -osis	CF R S	ear hardening condition of	A hardening condition of the ear characterized by progressive deafness
otoscope (ō′ tō-skōp)	ot/o -scope	CF S	ear instrument	An instrument used to examine the ear
oval window (ō′ văl wĭn′ dō)				Membrane in the middle ear into which fits the footplate of the stapes
perilymph (pĕr′ ĭ-lĭmf)	peri -lymph	P S	around serum, pale fluid	Serum fluid of the inner ear
presbycusis (prĕz″ bĭ-kū′ sĭs)	presby -cusis	R S	old hearing	Impairment of hearing in old age

MEDICAL WORD	WORD PARTS (WHEN APPLICABLE)			DEFINITION
	Part	Type	Meaning	
Rinne test (rĭn′ nē test)				A hearing test made with a tuning fork to compare bone conduction hearing with air conduction
stapedectomy (stā″ pē-dĕk′ tō-mē)	staped -ectomy	R S	stirrup excision	Surgical excision of the stapes in the ear
stapes (stā′ pēz)				The stirrup, the innermost of the ossicles
tinnitus (tĭn-ī′ tŭs)	tinnit -us	R S	a jingling pertaining to	A ringing or jingling sound in the ear. ✱ See Pathology Spotlight: Tinnitus.
tympanectomy (tĭm″ păn-ĕk tō-mē)	tympan -ectomy	R S	drum excision	Surgical excision of the tympanic membrane
tympanic (tĭm-păn′ ĭk)	tympan -ic	R S	drum pertaining to	Pertaining to the eardrum
tympanic thermometer (tĭm-păn′ ĭk thĕr-mŏm′ ĕ-tĕr)				An electronic thermometer that is used to determine core body temperature by measuring it from the tympanic membrane and its surrounding tissues. See Figure 13–3 and Figure 13–4.
tympanitis (tĭm-păn-ī′ tĭs)	tympan -itis	R S	drum inflammation	Inflammation of the eardrum
tympanoplasty (tĭm″ păn-ō-plăs′ tē)	tympan/o -plasty	CF S	drum surgical repair	Surgical repair of the tympanic membrane
utricle (ū′ trĭk-l)				A small, sac-like structure of the labyrinth of the inner ear
vertigo (ver′ tĭ-gō)				A feeling of dizziness, light-headedness, caused by a disturbance of the equilibrium organs in the labyrinth

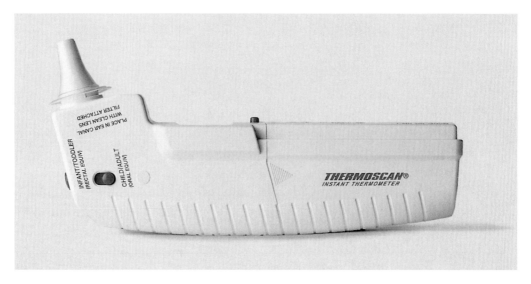

FIGURE 13–3

The Thermoscan Instant Thermometer. (Courtesy of Thermoscan, Inc., San Diego, CA.)

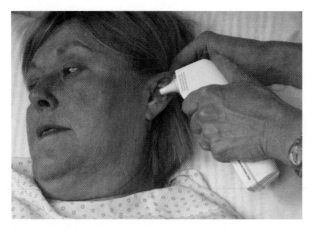

FIGURE 13–4

Using the tympanic thermometer to measure body temperature.

Terminology Translator

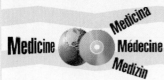

This feature, found on the accompanying CD-ROM, provides an innovative tool to translate medical words into Spanish, French, and German.

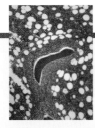

PATHOLOGY SPOTLIGHTS

Audiology

Audiology is the study of hearing disorders. Sustained noise over 85 decibels can cause permanent hearing loss. Risk doubles with each 5-decibel increase. About 2 in every 10 teens have lost some of their hearing ability from exposure to noise and are not aware of it, according to a study at the University of Florida. Standard hearing tests given to middle and high school students identified some hearing loss in 17 percent of the students. High-pitched sounds are the first to be affected by noise exposure. As hearing loss progresses, one can start to have difficulty hearing, particularly when there is noise in the background. Excessive noise can permanently damage the hair cell sensory receptors of the organ of Corti. These receptors are instrumental in transmitting sound to the brain.

In a study at the University of Florida, Alice Holmes, associate professor of communicative disorders, and her colleagues gave 42 students ages 10 to 20 audiologic exams that tested their ability to hear pure tones. Seventeen percent of the students did not hear one or more of the sounds in at least one ear.

Are you harming your hearing?	Above 85 decibels
Firecracker at 10 feet	160 decibels
Rock concert	125 decibels
Stereo headset, volume at six	115 decibels
Subway	100 decibels
Car horn	100 decibels
Garbage disposal	95 decibels
City traffic	90 decibels
Jet taking off at close range	120 decibels

Noise can get in the way of learning and cause stress. Research shows that noise can cause anger, aggression, poor performance, and insomnia. It may also be a factor in hypertension and cardiovascular and digestive problems. One study, at Germany's Max Planck Institute, showed that consistent exposure to 70 decibels of noise caused vascular constriction, a condition that can be dangerous for people with coronary artery disease. It is recommended that one wear earplugs or other sound protection when mowing the lawn, working with noisy equipment, riding a motorcycle, or attending a rock concert. If the noise around you is so loud that you have to raise your voice, then it is loud enough to hurt your hearing.

According to Tedd Mitchell, "MD HealthSmart: Here's to Ears," *USA Weekend,* one can use the word **sound** to remember things that can cause ear problems.

- *Sensory overload.* If you need to raise your voice above the background noise for others to hear you, then you need to either get away from the sound source or protect your ears.
- *Old age.* By age 55, 20% of people have hearing loss. By age 65, 33% are affected. Age-related hearing loss typically does not lead to complete deafness but does lead to auditory isolation. Everything that one does becomes more difficult when one can not hear. Simple conversations are a strain. Listening to the radio and watching TV becomes a chore. One doesn't hear doors closing, oven timers going off or air conditioners turning on or off. Fortunately, hearing loss is preventable for many people.
- *Undiagnosed tumors or under-treated infections.* These condition can cause hearing loss and should be addressed by a physician.
- *Non-functioning ear canal or bones.* Anything that blocks the ear canal impedes sound flow.

- *Damage from drugs, trauma or pressure.* Certain antibiotics, drugs for malaria, antiarrhythmics and even aspirin can have toxic effects on hearing. Also, trauma such as a hole in the eardrum, fracture to the skull, noise trauma (gunfire, fireworks) and pressure trauma (underwater diving or pressurized airplane cabins) can damage the ear and cause hearing loss.

Ménière's Disease

Ménière's disease is an abnormality of the inner ear causing a host of symptoms, including vertigo or severe dizziness, tinnitus or a roaring sound in the ears, fluctuating hearing loss, and the sensation of pressure or pain in the affected ear. The disorder usually affects only one ear and is a common cause of hearing loss. The disease is named after French physician Prosper Ménière who first described the syndrome in 1861.

The symptoms of Ménière's disease are associated with a change in fluid volume within the labyrinth portion of the inner ear. Many experts on Ménière's disease think that a rupture of the membranous labyrinth allows the endolymph to mix with perilymph, another inner ear fluid that occupies the space between the membranous labyrinth and the bony inner ear. This mixing, scientists believe, can cause the symptoms of Ménière's disease. Scientists are investigating several possible causes of the disease, including environmental factors, such as noise pollution and viral infections, as well as biological factors.

The symptoms of Ménière's disease occur suddenly and can arise daily or as infrequently as once a year. **Vertigo**, often the most debilitating symptom of Ménière's disease, typically involves a whirling dizziness that forces the sufferer to lie down. Vertigo attacks can lead to severe nausea, vomiting, and sweating and often come with little or no warning.

Some individuals with Ménière's disease have attacks that start with **tinnitus,** then a loss of hearing, and/or a full feeling or pressure in the affected ear. All of these symptoms are unpredictable. Typically, the attack is characterized by a combination of vertigo, tinnitus, and hearing loss lasting several hours. People experience these discomforts at varying frequencies, durations, and intensities. Other occasional symptoms of Ménière's disease include headaches, abdominal discomfort, and diarrhea. A person's hearing tends to recover between attacks but over time becomes worse.

There are currently approximately 615,000 individuals with diagnosed Ménière's disease in the United States and 45,500 newly diagnosed cases each year. Proper diagnosis of Ménière's disease entails several procedures, including a medical history interview and a physical examination by a physician, hearing and balance tests, and medical imaging with magnetic resonance imaging (MRI). Accurate measurement and characterization of hearing loss are of critical importance in the diagnosis of Ménière's disease.

Through the use of several types of hearing tests, physicians can characterize hearing loss as being sensory, arising from the inner ear, or neural, arising from the hearing nerve. Recording the auditory brain stem response, which measures electrical activity in the hearing nerve and brain stem, is useful in differentiating between these two types of hearing loss. **Electrocochleography**, recording the electrical activity of the inner ear in response to sound, helps confirm the diagnosis.

There is no cure for Ménière's disease. However, the symptoms of the disease are often controlled successfully by reducing the body's retention of fluids through dietary changes (such as a low-salt or salt-free diet and no caffeine or alcohol) or medication. Changes in medications that either control allergies or improve blood circulation in the inner ear may help. Eliminating tobacco use and reducing stress levels are more ways some people can lessen the severity of their symptoms.

Different surgical procedures have been advocated for patients with persistent, debilitating vertigo from Ménière's disease. **Labyrinthectomy** can effectively control vertigo, but sacrifices hearing and is reserved for patients with nonfunctional hearing in the affected ear. Recently, the administration of the antibiotic, gentamycin, directly into the middle ear space has gained popularity for the control of the vertigo of Ménière's disease.

Otitis Media

Otitis is an inflammation or infection of any part of the outer, middle, or inner ear. **Otitis media** is the most common type of otitis. This inflammation often begins when infections that cause sore throats, colds, or other respiratory or breathing problems spread to the middle ear. These can be viral or bacterial infections.

Children are more likely to suffer from otitis media than adults. Seventy-five percent of children experience at least one episode of otitis media by their third birthday. Almost half of these children will have three or more ear infections during their first three years. Although otitis media is primarily a disease of infants and young children, it can also affect adults.

There are many reasons why children are more likely to suffer from otitis media than adults. First, children have more trouble fighting infections. This is because their immune systems are still developing. Another reason has to do with the child's eustachian tube. It is shorter and straighter in the child than in the adult. It can contribute to otitis media in several ways. The eustachian tube is usually closed but opens regularly to ventilate or replenish the air in the middle ear. This tube also equalizes middle ear air pressure in response to air pressure changes in the environment. However, a eustachian tube that is blocked by swelling of its lining or plugged with mucus from a cold or for some other reason cannot open to ventilate the middle ear. The lack of ventilation may allow fluid from the tissue that lines the middle ear to accumulate. If the eustachian tube remains plugged, the fluid cannot drain and begins to collect in the normally air-filled middle ear.

One more factor that makes children more susceptible to otitis media is that adenoids in children are larger than they are in adults. Adenoids are composed largely of cells (lymphocytes) that help fight infections. They are positioned in the back of the upper part of the throat near the eustachian tubes. Enlarged adenoids can, because of their size, interfere with the eustachian tube opening. In addition, adenoids may themselves become infected, and the infection may spread into the eustachian tubes.

Bacteria reach the middle ear through the lining or the passageway of the eustachian tube and can then produce infection, which causes swelling of the lining of the middle ear, blocking of the eustachian tube, and migration of white cells from the bloodstream to help fight the infection. In this process the white cells accumulate, often killing bacteria and dying themselves, leading to the formation of pus, a thick yellowish-white fluid in the middle ear. As the fluid increases, the child may have trouble hearing because the eardrum and middle ear bones are unable to move as freely as they should. As the infection worsens, many children also experience severe ear pain. Too much fluid in the ear can put pressure on the eardrum and eventually tear it. Otitis media not only causes severe pain but may result in serious complications if it is not treated. An untreated infection can travel from the middle ear to the nearby parts of the head, including the brain. Although the hearing loss caused by otitis media is usually temporary, untreated otitis media may lead to permanent hearing impairment. Persistent fluid in the middle ear and chronic otitis media can reduce a child's hearing at a time that is critical for speech and language development. Children who have early hearing impairment from frequent ear infections are likely to have speech and language disabilities.

Otitis media is often difficult to detect because most children affected by this disorder do not yet have sufficient speech and language skills to tell someone what is bothering them. Common signs are:

- Unusual irritability
- Difficulty sleeping
- Tugging or pulling at one or both ears
- Fever
- Fluid draining from the ear

- Loss of balance
- Unresponsiveness to quiet sounds or other signs of hearing difficulty such as sitting too close to the television or being inattentive

Children who are cared for in group settings, as well as children who live with adults who smoke cigarettes, have more ear infections. Therefore, a child who is prone to otitis media should avoid contact with sick playmates and environmental tobacco smoke. Infants who nurse from a bottle while lying down also appear to develop otitis media more frequently. Children who have been breast-fed often have fewer episodes of otitis media. Research has shown that cold and allergy medications such as antihistamines and decongestants are not helpful in preventing ear infections.

Tinnitus

Tinnitus is a symptom associated with many forms of hearing loss. It can also be a symptom of other health problems. According to estimates by the American Tinnitus Association, at least 12 million Americans have tinnitus. Of these, at least 1 million experience it so severely that it interferes with their daily activities. People with severe cases of tinnitus may find it difficult to hear, work, or even sleep.

There are several possible causes of tinnitus:

- Hearing loss. Doctors and scientists have discovered that people with different kinds of hearing loss also have tinnitus.
- Loud noise. Too much exposure to loud noise can cause noise-induced hearing loss and tinnitus.
- Medicine. More than 200 medicines can cause tinnitus.
- Other health problems. Allergies, tumors, and problems in the heart and blood vessels, jaws, and neck can cause tinnitus.

A patient may be referred to an **otolaryngologist** for diagnosis, and/or an **audiologist**, who will test the patient's hearing. Although there is no cure for tinnitus, scientists and doctors have discovered several treatments that may provide some relief. Treatments can include:

- Hearing aids. Many people with tinnitus also have a hearing loss. Wearing a hearing aid makes it easier for some people to hear the sounds they need to hear by making them louder.
- Maskers. Maskers are small electronic devices that use sound to make tinnitus less noticeable. Maskers do not make tinnitus go away, but they make the ringing or roaring seem softer. For some people, maskers hide their tinnitus so well that they can barely hear it.
- Medicine or drug therapy. Medications such as antiarrhythmics and antidepressants may help suppress tinnitus.

✔PATHOLOGY CHECKPOINT

Following is a concise list of the pathology-related terms that you've seen in the chapter. Review this checklist to make sure that you are familiar with the meaning of each term before moving on to the next section.

Conditions and Symptoms

- ❏ cholesteatoma
- ❏ deafness
- ❏ labyrinthitis
- ❏ mastoidalgia
- ❏ mastoiditis
- ❏ Ménière's disease
- ❏ otitis
- ❏ otitis media
- ❏ otodynia
- ❏ otolith
- ❏ otomycosis
- ❏ otopyorrhea
- ❏ otosclerosis
- ❏ presbycusis
- ❏ tinnitus
- ❏ tympanitis
- ❏ vertigo

Diagnosis and Treatment

- ❏ audiogram
- ❏ audiometer
- ❏ audiometry
- ❏ audiphone
- ❏ electrocochleography
- ❏ fenestration
- ❏ labyrinthectomy
- ❏ labyrinthotomy
- ❏ myringectomy
- ❏ myringoplasty
- ❏ myringoscope
- ❏ myringotome
- ❏ myringotomy
- ❏ otoplasty
- ❏ otoscope
- ❏ Rinne test
- ❏ stapedectomy
- ❏ tympanectomy
- ❏ tympanic thermometer
- ❏ tympanoplasty

DRUG HIGHLIGHTS

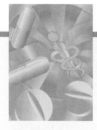

Drugs that are generally used for ear diseases and disorders include antibiotics and those used for vertigo.

Antibiotics	Used to treat infectious diseases. They may be natural or synthetic substances that inhibit the growth of or destroy microorganisms, especially bacteria.
Penicillins	Act by interfering with bacterial cell wall synthesis among newly formed bacterial cells. Penicillins are contraindicated in patients who are known to be allergic or hypersensitive to any of its varieties, or to any of the cephalosporins.

Examples: penicillin G, ampicillin, penicillin V, piperacillin, amoxicillin, and ticarcillin.

Cephalosporins	Are chemically and pharmacologically related to the penicillins. They act by inhibiting bacterial cell wall synthesis, thereby promoting the death of the developing microorganisms. Hypersensitivity to cephalosporins and/or penicillins may result in an allergic reaction.

Examples: Ancef (cefazolin sodium) Mandol (cefamandole nafate), Ceclor (cefaclor), Keflex (cephalexin), Suprax (cefixime), and Monocid (cefonicid).

Tetracyclines

Primarily bacteriostatic, and are active against a wide range of gram-negative and gram-positive microorganisms. They inhibit protein synthesis in the bacterial cell. **Contraindicated in children 8 years of age and younger. These drugs cause permanent discoloration of tooth enamel.**

Examples: Achromycin, Sumycin, Panmycin (tetracycline hydrochloride); Declomycin DMCT (demeclocycline HCl), and Doryx, Vibramycin (doxycycline).

Erythromycin

Works by inhibiting protein synthesis in susceptible bacteria. These drugs may be used for patients who are allergic to penicillin.

Examples: E-Mycin, Ilotycin, Ilosone, EES, EryPed, and Erythrocin.

Drugs Used in Vertigo

Vertigo is an illusion of movement. It may be caused by a lesion or other process affecting the brain, the eighth cranial nerve, or the labyrinthine system of the ear. Drugs that are used for vertigo may include anticholinergics, antihistamines, and antidopamines.

Examples: Dramamine (dimenhydrinate), Benadryl (diphenhydramine HCl), Antivert (meclizine HCl), Torecan (thiethylperazine maleate), Phenergan (promethazine HCl), Transderm-scop (scopolamine), and Torecan (thiethylperazine maleate).

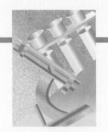

DIAGNOSTIC & LAB TESTS

TEST	DESCRIPTION
auditory evoked response (aw′ dĭ-tō rē ĕ-vōkd′ rē-spŏns)	The response to auditory stimuli (sound) that can be measured independent of the patient's subjective response. By using an electroencephalograph, the intensity of sound and presence of response can be determined. This test is useful for testing the hearing of children who are too young for standard tests, autistic, hyperkinetic, and/or retarded.
electronystagmography (ē-lĕk″ trō-nĭs tăg-mŏg′ ră-fē)	A recording of eye movement in response to specific stimuli, such as sound. It is used to determine the presence and location of a lesion in the vestibule of the ear, to help diagnose unilateral hearing loss of unknown origin, and to help identify the cause of vertigo, tinnitus, and dizziness.
falling test (fă′ lĭng test)	A test to observe the patient for marked swaying or falling. With eyes open, the patient is asked to stand on one foot, stand heel to toe, and then to walk forward. The patient is asked to repeat each of the above with the eyes closed. Marked swaying or falling may indicate vestibular and cerebellar dysfunction.
past-pointing test (păst-poynt′ ĭng test)	The patient is instructed to reach out and touch the examiner's index finger, which is held at shoulder level, then to lower the arm, close the eyes, and touch the finger again. The test is repeated using the finger of the examiner's opposite hand. The degree and direction of past-pointing is observed.
otoscopy (ō-tŏs′ kō-pē)	Visual examination of the external auditory canal and the tympanic membrane via an otoscope.

TEST	DESCRIPTION
tuning fork test (tn′ ĭng fork test)	A method of testing hearing by the use of a tuning fork. Two types of hearing loss (conductive and perceptive) may be distinguished through the use of this test.
tympanometry (tĭm″ păn-nŏm′ ĕ-trē)	Measurement of the movement of the tympanic membrane and pressure in the middle ear. It is used for detecting middle ear disorders.

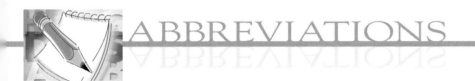

ABBREVIATIONS

ABBREVIATION	MEANING	ABBREVIATION	MEANING
AC	air conduction	EENT	eyes, ears, nose, throat
AD	auris dexter (right ear)	ETF	eustachian tube function
AS	auris sinistra (left ear)	HD	hearing distance
AU	auris unitas (both ears)	OM	otitis media
BC	bone conduction	oto	otology
CPS	cycles per second	PE tube	polyethylene tube
db, dB	decibel	SOM	serous otitis media
ENG	electronystagmography	UCHD	usual childhood diseases
ENT	ear, nose, and throat		

STUDY AND REVIEW

Anatomy and Physiology

Write your answers to the following questions. Do not refer to the text.

1. The ear is the site of the senses of _____ and _____.

2. Name the three divisions of the ear.

   a. _____   b. _____

   c. _____

3. The external ear consists of the a. _____, the b. _____,

   and the c. _____.

4. Which structure of the external ear collects sound waves? _____

5. State the two functions of cerumen.

   a. _____   b. _____

6. Name the three ossicles of the middle ear.

   a. _____   b. _____

   c. _____

7. State the function of the ossicles. _____

   _____

8. State the three functions of the middle ear.

   a. _____   b. _____

   c. _____

9. The bony labyrinth of the inner ear consists of the _____,

   _____, and the _____.

10. Name the three divisions of the membranous labyrinth.

    a. _____   b. _____

    c. _____

11. Located on the basilar membrane is the _____, containing hair cell
    sensory receptors for the sense of hearing.

12. The _____ is a bony structure located between the cochlea and the three semicircular canals.

13. The auditory nerve is also known as the _____.

14. The hair cells located in each ampulla of the semicircular canals sense changes in

_____ and report this information to the brain.

15. Name the two types of fluid found in the ear.

a. _____   b. _____

Word Parts

1. In the spaces provided, write the definitions of these prefixes, roots, combining forms, and suffixes. Do not refer to the listings of medical words. Leave blank those words you cannot define.

2. After completing as many as you can, refer to the medical word listings to check your work. For each word missed or left blank, write the word and its definition several times on the margins of these pages or on a separate sheet of paper.

3. To maximize the learning process, it is to your advantage to do the following exercises as directed. To refer to the word building section before completing these exercises invalidates the learning process.

PREFIXES

Give the definitions of the following prefixes:

1. end- _____   2. endo- _____

3. peri- _____   4. bin- _____

5. mon(o)- _____

ROOTS AND COMBINING FORMS

Give the definitions of the following roots and combining forms:

1. acoust _____   2. aud/i _____

3. audi/o _____   4. auditor _____

5. aur _____   6. chol/e _____

7. cochle/o _____   8. electr/o _____

9. labyrinth _____   10. labyrinth/o _____

11. laryng/o _____   12. log _____

13. mast _____   14. myc _____

15. myring _____   16. myring/o _____

17. neur/o _____   18. ot _____

19. ot/o _____   20. pharyng/e _____

21. phone _____   22. presby _____

23. py/o _____   24. rhin/o _____

25. scler _____   26. staped _____

27. steat _____   28. tinnit _____

29. tympan _____   30. aur/i _____

31. equ/i _____   32. libr/i _____

33. fenestrat _____   34. med _____

35. tympan/o _____

SUFFIXES

Give the definitions of the following suffixes:

1. -al _____   2. -algia _____

3. -cusis _____   4. -dynia _____

5. -ectomy _____   6. -gram _____

7. -graphy _____   8. -ic _____

9. -ist _____   10. -itis _____

11. -lith _____   12. -logy _____

13. -lymph _____   14. -meter _____

15. -metry _____   16. -oid _____

17. -oma _____   18. -osis _____

19. -plasty _____   20. -rrhea _____

21. -scope _____   22. -tome _____

23. -tomy _____   24. -us _____

25. -y _____   26. -cle _____

27. -um _____   28. -ion _____

29. -ia _____

Identifying Medical Terms

In the spaces provided, write the medical terms for the following meanings:

1. _____ One who specializes in disorders of hearing

2. _____ Measurement of the hearing sense

3. _____ Pertaining to the sense of hearing

4. _____ Pertaining to within the ear

5. _____ Inflammation of the labyrinth

6. _____ Surgical repair of the tympanic membrane

7. _____ An instrument used for cutting the eardrum

8. _____ Pain in the ear, earache

9. _____ The study of the ear and larynx

10. _____ Pertaining to the ear and pharynx

11. _____ An instrument used to examine the ear

12. _____ Serum fluid of the inner ear

13. _____ Surgical excision of the stapes of the ear

14. _____ Surgical excision of the tympanic membrane

15. _____ A ringing or jingling sound in the ear

Spelling

In the spaces provided, write the correct spelling of these misspelled words:

1. acostic _____   2. audilogy _____

3. cholestoma _____   4. electrochleography _____

5. labrinthitis _____   6. myringplasty _____

7. otomcosis _____   8. otosterosis _____

9. typanic _____   10. typanitis _____

Matching

Select the appropriate lettered meaning for each word listed below.

_____ 1. auricle

_____ 2. binaural

_____ 3. cerumen

_____ 4. equilibrium

_____ 5. fenestration

_____ 6. labyrinth

_____ 7. myringotomy

_____ 8. ossicle

_____ 9. tympanoplasty

_____10. vertigo

a. A state of balance
b. The inner ear
c. Small bone
d. Surgical repair of the tympanic membrane
e. Pertaining to both ears
f. A feeling of dizziness
g. Surgical operation in which a new opening is made in the labyrinth
h. The external portion of the ear
i. Earwax
j. Surgical incision of the tympanic membrane
k. Organ of hearing

Abbreviations

Place the correct word, phrase, or abbreviation in the space provided.

1. air conduction _____

2. right ear _____

3. AS _____

4. both ears _____

5. ENT _____

6. EENT _____

7. hearing distance _____

8. otology _____

9. SOM _____

10. usual childhood diseases _____

Diagnostic and Laboratory Tests

Select the best answer to each multiple choice question. Circle the letter of your choice.

1. The response to auditory stimuli that can be measured independent of the patient's subjective response.
   a. auditory evoked response
   b. electronystagmography
   c. falling test
   d. otoscopy

2. A recording of eye movement in response to specific stimuli.
   a. auditory evoked response
   b. electronystagmography
   c. falling test
   d. otoscopy

3. A test to observe the patient for marked swaying.
   a. auditory evoked response
   b. electronystagmography
   c. falling test
   d. past-pointing test

4. The visual examination of the external auditory canal and the tympanic membrane.
   a. tuning fork test
   b. tympanometry
   c. electronystagmography
   d. otoscopy

5. The measurement of the movement of the tympanic membrane.
   a. tuning fork tests
   b. tympanometry
   c. otoscopy
   d. past-pointing test

CASE STUDY

ACUTE OTITIS MEDIA

Read the following case study and then answer the questions that follow.

A 4-year-old female was seen by a physician and the following is a synopsis of the visit.

Present History: The mother states that her daughter has been complaining of an earache, ringing in the ears, and has been running a fever. She is irritable and doesn't want to eat.

Signs and Symptoms: Otodynia (otalgia), tinnitus, fever, irritability, and anorexia.

Diagnosis: Otitis media acute. The diagnosis was determined by a physical examination of the ear (otoscopy). A culture of the fluid taken from the ear showed the presence of bacteria—*Streptococcus pneumoniae.*

Treatment: The physician ordered an analgesic for pain (Tylenol) and an antibiotic (amoxicillin) for the infection.

Prevention: Since most middle ear infections are caused by an upper respiratory infection that has spread through the eustachian tube, URIs should be treated promptly.

CASE STUDY QUESTIONS

1. Signs and symptoms of otitis media include otodynia, _____ (ringing in the ears), fever, irritability, and anorexia.
2. The diagnosis was determined by a physical examination of the ear called an _____ and a culture of the fluid taken from the ear.
3. Tylenol is classified as an _____ and is given to relieve _____.
4. Amoxicillin is classified as an _____ and is given for the _____.
5. The medical word otodynia (otalgia) means _____.

MedMedia Wrap-Up

www.prenhall.com/rice

Additional interactive resources and activities for this chapter can be found on the Companion Website. For animations, videos, audio glossary, and review, access the accompanying CD-ROM in this book.

Audio Glossary
Medical Terminology Exercises & Activities
Pathology Spotlight
Terminology Translator
Animations
Videos

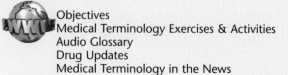

Objectives
Medical Terminology Exercises & Activities
Audio Glossary
Drug Updates
Medical Terminology in the News

SPECIAL SENSES: THE EYE

14

OUTLINE

On completion of this chapter, you will be able to:

- Describe the anatomical structures of the eye.
- Describe the external structures of the eye.
- Describe the internal structures of the eye.
- Analyze, build, spell, and pronounce medical words.
- Describe each of the conditions presented in the Pathology Spotlights.
- Complete the Pathology Checkpoint.
- Review Drug Highlights presented in this chapter.
- Provide the description of diagnostic and laboratory tests related to the eye.
- Identify and define selected abbreviations.
- Successfully complete the study and review section.

OBJECTIVES

MedMedia
www.prenhall.com/rice

Additional interactive resources and activities for this chapter can be found on the Companion Website. For Terminology Translator, animations, videos, audio glossary, and review, access the accompanying CD-ROM in this book.

Anatomy and Physiology Overview

|n this overview of the anatomy and physiology of the eye, a general description is offered as an aid to those learning the terminology associated with the functions of the eye.

The **eye** is composed of special anatomical structures that work together to facilitate sight. Light passes through the cornea, pupil, lens, and the vitreous body to stimulate sensory receptors (*rods and cones*) on the **retina** or innermost layer of the eye. **Vision** is made possible through the coordinated actions of nerves that control the movement of the eyeball, the amount of light admitted by the pupil, the focusing of that light on the retina by the lens, and the transmission of the resulting sensory impulses to the brain by the optic nerve.

EXTERNAL STRUCTURES

The orbit, the muscles of the eye, the eyelids, the conjunctiva, and the lacrimal apparatus make up the external structures of the eye.

The Orbit

The **orbit** is a cone-shaped cavity in the front of the skull that contains the *eyeball*. Formed by the combination of several bones, this cavity is lined with fatty tissue that cushions the eyeball and has several openings or **foramina** through which blood vessels and nerves pass. The largest of these is the optic foramen for the optic nerve and ophthalmic artery.

SPECIAL SENSES: THE EYE

Organ/Structure	Primary Functions
The Orbit	Contains the eyeball. Cavity is lined with fatty tissue that cushions the eyeball and has several openings through which blood vessels and nerves pass
The Muscles of the Eye	Six short muscles provide support and rotary movement of the eyeball
The Eyelids	Protect the eyeballs from intense light, foreign particles, and impact
The Conjunctiva	Acts as a protective covering for the exposed surface of the eyeball
The Lacrimal Apparatus	Produces, stores, and removes tears that cleanse and lubricate the eye
The Eyeball	Organ of vision
Sclera	The outer layer known as the "white" of the eye consists of the cornea, which bends light rays and helps to focus them on the surface of the retina
Choroid	Pigmented vascular membrane that prevents internal reflection of light
Ciliary body	Smooth muscle forming a part of the ciliary body that governs the convexity of the lens. The ciliary body secretes nutrient fluids that nourish the cornea, the lens, and surrounding tissues
Iris	Colored membrane attached to the ciliary body. It has a circular opening in its center, the pupil, and two muscles that contract to regulate the amount of light admitted by the pupil
Retina	Innermost layer. Contains photoreceptive cells that translate light waves focused on its surface into nerve impulses
The lens	Sharpens the focus of light on the retina (accommodation)

The Muscles of the Eye

Connecting the eyeball to the orbital cavity are *six short muscles* that provide it with support and rotary movement. Of the six, four are straight (*rectus*) muscles and two are slanted (*oblique*) muscles.

The Eyelids

Each eye has a pair of **eyelids** that protect the eyeball from intense light, foreign particles, and impact. Known as the *superior* and *inferior palpebrae*, those movable "curtains" join to form a **canthus** or angle at either corner of the eye. The slit between the eyelids is called the **palpebral fissure**, through which light reaches the inner eye. The edges of the eyelids contain *eyelashes* and *sebaceous glands*, which secrete an oily substance onto the eyelids.

The Conjunctiva

Lining the underside of each eyelid and reflected onto the anterior portion of the eyeball is a mucous membrane known as the **conjunctiva**. This membrane acts as a protective covering for the exposed surface of the eyeball.

The Lacrimal Apparatus

Included in the **lacrimal apparatus** are those structures that produce, store, and remove the tears that cleanse and lubricate the eye. These structures are the lacrimal gland, its ducts, the lacrimal canaliculi, the lacrimal sac, and the nasolacrimal duct, which empties into the nasal cavity (Fig. 14–1).

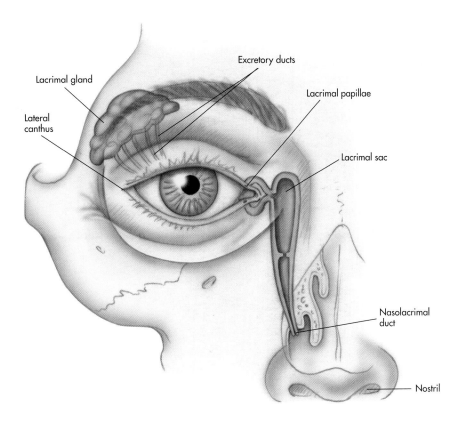

FIGURE 14–1

The lacrimal apparatus and its anatomic structures.

THE LACRIMAL GLAND

Located above the outer corner of the eye, the **lacrimal gland** secretes tears through approximately 12 ducts onto the surface of the conjunctiva of the upper lid. This fluid washes across the anterior surface of the eye and is collected by the *lacrimal canaliculi.*

THE LACRIMAL CANALICULI

The **lacrimal canaliculi** are the two ducts *(superior and inferior)* at the inner corner of the eye that collect tears and drain into the lacrimal sac.

THE LACRIMAL SAC

The enlargement of the upper portion of the lacrimal duct is known as the **lacrimal sac.** Tears secreted by the lacrimal glands are pulled into this sac and subsequently forced into the nasolacrimal duct by the blinking action of the eyelids. The sac is dilated and pulls in fluid as the muscles associated with blinking close the lids. The sac constricts, forcing the fluid down the nasolacrimal duct, as the lids are opened.

THE NASOLACRIMAL DUCT

The passageway draining lacrimal fluid into the nose is known as the **nasolacrimal duct.** The lacrimal sac is the enlarged upper portion of this duct.

INTERNAL STRUCTURES

The eyeball, its various structures, and the nerve fibers connecting it to the brain make up the internal eye (Fig. 14–2).

The Eyeball

The **eyeball** is the organ of vision. It is globe shaped and divided into two cavities. The space in front of the lens, called the **ocular cavity**, is further divided by the iris into **anterior** and **posterior chambers**, both filled with a watery fluid known as the **aqueous humor**. Behind the lens is a much larger cavity filled with a jelly-like material, the **vitreous humor**, which maintains the eyeball's spherical shape. The three layers forming the outer, middle, and inner surfaces of the eyeball are discussed, along with the lens and its functions.

THE OUTER LAYER

The eyeball's outer layer is composed of the **sclera** or white of the eye and the **cornea** or anterior transparent portion of the eye's fibrous outer surface. The curved surface of the cornea is important in that it bends light rays and helps to focus them on the surface of the retina.

THE MIDDLE LAYER

Known as the **uvea**, the middle layer of the eyeball, lying just below the sclera, consists of the **iris**, the **ciliary body**, and the **choroid** or pigmented vascular membrane that prevents internal reflection of light.

The Ciliary Body. The **ciliary body** is a thickened portion of the vascular membrane to which the iris is attached. Smooth muscle forming a part of the ciliary body governs the convexity of the lens. The ciliary body secretes nutrient fluids (the *aqueous humor*) that nourish the cornea, the lens, and the surrounding tissues.

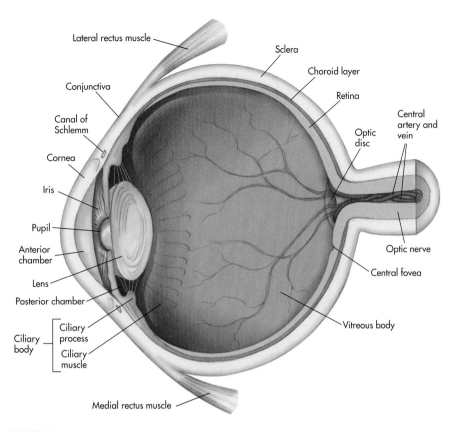

FIGURE 14-2

The eyeball and its anatomic structures.

The Iris.   The **iris** is a colored membrane attached to the ciliary body and suspended between the lens and the cornea in the aqueous humor. It has a circular opening in its center, the **pupil**, and two muscles that contract or dilate to regulate the amount of light admitted by the pupil.

THE INNER LAYER

The innermost layer, or **retina**, contains photoreceptive cells that translate light waves focused on its surface into nerve impulses. The photosensitive cells of the retina are the **rods** and **cones**. Most of the approximately 6 million cone cells are grouped into a small area called the **macula lutea**. In the center of the macula lutea is a small depression, the **fovea centralis**, containing only cone cells, which is the central focusing point within the eye. The eye contains approximately 120 million rods that are sensitive to dim light. They contain **rhodopsin**, a pigment necessary for night vision. The point at which nerve fibers from the retina converge to form the optic nerve is known as the **optic disk**. At this point, fibers of the optic nerve extend, through the optic chiasm, to the thalamus and on to the visual cortical areas of the brain. The absence of rods and cones in the area of the optic disk creates a blind spot in the visual field.

THE LENS

A colorless crystalline body, biconvex in shape and enclosed in a transparent capsule, the **lens** is suspended by ligaments just behind the iris. Contraction and relaxation of the ciliary muscle control the tension of the suspensory ligaments to change the shape of the lens. The function of the lens is to sharpen the focus of light on the retina. This process, called **accommodation**, is reflexive in nature and combines changes in the size of the pupil, the curvature of the lens, and the convergence of the optic axes to keep the image in the same place on both retinae. Accommodation occurs for both near and distant vision.

LIFE SPAN
CONSIDERATIONS

■ THE CHILD

The **eyes** begin to develop as an outgrowth of the fore-brain in the 4-week-old embryo. At 24 weeks the eyes are structurally complete. At 28 weeks eyebrows and eyelashes are present, and the eyelids open. The new-born can see, and **visual acuity** is estimated to be around 20/400. Most newborns appear cross-eyed because their eye muscles are not fully developed. At first, the eyes appear to be blue or gray. Permanent coloring becomes fixed between 6 and 12 months of age. Tears do not appear until approximately 1 to 3 months, because the lacrimal gland ducts are immature. Depth perception begins to develop around 9 months of age.

Visual acuity improves with age and by the age of 2 or 3 years, it is around 20/30 or 20/20. Children are farsighted until about 5 years of age.

Every minute that an infant is awake he or she is taking in the sights, sounds, smells, and feel of the surrounding world. For the 1- to 3-month-old, the human face is a favorite sight. By the second month, the baby's eye coordination has improved enough to follow something moving from one side of his or her face to the other. By the end of 3 months, brightly colored wall hangings or toys are favored.

■ THE OLDER ADULT

Sensory decline alters one's perception of the world. Smells become harder to distinguish and detect. Eyes may need corrective lenses to adjust for decreasing ability to focus. As the ciliary muscles weaken, pupil size is decreased, reducing light to the retina. The lens become stiff, thicker, and more opaque and begin to yellow. These changes make the older adult sensitive to glare, and the ability to focus is impaired; therefore, farsightedness, **presbyopia**, is common in the older adult. Night vision is impaired and driving at night is often very difficult for the older adult. The lens eventually may become opaque as **cataracts** develop. Vascular degeneration may affect the **retina**, which contains nerve cells for receiving images, and this condition causes permanent visual loss.

The leading cause of new cases of blindness in the older adult is age-related **macular degeneration**, a disease that affects the macula, the part of the eye that is responsible for sharp central vision. For the first time, researchers have linked gene defects to macular degeneration. The discovery may lead to identification of people at high risk for the disorder and perhaps ways to treat or prevent vision loss.

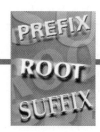

BUILDING YOUR MEDICAL VOCABULARY

This section provides the foundation for learning medical terminology. Medical words can be made up of four different types of word parts:

- Prefixes (P)
- Roots (R)
- Combining forms (CF)
- Suffixes (S)

By connecting various word parts in an organized sequence, thousands of words can be built and learned. In this text the word list is alphabetized so one can see the variety of meanings created when common prefixes and suffixes are repeatedly applied to certain word roots and/or combining forms. Words shown in pink are additional words related to the content of this chapter that are not built from word parts. These words are included to enhance your vocabulary. Note: an asterisk icon (✱) indicates words that are covered in the pathology spotlights section in this chapter.

MEDICAL WORD	WORD PARTS (WHEN APPLICABLE)			DEFINITION
	Part	**Type**	**Meaning**	
accommodation (ă-kŏm″ ō-dā′ shn)				The process whereby the eyes make adjustments for seeing objects at various distances
amblyopia (ăm″ blĭ-ō′ pĭ-ă)	ambly -opia	R S	dull vision	Dullness of vision
anisocoria (ăn-ĭ″ sō-kŏ′ rĭă)	anis/o cor -ia	CF R S	unequal pupil condition	A condition in which the pupils are unequal
aphakia (ă-fā′ kĭ-ă)	a phak -ia	P R S	lack of, without lentil, lens condition	A condition in which the crystalline lens is absent
astigmatism (ă-stĭg′ mă-tĭzm)	a stigmat -ism	P R S	lack of, without point condition of	A defect in the refractive powers of the eye in which a ray of light is not focused on the retina but is spread over an area
bifocal (bī-fō′ kăl)	bi foc -al	P R S	two focus pertaining to	Pertaining to having two foci, as in bifocal glasses
blepharitis (blĕf″ ăr-ī′ tĭs)	blephar -itis	R S	eyelid inflammation	Inflammation of the edges of the eyelids
blepharoptosis (blĕf″ ă-rō-tō′ sĭs)	blephar/o -ptosis	CF S	eyelid prolapse, drooping	A drooping of the upper eyelid(s)
cataract (kăt″ ə răkt′)				An opacity of the crystalline lens or its capsule; most often occurs in adults past middle age. ✱ See Pathology Spotlight: Cataract.
chalazion (kă-lā′ zĭ-ŏn)				A small, hard, painless cyst of a meibomian gland (one of the sebaceous follicles of the eyelids)
choroiditis (kō″ royd-ī′ tĭs)	choroid -itis	R S	choroid inflammation	Inflammation of the vascular coat of the eye
conjunctivitis (kŏn-jŭnk″ tĭ-vī′ tĭs)	conjunctiv -itis	R S	to join together inflammation	Inflammation of the conjunctiva caused by allergy, trauma, chemical injury, bacterial, viral, or rickettsial infection. The type called "pinkeye" is infectious and contagious. ✱ See Pathology Spotlight: Conjunctivitis.
corneal (kŏr′ nēə l)	corne -al	R S	cornea pertaining to	Pertaining to the cornea

MEDICAL WORD	WORD PARTS (WHEN APPLICABLE)			DEFINITION
	Part	**Type**	**Meaning**	
corneal transplant (kŏr′ nē-ăl trăns′ plănt)				The surgical process of transferring the cornea from a donor to a patient
cryosurgery (krī″ ō-sur′ jur-ē)	cry/o surgery	CF	cold surgery	A type of surgery that uses extreme cold for destruction of tissue or for production of well-demarcated areas of cell injury; may be used in the removal of cataracts and in the repair of retinal detachment
cycloplegia (sī″ klō-plē′ jĭ-ă)	cycl/o -plegia	CF S	ciliary body stroke, paralysis	Paralysis of the ciliary muscle
dacryoma (dăk″ rī-ō′ mă)	dacry -oma	R S	tear tumor	A tumor-like swelling caused by obstruction of the tear duct(s)
diplopia (dĭp-lō′ pĭ-ă)	dipl -opia	P S	double eye, vision	Double vision
electroretinogram (ē-lĕk″ trō-rĕt′ ĭ-nō-grăm)	electr/o retin/o -gram	CF CF S	electricity retina mark, record	A record of the electrical response of the retina to light stimulation
emmetropia (ĕm″ ĕ-trō′ pĭ-ă)	em metr -opia	P R S	in measure eye, vision	Normal or perfect vision. See Figure 14–3.
entropion (ĕn-trō-pē-ŏn)	en trop -ion	P R S	in turn process	The turning inward of the margin of the lower eyelid
enucleation (ē-nū″ klē-ā′ shŭn)	enucleat -ion	R S	to remove the kernel of process	A process of removing an entire part or mass without rupture, as the eyeball from its orbit
esotropia (ĕs″ ō-trō′ pĭ-ă)	eso trop -ia	P R S	inward turn condition	A condition in which the eye or eyes turn inward; *crossed eyes*
exotropia (ĕks″ ō-trō′ pē-ă)	ex (o) trop -ia	P R S	out turn condition of	The turning outward of one or both eyes
glaucoma (glaw-kō′ mă)				A disease characterized by increased intraocular pressure, which results in atrophy of the optic nerve and blindness. ✱ See Pathology Spotlight: Glaucoma.
gonioscope (gō′ nĭ-ō-skōp)	goni/o -scope	CF S	angle instrument	An instrument used to examine the angle of the anterior chamber of the eye

MEDICAL WORD	WORD PARTS (WHEN APPLICABLE)			DEFINITION
	Part	**Type**	**Meaning**	
hemianopia (hĕm″ ē-ă-nŏ′ pē-ă)	hemi an -opia	P P S	half lack of eye, vision	The inability (blindness) to see half the field of vision
hyperopia (hī″ pĕr-ō′ pĭ-ă)	hyper -opia	P S	beyond eye, vision	A defect in vision in which parallel rays come to a focus beyond the retina; *farsightedness.* See Figure 14–3.
intraocular (ĭn″ trăh-ŏk′ ū-lăr)	intra ocul -ar	P R S	within eye pertaining to	Pertaining to within the eye
iridectomy (ĭr″ ĭ-dĕk′ tō-mē)	irid -ectomy	R S	iris excision	Surgical excision of a portion of the iris
iridocyclitis (ĭr″ ĭd-ō-sī-klī′ tĭs)	irid/o cycl -itis	CF R S	iris ciliary body inflammation	Inflammation of the iris and ciliary body
keratitis (kĕr″ ă-tī′ tĭs)	kerat -itis	R S	cornea inflammation	Inflammation of the cornea
keratoconjunctivitis (kĕr″ ă-tō-kŏn-jŭnk″ tĭ-vī′ tĭs)	kerat/o conjunctiv -itis	CF R S	cornea to join together inflammation	Inflammation of the cornea and the conjunctiva
keratoplasty (kĕr′ ă-tō-plăs″ tē)	kerat/o -plasty	CF S	cornea surgical repair	Surgical repair of the cornea
lacrimal (lăk′ rĭm-ăl)	lacrim -al	R S	tear pertaining to	Pertaining to tears
laser (lā′ zĕr)				An acronym for **l**ight **a**mplification by **s**timulated **e**mission of **r**adiation. ✱ See Pathology Spotlight: Glaucoma for information about various types of laser eye surgery.
macular degeneration (măk′ ū-lăr dē′ gĕn-ēr″ ă-shŭn)				Degeneration of the macular area of the retina, an area important in the visualization of fine details. ✱ See Pathology Spotlight: Macular Degeneration.
microlens (mī′ krō-lĕns)				A small, thin corneal contact lens
miotic (mĭ-ŏt′ ĭk)	mi/o -tic	CF S	less, small pertaining to	Pertaining to an agent that causes the pupil to contract
mydriatic (mĭd″ rĭ-ăt′ ĭk)	mydriat -ic	R S	dilation, widen pertaining to	Pertaining to an agent that causes the pupil to dilate

MEDICAL WORD	WORD PARTS (WHEN APPLICABLE)			DEFINITION
	Part	**Type**	**Meaning**	
myopia (mī-ŏ' pĭ-ă)	my -opia	R S	to shut eye, vision	A defect in vision in which parallel rays come to a focus in front of the retina; *nearsightedness*. See Figure 14–3.
nyctalopia (nĭk" tă-lō' pĭ-ă)	nyctal -opia	R S	blind eye, vision	A condition in which the individual has difficulty seeing at night; night blindness
nystagmus (nĭs-tăg' mŭs)	nystagm -us	R S	to nod pertaining to	An involuntary, constant, rhythmic movement of the eyeball
ocular (ŏk' ū-lar)	ocul -ar	R S	eye pertaining to	Pertaining to the eye
ophthalmologist (ŏf" thăl-mŏl' ō-jĭst)	ophthalm/o log -ist	CF R S	eye study of one who specializes	One who specializes in the study of the eye
ophthalmology (ŏf" thăl-mŏl' ō-jē)	ophthalm/o -logy	CF S	eye study of	The study of the eye
ophthalmoscope (ŏf" thăl' mō-skōp)	ophthalm/o -scope	CF S	eye instrument	An instrument used to examine the interior of the eye
optic (op' tĭk)	opt -ic	R S	eye pertaining to	Pertaining to the eye
optician (ŏp-tĭsh' ăn)				One who specializes in the making of optical products and accessories. This person is not a physician.
optometrist (ŏp-tŏm' ě-trĭst)	opt/o metr -ist	CF R S	eye measure one who specializes	One who specializes in examining the eyes for refractive errors and providing appropriate corrective lenses. This person is not a physician but is trained and licensed as a Doctor of Optometry (OD).
optomyometer (ŏp" tō-mī-ŏm' ět-ěr)	opt/o my/o -meter	CF CF S	eye muscle instrument to measure	An instrument used to measure the strength of the muscles of the eye
orthoptics (or-thŏp' tĭks)	orth opt -ic (s)	R R S	straight eye pertaining to	The study and treatment of defective binocular vision resulting from defects in ocular musculature; also a technique of eye exercises for correcting defective binocular vision

MEDICAL WORD	WORD PARTS (WHEN APPLICABLE)			DEFINITION
	Part	**Type**	**Meaning**	
phacoemulsification (făk″ ō-ē′ mŭl′ sĭ-fĭ-kā″ shŭn)	phac/o emulsificat -ion	CF R S	lens disintegrate process	The process of using ultrasound to disintegrate a cataract. A needle is inserted through a small incision, and the disintegrated cataract is aspirated.
phacolysis (făk-ŏl″ ĭ-sĭs)	phac/o -lysis	CF S	lens destruction, to separate	Surgical destruction and removal of the crystalline lens in the treatment of cataract
phacosclerosis (făk″ ō-sklĕr-ō′ sĭs)	phac/o scler -osis	CF R S	lens hardening condition of	A condition of hardening of the crystalline lens
photocoagulation (fō″ tō-kō-ăg″ ū-lā′ shŭn)	phot/o coagulat -ion	CF R S	light to clot process	The process of altering proteins in tissue by the use of light energy such as the laser beam; used in the treatment of retinal detachment, retinal bleeding, intraocular tumors, and/or macular degeneration (wet)
photophobia (fō″ tō-fō′ bĭ-ă)	phot/o -phobia	CF S	light fear	Unusual intolerance of light
presbyopia (prĕz″ bĭ-ō′ pĭ-ă)	presby -opia	R S	old eye, vision	A defect in vision in which parallel rays come to a focus beyond the retina; occurs normally with aging; *farsightedness*
pupillary (pū′ pĭ-lĕr-ē)	pupill -ary	R S	pupil pertaining to	Pertaining to the pupil
radial keratotomy (rā′ dē-ăl kĕr-ă′ tŏt′ ō-mē)	rad/i -al kerat/o -tomy	CF S CF S	radiating out from a center pertaining to cornea incision	A surgical procedure that may be performed to correct nearsightedness *(myopia)*. Delicate spoke-like incisions are made in the cornea to flatten it, thereby shortening the eyeball so that light reaches the retina. Not all patients have their vision improved, and complications could lead to blindness.
retinal (rĕt′ ĭ-năl)	retin -al	R S	retina pertaining to	Pertaining to the retina
retinitis (rĕt″ ĭ-nī′ tĭs)	retin -itis	R S	retina inflammation	Inflammation of the retina
retinoblastoma (rĕt″ ĭ-nō-blăs-tō′ mă)	retin/o -blast -oma	CF S S	retina germ cell tumor	A malignant tumor arising from the germ cell of the retina

MEDICAL WORD	WORD PARTS (WHEN APPLICABLE)			DEFINITION
	Part	Type	Meaning	
retinopathy (rĕt″ ĭn-ŏp′ ă-thē)	retin/o -pathy	CF S	retina disease	Any disease of the retina
retrolental fibroplasia (RLF) (rĕt″ rō-lĕn-tăl fĭ-brō-plā-sē-ă)	retro lent -al fibr/o -plasia	P R S CF S	behind lens pertaining to fiber formation	A disease of the retinal vessels present in premature infants; may be caused by excessive use of oxygen in the incubator. Retinal detachment and blindness may occur.
scleritis (sklē-rī′ tĭs)	scler -itis	R S	sclera inflammation	Inflammation of the sclera
Snellen chart (snĕl′ ĕn chart)				A chart for testing visual acuity. It is printed with lines of black letters that are graduated in size from smallest, on the bottom to largest on the top (Fig. 14–4).
strabismus (stră-bĭz′ mŭs)	strabism -um	R S	a squinting tissue	A disorder of the eye in which the optic axes cannot be directed to the same object; *also called a squint*
sty(e) (stī)				Inflammation of one or more of the sebaceous glands of the eyelid; *also called a hordeolum*
tonography (tō-nŏg′ ră-fē)	ton/o -graphy	CF S	tone recording	Recording of intraocular pressure used in detecting glaucoma
tonometer (tŏn-ŏm′ ĕ-tĕr)	ton/o -meter	CF S	tone instrument to measure	An instrument used to measure intraocular pressure
trichiasis (trĭk-ī′ ăs-ĭs)	trich -iasis	R S	hair condition	A condition of ingrowing eyelids that rub against the cornea, causing a constant irritation to the eyeball
trifocal (trĭ-fō′ căl)	tri foc -al	P R S	three focus pertaining to	Pertaining to having three foci
uveal (ū′ vē-ăl)	uve -al	R S	uvea pertaining to	Pertaining to the second or vascular coat of the eye
uveitis (ū-vē-ī′ tĭs)	uve -itis	R S	uvea inflammation	Inflammation of the uvea

MEDICAL WORD	WORD PARTS (WHEN APPLICABLE)			DEFINITION
	Part	**Type**	**Meaning**	
xenophthalmia (zĕn″ ŏf-thăl′ mē-ă)	xen	R	foreign material	Inflamed eye condition caused by foreign material
	ophthalm	R	eye	
	-ia	S	condition	
xerophthalmia (zē-rŏf-thăl′ mē-ă)	xer	R	dry	An eye condition in which there is dryness of the conjunctiva
	ophthalm	R	eye	
	-ia	S	condition	

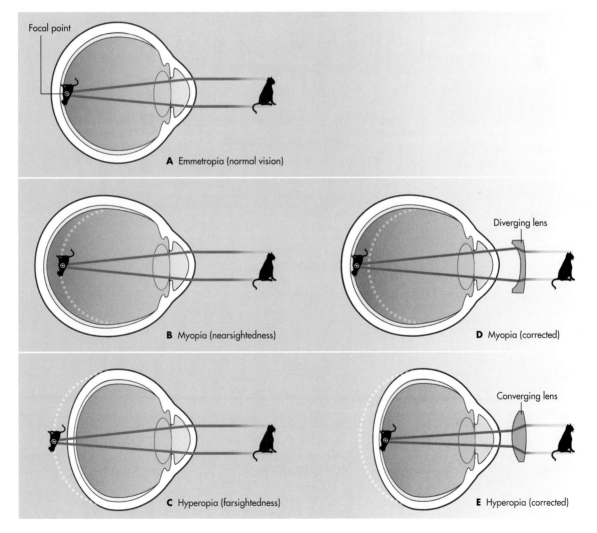

FIGURE 14–3

Visual abnormalities. (A) In normal vision, the lens focuses the visual image on the retina. Common problems with the accommodation mechanism involve (B) myopia, an inability to lengthen the focal distance enough to focus the image of a distant object on the retina, and (C) hyperopia, an inability to shorten the focal distance adequately for nearby objects. These conditions can be corrected by placing appropriately shaped lenses in front of the eyes. (D) A diverging lens is used to correct myopia, and (E) a converging lens is used to correct hyperopia.

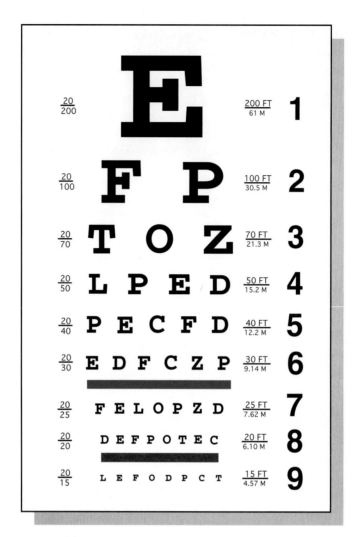

FIGURE 14–4

The Snellen eye chart. Individuals with normal vision can read line 8 of a full-sized chart at 20 feet (6.10 m).

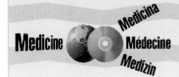

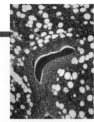

PATHOLOGY SPOTLIGHTS

Cataract

A **cataract** is a clouding of the eye's lens that can cause vision problems. In a normal eye, light passes through the lens and gets focused on the retina. To help produce a sharp image, the lens must remain clear. The lens is made mostly of water and protein. The protein is arranged to let light pass through and focus on the retina. Sometimes some of the protein clumps together. This can start to cloud small areas of the lens, blocking some light from reaching the retina and interfering with vision. This is a cataract.

In its early stages, a cataract may not cause a problem. The cloudiness may affect only a small part of the lens. However, over time, the cataract may grow larger and cloud more of the lens, making it harder to see. Because less light reaches the retina, the patient's vision may become dull and blurry. A cataract won't spread from one eye to the other, although many people develop cataracts in both eyes.

Following are the different types of cataracts:

- Age-related cataract: Most cataracts are related to aging. More than half of all Americans age 65 and older have a cataract.
- Congenital cataract: Some babies are born with cataracts or develop them in childhood, often in both eyes. These cataracts may not affect vision. If they do, they may need to be removed.
- Secondary cataract: Cataracts are more likely to develop in people who have certain other health problems, such as diabetes. Also, cataracts are sometimes linked to steroid use.
- Traumatic cataract: Cataracts can develop soon after an eye injury, or years later.

Although researchers are learning more about cataracts, no one knows for sure what causes them. Scientists think there may be several causes, including smoking, diabetes, and excessive exposure to sunlight.

The most common symptoms of a cataract are:

- Cloudy or blurry vision
- Problems with light. These can include headlights that seem too bright at night; glare from lamps or very bright sunlight; or a halo around lights
- Colors that seem faded
- Poor night vision
- Double or multiple vision (this symptom often goes away as the cataract grows)
- Frequent changes in eyeglass or contact lens prescription. When a cataract is small, the patient may not notice any changes in their vision. Cataracts tend to grow slowly, so vision gets worse gradually. Some people with a cataract find that their close-up vision suddenly improves, but this is temporary. Vision is likely to get worse again as the cataract grows.

For an early cataract, vision may improve by using different eyeglasses, magnifying lenses, or stronger lighting. If these measures don't help, surgery is the only effective treatment. The most common surgery to remove a cataract is **phacoemulsification**, or phaco. The physician makes a small incision on the side of the cornea, the clear, dome-shaped surface that covers the front of the eye. The doctor then inserts a tiny probe into the eye. This device emits ultrasound waves that soften and break up the cloudy center of the lens so it can be removed by suction. Most cataract surgery today is done by phaco, which is also called small incision cataract surgery.

Cataract removal is one of the most common operations performed in the United States today. It is also one of the safest and most effective. In about 90 percent of cases, people who have cataract surgery have better vision afterward.

Conjunctivitis

Conjunctivitis, often called "pink eye," is an inflammation of the conjunctiva, the tissue that lines the inside of the eyelid. This tissue helps keep the eyelid and eyeball moist. Conjunctivitis is one of the most common and treatable eye infections in children and adults.

Conjunctivitis can be caused by a virus, bacteria, irritating substances (shampoos, dirt, smoke and especially pool chlorine), allergens (substances that cause allergies) or sexually transmitted diseases (STDs). Types of pink eye caused by bacteria, viruses and STDs can spread easily from person to person, but are not a serious health risks if diagnosed promptly.

Following are the symptoms of conjunctivitis:

- Redness in the white of the eye or inner eyelid
- Increased amount of tears
- Thick yellow discharge that crusts over the eyelashes, especially after sleep (with conjunctivitis caused by bacteria)
- Other discharge from your eye (green or white)
- Itchy eyes (especially with conjunctivitis caused by allergies)
- Burning eyes (especially with conjunctivitis caused by chemicals and irritants)
- Blurred vision
- Increased sensitivity to light

An ophthalmologist or family physician will diagnose conjunctivitis by conducting an eye exam and may take a sample of fluid from the eyelid using a cotton swab. Bacteria or viruses that may have caused conjunctivitis, including STDs, can then be seen through a microscope.

Treatment is based on the cause. For example, antibiotic eye drops or ointments are used for conjunctivitis caused by a bacterial infection. If topical antibiotics do not solve the problem, then oral antibiotics are used. Eye drops containing antihistamines, nonsteroidal anti-inflammatory agents, or corticosteroids are used if allergies are the cause. Or, if foreign matter has caused the inflammation, this is removed.

Glaucoma

Glaucoma is a group of eye diseases characterized by increased intraocular pressure (IOP). The three major categories of glaucoma are: closed-angle (acute) glaucoma; open-angle (chronic) glaucoma; and congenital glaucoma. See Figure 14–5. Glaucoma occurs when the intraocular fluid accumulates in the anterior chamber of the eye and drains too slowly from the aqueous humor. This causes a buildup of intraocular pressure that is too high for the proper functioning of the optic nerve. When glaucoma is diagnosed early and managed properly, blindness may be prevented.

Approximately 80,000 people are totally blind from glaucoma, with approximately 250,000 people being blind in one eye and approximately 1.2 million more with some degree of visual loss from glaucoma. About 2 percent of the population aged 40 to 50 and 8 percent over age 70 have elevated intraocular pressure. Some 20 million people in the United States are susceptible to developing glaucoma. Glaucoma affects people of all ages and all races. Most patients have no symptoms from glaucoma; therefore, it is important to know the factors that predispose someone to glaucoma.

The predisposing factors for developing glaucoma include:

- Over 60 years of age
- African ancestry
- Someone in family has glaucoma or diabetes
- Previous eye injury
- Taking steroid medication

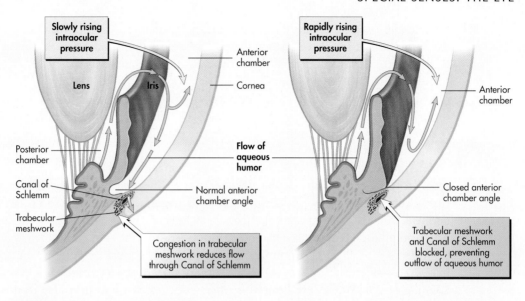

FIGURE 14–5

Forms of primary adult glaucoma: (A) In open-angle (chronic) glaucoma, the anterior chamber angle remains open, but drainage of aqueous humor through the canal of Schlemm is impaired; (B) in closed-angle (acute) glaucoma, the angle of the iris and anterior chamber narrows, obstructing the outflow of aqueous humor.

- Myopia
- Thyroid disease
- Diabetes
- Hypertension

Some examples of laser surgery that may be used in the treatment of glaucoma are:

1. Laser peripheral iridotomy (LPI), where a small hole is made in the iris that allows it to fall back from the fluid channel and helps the fluid drain

2. Argon laser trabeculoplasty (ALT), where the laser beam opens the fluid channels of the eye, helping the drainage system to work better

3. Selective laser trabeculoplasty (SLT), a type of laser surgery that uses a combination of frequencies allowing the laser to work at very low levels. It treats specific cells "selectively" and leaves untreated portions of the trabecular meshwork (the mesh-like drainage canals surrounding the iris) intact.

4. When medication and/or laser surgery does not lower the intraocular pressure of the eye, the doctor may recommend a procedure called **filtering microsurgery**. In this procedure, a tiny drainage hole is made in the sclera (sclerostomy). The new drainage hole allows fluid to flow out of the eye and thereby helps lower eye pressure. This prevents or reduces damage to the optic nerve.

Macular Degeneration

Macular degeneration is an incurable eye disease that affects more than 10 million Americans. It is the leading cause of blindness for those age 55 and older.

Macular degeneration is caused by the deterioration of the central portion of the retina, the inside back layer of the eye that records the images one sees and sends them via the optic nerve from the eye to the brain. The retina's central portion, known as the macula, is responsible for focusing central vision in the eye, and it controls the ability to read, drive a car, recognize faces or colors, and see objects in fine detail.

There are two basic types of macular degeneration: dry and wet. Approximately 85 percent to 90 percent of the cases of macular degeneration are the dry (atrophic) type.

In the dry type of macular degeneration, the deterioration of the retina is associated with the formation of small yellow deposits, known as drusen, under the macula. This phenomena leads to a thinning and drying out of the macula. The amount of central vision loss is directly related to the location and amount of retinal thinning caused by the drusen. This form of macular degeneration is much more common than the wet type of macular degeneration and it tends to progress more slowly than the wet type. However, a certain percentage of the dry type of macular degeneration turns to wet with the passage of time. There is no known treatment or cure for the dry type of macular degeneration.

Approximately 10 percent of the cases of macular degeneration are the wet (exudative) type. In the wet type of macular degeneration, abnormal blood vessels (known as subretinal neovascularization) grow under the retina and macula. These new blood vessels may then bleed and leak fluid, thereby causing the macula to bulge or lift up, thus distorting or destroying central vision. Under these circumstances, vision loss may be rapid and severe.

If vision is to be saved, immediate laser surgery should be done in the early stages of wet macular degeneration. However, laser surgery does not guarantee that vision will be saved. Existing laser therapies are limited in their effectiveness and may also lead to scarring of the macula and additional vision loss. The FDA has approved photodynamic laser therapy, which uses a light-activated drug called Visudyne. This treatment for wet macular degeneration works by sealing off leaking vessels while leaving healthy ones intact; thus it is a major improvement over previous laser treatments. Unfortunately, even the most successful treatments do not preclude reoccurrence, but various procedures can slow the rate of vision loss and hopefully preserve some sight.

Macular degeneration usually develops gradually and painlessly. The signs and symptoms of the disease may vary, depending on which of the two types of macular degeneration one has. With dry macular degeneration one may notice the following symptoms:

- The need for increasingly bright illumination when reading or doing close work
- Printed words that appear increasingly blurry
- Colors that seem washed out and dull
- Gradual increase in the haziness of overall vision
- A blind spot in the center of the visual field combined with a profound drop in central vision

With wet macular degeneration, the following symptoms may appear rapidly:

- Visual distortions, such as straight lines appearing wavy or crooked—a doorway or street sign that seems out of whack
- Decreased central vision
- Central blurry spot

In either form of macular degeneration, vision may falter in one eye while the other remains fine for years. One may not notice any or much change because the good eye compensates for the weak one. Vision and lifestyle begin to be dramatically affected when this condition develops in both eyes.

Stargardt's disease, also known as juvenile macular degeneration, contradicts the common belief that macular degeneration only happens to older people. It was discovered in 1997 that this disease has a strong genetic component. In September of that year, researchers announced that one in six people with age-related macular degeneration also have mutations of the gene that causes juvenile macular degeneration, although in different parts of the gene.

This inherited disease affects one in 10,000 people and usually manifests itself between the ages of 7 and 12. Scientists' current theory is that Stargardt's disease causes the eye's central vision to deteriorate because the rod cells just outside the macula erode and this eventually harms the retinal pigment epithelium (RPE). As the RPE fails, the disease may spread to the macula's cone cells, causing macular degeneration's characteristic loss of central vision. Peripheral vision generally remains.

Presently there is no cure for Stargardt's disease, nor is there any treatment that is proven to improve visual loss or to retard the progression of the disease. The degeneration process begins early, usually around the age of seven. Due to the young age of the patients, the disease can be hard to diagnose. The effect of the disease is loss of the central vision that is responsible for visual acuity and color perception. Vision loss is usually slow until the 20/40 level, then rapidly progresses to the 20/200 level. Unfortunately, in some cases, vision can degenerate to 10/200 in a period of months.

Historically, macular degeneration was thought to be a single disease that caused central vision loss in older people. This misconception is changing. Macular degeneration is a group of diseases that have one feature in common—a loss of central vision—which may affect people of any age.

✔ PATHOLOGY CHECKPOINT

Following is a concise list of the pathology-related terms that you've seen in the chapter. Review this checklist to make sure that you are familiar with the meaning of each term before moving on to the next section.

Conditions and Symptoms

- ❏ amblyopia
- ❏ anisocoria
- ❏ aphakia
- ❏ astigmatism
- ❏ blepharitis
- ❏ blepharoptosis
- ❏ cataract
- ❏ chalazion
- ❏ choroiditis
- ❏ conjunctivitis
- ❏ cycloplegia
- ❏ dacryoma
- ❏ diplopia
- ❏ entropion
- ❏ esotropia
- ❏ exotropia
- ❏ glaucoma
- ❏ hemianopia
- ❏ hyperopia
- ❏ iridocyclitis
- ❏ keratitis

- ❏ keratoconjunctivitis
- ❏ macular degeneration
- ❏ myopia
- ❏ nyctalopia
- ❏ nystagmus
- ❏ phacosclerosis
- ❏ photophobia
- ❏ presbyopia
- ❏ retinitis
- ❏ retinoblastoma
- ❏ retinopathy
- ❏ retrolental fibroplasia (RLF)
- ❏ scleritis
- ❏ strabismus
- ❏ sty(e)
- ❏ trichiasis
- ❏ uveitis
- ❏ xenophthalmia
- ❏ xerophthalmia

Diagnosis and Treatment

- ❏ bifocal
- ❏ corneal transplant

- ❏ cryosurgery
- ❏ electroretinogram
- ❏ enucleation
- ❏ gonioscope
- ❏ iridectomy
- ❏ keratoplasty
- ❏ laser
- ❏ microlens
- ❏ miotic
- ❏ mydriatic
- ❏ ophthalmoscope
- ❏ optomyometer
- ❏ orthoptics
- ❏ phacoemulsification
- ❏ phacolysis
- ❏ photocoagulation
- ❏ radial keratotomy
- ❏ Snellen chart
- ❏ tonography
- ❏ tonometer
- ❏ trifocal

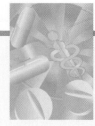

DRUG HIGHLIGHTS

DRUG HIGHLIGHTS

Drugs that are generally used for the eye include those that are used for glaucoma, during diagnostic examination of the eye, and in intraocular surgery. Antibiotics, antifungal, and antiviral drugs are used in the treatment of eye infections.

Drugs Used to Treat Glaucoma

Either increase the outflow of aqueous humor, decrease its production, or produce both of these actions.

Prostaglandin analogues

Work by increasing the drainage of intraocular fluid, thereby decreasing intraocular pressure.

Examples: Travatan (travoprost ophthalmic solution 0.004%), Lumigan (bimatoprost ophthalmic solution 0.03%), and Xalatan (latanoprost).

Adrenergic drugs

Increase drainage of intraocular fluid.

Examples: Epifin sterile ophthalmic solution and Propine ophthalmic solution, USP, 0.1% (epinephrine), and Dipivefin ophthalmic solution USP, 0.1%.

Alpha antagonist

Works to both decrease production of fluid and increase drainage.

Example: Alphagan (brimonide tartrate ophthalmic solution 0.2%).

Beta blockers

Decrease production of intraocular fluid.

Examples: Akbeta (levobunolol HCl ophthalmic solution, USP), Carteleolo HCl (carteolo HCl ophthalmic solution), Timolol Maleate, Betoptic S (betaxolol HCl 0.25%), Betaxon (levobetaxolo ophthalmic suspension 0.5%), Betagan Liquifilm Sterile Ophthalmic Solution (levobunolol), OptiPranolol (metipranolol), Timoptic-XE (timolol maleate ophthalmic gel forming solution), Betimol (timolol hemihydrate), and Ocupress (carteolol HCl).

Carbonic anhydrase inhibitors

Decrease production of intraocular fluid.

Examples: Azopt (brinzolamide ophthalmic suspension 1%), Diamox Sequels Sustained Release Capsules (acetazolomide), Trusopt (dorzolamide), and Neptazane (methazolamide).

Cholinergic (miotic)

Increases drainage of intraocular fluid.

Examples: Ocusert Pilo-20 and Pilo-40 Ocular Therapeutic Systems (pilocarpine), and Pilocarpine HCl Ophthalmic Solution.

Cholinesterase

Increases drainage of intraocular fluid.

Example: Phospholine Iodide (echothiophate).

Combination of beta blocker and carbonic anhydrase inhibitor

Decreases production of intraocular fluid.

Example: Cosopt (dorzolomide HCl timolol maleate ophthalmic solution).

Mydriatics

Agents that are used to produce dilation of the pupil (mydriasis) may be anticholinergics or sympathomimetics.

Anticholinergics

Produce dilation of the pupil and interfere with the ability of the eye to focus properly (cycloplegia). They are used primarily as an aid in refraction, during internal examination of the eye, in intraocular surgery, and in the treatment of anterior uveitis and secondary glaucomas.

Examples: Atropisol (atropine sulfate), Hyoscine (scopolamine HBr), Mydriacyl (tropicamide).

Sympathomimetics

Produced mydriasis without cycloplegia. Pupil dilation is obtained as the drug causes contraction of the dilator muscle of the iris. They also affect intraocular pressure by decreasing production of aqueous humor while increasing its outflow from the eye.

Examples: Propine (dipivefrin HCl), Naphcon (naphazoline HCl), Glaucon (epinephrine HCl), and neo-synephrine (phenylephrine HCl).

Antibiotics

Used to treat infectious diseases. Those that are used for the eye may be in the form of an ointment, cream, or solution.

Examples: Aureomycin Ophthalmic (chlortetracycline HCl) ointment 1%, erythromycin, bacitracin, tetracycline HCl, chloramphenicol, and polymyxin B sulfate.

Antifungal Agent

Natacyn (natamycin) is used in treating fungal infections of the eye, such as blepharitis, conjunctivitis, and keratitis.

Antiviral Agents

Stoxil, Herplex (idoxuridine) are potent antiviral agents used in the treatment of keratitis caused by the herpes simplex virus. *Vira-A (vidarabine)* and *Viroptic (trifluridine)* are also used to treat viral infections of the eye and are effective in the treatment of herpes simplex infections.

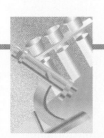

DIAGNOSTIC & LAB TESTS

TEST	DESCRIPTION
color vision tests (kul′ or vĭzh′ ŭn test)	The use of polychromatic plates or an anomaloscope to assess the ability to recognize differences in color.
exophthalmometry (ĕk″ sŏf-thăl-mŏm′ ĕ-trē)	Measurement of the forward protrusion of the eye via an exophthalmometer; used to evaluate an increase or decrease in exophthalmos.
gonioscopy (gō″ nē-ŏs′ kō-pē)	Examination of the anterior chamber of the eye via a gonioscope; used for determining ocular motility and rotation.
keratometry (kĕr″ ă-tŏm′ ĕ-trē)	Measurement of the cornea via a keratometer.
ocular ultrasonography (ŏk′ ū lăr ŭl-tră-sŏn-ŏg ră-fē)	The use of high-frequency sound waves (via a small probe placed on the eye) to measure for intraocular lenses and to detect orbital and periorbital lesions; also used to measure the length of the eye and the curvature of the cornea in preparation for surgery.
ophthalmoscopy (ŏf-thăl-mŏs′ kō-pē)	Examination of the interior of the eyes via an ophthalmoscope; used to identify changes in the blood vessels in the eye and to diagnose systemic diseases.
tonometry (tōn-ŏm′ ĕ-trē)	Measurement of the intraocular pressure of the eye via a tonometer; used to screen for and detect glaucoma.
visual acuity (vĭzh′ ū-ăl ă-kū′ ĭ-tē)	Measurement of the acuteness or sharpness of vision. A Snellen eye chart may be used, and the patient reads letters of various sizes from a distance of 20 feet. Normal vision is 20/20.

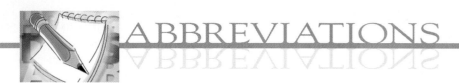

ABBREVIATIONS

ABBREVIATION	MEANING	ABBREVIATION	MEANING
Acc	accommodation	NVA	near visual acuity
ALT	argon laser trabeculoplasty	OD	oculus dexter (right eye)
D	diopter	OS	oculus sinister (left eye)
DVA	distance visual acuity	OU	oculus uterque (each eye);
ECCE	extracapsular cataract		oculi unitas (both eyes)
	extraction	PERRLA	pupils equal, regular, react to
EM	emmetropia		light and accommodation
EOM	extraocular movement;	RE	right eye
	extraocular muscles	REM	rapid eye movement
HT	hypermetropia (hyperopia)	RPE	retinal pigment epithelium
ICCE	intracapsular cataract	SLT	selective laser trabeculoptasty
	cryoextraction	SMD	senile macular degeneration
IOL	intraocular lens	ST	esotropia
IOP	intraocular pressure	VA	visual acuity
L & A	light and accommodation	VF	visual field
LE	left eye	XT	exotropia
LPI	laser peripheral iridotomy	+	plus or convex
MY	myopia	–	minus or concave

STUDY AND REVIEW

Anatomy and Physiology

Write your answers to the following questions. Do not refer to the text.

1. The external structures of the eye are the _____, _____,

   _____, _____, and the _____ _____.

2. The orbit is lined with _____ _____, which cushions the eyeball.

3. The optic foramen is an opening for the _____ _____ and

   _____ _____.

4. State the functions of the muscles of the eye.

   a. _____

   b. _____

5. Each eye has a pair of eyelids that function to protect the eyeball from

   _____ _____, _____ _____, and

   _____.

6. Describe the conjunctiva and state its function. _____

   _____

7. Define lacrimal apparatus. _____

   _____

8. The internal structures of the eye are the _____, _____,

   and the _____ _____.

9. The eyeball is the organ of _____.

10. The point at which nerve fibers from the retina converge to form the optic nerve

    is known as the _____ _____.

11. Define accommodation. _____

    _____

12. Match the following terms and definitions by placing the correct letter on the line provided.

_____ 1. Aqueous humor

_____ 2. Vitreous humor

_____ 3. Iris

_____ 4. Sclera

_____ 5. Uvea

_____ 6. Pupil

_____ 7. Retina

_____ 8. Rods and cones

_____ 9. Lens

_____ 10. Cornea

a. White of the eye
b. Colored membrane attached to the ciliary body
c. Watery fluid
d. Opening in the center of the iris
e. Jelly-like material
f. Middle layer of the eyeball
g. Anterior transparent portion of the eyeball
h. Innermost layer of the eyeball
i. Photoreceptive cells
j. Colorless crystalline body

Word Parts

1. In the spaces provided, write the definitions for the following prefixes, roots, combining forms, and suffixes. Do not refer to the listings of medical words. Leave blank those words you cannot define.

2. After completing as many as you can, refer to the medical word listings to check your work. For each word missed or left blank, write the word and its definition several times on the margins of these pages or on a separate sheet of paper.

3. To maximize the learning process, it is to your advantage to do the following exercises as directed. To refer to the word building section before completing these exercises invalidates the learning process.

PREFIXES

Give the definitions of the following prefixes:

1. a- _____

2. bi- _____

3. dipl- _____

4. en- _____

5. em- _____

6. eso- _____

7. hyper- _____

8. intra- _____

9. tri- _____

10. ex(o)- _____

11. hemi- _____

12. an- _____

13. retro- _____

ROOTS AND COMBINING FORMS

Give the definitions of the following roots and combining forms:

1. ambly _____

2. conjunctiv _____

3. anis/o _____

4. blephar _____

5. blephar/o _____

6. choroid _____

7. cry/o _____

8. cor _____

9. corne _____

10. cycl _____

11. cycl/o _____

12. enucleat _____

13. dacry _____

14. mi/o _____

15. electr/o _____

16. foc _____

17. goni/o _____

18. irid _____

19. irid/o _____

20. kerat _____

21. kerat/o _____

22. lacrim _____

23. log _____

24. metr _____

25. my _____

26. my/o _____

27. nyctal _____

28. ocul _____

29. ophthalm _____

30. ophthalm/o _____

31. opt _____

32. opt/o _____

33. phac/o _____

34. phak _____

35. phot/o _____

36. presby _____

37. pupill _____

38. retin _____

39. retin/o _____

40. scler _____

41. stigmat _____

42. ton/o _____

43. trop _____

44. uve _____

45. xen _____

46. xer _____

47. mydriat _____

48. nystagm _____

49. orth _____

50. emulsificat _____

51. coagulat _____

52. rad/i _____

53. lent _____

54. fibr/o _____

55. strabism _____

56. trich _____

SUFFIXES

Give the definitions of the following suffixes:

1. -al _____   2. -ar _____

3. -ary _____   4. -blast _____

5. -iasis _____   6. -ectomy _____

7. -gram _____   8. -graphy _____

9. -ia _____   10. -ic _____

11. -ion _____   12. -ism _____

13. -ist _____   14. -itis _____

15. -logy _____   16. -lysis _____

17. -plasia _____   18. -meter _____

19. -oma _____   20. -opia _____

21. -osis _____   22. -pathy _____

23. -phobia _____   24. -plasty _____

25. -plegia _____   26. -ptosis _____

27. -scope _____   28. -tic _____

29. -tomy _____   30. -um _____

Identifying Medical Terms

In the spaces provided, write the medical terms for the following meanings:

1. _____ Dullness of vision

2. _____ Pertaining to having two foci

3. _____ A drooping of the upper eyelid

4. _____ Pertaining to the cornea

5. _____ A tumor-like swelling caused by obstruction of the tear duct

6. _____ Double vision

7. _____ Normal or perfect vision

8. _____ Pertaining to within the eye

9. _____ Inflammation of the cornea

10. _____ Surgical repair of the cornea

11. _____ Pertaining to tears

12. _____ Pertaining to the eye

13. _____ Unusual intolerance of light

Spelling

In the spaces provided, write the correct spelling of these misspelled words:

1. atigmatism _____

2. cyloplegia _____

3. irdectomy _____

4. opthalmologist _____

5. pacosclerosis _____

6. pupilary _____

7. retinblastoma _____

8. sleritis _____

9. tonmeter _____

10. ueal _____

Matching

Select the appropriate lettered meaning for each word listed below.

_____ 1. anomaloscope

_____ 2. entropion

_____ 3. epiphora

_____ 4. hemianopia

_____ 5. phacoemulsification

_____ 6. photocoagulation

_____ 7. radial keratotomy

_____ 8. retrolental fibroplasia

_____ 9. strabismus

_____ 10. sty(e)

a. A squint

b. A disease of the retinal vessels present in premature infants

c. The process of using ultrasound to disintegrate a cataract

d. The use of a laser to treat retinal detachment and/or retinal bleeding

e. An instrument used for detecting color blindness

f. The turning inward of the margin of the lower eyelid

g. A surgical procedure that may be performed to correct myopia

h. The inability to see half the field of vision

i. A hordeolum

j. The abnormal downpour of tears

k. A disease characterized by increased intraocular pressure

Abbreviations

Place the correct word, phrase, or abbreviation in the space provided.

1. distance visual acuity _____

2. EM _____

3. HT _____

4. intraocular lens _____

5. light and accommodation _____

6. MY _____

7. OD _____

8. left eye _____

9. each eye _____

10. XT _____

Diagnostic and Laboratory Tests

Select the best answer to each multiple choice question. Circle the letter of your choice.

1. The measurement of the forward protrusion of the eye.
   a. gonioscopy
   b. keratometry
   c. exophthalmometry
   d. tonometry

2. The measurement of the cornea.
   a. gonioscopy
   b. keratometry
   c. exophthalmometry
   d. tonometry

3. Used to identify changes in the blood vessels in the eye and to diagnose systemic diseases.
   a. exophthalmometry
   b. gonioscopy
   c. ophthalmoscopy
   d. tonometry

4. The measurement of the intraocular pressure of the eye.
   a. exophthalmometry
   b. gonioscopy
   c. ophthalmoscopy
   d. tonometry

5. The measurement of the acuteness or sharpness of vision.
   a. color vision tests
   b. ultrasonography
   c. tonometry
   d. visual acuity

CASE STUDY   CATARACTS

Read the following case study and then answer the questions that follow.

A 67-year-old male was seen by a physician, and the following is a synopsis of the visit.

Present History: The patient states that he has trouble driving at night, bright lights hurt his eyes, his vision seems to blur while watching television, he feels as though his glasses are dirty and there is a film over his eyes, and on occasion he has seen halos around lights. His ophthalmologist previously told him that he was developing cataracts and when the condition began to interfere with his lifestyle he would be a candidate for surgery. He is back in for his yearly eye examination and to talk to his physician about eye surgery. He would like to have his right eye done first.

Signs and Symptoms: Trouble driving at night, photophobia, blurred vision, feels like there is a film over his eyes, and sees halos around lights.

Diagnosis: Cataracts. The diagnosis was determined by a complete eye examination.

Treatment: Surgical procedure—phacoemulsification. Phacoemulsification is the process of using an ultrasonic device to disintegrate the cataract, which is then aspirated and removed. After surgery, the patient is advised not to lift any heavy objects, run, jog, or ride a horse. The patient should avoid sleeping on the operative side, rubbing the eyes, squeezing the eyelids shut, straining at bowel movement, getting soap in the eyes, sexual relations, driving, coughing, sneezing, vomiting, and bending head down below waist. The patient is advised to report any unusual symptoms such as pain, changes in vision, persistent headache, and discharge from the eye to his physician.

Prevention: Since most cataracts occur as part of the aging process, there are no known preventive measures.

CASE STUDY QUESTIONS

1. Signs and symptoms of cataracts include trouble driving at night, _____, blurred vision, film over the eyes, and seeing halos around lights.

2. The diagnosis was determined by a _____ eye examination.

3. Treatment included a surgical procedure known as phacoemulsification where an _____ device is used to disintegrate the cataract.

4. After the cataract is disintegrated, how is it removed?

5. The medical word *photophobia* means _____ _____.

MedMedia Wrap-Up
www.prenhall.com/rice

Additional interactive resources and activities for this chapter can be found on the Companion Website. For animations, videos, audio glossary, and review, access the accompanying CD-ROM in this book.

Audio Glossary
Medical Terminology Exercises & Activities
Pathology Spotlights
Terminology Translator
Animations
Videos

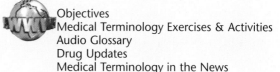

Objectives
Medical Terminology Exercises & Activities
Audio Glossary
Drug Updates
Medical Terminology in the News

THE FEMALE REPRODUCTIVE SYSTEM

15

OBJECTIVES

On completion of this chapter, you will be able to:

- Describe the uterus and state its functions.
- Describe the fallopian tubes and state their functions.
- Describe the ovaries and state their functions.
- Describe the vagina and state its functions.
- Describe the breast.
- Describe the menstrual cycle.
- Analyze, build, spell, and pronounce medical words.
- Describe each of the conditions presented in the Pathology Spotlights.
- Complete the Pathology Checkpoint.
- Review Drug Highlights presented in this chapter.
- Provide the description of diagnostic and laboratory tests related to the female reproductive system.
- Identify and define selected abbreviations.
- Successfully complete the study and review section.

MedMedia
www.prenhall.com/rice

Additional interactive resources and activities for this chapter can be found on the Companion Website. For Terminology Translator, animations, videos, audio glossary, and review, access the accompanying CD-ROM in this book.

Anatomy and Physiology Overview

The female reproductive system consists of the left and right **ovaries,** which are the female's primary sex organs, and the following accessory sex organs: two **fallopian tubes,** the **uterus,** the **vagina,** the **vulva,** and two **breasts.** The vital function of the female reproductive system is to perpetuate the species through sexual or germ cell reproduction.

THE UTERUS

The **uterus** is a muscular, hollow, pear-shaped organ having three identifiable areas: the **body** or upper portion, the **isthmus** or central area, and the **cervix,** which is the lower cylindrical portion or neck. The **fundus** is the bulging surface of the body of the uterus extending from the internal os (*mouth*) of the cervix upward above the fallopian tubes. The uterus is suspended in the anterior part of the pelvic cavity, halfway between the sacrum and the symphysis pubis, above the bladder, and in front of the rectum. A number of ligaments support the uterus and hold it in position. These are two broad ligaments, two round ligaments, two uterosacral ligaments, and the ligaments that are attached to the bladder. The normal position of the uterus is with the cervix pointing toward the lower end of the sacrum and the fundus toward the suprapubic region. An average, normal uterus is about 8 cm long, 5 cm wide, and 2.5 cm thick (Figs. 15–1 and 15–2).

THE FEMALE REPRODUCTIVE SYSTEM

Organ/Structure	Primary Functions
The Uterus	Organ of the cyclic discharge of menses; provides place for the nourishment and development of the fetus; contracts during labor to help expel the fetus
The Fallopian Tubes	Serve as a duct for the conveyance of the ovum from the ovary to the uterus; serve as ducts for the conveyance of spermatozoa from the uterus toward the ovary
The Ovaries	Production of ova and hormones
The Vagina	Female organ of copulation; serves as a passageway for the discharge of menstruation; serves as a passageway for the birth of the fetus
The Vulva	External female genitalia
Mons pubis	Provides pad of fatty tissue
Labia majora	Provides two folds of adipose tissue
Labia minora	Lies within the labia majora and encloses the vestibule
Vestibule	Opening for the urethra, the vagina, and two excretory ducts of Bartholin's glands
Clitoris	Erectile tissue that is homologous to the penis of the male; produces pleasurable sensations during the sexual act
The Breast	Following childbirth, mammary glands produce milk

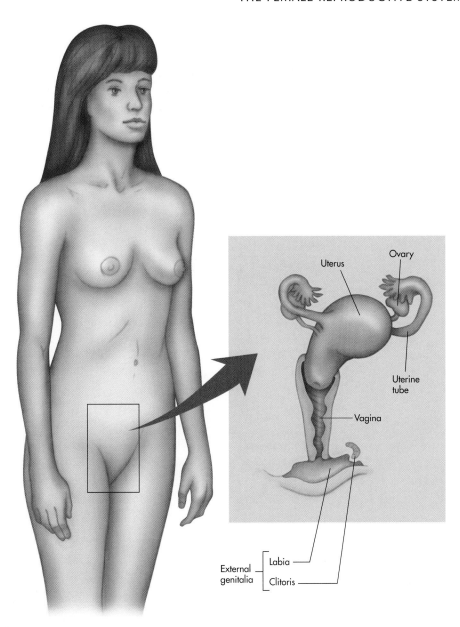

FIGURE 15–1

The female reproductive system.

The Uterine Wall

The wall of the uterus consists of three layers: the **peritoneum** or outer layer, the **myometrium** or muscular middle layer, and the **endometrium,** which is the mucous membrane lining the inner surface of the uterus. The endometrium is composed of columnar epithelium and connective tissue and is supplied with blood by both straight and spiral arteries. It undergoes marked changes in response to hormonal stimulation during the menstrual cycle. These changes are discussed in the last section of this overview.

Functions of the Uterus

There are three primary functions associated with the uterus:

- It is the organ of the cyclic discharge of a bloody fluid from the uterus and the changes that occur to its endometrium.

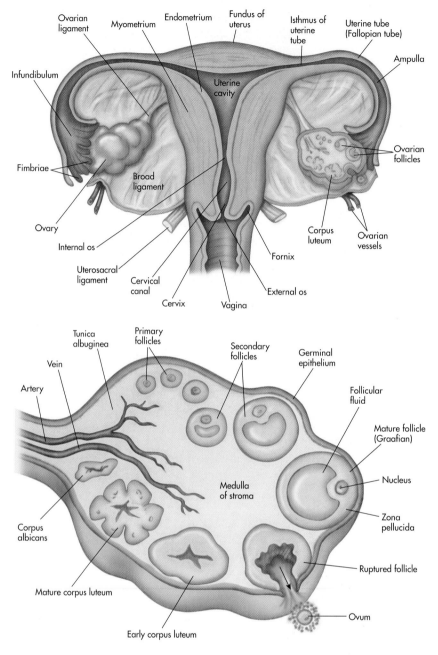

FIGURE 15–2

The uterus, ovaries, and associated structures, with an expanded view of a mammalian ovary showing stages of graafian follicle and ovum development.

- It functions as a place for the protection and nourishment of the fetus during pregnancy.
- During labor, the muscular uterine wall contracts rhythmically and powerfully to expel the fetus from the uterus.

Abnormal Positions of the Uterus

The uterus may become malpositioned because of weakness of any of its supporting ligaments. Trauma, disease processes of the uterus, or multiple pregnancies may contribute to the weakening of the supporting ligaments. The following terms describe some of the abnormal positions of the uterus:

Anteflexion. The process of bending forward of the uterus at its body and neck

Retroflexion. The process of bending the body of the uterus backward at an angle with the cervix usually unchanged from its normal position

Anteversion. The process of turning the fundus forward toward the pubis, with the cervix tilted up toward the sacrum

Retroversion. The process of turning the uterus backward, with the cervix pointing forward toward the symphysis pubis

THE FALLOPIAN TUBES

Also called the **uterine tubes** or **oviducts**, the **fallopian tubes** extend laterally from either side of the uterus and end near each ovary. An average, normal fallopian tube is about 11.5 cm long and 6 mm wide. Its wall is composed of three layers: the **serosa** or outermost layer, composed of connective tissue; the **muscular layer**, containing inner circular and outer longitudinal layers of smooth muscle; and the **mucosa** or inner layer, consisting of simple columnar epithelium.

Anatomical Features of the Fallopian Tubes

The **isthmus** is the constricted portion of the tube nearest the uterus (see Fig. 15–2). From the isthmus, the tube continues laterally and widens to form a section called the **ampulla**. Beyond the ampulla, the tube continues to expand and ends as a funnel-shaped opening. This end of the tube is called the **infundibulum**, and its opening is the **ostium**. Surrounding each ostium are **fimbriae** or **finger-like processes** that work to propel the discharged ovum into the tube, where ciliary action aids in moving it toward the uterus. Should the ovum become impregnated by a spermatozoon while in the tube, the process of **fertilization** occurs.

Functions of the Fallopian Tubes

The two basic functions of the fallopian tubes are as follows:

- Each tube serves as a duct for the conveyance of the ovum from the ovary to the uterus.

- The tubes serve as ducts for the conveyance of spermatozoa from the uterus toward each ovary.

THE OVARIES

Located on either side of the uterus, the **ovaries** are almond-shaped organs attached to the uterus by the ovarian ligament and lie close to the fimbriae of the fallopian tubes. The anterior border of each ovary is connected to the posterior layer of the broad ligament by the **mesovarium**. Each ovary is attached to the side of the pelvis by the **suspensory ligaments**. An average, normal ovary is about 4 cm long, 2 cm wide, and 1.5 cm thick.

Microscopic Anatomy

Each ovary consists of two distinct areas: the **cortex** or outer layer and the **medulla** or inner portion. The cortex contains small secretory sacs or follicles in three stages of development. These stages are known as **primary**, **growing**, and **graafian**, which is the follicles' mature stage (see Fig. 15–2). The ovarian medulla contains connective tissue, nerves, blood and lymphatic vessels, and some smooth muscle tissue in the region of the hilus.

Function of the Ovaries

The functional activity of the ovary is primarily controlled by the anterior lobe of the pituitary gland, which produces the *gonadotropic hormones* FSH and LH. These abbreviations are for follicle-stimulating hormone, instrumental in the development of the ovarian follicles, and luteinizing hormone, which stimulates the development of the **corpus luteum**, a small yellow mass of cells that develops within a ruptured ovarian follicle.

Two functions have been identified for the ovary: the production of ova or female reproductive cells and the production of hormones.

THE PRODUCTION OF OVA

Each month a *graafian follicle* ruptures on the ovarian cortex, and an **ovum** (singular of ova) discharges into the pelvic cavity, where it enters the fallopian tube. This process is known as **ovulation**. In an average, normal woman more than 400 ova may be produced during her reproductive years (see Fig. 15–2).

THE PRODUCTION OF HORMONES

The ovary is also an endocrine gland, producing **estrogen** and **progesterone**. Estrogen is the female sex hormone secreted by the follicles. Progesterone is a steroid hormone secreted by the corpus luteum. These hormones are essential in promoting growth, development, and maintenance of the female secondary sex organs and characteristics. They also prepare the uterus for pregnancy, promote development of the mammary glands, and play a vital role in a woman's emotional well-being and sexual drive.

THE VAGINA

The **vagina** is a musculomembranous tube extending from the vestibule to the uterus (Fig. 15–2). It is 10 to 15 cm in length and is situated between the bladder and the rectum. It is lined by mucous membrane made up of *squamous epithelium*. A fold of mucous membrane, the **hymen**, partially covers the external opening of the vagina.

Functions of the Vagina

The vagina has three basic functions:

- It is the female organ of copulation. The vagina receives the seminal fluid from the male penis.
- It serves as a passageway for the discharge of menstruation.
- It serves as a passageway for the birth of the fetus.

THE VULVA

The **vulva** consists of the following five organs that comprise the external female genitalia (Fig. 15–3):

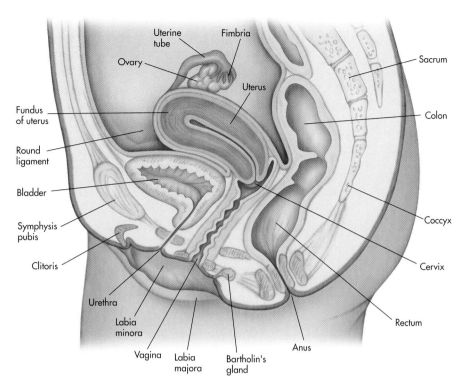

FIGURE 15–3

Sagittal section of the female pelvis showing organs of the reproductive system.

Mons pubis. A pad of fatty tissue of triangular shape and, after puberty, covered with pubic hair. It may be referred to as the mons veneris or "mound of Venus," and is the rounded area over the symphysis pubis.

Labia majora. The two folds of adipose tissue, which are large lip-like structures, lying on either side of the vaginal opening.

Labia minora. Two thin folds of skin that lie within the labia majora and enclose the vestibule.

Vestibule. The cleft between the labia minora. It is approximately 4 to 5 cm long and 2 cm wide. Four major structures open into it: the urethra, the vagina, and two excretory ducts of the Bartholin glands.

Clitoris. A small organ consisting of sensitive erectile tissue that is homologous to the penis of the male.

Between the vulva and the anus is an external region known as the **perineum.** It is composed of muscle covered with skin. During the second stage of labor, a decision is made by the attending physician as to the need to perform an **episiotomy,** a surgical procedure to prevent tearing of the perineum and to facilitate delivery of the fetus.

THE BREAST

The **breasts** or mammary glands are compound *alveolar structures* consisting of 15 to 20 glandular tissue lobes separated by septa of connective tissue. Most women have two breasts that lie anterior to the pectoral muscles and curve outward from the lateral margins of the sternum to the anterior border of the axilla. The size of the breast may greatly vary according to age, heredity, and adipose (*fatty*) tissue present. The **areola** is the dark, pigmented area found in the skin over each breast, and the nipple is the elevated area in the center of the areola. During pregnancy, the areola changes from its pinkish color to a dark brown or reddish color. The areola is supplied with a row of small sebaceous glands that secrete an oily substance to keep it resilient. The *lactiferous glands* consist of 20 to 24 glands in the areola of the nipple and, during lactation, secrete and convey milk to a suckling infant (Fig. 15–4). The hormone **prolactin**, which is produced by the anterior lobe of the pituitary, stimulates the mammary glands to produce milk after childbirth. Other hormones playing a role in milk production are insulin and glucocorticoids. **Colostrum**, a thin yellowish secretion, is the "first milk" and contains mainly serum and white blood cells. Suckling stimulates the production of **oxytocin** by the posterior lobe of the pituitary gland. It acts on the mammary glands to stimulate the release of milk and stimulates the uterus to contract during parturition. See Figure 15–5.

Breast Feeding

Among the natural advantages of breast feeding are the following:

- It provides an ideal food for most newborn babies.
- The milk provides essential nutrients for growth and development.

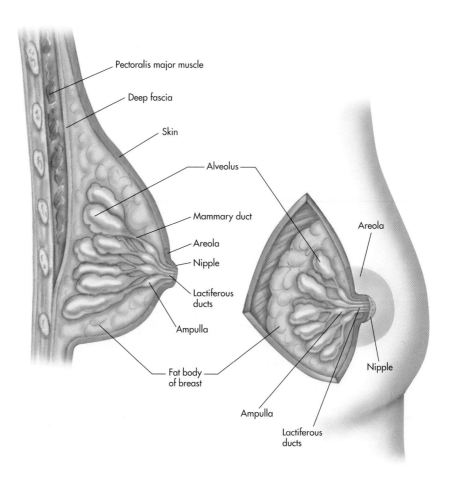

FIGURE 15–4

The breast.

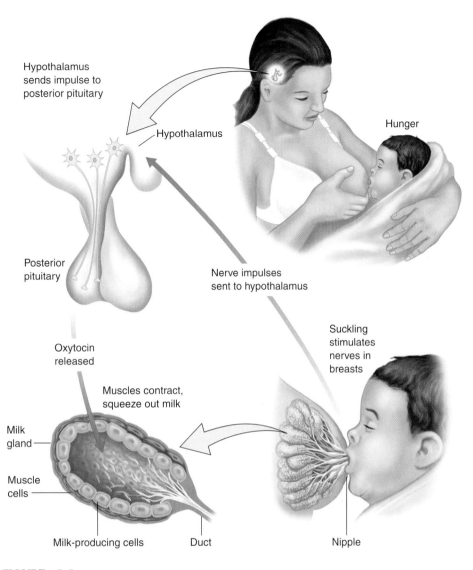

FIGURE 15–5

Oxytocin and breastfeeding. (Source: Pearson Education/PH College.)

- The milk is virtually free from harmful bacteria.
- It is easier for babies to digest.
- It does not need to be prepared.
- It costs nothing to make and is in ready supply.
- It is good for the environment since there are no bottles, cans, and boxes to put in the garbage.

After the first 2 weeks, the nursing mother may produce 1 or more pints of milk per day. Milk production may be affected by emotions, food, fluids, physical health, and medications. The nursing mother will usually have a supply of milk for her suckling infant for a period of 6 to 9 months. The nursing process is usually a satisfying experience for both mother and infant. For the mother, the nursing causes contractions of the muscles of the uterus, which aid in its rapid return to normal size. For the infant, breast milk is a natural substance that provides almost everything needed for the first months of life.

THE MENSTRUAL CYCLE

The onset of the **menstrual cycle** occurs at the age of **puberty** and its cessation is at **menopause**. It is a periodic recurrent series of changes occurring in the uterus, ovaries, vagina, and breasts approximately every 28 days. The menstrual cycle is divided into four phases, each of which is described for you. See Figure 15–6.

Menstruation Phase

The **menstruation phase** is characterized by the discharge of a bloody fluid from the uterus accompanied by a shedding of the endometrium. This phase averages 4 to 5 days and is considered to be the first to the fifth days of the cycle.

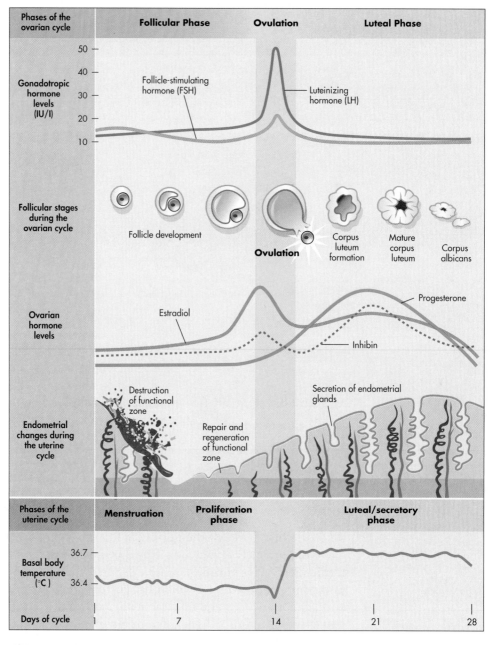

FIGURE 15–6

The hormonal regulation of the female reproductive cycle.

Proliferation Phase

The **proliferation phase** is characterized by the stimulation of estrogen, the thickening and vascularization of the endometrium, along with the maturing of the ovarian follicle. This phase begins about the fifth day and ends at the time of rupture of the graafian follicle—about 14 days before the onset of menstruation.

Luteal or Secretory Phase

The **luteal phase** is characterized by continued thickening of the endometrium, by the glands within the endometrium becoming tortuous, and by the appearance of coiled arteries in its tissues. The endometrium becomes edematous, and the stroma becomes compact. During this phase, the corpus luteum in the ovary is developing and secreting progesterone. The progesterone level is highest during this phase as the estrogen level decreases. This phase lasts about 10 to 14 days.

Premenstrual or Ischemic Phase

During the **premenstrual phase**, the coiled arteries become constricted, the endometrium becomes anemic and begins to shrink, and the corpus luteum decreases in functional activity. This phase lasts about 2 days and ends with the occurrence of menstruation. See Premenstrual Syndrome (PMS) in Pathology Spotlights for information about a common condition that occurs during this phase.

LIFE SPAN
CONSIDERATIONS

■ THE CHILD

The sex of the child is determined at the time of **fertilization**. When a spermatozoon carrying the X sex chromosome fertilizes the X-bearing ovum, the result is a female child (X + X = female). When the X-bearing ovum is fertilized by the Y-bearing spermatozoon, a male child is produced (X + Y = male). Sex differentiation occurs early in the embryo. At 16 weeks the external **genitals** of the fetus are recognizably male or female. This difference may be seen during ultrasonography. See Figure 15–7.

The genitals of the newborn are not fully developed at birth. They may be slightly swollen, and in the female infant, blood-tinged mucus may be discharged from the vagina. This is due to hormones transmitted from the mother to the infant. The labia minora may protrude beyond the labia majora.

The sex organs do not mature until the onset of **puberty**. At puberty the female experiences breast development, vaginal secretions, and menarche. A study published in the *Journal of Pediatrics*, April 1997, revealed that many girls begin to develop sexually by age 8. This study involved 17,000 American girls ages 3 to 12, who were seen in 65 pediatric practices nationwide. At age 8, 48.3% of African American girls and 14.7% of white girls had begun developing breasts, pubic hair, or both. Among African American girls, menstruation began on average at 12.16 years; among white girls, the average was 12.88 years. The study raised questions about whether environmental estrogens, chemicals that mimic the female hormone estrogen, are bringing on puberty at an earlier age. The study also suggested that sex education should begin sooner than it often does.

■ THE OLDER ADULT

At about 50 years of age, men and women begin experiencing bodily changes that are directly related to **hormonal** production. In women, the ovaries cease to produce estrogen and progesterone. With decreased production of the female hormones, estrogen and progesterone, women enter the phase of life known as

menopause. Natural menopause will occur in 25 percent of women by age 47, in 50 percent by age 50, 75 percent by age 52, and in 95 percent by age 55.

The symptoms of menopause vary from being hardly noticeable to being severe. Symptoms may include irregular periods, hot flashes, vaginal dryness, insomnia, joint pain, headache, emotional instability, irritability, and depression. Breast tissue may lose its firmness, and pubic and axillary hair becomes sparse. Without estrogen, the uterus becomes smaller, the vagina shortens and vaginal tissues become drier. There may be loss of bone mass leading to **osteoporosis**.

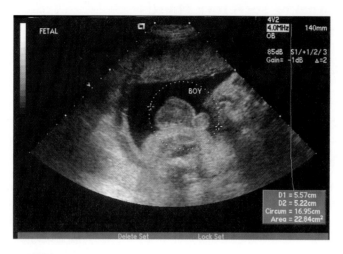

FIGURE 15–7

Ultrasonogram showing a male fetus. (Courtesy of Nancy West.)

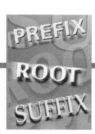

BUILDING YOUR MEDICAL VOCABULARY

This section provides the foundation for learning medical terminology. Medical words can be made up of four different types of word parts:

- Prefixes (P)
- Roots (R)
- Combining forms (CF)
- Suffixes (S)

By connecting various word parts in an organized sequence, thousands of words can be built and learned. In this text the word list is alphabetized so one can see the variety of meanings created when common prefixes and suffixes are repeatedly applied to certain word roots and/or combining forms. Words shown in pink are additional words related to the content of this chapter that are not built from word parts. These words are included to enhance your vocabulary. Note: an asterisk icon (✱) indicates words that are covered in the Pathology Spotlights section in this chapter.

MEDICAL WORD	WORD PARTS (WHEN APPLICABLE)			DEFINITION
	Part	**Type**	**Meaning**	
abortion (ă-bōr′ shŭn)	abort -ion	R S	to miscarry process	The process of miscarrying
amenorrhea (ă-měn″ ō-rē′ ă)	a men/o -rrhea	P CF S	lack of month flow	A lack of the monthly flow or menstruation
amniocentesis (ăm″ nĭ-ō-sĕn-tē′ sĭs)	amni/o -centesis	CF S	lamb surgical puncture	Surgical puncture of the amniotic sac to obtain a sample of amniotic fluid from which it can be determined if the fetus has Down syndrome, neural tube defects, Tay-Sachs disease, or other genetic defects
ante partum (ăn′ tē pär′ tŭm)	ante partum	P R	before labor	The time before the onset of labor
bartholinitis (bar″ tō-lĭn-ī′ tĭs)	bartholin -itis	R S	Bartholin's glands inflammation	Inflammation of Bartholin's glands
biotics (bī-ōt′ ĭks)	bi/o -tic (s)	CF S	life pertaining to	The science of living organisms and the sum of knowledge regarding the life process
blastocyst (blăs′ tō-sĭst)	blast/o -cyst	CF S	germ cell sac	An embryonic cell mass that attaches to the uterus wall and is a stage in the development of a mammalian embryo
cervicitis (sěr-vĭ-sī′ tĭs)	cervic -itis	R S	cervix inflammation	Inflammation of the uterine cervix
colposcope (kŏl′ pō-skōp)	colp/o -scope	CF S	vagina instrument	An instrument used to examine the vagina and cervix by means of a magnifying lens
conception (kŏn-sěp′ shŭn)	con cept -ion	P R S	together receive process	Process of the union of the male's sperm and the female's ovum; *fertilization*
contraception (kŏn″ tră-sěp′ shŭn)	contra cept -ion	P R S	against receive process	Process of preventing conception
culdocentesis (kŭl″ dō-sĕn-tē′ sĭs)	culd/o -centesis	CF S	cul-de-sac surgical puncture	Surgical puncture of the cul-de-sac for removal of fluid
cystocele (sĭs′ tō-sēl)	cyst/o -cele	CF S	bladder hernia	A hernia of the bladder that protrudes into the vagina

MEDICAL WORD	WORD PARTS (WHEN APPLICABLE)			DEFINITION
	Part	**Type**	**Meaning**	
diagnostic ultrasound (dĭ″ ăg-nŏs′ tĭk ŭl′ tră-sŏund)				The use of extremely high-frequency sound waves for the purpose of diagnosing genetic defects and hydrocephalic conditions in the unborn fetus
Doppler ultrasound (däp′ lər ŭl′ trăh-sŏund)				A procedure using an audio transformation of high-frequency sounds to monitor the fetal heartbeat
dysmenorrhea (dĭs″ mĕn-ō-rē′ ă)	dys men/o -rrhea	P CF S	difficult, painful month flow	Difficult or painful monthly flow
dyspareunia (dĭs′ pă-rū′ nĭ-ă)	dys par eunia	P P R	difficult, painful beside a bed	Difficult or painful sexual intercourse
dystocia (dĭs-tō′ sĭ-ă)	dys toc -ia	P R S	difficult, painful birth condition	The condition of a difficult and painful childbirth
eclampsia (ĕ-klămp′sē-ă)	ec lamp (s) -ia	P R S	out to shine condition of	A complication of severe preeclampsia that involves seizures. ✱ See Pathology Spotlight: Preeclampsia and Eclampsia.
ectopic pregnancy (ĕk-tŏp′ ĭk prĕg′ năn-sē)	ectop -ic	R S	displaced pertaining to	A pregnancy that occurs when the fertilized egg is implanted in one of the fallopian tubes; also referred to as a "tubal" pregnancy. This type of pregnancy is life-threatening to the mother, and almost always fatal to her fetus. It is the leading cause of pregnancy-related death in African American women.
endometriosis (ĕn″ dō-mē″ trĭ-ō′ sĭs)	endo metr/i -osis	P CF S	within uterus condition of	A condition in which endometrial tissue occurs in various sites in the abdominal or pelvic cavity. ✱ See Pathology Spotlight: Endometriosis.
episiotomy (ĕ-pĭs″ ĭ-ŏt′ ō-mē)	episi/o -tomy	CF S	vulva, pudenda incision	Incision of the perineum to prevent tearing of the perineum and to facilitate delivery
fetus (fē′ tŭs)				The developing young in the uterus from the third month to birth
fibroma (fī-brō′ mă)	fibr -oma	R S	fibrous tissue tumor	A fibrous tissue tumor

MEDICAL WORD	WORD PARTS (WHEN APPLICABLE)			DEFINITION
	Part	**Type**	**Meaning**	
gamete intrafallopian transfer (GIFT) (găm′ ēt ĭn″ tră-fă-lō′ pē-ăn)				A procedure that places the sperm (*spermatozoa*) and eggs (*oocytes*) directly in the fimbriated end of the fallopian tube via a laparoscope
genetics (jĕn-ĕt′ ĭks)	genet -ic (s)	R S	formation, produce pertaining to	The science of biology that studies the phenomenon of heredity and the laws governing it
genitalia (jĕn-ĭ-tăl′ ĭ-ă)	genital -ia	R S	belonging to birth condition	The male or female reproductive organs
gynecologist (gī″ nĕ-kōl′ ō-jĭst)	gynec/o log -ist	CF R S	female study of one who specializes	One who specializes in the study of the female
gynecology (gī″ nĕ-kōl′ ō-jē)	gynec/o -logy	CF S	female study of	The study of the female
hymenectomy (hī″ mĕn-ĕk′ tō-mē)	hymen -ectomy	R S	hymen excision	Surgical excision of the hymen
hysterectomy (hĭs″ tĕr-ĕk′ tō-mē)	hyster -ectomy	R S	womb, uterus excision	Surgical excision of the uterus. ✱ See Pathology Spotlight: Hysterectomy.
hysteroscope (hĭs′ tĕr-ō-skōp)	hyster/o -scope	CF S	womb, uterus instrument	An instrument used in the biopsy of uterine tissue before 12 weeks of gestation. This tissue is then analyzed for chromosome arrangement, DNA sequence, and genetic defects.
hysterotomy (hĭs″ tĕr-ŏt′ ō-mē)	hyster/o -tomy	CF S	womb, uterus incision	Incision into the uterus; also called a cesarean section
intrauterine (ĭn′ tră-ū′ tĕr-ĭn)	intra uter -ine	P R S	within uterus pertaining to	Pertaining to within the uterus
laser ablation (lā′ zĕr ăb-lā′ shŭn)				A procedure that uses a laser to destroy the uterine lining. A biopsy is performed before the procedure to make sure no cancer is present. This procedure may be used for disabling menstrual bleeding. *It does cause sterility.*

MEDICAL WORD	WORD PARTS (WHEN APPLICABLE)			DEFINITION
	Part	**Type**	**Meaning**	
laser laparoscopy (lā′ zĕr lăp-ăr-ŏs′ kō-pē)				A procedure that uses a long, telescope-like instrument equipped with a laser, lights, and a tiny video camera. It may be used to explore the abdominal area and to treat ectopic pregnancy.
laser lumpectomy (lā-zĕr lŭm-pĕk′ tō-mē)				The use of a contact Yag laser to remove a tumor from the breast. It appears to cause less pain for the patient, and discharge time from the hospital is sooner.
lumpectomy (lŭm-pĕk′ tō-mē)	lump -ectomy	R S	lump excision	The surgical removal of a tumor from the breast. In this procedure, no other tissue or lymph nodes are removed, only the tumor; usually not considered for large tumors, although the latest strategy involves shrinking large tumors with chemotherapy so that they become small enough to be removed by this method
mammoplasty (măm′ ō-plăs″ tē)	mamm/o -plasty	CF S	breast surgical repair	Surgical repair of the breast
mastectomy (măs-tĕk′ tō-mē)	mast -ectomy	R S	breast excision	Surgical excision of the breast
mastitis (măs-tī′ tĭs)	mast -itis	R S	breast inflammation	Inflammation of the breast
menarche (mĕn-ar′ kē)	men arche	R R	month beginning	The beginning of the monthly flow; *menses*
menopause (mĕn′ ō-pawz)	men/o pause	CF R	month cessation	Cessation of the monthly flow; *also called climacteric*
menorrhagia (mĕn″ ō-rā′ jĭ-ă)	men/o -rrhagia	CF S	month to burst forth	Excessive bursting forth of blood at the time of the monthly flow
menorrhea (mĕn″ ō-rē′ ă)	men/o -rrhea	CF S	month flow	A normal monthly flow
mittelschmerz (mĭt′ ĕl-shmārts)				Abdominal pain that occurs midway between the menstrual periods at ovulation
multipara (mŭl-tĭp′ ă-ră)	multi para	P R	many to bear	A woman who has borne more than one child

MEDICAL WORD	WORD PARTS (WHEN APPLICABLE)			DEFINITION
	Part	Type	Meaning	
myometritis (mī″ ō-mē-trī′ tĭs)	my/o	CF	muscle	Inflammation of the muscular wall of the uterus
	metr	R	womb, uterus	
	-itis	S	inflammation	
neonatal (nē″ ō-nā′ tăl)	neo	P	new	Pertaining to the first 4 weeks after birth
	nat	R	birth	
	-al	S	pertaining to	
nonstress test (nŏn′ strĕs tĕst)				A diagnostic procedure, often done in a physician's office, wherein a monitor is placed on the mother's abdomen and fetal heartbeats are recorded. The fetal heartbeats should accelerate if the fetus moves.
nullipara (nŭl-ĭp′ ă-ră)	nulli	P	none	A woman who has borne no offspring
	para	R	to bear	
oligomenorrhea (ŏl″ ĭ-gō-mĕn″ ō-rē′ ă)	oligo	P	scanty	A scanty monthly flow
	men/o	CF	month	
	-rrhea	S	flow	
oogenesis (ō″ ō-jĕn′ ĕ-sĭs)	o/o	CF	ovum, egg	Formation of the ovum
	-genesis	S	formation, produce	
oophorectomy (ō″ ŏf-ō-rĕk′ tō-mē)	oophor	R	ovary	Surgical excision of an ovary
	-ectomy	S	excision	
ovulation (ŏv″ ū-lā′ shŭn)	ovulat	R	little egg	The process in which an ovum is discharged from the cortex of the ovary
	-ion	S	process	
ovum transfer (ō′ vum trăns′ fer)				A method of fertilization for women who cannot conceive children. A donor ovum is impregnated within the donor's body by artificial insemination and later transferred to the recipient female.
parturition (par″ tū-rĭsh′ ŭn)	parturit	R	in labor	The act of giving birth; *also known as childbirth or delivery*
	-ion	S	process	
pelvic inflammatory disease (PID) (pĕl′ vĭk ĭn-flăm′ ă-tŏr′ ē dĭ-zēz)				An infection of the upper genital area. PID can affect the uterus, ovaries, and fallopian tubes. ✱ See Pathology Spotlight: Pelvic Inflammatory Disease (PID).
pelvimetry (pĕl-vĭm′ ĕt-rē)	pelv/i	CF	pelvis	Measurement of the pelvis to determine its capacity and diameter
	-metry	S	measurement	

MEDICAL WORD	WORD PARTS (WHEN APPLICABLE)			DEFINITION
	Part	**Type**	**Meaning**	
perimenopause (pĕr-ĭ-mĕn′ ō-pawz)	peri men/o pause	P CF R	around month cessation	The period of gradual changes that lead into menopause. It affects a woman's hormones, body, and feelings. It can be a stop-start process that may take months or years. Hormone levels fluctuate, thereby causing changes in the menstrual cycle, which becomes irregular.
perinatology (pĕr″ ĭ-nă-tŏl′ ō-jē)	peri nat/o -logy	P CF S	around birth study of	Study of the fetus and infant from 20 to 29 weeks of gestation to 1 to 4 weeks after birth
postcoital (pōst-kō′ ĭt-ăl)	post coit -al	P R S	after a coming together pertaining to	Pertaining to after sexual intercourse
postpartum (pōst păr′ tŭm)	post partum	P R	after labor	Pertaining to after childbirth
preeclampsia (prē″ ē-klămp′ sē-ă)	pre ec lamp (s) -ia	P P R S	before out to shine condition of	A complication of pregnancy characterized by increasing hypertension, proteinuria, and edema. ✷ See Pathology Spotlight: Preeclampsia and Eclampsia.
pregnancy (prĕg′ năn-sē)				A temporary condition that occurs within a woman's body from the time of conception through the embryonic and fetal periods to birth. It lasts approximately 280 days (40 weeks; 10 lunar months; 9 1/3 calendar months).
premenstrual syndrome (PMS) (prē-mĕn-stroo-ăl sĭn-drŏm)				A condition that affects certain women and may cause distressful symptoms such as constipation, diarrhea, nausea, appetite cravings, headache, backache, muscular aches, edema, insomnia, clumsiness, irritability, indecisiveness, mental confusion, and depression. ✷ See Pathology Spotlight: Premenstrual Syndrome (PMS).
prenatal (prē-nā′ tl)	pre nat -al	P R S	before birth pertaining to	Pertaining to before birth
primigravida (prī-mī-grăv′ ĭ-dă)	primi gravida	P R	first pregnant	Refers to a woman during her first pregnancy

MEDICAL WORD	WORD PARTS (WHEN APPLICABLE)			DEFINITION
	Part	Type	Meaning	
primipara (prī-mĭp′ ă-ră)	primi para	P R	first to bear	A woman who is bearing her first child
pseudocyesis (sū″ dō-sī-ē′ sĭs)	pseudo -cyesis	P S	false pregnancy	A false pregnancy
pudendal (pū-dĕn′ dăl)	pudend -al	R S	external genitals pertaining to	Pertaining to the external female genitalia
puerperium (pū″ ĕr-pē′ rĭ-ŭm)				The 4 to 6 weeks after childbirth when the female generative organs usually return to a normal state
quickening (kwĭk′ ĕn-ĭng)				The first movement of the fetus felt in the uterus, occurring during the 16th to 20th week of pregnancy
rectovaginal (rĕk″ tō-văj′ ĭ-năl)	rect/o vagin -al	CF R S	rectum vagina pertaining to	Pertaining to the rectum and vagina
retroversion (rĕt″ rō-vur′ shŭn)	retro vers -ion	P R S	backward turning process	The process of being turned backward, such as the displacement of the uterus with the cervix pointed forward
salpingectomy (săl″ pĭn-jĕk′ tō-mē)	salping -ectomy	R S	tube excision	Surgical excision of a fallopian tube
salpingitis (săl″ pĭn-jī′ tĭs)	salping -itis	R S	tube inflammation	Inflammation of a fallopian tube
salpingo-oophor-ectomy (săl′ pĭng″ gō-ō″ ŏf-ō-rĕk′ tō-mē)	salping/o oophor -ectomy	CF R S	tube ovary excision	Surgical excision of an ovary and a fallopian tube
secundines (sĕk′ ŭn-dīnz)	secund -ine(s)	R S	second pertaining to	The afterbirth, consisting of the placenta, umbilical cord, and fetal membranes
sonogram (sō′ nŏ-grăm)	son/o -gram	CF S	sound record	A procedure using high-frequency sound waves to display a visual echo image of the fetus; used to determine size of the fetus and to diagnose genetic defects
surrogate mother (sur′ ō-gāt mŭth′ ēr)	surrog -ate	R S	substituted use	A female who contracts to bear a child for another. Pregnancy may occur as a result of artificial insemination

MEDICAL WORD	WORD PARTS (WHEN APPLICABLE)			DEFINITION
	Part	**Type**	**Meaning**	
"test-tube baby" (těs' tūb bā' bē)				An in vitro fertilization technique whereby the ovum is fertilized outside the body and later implanted in the host female
toxic shock syndrome (tŏk' sĭk shŏk sĭn' drōm)				A poisonous *Staphylococcus aureus* infection that may strike young, menstruating women
trimester (trī-měs' těr)	tri mester	P R	three month	A period of 3 months
uterine fibroid (ū' těr-ĭn fī-broyd)	uter -ine fibr -oid	R S R S	uterus pertaining to fiber resemble	A benign fibrous tumor of the uterus, made up of muscle cells and other tissues, that grow within the wall of the uterus. The synonym for uterine fibroid is *uterine leiomyoma.* ✱ See Pathology Spotlight: Uterine Fibroids.
vaginitis (vǎj" ĭn-ī' tĭs)	vagin -itis	R S	vagina inflammation	Inflammation of the vagina
venereal (vē-nē' rē-ăl)	venere -al	R S	sexual intercourse pertaining to	Pertaining to or resulting from sexual intercourse
zygote (zī' gōt)				The fertilized ovum. The zygote is produced by the union of two gametes.

Terminology Translator

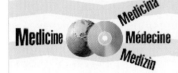

This feature, found on the accompanying CD-ROM, provides an innovative tool to translate medical words into Spanish, French, and German.

PATHOLOGY SPOTLIGHTS

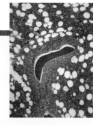

Endometriosis

The endometrium is the tissue that lines the inside of the uterus. **Endometriosis** occurs when this tissue travels outside the uterus.

The female hormones estrogen and progesterone encourage the growth of endometrial tissue during a woman's monthly cycle. If no fertilized egg implants itself in this lining, it is shed as menstrual flow. In a woman with endometriosis, endometrial tissue is found outside the uterus. This tissue most often appears in the pelvis or abdominal cavity and rarely in distant areas such as the lungs or brain. This tissue also responds to cyclic hormonal signals. Since it is outside of the uterus and cannot be cast off each month, the tissue causes bleeding, with the formation of scars and adhesions. This is generally what causes daily or monthly cyclic pain.

Symptoms of endometriosis may include: blood in the urine, difficulty in urinating, **dyspareunia** (painful intercourse), heavy menstrual bleeding, irregular or more frequent periods, nausea and vomiting, pain with bowel movements, pelvic pain after intercourse or exercise, and spotty bleeding just before the period starts. The most common symptom of endometriosis is increasingly painful periods, or **dysmenorrhea**. The woman may experience a steady dull or severe pain in the lower abdomen, vagina, and/or back. This pain can begin 5 to 7 days before a period. After **menopause**, the symptoms subside as the abnormal tissue shrinks.

The cause of endometriosis is unknown. Several theories have been proposed such as delayed childbearing increases the risk for endometriosis and during menstruation, some of the endometrial tissue backs up through the fallopian tubes into the abdomen. Genetics may also play a role, with some women being more prone to endometriosis.

Diagnosis of endometriosis begins with a complete medical history and physical exam, including a pelvic exam. A **laparoscopy** may be performed to confirm the diagnosis.

Many women with endometriosis have no long-term problems. Others may have the following conditions: bowel obstruction, constant bladder or rectal pain, constant pelvic pain, damage to the kidneys and ureters, irritable bowel syndrome, and pelvic or abdominal adhesions. Thirty to 40 percent of women with endometriosis face infertility. Less than 1 percent of women with endometriosis develop endometrial cancer.

Early diagnosis and treatment may limit cell growth and help prevent adhesions, while pregnancy, oral contraceptives, and other hormones seem to delay its onset. Treatment with medications may focus on several strategies. Analgesic therapy, treating the discomfort of the disease only, may be indicated for women with mild to moderate premenstrual pain, with no pelvic examination abnormalities, and with no immediate desire to become pregnant.

Surgery (either laparoscopy or laparotomy) is usually reserved for women with severe endometriosis. Conservative surgery attempts to remove or destroy all of the outside endometriotic tissue, remove adhesions, and restore the pelvic anatomy to as close to normal as possible. More extensive surgery may be necessary for the woman with severe symptoms or disease, and no desire for future childbearing. This type of surgery involves surgical removal of the uterus (**hysterectomy**), both ovaries, both fallopian tubes, and any remaining adhesions or endometriotic implants. Hormonal replacement therapy may be used after removal of the ovaries.

Hysterectomy

A **hysterectomy** is a surgical procedure to remove a woman's uterus. Sometimes the fallopian tubes, ovaries, and cervix are removed at the same time the uterus is removed. If a woman hasn't yet reached menopause, a hysterectomy will stop her monthly bleeding (periods). She also won't be able to get pregnant.

There are several types of hysterectomy:

- A *complete* or *total hysterectomy* removes the cervix as well as the uterus. This is the most common type of hysterectomy.
- A *partial* or *subtotal hysterectomy* (also called a *supracervical hysterectomy*) removes the upper part of the uterus and leaves the cervix in place.
- A *radical hysterectomy* removes the uterus, the cervix, the upper part of the vagina, and supporting tissues. This is done in some cases of cancer.

Often one or both ovaries and fallopian tubes are removed at the same time a hysterectomy is done. When both ovaries and both tubes are removed, it is called a *bilateral salpingo-oophorectomy*.

If the ovaries are removed in a woman before she reaches menopause, the sudden loss of her main source of female hormones will cause her to suddenly enter menopause (*surgical menopause*). This can cause more severe symptoms than a natural menopause.

Hysterectomy is the second most common major surgery among women in the United States. (The most common major surgery that women have is cesarean section delivery.) Each year, more than 600,000 hysterectomies are done. About one third of women in the United States have had a hysterectomy by age 60.

Hysterectomies are done through a cut in the abdomen (abdominal hysterectomy) or the vagina (vaginal hysterectomy). Sometimes a laparoscope is used to view inside the abdomen. The type of surgery that is done depends on the reason for the surgery. Abdominal hysterectomies are more common than vaginal hysterectomies and usually require a longer recovery time. Hysterectomies are most often done for the following reasons:

- *Uterine fibroids*. Fibroids are common, benign (noncancerous) tumors that grow in the muscle of the uterus. More hysterectomies are done because of fibroids than any other problem of the uterus. Fibroids often cause no symptoms and need no treatment, and they usually shrink after menopause. But sometimes fibroids cause heavy bleeding or pain. There are alternatives to hysterectomy to treat fibroids, which may be especially important for younger women who hope to have children. Sometimes fibroids are treated with medicine or other treatments designed to shrink the fibroids. But, this is only temporary—when the medicine is stopped, the fibroids will grow again. A type of surgery to remove only the fibroids without removing the uterus is called a *myomectomy*.
- *Endometriosis*. This is another benign condition that affects the uterus. Endometriosis is the second leading reason for hysterectomies. It is most common in women in their thirties and forties, especially in women who have never been pregnant. It occurs when *endometrial* tissue begins to grow on the outside of the uterus and on nearby organs. Women with endometriosis are often treated with hormones and medicines that lower their levels of estrogen. A hysterectomy is generally not done unless other treatment has failed.

Cancers affecting the pelvic organs account for only about 10 percent of all hysterectomies. Endometrial cancer, uterine sarcoma, cervical cancer, and cancer of the ovaries or fallopian tubes often require hysterectomy. Depending on the type and extent of the cancer, other kinds of treatment such as radiation or hormonal therapy may be used as well.

Other reasons for hysterectomies include chronic pelvic pain, heavy bleeding during or between periods, and chronic pelvic inflammatory disease.

Pelvic Inflammatory Disease

Aside from AIDS, the most common and serious complication of sexually transmitted diseases (STDs) among women is **pelvic inflammatory disease** (PID). This condition is an infection of the upper genital area and occurs when disease-causing organisms migrate upward from the urethra and cervix into the upper genital area. PID can affect the uterus, ovaries, and fallopian tubes. If untreated this disease can cause scarring which can lead to infertility, tubal pregnancy, chronic pelvic pain, and other serious consequences. Women with recurrent episodes of PID are more likely than women with a single episode to suffer scarring of the fallopian tubes that leads to infertility, ectopic pregnancy, or chronic pelvic pain. Infertility occurs in approximately 20 percent of women who have had PID.

A woman who has had PID has a six- to tenfold increased risk of tubal pregnancy. In addition, untreated PID can cause chronic pelvic pain and scarring in about 20 percent of patients. These conditions are difficult to treat but are sometimes improved with surgery.

Another complication of PID is the risk of repeated attacks of PID. As many as one-third of women who have had PID will have the disease at least one more time. With each episode of reinfection, the risk of infertility is increased.

Each year in the United States, more than 1 million women experience an episode of acute PID, with the rate of infection highest among teenagers. More than 100,000 women become infertile each year as a result of this condition, and a large proportion of the 70,000 **ectopic** pregnancies occurring every year are due to the consequences of PID.

Many different organisms can cause PID, but most cases are associated with gonorrhea and genital chlamydial infections, two very common STDs. Scientists have found that bacteria normally present in small numbers in the vagina and cervix also may play a role.

Researchers are learning more about how these organisms cause PID. The gonococcus, *Neisseria gonorrhea*, probably travels to the fallopian tubes, where it causes sloughing (casting out) of some cells and invades others. Researchers think it multiplies within and beneath these cells. The infection then may spread to other organs, resulting in more inflammation and scarring. *Chlamydia trachomatis* and other bacteria may behave in a similar manner.

The major symptoms of PID are lower abdominal pain and abnormal vaginal discharge. Other symptoms such as fever, pain in the right upper abdomen, painful intercourse, and irregular menstrual bleeding can occur as well. PID, particularly when caused by chlamydial infection, may produce only minor symptoms or no symptoms at all, even though it can seriously damage the reproductive organs.

PID can be difficult to diagnose. If symptoms such as lower abdominal pain are present, the physician will perform a physical exam to determine the nature and location of the pain. The physician will also check the patient for fever, abnormal vaginal or cervical discharge, and evidence of cervical chlamydial infection or gonorrhea. If the findings of this exam suggest that PID is likely, current guidelines advise that treatment should be initiated.

To distinguish between PID and other serious problems that may mimic PID, other tests such as a sonogram, endometrial biopsy, or laparoscopy are ordered. Because cultures of specimens from the upper genital area are difficult to obtain and because multiple organisms may be responsible for an episode of PID, the physician will prescribe at least two antibiotics that are effective against a wide range of infectious agents. The symptoms may go away before the infection is cured. Even if symptoms do go away, patients should finish taking all of the medicine. Patients should be reevaluated by their physicians two to three days after treatment is begun to be sure the antibiotics are working to cure the infection.

About one-fourth of women with suspected PID must be hospitalized. The physician may recommend this if the patient is severely ill; if she cannot take oral medication and needs intravenous antibiotics; if she is pregnant or is an adolescent; if the diagnosis is uncertain and may include an abdominal emergency such as appendicitis; or if she is infected with HIV.

Many women with PID have sex partners who have no symptoms, although their sex partners may be infected with organisms that can cause PID. Because of the risk of reinfection, however, sex partners should be treated even if they do not have symptoms.

Women can play an active role in protecting themselves from PID by taking the following steps:

- Signs of discharge with odor or bleeding between cycles could mean infection. Early treatment may prevent the development of PID.

- If used correctly and consistently, male latex condoms will prevent transmission of gonorrhea and partially protect against chlamydial infection.

Preeclampsia and Eclampsia

Preeclampsia is a complication of pregnancy characterized by increasing hypertension, proteinuria, and edema. Preeclampsia develops in approximately 5 percent of pregnant women and usually occurs after the 20th week of pregnancy. This condition may be mild or severe.

Some experts believe that a problem with the placenta causes preeclampsia. The mother has spasms of the blood vessels, which increase her blood pressure. The blood flow to the placenta is impaired. If the blood pressure is not controlled, it can damage the placenta and cause death of the fetus. The high blood pressure can also affect the brain, kidneys, liver, and lungs. If the woman develops seizures or coma, the condition is known as eclampsia.

The symptoms of preeclampsia may include: agitation and confusion, changes in mental status, decreased urine output, headaches, nausea and vomiting, pain in the right upper part of the abdomen, shortness of breath, sudden weight gain over 1 to 2 days, swelling of the face or hands, visual impairment, and weight gain of more than 2 pounds per week.

Following are factors that increase a woman's risk of preeclampsia: African American ethnicity, age younger than 20 or older than 35, first pregnancy, low socioeconomic status, and multiple gestation such as twins or triplets.

Additional factors that increase the risk of preeclampsia are as follows: preeclampsia or eclampsia in previous pregnancies, diabetes, high blood pressure before pregnancy, underlying kidney disease, and if the mother or the baby's father was born of a pregnancy with preeclampsia or eclampsia.

There are no known ways to prevent preeclampsia. All pregnant women should have early prenatal care and blood pressure changes should be watched closely.

Eclampsia is a complication of severe preeclampsia that involves seizures. One in 200 pregnant women who have preeclampsia will develop eclampsia. Usually the seizures of eclampsia start before the baby is born. However, about 20 to 25 percent of the time, seizures begin within the first 24 hours after the baby is born. A few women develop seizures later, up to 3 weeks after the birth.

Women who have the symptoms of preeclampsia are at high risk for eclampsia. Usually there are no clues or warning signs before a seizure. A woman with eclampsia may have one or many seizures. The seizures cause muscle spasms, loss of consciousness, and short-term memory problems. Afterward, the woman may breathe very rapidly to make up for the lack of oxygen during the seizure itself. A fever at this point is a sign of serious trouble.

During or after a seizure, a woman may: bite her tongue, break bones, breathe fluids into her lungs, develop fluid and swelling in her lungs that make it hard to breathe, experience a detached retina in the eye, or harm her head.

It is not known why some women with preeclampsia develop the seizures associated with eclampsia. Theories about why seizures might occur in pregnancy involve: small clots that block blood vessels in the brain and restrict oxygen, narrowing of tiny arteries in the brain, areas of bleeding in the brain, high blood pressure, dietary risks, genetic risks, or a problem with the brain or nervous system.

Premenstrual Syndrome (PMS)

Premenstrual syndrome (PMS) is a condition that affects certain women and may cause distressful symptoms such as constipation, diarrhea, nausea, anorexia, appetite cravings, headache, backache, muscular aches, edema, insomnia, clumsiness, malaise, irritability, indecisiveness, mental confusion, and depression. These symptoms may begin 2 weeks before the onset of menstruation. Although the exact cause of this syndrome has not been determined, it may be due to the amount of prostaglandin produced, a deficient or excessive amount of estrogen or progesterone, or an interrelationship between these factors. See Figure 15–8.

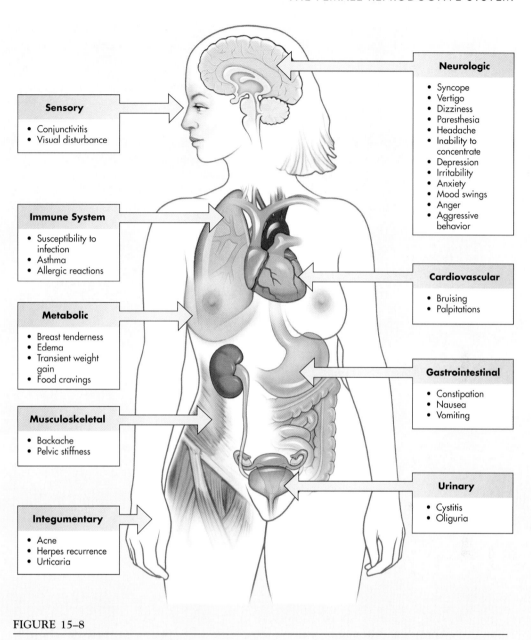

Sensory

- Conjunctivitis
- Visual disturbance

Immune System

- Susceptibility to infection
- Asthma
- Allergic reactions

Metabolic

- Breast tenderness
- Edema
- Transient weight gain
- Food cravings

Musculoskeletal

- Backache
- Pelvic stiffness

Integumentary

- Acne
- Herpes recurrence
- Urticaria

Neurologic

- Syncope
- Vertigo
- Dizziness
- Paresthesia
- Headache
- Inability to concentrate
- Depression
- Irritability
- Anxiety
- Mood swings
- Anger
- Aggressive behavior

Cardiovascular

- Bruising
- Palpitations

Gastrointestinal

- Constipation
- Nausea
- Vomiting

Urinary

- Cystitis
- Oliguria

FIGURE 15–8

Multisystem effects of premenstrual syndrome.

PMS is estimated to affect 85 percent of women who menstruate. However, only 5 percent to 10 percent of menstruating women are severely impaired by PMS. It is not known what makes PMS so severe in some women and mild in others.

The following lifestyle recommendations may help prevent PMS or relieve some of the symptoms:

- Eat a healthful diet which limits foods that are high in sodium, fat, caffeine, alcohol, and simple sugars.
- Get aerobic exercise on a regular basis.
- Get enough vitamins and minerals, especially the B vitamins, calcium, and magnesium.
- Use relaxation therapy and other stress management techniques.

Several herbal remedies, such as chasteberry and black cohosh, have been reported to relieve PMS. Women should discuss these options with their healthcare providers.

Medications used to treat PMS include the following:

- Antidepressant medicines, such as fluoxetine, that increase serotonin production
- Benzodiazepine medicines, such as alprazolam, that lower anxiety
- Danazol, a modified male hormone, which can decrease breast pain
- Diuretics, such as spironolactone and metolazone, which help the body excrete excess water and salts
- Hormones, such as nafarelin and leuprolide, which block the release of eggs from the ovaries
- Medicines that affect high prostaglandin levels, such as mefenamic acid, ibuprofen, and naproxen

Uterine Fibroids

Uterine fibroids are benign tumors or growths, made up of muscle cells and other tissues that grow within the wall of the uterus. Fibroids can grow as a single growth or in clusters (or groups). Their size can vary from small, like an apple seed (or less than one inch), to even larger than a grapefruit, or eight inches across or more.

Uterine fibroids are the most common, benign tumors in women of childbearing age, but no one knows exactly what causes them. They can be frustrating to live with because there are limited treatment options, and they are the cause of many hysterectomies.

Fibroids are classified into three groups based on where they grow, such as just underneath the lining of the uterus, in between the muscles of the uterus, or on the outside of the uterus. Most fibroids grow within the wall of the uterus. Some fibroids grow on stalks (called peduncles) that grow out from the surface of the uterus, or into the cavity of the uterus.

Most fibroids do not cause any symptoms, but some women with fibroids can have:

- Heavy bleeding or painful periods
- Bleeding between periods
- Feeling of fullness in the pelvic area (lower abdomen)
- Frequent urination
- Pain during sex
- Lower back pain
- Reproductive problems, such as infertility, or having early onset of labor during pregnancy

It is not known for sure what causes fibroids. Researchers have some theories, but most likely, fibroids are the result of many factors interacting with each other. These factors could be hormonal, genetic, environmental, or a combination of all three. For the most part, fibroids stop growing or shrink after menopause. But this is not true for all women with fibroids.

Fibroids are almost always benign, or not cancerous, and they rarely turn into cancer (less than 0.1 percent of cases). Having fibroids does not increase a woman's chances of getting cancer of the uterus.

Most of the time, fibroids grow in women of childbearing age. While no one knows for sure what will increase a woman's chances of getting fibroids, researchers have found that African American women are 2 to 3 times more likely to get them than are women of other racial groups. African American women also tend to get fibroids at an earlier age than do other women with fibroids. Women who are overweight or obese also are at a slightly higher risk for fibroids than women who are not overweight. Women who have given birth appear to be at a lower risk for fibroids.

Treatment for women with fibroids who have mild symptoms may only involve pain medication. Over-the-counter anti-inflammatory drugs (like Advil or Motrin) or other medications (like Tylenol) can be used for mild pain. Other drugs used to treat fibroids are called *gonadotropin releasing hormone agonists (GnRHa)*. These drugs can decrease the size of the fibroids. Sometimes they are used before surgery, to shrink the fibroids, making them easier to remove. Side effects can include hot flashes, depression, not being able to sleep, decreased sex drive, and joint pain. *Anti-hormonal agents*, such as a drug called mifepristone, also can stop or slow the growth of fibroids. These drugs only offer temporary relief from the symptoms of fibroids; once the drug therapy is discontinued, the fibroids often grow back.

Following are the types of surgery used to treat fibroids:

- *Myomectomy* is a surgery to remove fibroids without taking out the healthy tissue of the uterus. There are many ways a surgeon can perform this procedure. It can be major surgery (with an abdominal incision) or minor surgery. The type, size, and location of the fibroids will determine what type of procedure will be done.

- *Hysterectomy* is a surgery to remove the uterus, and is the only sure way to cure uterine fibroids. This surgery is used when a woman's fibroids are large, or if she has heavy bleeding, and is either near or past menopause and does not want children.

✓PATHOLOGY CHECKPOINT

Following is a concise list of the pathology-related terms that you've seen in the chapter. Review this checklist to make sure that you are familiar with the meaning of each term before moving on to the next section.

Conditions and Symptoms

- ❑ abortion
- ❑ amenorrhea
- ❑ bartholinitis
- ❑ cervicitis
- ❑ cystocele
- ❑ dysmenorrhea
- ❑ dyspareunia
- ❑ dystocia
- ❑ eclampsia
- ❑ ectopic pregnancy
- ❑ endometriosis
- ❑ fibroma
- ❑ mastitis
- ❑ menarche
- ❑ menorrhagia
- ❑ menorrhea
- ❑ mittelschmerz
- ❑ myometritis
- ❑ oligomenorrhea
- ❑ ovulation
- ❑ parturition

- ❑ pelvic inflammatory disease (PID)
- ❑ preeclampsia
- ❑ premenstrual syndrome (PMS)
- ❑ pseudocyesis
- ❑ quickening
- ❑ retroversion
- ❑ salpingitis
- ❑ secundines
- ❑ toxic shock syndrome
- ❑ uterine fibroid
- ❑ vaginitis
- ❑ venereal

Diagnosis and Treatment

- ❑ amniocentesis
- ❑ colposcope
- ❑ contraception
- ❑ culdocentesis
- ❑ diagnostic ultrasound
- ❑ Doppler ultrasound

- ❑ episiotomy
- ❑ gamete intrafallopian transfer (GIFT)
- ❑ genetics
- ❑ hymenectomy
- ❑ hysterectomy
- ❑ hysteroscope
- ❑ hysterotomy
- ❑ laser ablation
- ❑ laser laparoscopy
- ❑ laser lumpectomy
- ❑ lumpectomy
- ❑ mammoplasty
- ❑ mastectomy
- ❑ nonstress test
- ❑ oophorectomy
- ❑ ovum transfer
- ❑ pelvimetry
- ❑ salpingectomy
- ❑ salpingo-oophorectomy
- ❑ sonogram

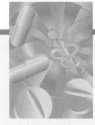

DRUG HIGHLIGHTS

Drugs that are generally used for the female reproductive system include hormones, contraceptives, and those used during labor and delivery.

Female Hormones

Estrogens

Are used for a variety of conditions. They may be used in the treatment of amenorrhea, dysfunctional bleeding, and hirsutism and in palliative therapy for breast cancer in women and prostatic cancer in men. They are also used as replacement therapy in the treatment of uncomfortable symptoms that are related to menopause.

Examples: Premarin (conjugated estrogens, USP), DES (diethylstilbestrol), Estrace (estradiol), Estraderm (estradiol) transdermal system, Ogen (estropipate), and Menest (esterified estrogens).

Progestogens/progestins

Synthetic preparations of progesterone. They are used to prevent uterine bleeding and are combined with estrogen for treatment of amenorrhea. They may be used in cases of infertility and threatened or habitual miscarriage. Progesterone is responsible for changes in the uterine endometrium during the second half of the menstrual cycle, development of maternal placenta after implantation, and development of mammary glands.

Examples: Provera (medroxyprogesterone acetate), Norlutin and Norlutate (norethindrone acetate), Ovrette (norgestrel) and Prometrium (natural progesterone).

Contraceptives

Oral

Nearly 100 percent effective when used as directed. These pills contain mixtures of estrogen and progestin in various levels of strength. The estrogen in the pill inhibits ovulation and the progestin inhibits pituitary secretion of luteinizing hormone (LH), causes changes in the cervical mucus that renders it unfavorable to penetration by sperm, and alters the nature of the endometrium.

Examples: Ortho-Novum 10/11, Triphasil, Micronor, Brevicon, Demulen, Lo/Ovral, Ovrette, Nelova 10/11, Alesse, and Nor-QD.

Birth Control Patch

Ortho Evra is the first transdermal birth control patch that continuously delivers two synthetic hormones, progestin (norelgestromin) and estrogen (ethinyl estradiol). The patch impedes pregnancy by preventing the ovaries from releasing eggs (ovulation) and it also thickens the cervical mucus. The patch is applied directly to the skin (buttocks, abdomen, upper torso or upper outer arm) and has an effectiveness rate of 95 percent.

Injectable

Depo-Provera is an injectable contraceptive that is given four times a year. It contains medroxyprogesterone acetate, a synthetic drug that's similar to progesterone. Depo-Provera prevents pregnancy by preventing the ovaries from releasing eggs (ovulation) and it also thickens the cervical mucus. When used correctly, it may prevent pregnancy more than 99 percent of the time.

Uterine Stimulants

Oxytocic agents (uterine stimulants) may be used in obstetrics to induce labor at term. They are also used to control postpartum hemorrhage and to induce therapeutic abortion.

Examples: Ergotate Maleate (ergonovine maleate), Pitocin (oxytocin), and Methergine (methylergonovine maleate).

Uterine Relaxants   May be administered to delay labor until the fetus has gained sufficient maturity as to be likely to survive outside the uterus.

Examples: Ethanol (ethyl alcohol) and Yutopar (ritodrine HCl).

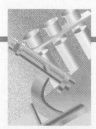

DIAGNOSTIC & LAB TESTS

TEST	DESCRIPTION
amniotic fluid analysis (ăm-nē-ŏt′ ĭk floo′ ĭd ă-năl′ ĭ-sĭs)	A procedure that involves the removal of amniotic fluid via a large needle. Ultrasound is used to give the location of the fetus, and then the needle is inserted into a suprapubic site of the mother. Abnormal results can indicate spina bifida, Down syndrome, hemophilia, hemolytic disease, and/or poor fetal maturity.
breast examination (brest ĕks-ăm″ ĭ-nā′ shŭn)	Visual inspection and manual examination of the breast for changes in contour, symmetry, "dimpling" of skin, retraction of the nipple(s), and for the presence of lumps.
chorionic villus sampling (CVS) (kō-rē-ŏn′ ĭk vĭl ŭs sam′ plĭng)	A procedure that involves the insertion of a catheter into the cervix and into the outer portion of the membranes surrounding the fetus. A sample of the chorionic villi can be examined for the chromosomal abnormalities and biochemical disorders. This procedure can be done 8 weeks into pregnancy.
colposcopy (kŏl-pŏs′ kō-pē)	Visual examination of the vagina and cervix via a colposcope. Abnormal results may indicate cervical or vaginal erosion, tumors, and dysplasia.
culdoscopy (kŭl-dŏs′ kō-pē)	Visual examination of the viscera of the female pelvis via a culdoscope. May be used in suspected ectopic pregnancy and unexplained pelvic pain, and to check for pelvic masses.
estrogens (es′ trō-jĕns)	A urine test or blood serum test to determine the level of estrone, estradiol, and estriol.
human chorionic gonadotropin (HCG) (hū′ măn kō-rē-ŏn′ ĭk gŏn″ ă-dō-trō′ pĭn)	A urine test or blood serum test to determine the presence of HCG. A positive result may indicate pregnancy.
hysterosalpingography (hĭs″ tĕr-ō-săl″ pĭn-gŏg′ ră-fē)	X-ray of the uterus and fallopian tubes after the injection of a radiopaque substance. Size and structure of the uterus and fallopian tubes can be evaluated. Uterine tumors, fibroids, tubal pregnancy, and tubal occlusion may be observed. Also used for treatment of an occluded fallopian tube.
laparoscopy (lăp-ăr-ŏs′ kō-pē)	Visual examination of the abdominal cavity via a laparoscope. Used to examine the ovaries and fallopian tubes.
mammography (măm-ŏg′ ră-fē)	The process of obtaining pictures of the breast by use of x-rays. This procedure is able to locate breast tumors before they grow to 1 cm. It is the most effective means of detecting early breast cancers.

TEST	DESCRIPTION
Papanicolaou (Pap smear) (păp′ ăh-nĭk″ ō-lă′ oo)	A screening technique to aid in the detection of cervical/uterine cancer and cancer precursors. It is not a diagnostic procedure. Both false-positive and false-negative results have been experienced with Pap smears. Any lesion should be biopsied unless not indicated clinically. The Pap smear should not be used as a sole means to diagnose or exclude malignant and premalignant lesions. It is a screening procedure only.
	Pap smear results are generally reported as: within normal limits (WNL); abnormal squamous cells of undetermined significance (Ascus); mild dysplasia (CIN I); moderate dysplasia (CIN II); and severe dysplasia and/or carcinoma-in-situ (CIN III).
pregnanediol (prĕg″ nān-dī-ŏl)	A urine test that determines menstrual disorders or possible abortion.
wet mat or wet-prep (wĕt măt or wĕt-prĕp)	Examination of vaginal discharge for the presence of bacteria and yeast. A vaginal smear is placed on a microscopic slide, wet with normal saline, and then viewed under a microscope by the physician.

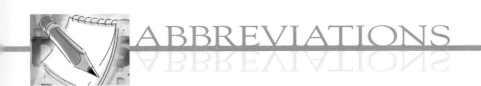

ABBREVIATIONS

ABBREVIATION	MEANING	ABBREVIATION	MEANING
AB	abortion	Gyn	gynecology
AFP	alpha-fetoprotein	HCG	human chorionic gonadotropin
AH	abdominal hysterectomy		
Ascus	atypical squamous cells of undetermined significance	HPV	human papillomavirus
		HRT	hormone replacement therapy
BBT	basal body temperature	HSG	hysterosalpingography
C-section	cesarean section	IUD	intrauterine device
CIN	cervical intraepithelial neoplasia	LH	luteinizing hormone
		LMP	last menstrual period
CIS	carcinoma-in-situ	MH	marital history
CS	cesarean section	OB	obstetrics
CVS	chorionic villus sampling	OC	oral contraceptive
D&C	dilation (dilatation) and curettage	Pap	Papanicolaou (smear)
		PID	pelvic inflammatory disease
DES	diethylstilbestrol	PMP	previous menstrual period
DUB	dysfunctional uterine bleeding	PMS	premenstrual syndrome
EDC	estimated date of confinement	TSS	toxic shock syndrome
FSH	follicle-stimulating hormone	UC	uterine contractions
GIFT	gamete intrafallopian transfer	WNL	within normal limits
grav I	pregnancy one		

STUDY AND REVIEW

Anatomy and Physiology

Write your answers to the following questions. Do not refer to the text.

1. List the primary and accessory sex organs of the female reproductive system.

   a. _____

   b. _____

   c. _____

   d. _____

   e. _____

   f. _____

2. State the vital function of the female reproductive system. _____

   _____

3. Name the three identifiable areas of the uterus.

   a. _____

   b. _____

   c. _____

4. Define fundus. _____

   _____

5. Name the ligaments that support the uterus and hold it in position.

   a. _____

   b. _____

   c. _____

   d. _____

6. Name the three layers of the uterine wall.

   a. _____

   b. _____

   c. _____

7. State the three primary functions associated with the uterus.

   a. _____

   b. _____

   c. _____

8. Define the following terms:

   a. Anteflexion _____

   _____

   b. Retroflexion _____

   _____

   c. Anteversion _____

   _____

   d. Retroversion _____

   _____

9. The fallopian tubes are also called the _____ _____

   or _____.

10. Name the three layers of the fallopian tubes.

   a. _____   b. _____

   c. _____

11. Define fimbriae. _____

   _____

12. Should the ovum become impregnated by a spermatozoon while in the fallopian

   tube, the process of _____ occurs.

13. State two functions of the fallopian tubes.

   a. _____   b. _____

   c. _____

14. Describe the ovaries. _____

   _____

15. Name the three stages of an ovarian follicle.

   a. _____   b. _____

   c. _____

16. The functional activity of the ovary is controlled by the _____.

17. State the two functions of the ovary.

   a. _____   b. _____

18. The vagina is a _____ tube extending from the _____ to the uterus.

19. State the three functions of the vagina.

    a. _____   b. _____

    c. _____

20. Name the organs that comprise the external female genitalia.

    a. _____   b. _____

    c. _____   d. _____

    e. _____

21. Between the vulva and the anus is an external region known as the

    _____.

22. Define episiotomy. _____

    _____

23. The breasts or _____ _____ are compound alveolar struc-
    tures.

24. The _____ is the dark pigmented area found in the skin over each

    breast and the _____ is the elevated area in its center.

25. Name the three hormones that play a role in milk production.

    a. _____   b. _____

    c. _____

26. Define colostrum. _____

    _____

27. Name the four phases of the menstrual cycle.

    a. _____   b. _____

    c. _____   d. _____

28. Define premenstrual syndrome. _____

    _____

    _____

Word Parts

1. In the spaces provided, write the definitions of these prefixes, roots, combining forms, and suffixes. Do not refer to the listings of medical words. Leave blank those words you cannot define.

2. After completing as many as you can, refer to the medical word listings to check your work. For each word missed or left blank, write the word and its definition several times on the margins of these pages or on a separate sheet of paper.

3. To maximize the learning process, it is to your advantage to do the following exercises as directed. To refer to the word building section before completing these exercises invalidates the learning process.

PREFIXES

Give the definitions of the following prefixes:

1. a- _____

2. ec- _____

3. ante- _____

4. con- _____

5. contra- _____

6. dys- _____

7. endo- _____

8. intra- _____

9. multi- _____

10. neo- _____

11. nulli- _____

12. oligo- _____

13. par- _____

14. peri- _____

15. post- _____

16. pre- _____

17. primi- _____

18. pseudo- _____

19. retro- _____

20. tri- _____

ROOTS AND COMBINING FORMS

Give the definition of the following roots and combining forms:

1. abort _____

2. amni/o _____

3. bartholin _____

4. cept _____

5. cervic _____

6. coit _____

7. colp/o _____

8. culd/o _____

9. cyst/o _____

10. episi/o _____

11. eunia _____

12. fibr _____

13. genital_____

14. gynec/o _____

15. bi/o _____

16. hymen _____

17. hyster _____

18. hyster/o _____

19. log _____

20. mamm/o _____

21. mast _____

22. men _____

23. men/o_____

24. mester _____

25. metr _____

26. metr/i _____

27. my/o _____

28. nat _____

29. nat/o _____

30. o/o _____

31. oophor _____

32. ovulat_____

33. para_____

34. partum_____

35. pause_____

36. pelv/i _____

37. blast/o_____

38. lamp(s)_____

39. rect/o _____

40. salping _____

41. salping/o _____

42. ectop _____

43. genet_____

44. uter_____

45. vagin _____

46. venere _____

47. vers _____

48. lump_____

49. arche_____

50. parturit_____

51. gravida _____

52. pudend _____

53. secund _____

54. son/o _____

55. surrog _____

SUFFIXES

Give the definitions of the following suffixes:

1. -al_____

2. -ate_____

3. -cele_____

4. -centesis_____

5. -cyesis _____

6. -ectomy_____

7. -genesis_____

8. -gram_____

9. -ia_____

10. -ine _____

11. -ion _____

12. -ist_____

13. -itis_____

14. -logy_____

15. -metry_____

16. -oma_____

17. -osis_____

18. -plasty _____

19. -rrhagia_____

20. -cyst _____

21. -rrhea _____

22. -scope _____

23. -ic_____

24. -tomy_____

25. -oid _____

26. -tic(s) _____

Identifying Medical Terms

In the spaces provided, write the medical terms for the following meanings:

1. _____ The process of miscarrying

2. _____ The time before the onset of labor

3. _____ Inflammation of the uterine cervix

4. _____ A difficult or painful monthly flow

5. _____ A fibrous tissue tumor

6. _____ The study of the female

7. _____ Surgical excision of the hymen

8. _____ Surgical repair of the breast

9. _____ A normal monthly flow

10. _____ Pertaining to the first 4 weeks after birth

11. _____ Formation of the ovum

12. _____ Pertaining to after childbirth

Spelling

In the spaces provided, write the correct spelling of these misspelled words:

1. amiocentesis _____

2. bartolinitis _____

3. dytocia _____

4. epsiotomy _____

5. hystrotomy_____

6. menorhagia_____

7. oophritis_____

8. salpinitis_____

9. vajinitis _____

10. veneral_____

Matching

Select the appropriate lettered meaning for each word listed below.

_____ 1. gamete intrafallopian transfer

_____ 2. laser ablation

_____ 3. lumpectomy

_____ 4. menarche

_____ 5. mittelschmerz

_____ 6. morula

_____ 7. ovulation

_____ 8. parturition

_____ 9. pudendal

_____10. quickening

a. A solid mass of cells resulting from cell division after fertilization of an ovum

b. Pertaining to the external female genitalia

c. The beginning of the monthly flow; menses

d. Surgical removal of a tumor from the breast

e. Abdominal pain that occurs midway between the menstrual periods at ovulation

f. A procedure that places the sperm and eggs directly in the fimbriated end of the fallopian tube

g. The process in which an ovum is discharged from the cortex of the ovary

h. The act of giving birth

i. The first movement of the fetus felt in the uterus, occurring during the 16th to 20th week of pregnancy

j. A procedure that uses a laser to destroy the uterine lining

k. The fertilized ovum

Abbreviations

Place the correct word, phrase, or abbreviation in the space provided.

1. AB _____

2. alpha-fetoprotein _____

3. AH _____

4. cesarean section _____

5. DES _____

6. estimated date of confinement _____

7. grav I _____

8. Gyn _____

9. intrauterine device _____

10. pelvic inflammatory disease _____

Diagnostic and Laboratory Tests

Select the best answer to each multiple choice question. Circle the letter of your choice.

1. A procedure that involves the insertion of a catheter into the cervix and into the outer portion of the membranes surrounding the fetus.
   a. amniotic fluid analysis
   b. chorionic villus sampling
   c. colposcopy
   d. culdoscopy

2. A positive result may indicate pregnancy.
   a. colposcopy
   b. culdoscopy
   c. HCG
   d. laparoscopy

3. X-ray of the uterus and fallopian tubes after the injection of a radiopaque substance.
   a. hysterosalpingography
   b. laparoscopy
   c. culdoscopy
   d. mammography

4. Used to examine the ovaries and fallopian tubes.
   a. colposcopy
   b. culdoscopy
   c. laparoscopy
   d. mammography

5. The process of obtaining pictures of the breast by use of x-rays.
   a. colposcopy
   b. culdoscopy
   c. laparoscopy
   d. mammography

CASE STUDY   MENOPAUSE

Read the following case study and then answer the questions that follow.

A 52-year-old female was seen by a physician and the following is a synopsis of the visit.

Present History: The patient states that her periods have become very irregular, that she has hot flashes and trouble sleeping, that sex with her husband has become uncomfortable, and that she is very moody.

Signs and Symptoms: Irregular periods, hot flashes, insomnia, dyspareunia, and emotional instability.

Diagnosis: Menopause. The diagnosis was determined by a complete gynecologic examination.

Treatment: The patient was given the opportunity to receive hormone replacement therapy or to try a non-prescription treatment regimen. She decided to try the nonprescription treatment and then to be reevaluated in six months.

Nonprescription Regimen

- **Exercise.** Aerobic, weight bearing, and/or stretching exercises at least thirty minutes to an hour, four to five times a week.
- **Diet.** High in fruits and vegetables and low in saturated fat. To include four to six servings of soy products, foods such as soybeans, tofu, soymilk and roasted soy nuts daily. Soy contains phytoestrogens which are similar to estrogen and isoflavones. Blueberries and cherries also contain bioflavonoids which are a source of phytoestrogens. Flaxseeds and flaxseed oil are lignans—also phytoestrogens—and can help relieve hot flashes and vaginal dryness. These lignans also can have a stabilizing effect on hormone-related mood swings. It is also recommended that she reduce the intake of caffeine, alcohol, hot beverages, and spicy foods.
- **FYI: Phyto is the combining form for plant.** The phytoestrogens, isoflavones, and lignans are important secondary nutrients contained in soybeans and linseed. Isoflavones are a type of phytoestrogen, compounds that have weak estrogenic activity.

There are many types of phytoestrogens and not all are in edible plants. Isoflavones are found in chickpeas and legumes. The legume soy has the most concentrated amount. Lignans are often considered a type of fiber, but are more appropriately considered as a type of phytoestrogen or a plant compound with estrogen-like activity. Bioflavonoids refers to a class of water-soluble plant pigments believed to have favorable medicinal qualities.

- **Vaginal products.** As a lubricant for intercourse and moisturizer for vaginal dryness, she may use over-the-counter creams that do not contain estrogen.
- **Herbal treatments.** If so desired, to see an herbalist for herbal products rich in phytoestrogens.
- **Dietary supplements.** Take a multivitamin and mineral complex that contains 400 micrograms of folic acid. Also take 1200 milligrams of calcium daily and an antioxidant.
- **Not smoking.**
- **Reduce weight as needed.**

Prevention: There are no known preventive measures.

CASE STUDY QUESTIONS

1. Symptoms of menopause include irregular periods, hot flashes, insomnia, _____, and emotional instability.
2. The diagnosis was determined by a complete _____ examination.
3. The patient choose a nonprescription treatment regimen which included exercise, _____, vaginal products, and _____.
4. What product does soy contain that is similar to estrogen? _____
5. What effect can lignans have on hormone-related mood swings? _____

MedMedia
Wrap-Up
www.prenhall.com/rice

Additional interactive resources and activities for this chapter can be found on the Companion Website. For animations, videos, audio glossary, and review, access the accompanying CD-ROM in this book.

Audio Glossary
Medical Terminology Exercises & Activities
Pathology Spotlight
Terminology Translator
Animations
Videos

Objectives
Medical Terminology Exercises & Activities
Audio Glossary
Drug Updates
Medical Terminology in the News

THE MALE REPRODUCTIVE SYSTEM

16

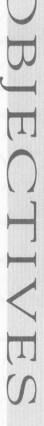

OBJECTIVES

On completion of this chapter, you will be able to:

- Describe the male's external organs of reproduction.
- Describe and state the functions of the testes, epididymis, ductus deferens, seminal vesicles, prostate gland, bulbourethral glands, and urethra.
- Analyze, build, spell, and pronounce medical words.
- Describe each of the conditions presented in the Pathology Spotlights.
- Complete the Pathology Checkpoint.
- Review Drug Highlights presented in this chapter.
- Provide the description of diagnostic and laboratory tests related to the male reproductive system.
- Identify and define selected abbreviations.
- Successfully complete the study and review section.

MedMedia
www.prenhall.com/rice

Additional interactive resources and activities for this chapter can be found on the Companion Website. For Terminology Translator, animations, videos, audio glossary, and review, access the accompanying CD-ROM in this book.

Anatomy and Physiology Overview

The male reproductive system consists of the **testes, various ducts,** the **urethra,** and the following accessory glands: **bulbourethral, prostate,** and the **seminal vesicles.** The supporting structures and accessory sex organs are the **scrotum** and the **penis** (Fig. 16–1). The vital function of the male reproductive system is to provide the sperm cells necessary to fertilize the ovum, thereby perpetuating the species. The following is a general overview of the organs and functions of this system.

EXTERNAL ORGANS

In the male, the scrotum and the penis are the external organs of reproduction.

The Scrotum

The **scrotum** is a pouch-like structure located behind the penis. It is suspended from the perineal region and is divided by a septum into two sacs, each containing one of the testes along with its connecting tube called the **epididymis**. Within the tissues of the scrotum are fibers of smooth muscle that contract in the absence of sufficient heat, giving the scrotum a wrinkled appearance. This contractile action brings the testes closer to the perineum where they can absorb sufficient body heat to maintain the viability of the **spermatozoa**. Under normal conditions, the walls of the scrotum are generally free of wrinkles, and it hangs loosely between the thighs (Fig. 16–1).

The Penis

The **penis** is the external male sex organ and is composed of erectile tissue covered with skin. The size and shape of the penis varies, with an average erect penis being 15 to 20

THE MALE REPRODUCTIVE SYSTEM

Organ/Structure	Primary Functions
Scrotum	Contains testes and connecting tubes; contractile action brings the testes closer to the perineum, where they can absorb sufficient body heat to maintain the viability of the spermatozoa
Penis	Male organ of copulation; site of the orifice for the elimination of urine and semen from the body
Testes	Contains seminiferous tubules that are the site of the development of spermatozoa; cells within the testes also produce the male sex hormone, testosterone
Epididymis	Storage site for the maturation of sperm
Ductus Deferens or Vas Deferens	Excretory duct of the testis
Seminal Vesicles	Produce a slightly alkaline fluid that becomes a part of the seminal fluid or semen
Prostate Gland	Secretes an alkaline fluid that aids in maintaining the viability of spermatozoa
Bulbourethral or Cowper's Glands	Produce a mucous secretion before ejaculation, which becomes a part of the semen
Urethra	Transmits urine and semen out of the body

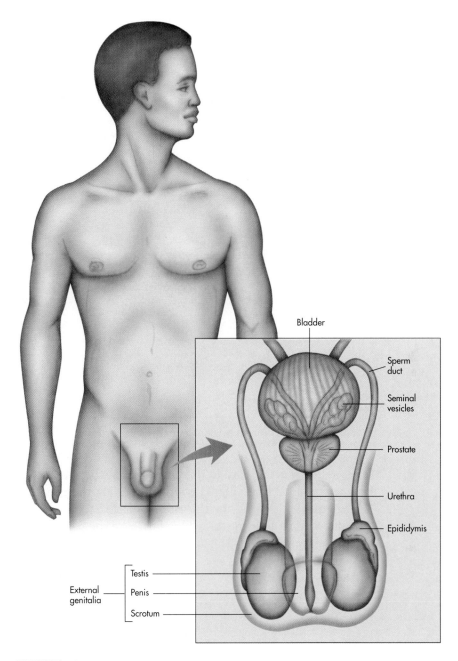

FIGURE 16–1

The male reproductive system: seminal vesicles, prostate, urethra, sperm duct, epididymis, and external genitalia.

cm in length. The penis has three longitudinal columns of erectile tissue that are capable of significant enlargement when engorged with blood, as is the case during sexual stimulation. Two of these columns, located side by side, form the greater part of the penis. These columns are known as the *corpora cavernosa penis*. The third longitudinal column, the *corpus spongiosum,* has the same function as the first two columns but is transversed by the penile portion of the urethra and tends to be more elastic when in an erectile state. The *corpus spongiosum,* at its distal end, expands to form the *glans penis*. The glans penis is the cone-shaped head of the penis and is the site of the urethral orifice. It is covered with loose skin folds called the **foreskin** or prepuce. See Figure 16–2. The foreskin contains glands that secrete a lubricating fluid called *smegma*. The foreskin may be removed by a surgical procedure known as **circumcision**.

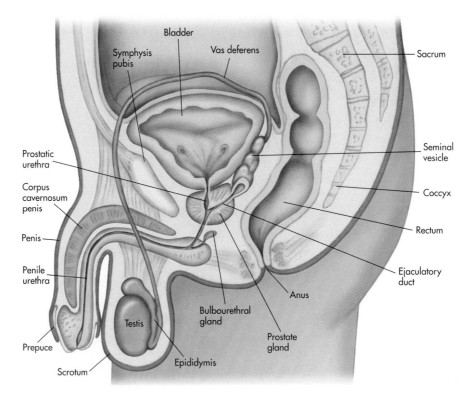

FIGURE 16–2

Sagittal section of the male pelvis, showing the organs of the reproductive system.

The erectile state in the penis results when sexual stimulation causes large quantities of blood from dilated arteries supplying the penis to fill the cavernous spaces in the erectile tissue. When the arteries constrict, the pressure on the veins in the area is reduced, thus allowing more blood to leave the penis than enters, and the penis returns to its normal state. The functions of the penis are to serve as the male organ of **copulation** and as the site of the orifice for the elimination of urine and semen from the body.

THE TESTES

The male has two ovoid-shaped organs, the **testes**, located in the scrotum. Each testis is about 4 cm long and 2.5 cm wide. The interior of each testis is divided into about 250 wedge-shaped lobes by fibrous tissues. Coiled within each lobe are one to three small tubes called the **seminiferous tubules**. These tubules are the site of the development of male reproductive cells, the **spermatozoa**. Cells within the testes also produce the male sex hormone, **testosterone**, which is responsible for the development of secondary male characteristics during puberty. Testosterone is essential for normal growth and development of the male accessory sex organs. It plays a vital role in the erection process of the penis, and thus, is necessary for the reproductive act, copulation. Additionally, it affects the growth of hair on the face, muscular development, and vocal timbre. The *seminiferous tubules* form a plexus or network called the rete testis from which 15 to 20 small ducts, the efferent ductules, leave the testis and open into the epididymis (Figs. 16–1 and 16–2).

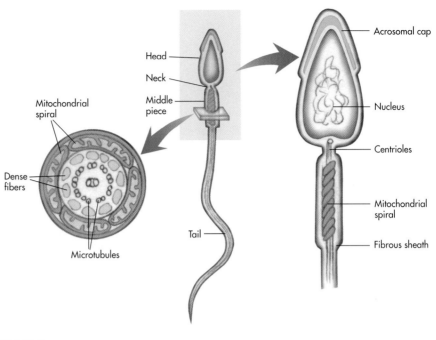

FIGURE 16–3

The basic structure of a spermatozoon (sperm).

THE EPIDIDYMIS

Each testis is connected by efferent ductules to an **epididymis**, which is a coiled tube lying on the posterior aspect of the testis. The epididymis is between 13 and 20 feet in length but is coiled into a space less than 2 inches (5 cm) long and ends in the ductus deferens. Each epididymis functions as a storage site for the maturation of **sperm** (Fig. 16–3) and as the first part of the duct system through which sperm pass on their journey to the urethra (see Figs. 16–1 and 16–2).

THE DUCTUS DEFERENS OR VAS DEFERENS

The **ductus deferens** is a slim muscular tube, about 45 cm in length, and is a continuation of the epididymis. It has been described as the *excretory duct* of the testis and extends from a point adjacent to the testis to enter the abdomen through the inguinal canal. It is later joined by the duct from the seminal vesicle. Between the testis and the part of the abdomen known as the internal inguinal ring, the ductus deferens is contained within a structure known as the **spermatic cord**. The spermatic cord also contains arteries, veins, lymphatic vessels, and nerves (see Fig. 16–4).

THE SEMINAL VESICLES

There are two **seminal vesicles**, each connected by a narrow duct to a ductus deferens, which then forms a short tube, the **ejaculatory duct**, that penetrates the base of the prostate gland and opens into the prostatic portion of the urethra. The seminal vesicles

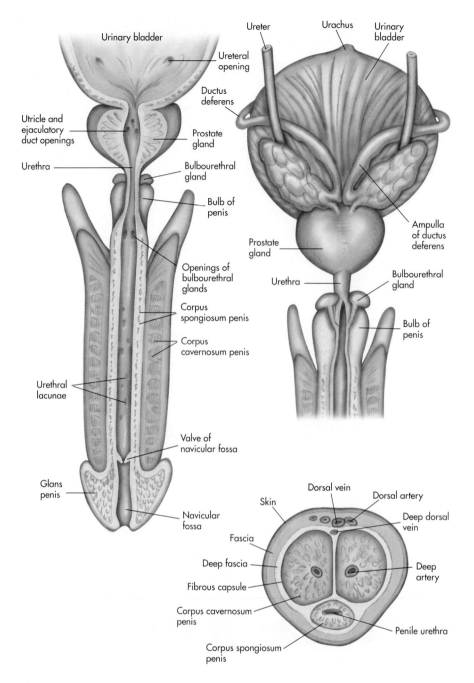

FIGURE 16–4

The structures of the bladder, prostate gland, and penis.

produce a slightly alkaline fluid that becomes a part of the seminal fluid or semen (see Fig. 16–4).

THE PROSTATE GLAND

The **prostate gland** is about 4 cm wide and weighs about 20 g. It is composed of glandular, connective, and muscular tissue and lies behind the urinary bladder. It surrounds the first 2.5 cm of the urethra and secretes an alkaline fluid that aids in maintaining the viability of spermatozoa. Enlargement of the prostate (**benign prostatic hyperplasia**) is a condition that sometimes occurs in older men. In this condition, the prostate obstructs the urethra and causes interference with the normal passage of urine. When this occurs, a **prostatectomy** may be performed to remove a part of the gland. The prostate gland may also be a site for cancer in older men (see Fig. 16–4).

THE BULBOURETHRAL OR COWPER'S GLANDS

The **bulbourethral glands** are two small pea-sized glands located below the prostate and on either side of the urethra. A duct about 2.5 cm long connects them with the wall of the urethra. The bulbourethral glands produce a mucous secretion before ejaculation, which becomes a part of the semen (see Fig. 16–4).

THE URETHRA

The male **urethra** is approximately 20 cm long and is divided into three sections: prostatic, membranous, and penile. It extends from the urinary bladder to the external urethral orifice at the head of the penis. It serves the function of transmitting urine and semen out of the body (see Fig. 16–4).

LIFE SPAN CONSIDERATIONS

■ THE CHILD

In the newborn, the **testicles** may appear large at birth. They may fail to descend into the scrotum, causing a condition, **cryptorchism.** The foreskin of the penis may be tight at birth, causing **phimosis,** a condition of narrowing of the opening of the prepuce wherein the foreskin cannot be drawn back over the glans penis.

Puberty is defined as a period of rapid change in the lives of boys and girls during which time the reproductive systems mature and become functionally capable of reproduction. In the male, puberty begins around 12 years of age, when the genitals start to increase in size and the shoulders broaden and become muscular. As testosterone is released, secondary sexual characteristics develop, such as pubic and axillary hair, increase in size of the penis and testes, voice changes, facial hair, erections, and nocturnal emissions.

■ THE OLDER ADULT

With aging, the **prostate gland** enlarges and its glandular secretions decrease, the **testes** become smaller and more firm, there is a gradual decrease in the production of **testosterone,** and pubic hair becomes sparser and stiffer. This period of change in the male has been referred to as the "male climacteric" and may be associated with symptoms such as hot flashes, feelings of suffocation, insomnia, irritability, and emotional instability. Testosterone replacement therapy may be recommended for the male climacteric.

In a healthy, normal male, **spermatogenesis** and the ability to have erections lasts a lifetime. However, sexual arousal may be slowed, with a longer refractory period between erections. In men, a "refractory period" is a time after one orgasm during which they are not physically able to have another one. See Pathology Spotlight: Erectile Dysfunction for more information.

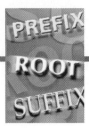

BUILDING YOUR MEDICAL VOCABULARY

This section provides the foundation for learning medical terminology. Medical words can be made up of four different types of word parts:

- Prefixes (P)
- Roots (R)
- Combining forms (CF)
- Suffixes (S)

By connecting various word parts in an organized sequence, thousands of words can be built and learned. In this text the word list is alphabetized so one can see the variety of meanings created when common prefixes and suffixes are repeatedly applied to certain word roots and/or combining forms. Words shown in pink are additional words related to the content of this chapter that are not built from word parts. These words are included to enhance your vocabulary. Note: an asterisk icon (✱) indicates words that are covered in the Pathology Spotlights section in this chapter.

MEDICAL WORD	WORD PARTS (WHEN APPLICABLE)			DEFINITION
	Part	**Type**	**Meaning**	
anorchism (ăn-ōr′ kĭzm)	an	P	lack of	A condition in which there is a lack of one or both testes
	orch	R	testicle	
	-ism	S	condition of	
artificial insemination (ăr″ tĭ-físh′ ăl ĭn-sĕm″ ĭn-ā′ shŭn)	artific/i	CF	not natural	The process of artificial placement of semen into the vagina so that conception may take place
	-al	S	pertaining to	
	in	P	into	
	seminat	R	seed	
	-ion	S	process	
aspermia (ă-spĕr′ mē-ă)	a	P	lack of	A condition in which there is a failure to form semen
	sperm	R	seed	
	-ia	S	condition of	
azoospermia (ă-zō″ ō-spĕr′ mē-ă)	a	P	lack of	A condition in which there is a lack of spermatozoa in the semen
	zo/o	CF	animal	
	sperm	R	seed	
	-ia	S	condition	
balanitis (băl″ ă-nī′ tĭs)	balan	R	glans	Inflammation of the glans penis
	-itis	S	inflammation	
benign prostatic hyperplasia (bē-nīn′ prŏs-tăt′-ĭk hī″ pĕr-plā′zē-ă)				An enlargement of the prostate gland. ✱ See Pathology Spotlight: Benign Prostatic Hyperplasia.

MEDICAL WORD	WORD PARTS (WHEN APPLICABLE)			DEFINITION
	Part	**Type**	**Meaning**	
castrate (kăs′ trāt)	castr -ate	R S	to prune use	To remove the testicles or ovaries; *to geld, to spay*
circumcision (sĕr″ kŭm-sĭ′ shŭn)	circum cis -ion	P R S	around to cut process	The surgical process of removing the foreskin of the penis
cloning (klōn′ ing)				The process of creating a genetic duplicate of an individual organism through asexual reproduction
coitus (kō′ ĭ-tŭs)				Sexual intercourse between a man and a woman
condom (kŏn′ dŭm)				A thin, flexible protective sheath, usually rubber, worn over the penis during copulation to help prevent impregnation or venereal disease
condyloma (kŏn″ dĭ-lō′ mă)				A wart-like growth of the skin, most often seen on the external genitalia; is either viral or syphilitic in origin
cryptorchism (krĭpt-ōr′ kĭzm)	crypt orch -ism	R R S	hidden testicle condition of	A condition in which the testes fail to descend into the scrotum
ejaculation (ē-jăk″ ū-lā′ shŭn)	ejaculat -ion	R S	to throw out process	The process of expulsion of seminal fluid from the male urethra
epididymectomy (ĕp″ ĭ-dĭd″ ĭ-mĕk′ tō-mē)	epi didym -ectomy	P R S	upon testis excision	Surgical excision of the epididymis
epididymitis (ĕp″ ĭ-dĭd″ ĭ-mī′ tĭs)	epi didym -itis	P R S	upon testis inflammation	Inflammation of the epididymis
epispadias (ĕp″ ĭ-spā′ dĭ-ăs)	epi spadias	P R	upon a rent, an opening	A congenital defect in which the urethra opens on the dorsum of the penis. See Figure 16–5.
erectile dysfunction (ĕ-rĕk′ tīl dĭs-fŭnk′ shŭn)				Involves the inability to achieve and maintain penile erection sufficient to complete satisfactory intercourse. ✱ See Pathology Spotlight: Erectile Dysfunction.

MEDICAL WORD	WORD PARTS (WHEN APPLICABLE)			DEFINITION
	Part	Type	Meaning	
Ericsson sperm separation method (er' ik-son sperm sĕp" ă-rā' shŭn mĕth od)				A process of separating the Y-chromosome sperm from the X-chromosome sperm. A sperm sample is taken and placed in a tube of albumin. Those that survive are Y-chromosome sperm, which make male babies. Women inseminated with these sperm have a 75 to 80% chance of producing a male child.
eugenics (ū-jĕn' ĭks)	eu -genic(s)	P S	good formation, produce	The study and control of the bringing forth of offspring as a means of improving genetic characteristics of future generations
eunuch (ū' nŭk)				A male who has been castrated, i.e., had his testicles removed
gamete (găm' ēt)				A mature reproductive cell of the male or female; *a spermatozoon or ovum*
gonorrhea (gŏn" ŏ-rē' ă)	gon/o -rrhea	CF S	genitals flow	A highly contagious venereal disease of the genital mucous membrane of either sex; the infection transmitted by the gonococcus *Neisseria gonorrhoeae*
gynecomastia (jī" nĕ-kō-măs' tĭ-ă)	gynec/o mast -ia	CF R S	female breast condition of	A condition of excessive development of the mammary glands in the male
herpes genitalis (hĕr' pēz jĕn-ĭ-tăl' ĭs)				A highly contagious venereal disease of the genitalia of either sex; caused by herpes simplex virus-2 (HSV-2)
heterosexual (hĕt" ĕr-ō-sĕk' shū-ăl)	hetero sexu -al	P R S	different sex pertaining to	Pertaining to the opposite sex; refers to an individual who has a sexual preference for the opposite sex
homosexual (hō" mō-sĕks' ū-ăl)	homo sexu -al	P R S	similar, same sex pertaining to	Pertaining to the same sex; refers to an individual who has a sexual preference for the same sex
hydrocele (hī' drō-sēl)	hydro -cele	P S	water hernia	A collection of serous fluid in a sac-like cavity, specifically the tunica vaginalis testis
hypospadias (hī" pō-spă' dĭ-ăs)	hypo spadias	P R	under a rent, an opening	A congenital defect in which the urethra opens on the underside of the penis

MEDICAL WORD	WORD PARTS (WHEN APPLICABLE)			DEFINITION
	Part	Type	Meaning	
infertility (ĭn″ fĕr-tĭl′ ĭ-tē)				The inability to produce a viable offspring
mitosis (mī-tō′ sĭs)	mit -osis	R S	thread condition of	The ordinary condition of cell division
oligospermia (ŏl″ ĭ-gō-spĕr′ -mĭ-ă)	oligo sperm -ia	P R S	scanty seed condition	A condition in which there is a scanty amount of spermatozoa in the semen
orchidectomy (or″ kĭ-dĕk′ tō-mē)	orchid -ectomy	R S	testicle excision	Surgical excision of a testicle
orchidotomy (or″ kĭd-ŏt′ ō-mē)	orchid/o -tomy	CF S	testicle incision	Incision into a testicle
orchitis (or-kī′ tĭs)	orch -itis	R S	testicle inflammation	Inflammation of a testicle
parenchyma (păr-ĕn′ kĭ-mă)	par enchyma	P R	beside to pour	The essential cells of a gland or organ that are concerned with its function
penitis (pē-nī′ tĭs)	pen -itis	R S	penis inflammation	Inflammation of the penis
phimosis (fī-mō′ sĭs)	phim -osis	R S	a muzzle condition of	A condition of narrowing of the opening of the prepuce wherein the foreskin cannot be drawn back over the glans penis
prepuce (prē′ pūs)				The foreskin over the glans penis in the male
prostate cancer (prŏs′ tāt kăn′ sĕr)				A malignant tumor of the prostate gland. ✱ See Pathology Spotlight: Prostate Cancer.
prostatectomy (prŏs″ tă-tĕk′ tō-mē)	prostat -ectomy	R S	prostate excision	Surgical excision of the prostate
prostatitis (prŏs″ tă-tī′ tĭs)	prostat -itis	R S	prostate inflammation	Inflammation of the prostate
puberty (pū′ ber-tē)				The stage of development in the male and female when secondary sex characteristics begin to develop and become functionally capable of reproduction
semen (sē′ mĕn)				The fluid-transporting medium for spermatozoa discharged during ejaculation

MEDICAL WORD	WORD PARTS (WHEN APPLICABLE)			DEFINITION
	Part	**Type**	**Meaning**	
spermatoblast (spĕr-măt′ ō-blăst)	spermat/o -blast	CF S	seed, sperm immature cell, germ cell	The sperm germ cell
spermatogenesis (spĕr″ măt-ō-jĕn′ ĕ-sĭs)	spermat/o -genesis	CF S	seed, sperm formation, produce	Formation of spermatozoa
spermatozoon (spĕr″ măt-ō-zō′ ŏn)	spermat/o zoon	CF R	seed, sperm life	The male sex cell. *The plural form is spermatozoa.*
spermicide (spĕr′ mĭ-sīd)	sperm/i -cide	CF S	seed, sperm to kill	An agent that kills sperm
syphilis (sĭf′ ĭ-lĭs)				A chronic infectious venereal disease caused by *Treponema pallidum,* which is transmitted sexually
testicular (tĕs-tĭk′ ū-lar)	testicul -ar	R S	testicle pertaining to	Pertaining to a testicle
trisomy (trī′ sōm-ē)	tri som -y	P R S	three body pertaining to	A genetic condition of having three chromosomes instead of two. The condition causes various birth defects.
varicocele (văr′ ĭ-kō-sēl)	varic/o -cele	CF S	twisted vein hernia	An enlargement and twisting of the veins of the spermatic cord
vasectomy (văs-ĕk′ tō-mē)	vas -ectomy	R S	vessel excision	Surgical excision of the vas deferens. ✱ See Pathology Spotlight: Vasectomy.
vesiculitis (vĕ-sĭk″ ū-lī′ tĭs)	vesicul -itis	R S	vesicle inflammation	Inflammation of a vesicle; in particular, the seminal vesicle

Terminology Translator

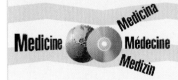

This feature, found on the accompanying CD-ROM, provides an innovative tool to translate medical words into Spanish, French, and German.

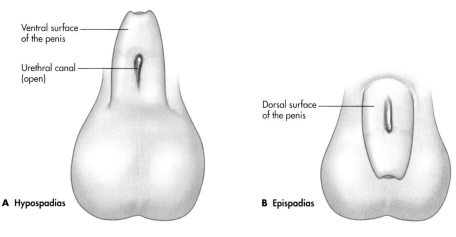

A Hypospadias

Ventral surface
of the penis

Urethral canal
(open)

B Epispadias

Dorsal surface
of the penis

FIGURE 16–5

Hypospadias and epispadias. (A) In hypospadias the urethral canal is open on the ventral surface of the penis. (B) In epispadias the canal is open on the dorsal surface.

PATHOLOGY SPOTLIGHTS

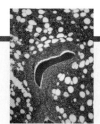

Benign Prostatic Hyperplasia

Benign prostatic hyperplasia (BPH) is an enlargement of the prostate gland that may occur in men who are 50 years of age and older. By age 60, four out of five men may have an enlarged prostate. As the prostate enlarges, it compresses the urethra, thereby restricting the normal flow of urine. See Figure 16–6. This restriction generally causes a number of symptoms and can be referred to as prostatism. Prostatism is any condition of the prostate gland that interferes with the flow of urine from the bladder. Symptoms usually include:

- A weak or hard-to-start urine stream
- A feeling that the bladder is not empty
- A need to urinate often, especially at night
- A feeling of urgency (a sudden need to urinate)
- Abdominal straining; a decrease in size and force of the urinary stream

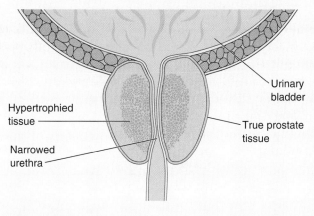

Hypertrophied
tissue

Narrowed
urethra

Urinary
bladder

True prostate
tissue

FIGURE 16–6

Benign prostatic hyperplasia.

- Interruption of the stream
- Acute urinary retention
- Recurrent urinary infections

Treatment for benign prostatic hyperplasia may include drug therapy, nonsurgical procedures and/or surgery.

- **Drug therapy**. Over the years, researchers have tried to find a way to shrink or at least stop the growth of the prostate without using surgery. The Food and Drug Administration (FDA) has approved four drugs to treat BPH. One of the first drugs so approved is Proscar (finasteride), an oral medication prescribed to help relieve the symptoms of BPH. It lowers the levels of dihydrotestosterone (DHT), which is a major factor in enlargement of the prostate. Lowering of DHT leads to shrinkage of the enlarged prostate gland in most men. Although this can lead to gradual improvement in urine flow and symptoms, it does not work for all cases. Other medications include terazosin (Hytrin), doxazosin (Cardura), and tamsulosin (Flomax). All three drugs act by relaxing the smooth muscle of the prostate and bladder neck to improve urine flow and to reduce bladder outlet obstruction.

- **Nonsurgical treatment**. Because drug therapy is not effective in all cases, researchers in recent years have developed a number of procedures that relieve the symptoms of BPH, and are less invasive than surgery. Two of these procedures are:
  1. **Transurethral microwave**. This procedure uses a device, Prostatron, that uses microwaves to heat and destroy excess prostate tissue. In the procedure called transurethral microwave thermotherapy (TUMT), the Prostatron sends computer-regulated microwaves through a catheter to heat selected portions of the prostate to at least 111 degrees Fahrenheit. A cooling system protects the urinary tract during the procedure. Another microwave device is the Targis System, which delivers microwaves to destroy selected portions of the prostate and uses a cooling system to protect the urethra. A heat-sensing device inserted in the rectum helps monitor the therapy. Both procedures take about 1 hour and can be performed on an outpatient basis without general anesthesia. Neither procedure has been reported to lead to impotence or incontinence.
  2. **Transurethral needle ablation**. The transurethral needle ablation (TUNA) system is a minimally invasive treatment for BPH. It delivers low-level radiofrequency energy through twin needles to burn away a well defined region of the enlarged prostate. Shields protect the urethra from heat damage. The TUNA System improves urine flow and relieves symptoms with fewer side effects when compared with transurethral resection of the prostate (TURP). No incontinence or impotence has been observed.

- **Surgery**
  1. **Transurethral resection of the prostate** (TURP or TUR). The most common form of surgery used for benign prostatic hyperplasia. During this procedure, an endoscopic instrument that has ocular and surgical capabilities is introduced directly through the urethra to the prostate and small pieces of the prostate gland are removed by using an electrical cutting loop.
  2. **Transurethral incision of the prostate** (TUIP). Used to widen the urethra by making a few small cuts in the bladder neck, where the urethra joins the bladder, and in the prostate gland itself.
  3. **Open surgery**. This type of surgery is used when a transurethral procedure cannot be done. It is often done when the gland is greatly enlarged, when there are complicating factors, or when the bladder has been damaged and needs to be repaired.
  4. **Laser surgery**. This type of surgery employs side-firing laser fibers and ND: YAG (Neodimium Doped Yttrium Aluminum Garnet) lasers to vaporize obstructing prostate tissue.

Erectile Dysfunction (ED)

Erectile dysfunction is the inability to achieve or maintain an erection sufficient for sexual intercourse. It occurs when not enough blood is supplied to the penis, when the smooth muscle in the penis fails to relax, or when the penis does not retain the blood that flows into it. According to studies by the NIH, 5 percent of men have some degree of erectile dysfunction at age 40 and approximately 15 to 25 percent at age 65 or older. Although the likelihood of erectile dysfunction increases with age, it is not an inevitable part of aging. About 80 percent of erectile dysfunction has a physical cause. See Table 16–1 for physical causes of erectile dysfunction.

Risk factors for ED include hypertension, hyperlipidemia, endocrine disorders, low testosterone (such as patients receiving hormonal therapy for prostate cancer or patients with hypogonadotropic hypogonadism), thyroid disease, diabetes, coronary artery disease, peripheral vascular disease, anemia, medications, smoking, alcohol abuse, surgical procedures, vascular surgeries, radical prostatectomy, neurological conditions, psychiatric illness, anxiety disorder depression, obsessive-compulsive disorder, and injury.

Erectile dysfunction can affect relationships and men should discuss the issue with their partners and seek medical advice. A medical evaluation is done when a man expresses concerns about his condition with his physician. Any underlying condition causing the problem should be treated.

Treatment may include counseling or sex therapy for men whose erectile dysfunction stems from emotional problems. Treatments for physical causes are based upon the cause. For example, if ED is caused by a medication, the man should consult with his physician about changing medications. Mixing medications and/or not following instructions are common causes of ED.

There are many treatment options for ED today. These include the vacuum constriction device (VCD), oral medications, medication patches and gels, urethral and penile injection therapies and surgical therapies, including penile prosthesis.

Viagra (sildenafil citrate) is an oral medication that may be prescribed for erectile dysfunction. It increases the body's ability to achieve and maintain an erection during sexual stimulation. It does not protect one from getting sexually transmitted diseases, including HIV. There is a potential for cardiac risk during sexual activity in patients with preexisting cardiovascular disease. Therefore, treatments for erectile dysfunction, including Viagra, generally should not be used in men for whom sexual activity is inadvisable because of their underlying cardiovascular status. The drug is potentially hazardous in those with acute coronary ischemia who are not on nitrates, those who have congestive heart failure, and those with borderline low blood pressure.

TABLE 16–1 SOME PHYSICAL CAUSES OF ERECTILE DYSFUNCTION

Vascular Diseases	Arteriosclerosis, hypertension, high cholesterol, and other medical conditions can obstruct blood flow and cause erectile dysfunction
Diabetes	Can alter nerve function and blood flow to the penis and cause erectile dysfunction
Prescription Drugs	Certain antihypertensive and cardiac medications, antihistamines, psychiatric medications, and other prescription drugs can cause erectile dysfunction
Substance Abuse	Excessive smoking, alcohol, and illegal drugs constrict blood vessels and can cause erectile dysfunction
Neurologic Diseases	Multiple sclerosis, Parkinson's disease, and other diseases can interrupt nerve impulses to the penis and cause erectile dysfunction
Surgery	Prostate, colon, bladder, and other types of pelvic surgery may damage nerves and blood vessels and cause erectile dysfunction
Spinal Injury	Interruptions of nerve impulses from the spinal cord to the penis can cause erectile dysfunction
Other	Hormonal imbalance, kidney failure, dialysis, and reduced testosterone levels can cause erectile dysfunction

Prostate Cancer

Prostate cancer is a malignant tumor that grows in the prostate gland. It is the most common type of cancer found in American men. By age 50, up to one in four men have some cancerous cells in the prostate gland. By age 80, the ratio increases to one in two. In the United States, the average age at diagnosis is 70.

Prostate cancer is the second leading cause of cancer death in men, exceeded only by lung cancer. While 1 man in 6 will get prostate cancer during his lifetime, only 1 man in 32 will die of this disease. One is more likely to die *with* prostate cancer than one is to die from prostate cancer. African American men are more likely to have prostate cancer and to die of it than are white or Asian men. The reasons for this are not known.

In some cases, prostate cancer can grow slowly for many years. Other times, it may grow rapidly and spread swiftly to other parts of the body. It may also spread its cells throughout the lymph system or bloodstream and along nerve pathways.

Some men with prostate cancer have no symptoms. Others notice symptoms such as dull pain in the lower pelvic area; general pain in the lower back, hips, or upper thighs; blood in the urine or semen; dribbling when urinating; erectile dysfunction; frequent urination, especially at night; painful urination and/or ejaculation; a smaller stream of urine and/or an urgent need to urinate; loss of appetite and weight.

If the cancer has spread to other parts of the body, such as the bones, the man may have persistent bone pain. He may also have occasional nerve paralysis or loss of bladder function.

Following are some of the risk factors associated with prostate cancer.

- Advanced age. Prostate cancer is seen mostly in men over the age of 55.
- Diet. Some evidence suggests that a diet high in animal fat may increase the risk of prostate cancer. Fruits, vegetables, and fatty fish may lower a man's risk for prostate cancer.
- Ethnic background. Prostate cancer occurs more often in African and northern European ethnic groups. It is less common in American Indian and Asian men.
- Family history of cancer. A man's risk is higher if his father or brother had prostate cancer.
- Men who have had a vasectomy, who smoke, or who have been exposed to a metal called cadmium may also be at an increased risk.

As yet, prostate cancer cannot be completely prevented. Prostate screening with exams and blood tests help with early diagnosis. The American Cancer Society (ACS) recommends that a digital rectal exam be offered every year to men 50 years of age or older who have a life expectancy of at least 10 years.

The ACS also recommends that a prostate-specific antigen test, also called a PSA blood test, be offered every year to men 50 years of age or older who have a life expectancy of at least 10 years. ACS recommends that screening start at the age of 45 years for African American men or men with a family history of prostate cancer.

Diagnosis of prostate cancer begins with a medical history and physical exam. The physician will perform a digital rectal exam. The physician will insert a lubricated, gloved finger into the rectum and feel the prostate through the rectal wall to check for hard or lumpy areas.

The PSA may help in diagnosing prostate cancer. The level of PSA may rise in men who have prostate cancer, BPH, or prostate infection. A new study suggests lowering the threshold of the PSA test for biopsy to 2.6 ng/mL in men younger than 60 would double the cancer-detection rate from 18 percent to 36 percent. Researchers say under the current guidelines, if a PSA test level of greater than 4.1 ng/mL was used to determine who underwent a biopsy, 82 percent of cancers in younger men and 65 percent of cancers in older men would be missed.

If test results suggest that cancer may be present, the man will need to have a biopsy. During a biopsy, the physician removes tissue samples from the prostate, usually with a needle, and sends them to pathology for evaluation.

Prostate cancer is graded and staged for aggressiveness based on how far it has spread throughout the body. CT scans and bone scans help in staging. Sometimes staging only becomes clear at the time of surgery. Following are the stages of prostate cancer:

- Stages A and B are cancers confined to the prostate gland.
- Stage C cancer has spread to other tissues near the prostate gland.
- Stage D cancer has spread to lymph nodes or sites in the body a distance away from the prostate.

The proper management of the many stages of prostate cancer is controversial. Depending on the grade and stage of the cancer, some options are as follows:

- Chemotherapy
- Cryosurgery to freeze cancer cells
- External radiation to the prostate and pelvis
- Hormone therapy
- Radioactive implants put directly into the prostate, which slowly kill cancer cells
- Surgery to remove part or all of the prostate and surrounding tissue
- Surgical removal of the testicles to block testosterone production
- Watchful waiting and monitoring only

Hormone therapy or chemotherapy is used mostly for men with advanced stage D disease. Hormone therapy includes use of the following: antiandrogens, such as flutamide and bicalutamide, that block the action of testosterone; corticosteroids, such as prednisone; GnRH agonists, also known as LH-RH (luteinizing hormone-releasing hormone) agonists, such as goserelin, leuprolide, and buserelin, which reduce the body's production of testosterone and/or medicines that stop the production of testosterone, such as ketoconazole and amino-glutethimide.

A significant number of prostate cancer patients use complementary and alternative medicines (CAM) as part of their treatment, according to a new study. But many of those men don't tell their doctors about these therapies, which could have a negative effect on their care.

CAM therapies—everything from acupuncture to vitamin supplements—have become increasingly popular in the United States over the past decade, both among the general public and among cancer patients. For example, studies suggest that 30 to 40 percent of breast cancer patients use some type of complementary or alternative medicine to supplement their treatment.

Vasectomy

A **vasectomy** is a surgery in which the vas deferens are tied off and cut apart which causes permanent sterility by preventing transport of sperm out of the testes. A vasectomy is usually done in the surgeon's office while the patient is awake, using local anesthesia. After the surgery, the patient is able to return home immediately. The patient can return to work the next day (if the job is sedentary) and can resume strenuous physical activity in 3–7 days.

This surgery does not affect the man's ability to achieve orgasm, ejaculate, or achieve erections. There is still a fluid ejaculate, but no sperm is in this fluid, so the man cannot impregnate his partner.

Vasectomy provides permanent sterilization. It is not recommended as a temporary or reversible procedure. After vasectomy, the sperm count gradually decreases. After 4 to 6 weeks, sperm are no longer present in the semen. A semen specimen must be examined and found to be totally free of sperm a month or more after vasectomy before the patient can rely on the vasectomy for birth control. Continued use of contraception is recommended until 2 to 3 sperm count tests are negative, indicating that the patient is sterile.

✔PATHOLOGY CHECKPOINT

Following is a concise list of the pathology-related terms that you've seen in the chapter. Review this checklist to make sure that you are familiar with the meaning of each term before moving on to the next section.

Conditions and Symptoms

- ❑ anorchism
- ❑ aspermatism
- ❑ azoospermia
- ❑ balanitis
- ❑ benign prostatic hyperplasia (BPH)
- ❑ condyloma
- ❑ cryptorchism
- ❑ epididymitis
- ❑ epispadias
- ❑ erectile dysfunction (ED)
- ❑ eunuch
- ❑ gonorrhea
- ❑ gynecomastia
- ❑ herpes genitalis
- ❑ heterosexual
- ❑ homosexual
- ❑ hydrocele
- ❑ hypospadias
- ❑ infertility
- ❑ oligospermia
- ❑ orchitis
- ❑ penitis
- ❑ phimosis
- ❑ prostate cancer
- ❑ prostatitis
- ❑ puberty
- ❑ syphilis
- ❑ trisomy
- ❑ varicocele
- ❑ vesiculitis

Diagnosis and Treatment

- ❑ artificial insemination
- ❑ castrate
- ❑ circumcision
- ❑ epididymectomy
- ❑ Ericsson sperm separation method
- ❑ eugenics
- ❑ orchidectomy
- ❑ orchidotomy
- ❑ prostatectomy
- ❑ spermicide

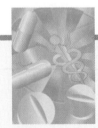

DRUG HIGHLIGHTS
DRUG HIGHLIGHTS

Drugs that are generally used for the male reproductive system include androgenic hormones. Testosterone is the most important androgen and adequate secretions of this hormone are necessary to maintain normal male sex characteristics, the male libido, and sexual potency.

Testosterone Is responsible for growth, development, and maintenance of the male reproductive system, and secondary sex characteristics.

Therapeutic use As replacement therapy in primary hypogonadism, and to stimulate puberty in carefully selected males. It may be used to relieve male menopause symptoms due to androgen deficiency. It may also be used to help stimulate sperm production in oligospermia and in impotence due to androgen deficiency. It may be used when there is advanced inoperable metastatic breast cancer in women who are 1 to 5 years postmenopausal.

Examples: Andro 100 and AndroGel (testosterone), DepoTestosterone (testosterone cypionate in oil), Delatestryl (testosterone enanthate in oil), Testex (testosterone propionate in oil), and Testoderm and Androderm (testosterone transdermal systems).

Patient teaching	Educate the patient to be aware of possible adverse reactions and report any of the following to the physician. *All patients:* nausea, vomiting, jaundice, edema. *Males:* frequent or persistent erection of the penis. Adolescent males: signs of premature epiphyseal closure. Should have bone development checked every 6 months. *Females:* hoarseness, acne, changes in menstrual periods, growth of hair on face and/or body.
Special considerations	In diabetic patients, the effects of testosterone may decrease blood glucose and insulin requirements.
	Testosterone may decrease the anticoagulant requirements of patients receiving oral anticoagulants. These patients require close monitoring when testosterone therapy is begun and then when it is stopped.
	Anabolic steroids (testosterone) may be abused by individuals who seek to increase muscle mass, strength, and overall athletic ability. This form of use is illegal and signs of abuse may include flu-like symptoms, headaches, muscle aches, dizziness, bruises, needle marks, increased bleeding (nosebleeds, petechiae, gums, conjunctiva), enlarged spleen, liver, and/or prostate, edema, and in the female increased facial hair, menstrual irregularities, and enlarged clitoris.

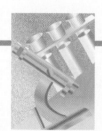

DIAGNOSTIC & LAB TESTS

DIAGNOSTIC & LAB TESTS

TEST	DESCRIPTION
fluorescent treponemal antibody absorption (floo-ō-rĕs′ ĕnt trĕp″ ō-nē măl ăn′ tĭ-bŏd″ ē ab-sorp′ shŭn)	A test performed on blood serum to determine the presence of *Treponema pallidum*. Used to detect syphilis.
paternity (pă-tĕr′ nĭ-tē)	A test to determine whether a certain man could be the father of a specific child. The test can indicate only who is not the father. Types of tests that may be used are blood type, human leukocyte antigen (HLA), white blood cell, enzyme and protein, and genetic. The blood type of the child and accused father are analyzed for compatibility. For example, a parent with type O blood cannot be the parent of a child with type AB blood. The HLA looks at the body's tissue compatibility system, and the white blood cell test looks at chemical markers (antigens) on the surface of the white blood cells. Enzyme and protein looks at red blood cell enzymes, and a new genetic test is being developed that uses molecular and protein biology to look at family-related patterns among genes.
prostate-specific antigen (PSA) immunoassay (prŏs′ tāt-spĕ-sĭf′ ĭk ăn′ tĭ-jĕn ĭm″ ū-nō-ăs′ sā)	A blood test that measures concentrations of a special type of protein known as prostate-specific antigen. Increased level indicates prostate disease or possibly prostate cancer.

TEST	DESCRIPTION
semen (sē′ mĕn)	A test performed on semen that looks at the volume, pH, sperm count, sperm motility, and morphology. Used to evaluate infertility in men.
testosterone toxicology (tĕs-tŏs′ tĕr-ōn tŏks″ ĭ-kŏl′ ō-jē)	A test performed on blood serum to identify the level of testosterone. Increased level may indicate benign prostatic hyperplasia. Decreased level may indicate hypogonadism, testicular hypofunction, hypopituitarism, and/or orchidectomy.
venereal disease research laboratory (vĕ-nē′ rē-ăl dĭ-zēz rē′ sĕrch lăb′ ră-tor″ ē)	A test performed on blood serum to determine the presence of *Treponema pallidum*. Used to detect syphilis.

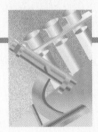

SEXUALLY TRANSMITTED DISEASES (STDs)

Sexually transmitted diseases can occur in men, women, and children. They are passed from person to person through sexual contact or from mother to child. The following is a summary of the most common sexually transmitted diseases:

DISEASE	CAUSE	SYMPTOMS	TREATMENT
Chlamydia (klă-mĭd′ ē-ă)	*Chlamydia trachomatis* (bacterium)	**MAY BE ASYMPTOMATIC OR** **MALE:** Mucopurulent discharge from penis, burning, itching in genital area, dysuria, swollen testes. Can lead to sterility. **FEMALE:** Mucopurulent discharge from vagina, cystitis, pelvic pain, cervicitis. Can lead to pelvic inflammatory disease (PID) and sterility. **NEWBORN:** Eye infection, pneumonia. Can cause death.	Antibiotics—tetracycline or erythromycin
Genital warts (jĕn′ ĭ-tăl wŏrts)	Human papilloma-virus (HPV)	**MALE:** Cauliflower-like growths on the penis and perianal area **FEMALE:** Cauliflower-like growths around vagina and perianal area	Laser surgery, chemotherapy, cryosurgery, cauterization
Gonorrhea (gŏn″ ŏ-rē′ ā)	*Neisseria gonorrhoeae* (bacterium)	**MALE:** Purulent urethral discharge, dysuria, urinary frequency **FEMALE:** Purulent vaginal discharge, dysuria, urinary frequency, abnormal menstrual bleeding, abdominal tenderness. Can lead to PID and sterility. **NEWBORN:** Gonorrheal ophthalmia neonatorum, purulent eye discharge. Can cause blindness.	Antibiotics—penicillin or tetracycline

DISEASE	CAUSE	SYMPTOMS	TREATMENT
Herpes genitalis (hĕr′ pēz jĕn-ĭ-tāl′ ĭs)	Herpes simplex virus-2 (HSV-2)	**ACTIVE PHASE MALE:** Fluid-filled vesicles (blisters) on penis. Rupture causes acute pain and itching. **FEMALE:** Blisters in and around vagina **NEWBORN:** Can be infected during vaginal delivery. Severe infection, physical and mental damage. **GENERALIZED:** "Flu-like" symptoms, fever, headache, malaise, anorexia, muscle pain	**NO CURE:** Antiviral drug acyclovir (Zovirax) may be used to relieve symptoms during acute phase
Syphilis (sĭf′ ĭ-lĭs)	*Treponema pallidum* (bacterium)	**PRIMARY**—1st stage Chancre at point of infection. See Figures 16–7 and 16–8. **Male**—penis, anus, rectum. **Female**—vagina, cervix. **Both**—lips, tongue, fingers, or nipples **SECONDARY**—2nd stage "Flu-like" symptoms with a skin rash over moist, fatty areas of the body. See Figure 16–9. **TERTIARY**—latent-3rd stage. No symptoms—damage to internal organs. **NEWBORN:** Congenital syphilis—may have a heart defect, bone deformity, or other deformities.	Antibotics—penicillin, tetracycline, or erythromycin
Trichomoniasis (trĭk″ ō-mō-nī′ ă-sĭs)	*Trichomonas* (parasitic protozoa)	**MALE:** Usually asymptomatic. Can lead to cystitis, urethritis, prostatitis. **FEMALE:** White frothy vaginal discharge, burning and itching of vulva. Can lead to cystitis, urethritis, vaginitis.	Metronidazole (Flagyl)

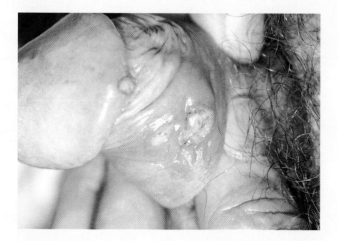

FIGURE 16–7

Chancre. (Courtesy of Jason L. Smith, MD.)

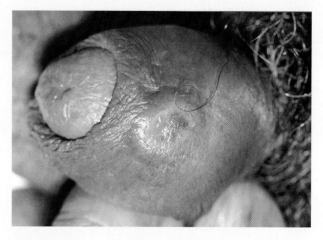

FIGURE 16–8

Chancre. (Courtesy of Jason L. Smith, MD.)

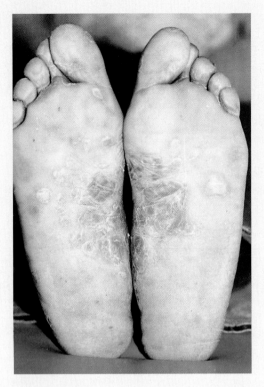

FIGURE 16–9

Secondary syphilis. (Courtesy of Jason L. Smith, MD.)

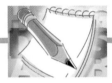 # ABBREVIATIONS

ABBREVIATION	MEANING
AIH	artificial insemination homologous
BPH	benign prostatic hyperplasia
CAM	complementary and alternative medicines
DHT	dihydrotestosterone
ED	erectile dysfunction
FTA-ABS	fluorescent treponemal antibody absorption
GC	gonorrhea
HLA	human leukocyte antigen
HPV	human papillomavirus
HSV-2	herpes simplex virus-2
LH-RH	luteinizing hormone-releasing hormone
NPT	nocturnal penile tumescence
PSA	prostate-specific antigen
SPP	suprapubic prostatectomy

ABBREVIATION	MEANING
STDs	sexually transmitted diseases
STS	serologic test for syphilis
TPA	*Treponema pallidum* agglutination
TUIP	transurethral incision of the prostate
TUMT	transurethral microwave thermotherapy
TUNA	transurethral needle ablation
TUR	transurethral resection
TURP	transurethral resection of the prostate
UG	urogenital
VCD	vacuum constriction device
VD	venereal disease
VDRL	venereal disease research laboratory

STUDY AND REVIEW

Anatomy and Physiology

Write your answers to the following questions. Do not refer to the text.

1. List the primary and accessory glands of the male reproductive system.

   a. _____   b. _____

   c. _____   d. _____

   e. _____   f. _____

2. Name the supporting structure and accessory sex organs of the male reproductive system.

   a. _____   b. _____

3. State the vital function of the male reproductive system. _____

   _____

4. Describe the scrotum. _____

   _____

5. The _____ _____ _____ and the

   _____ _____ are names of the three longitudinal columns

   of erectile tissue in the penis.

6. The average erect penis measures _____ to _____ cm in length.

7. The _____ _____ is the cone-shaped head of the penis.

8. Define prepuce. _____

   _____

9. Define smegma. _____

10. State two functions of the penis.

    a. _____   b. _____

11. Describe the testes. _____

    _____

    _____

12. _____ _____ are the site of the development of
    spermatozoa.

13. List five effects of testosterone regarding male development.

    a. _____   b. _____

    c. _____   d. _____

    e. _____

14. Name the plexus that the seminiferous tubules form. _____

15. Describe the epididymis. _____

    _____

16. State two functions of the epididymis.

    a. _____   b. _____

17. The excretory duct of the testes is known by two names, _____

    _____ or _____ _____.

18. The spermatic cord contains five types of structures and connects the testes with
    organs in the abdomen. Name these five structures.

    a. _____   b. _____

    c. _____   d. _____

    e. _____

19. State the function of the seminal vesicles. _____

    _____

20. Describe the prostate gland. _____

    _____

21. Define the condition known as benign prostatic hyperplasia. _____

    _____

22. The two small pea-sized glands located below the prostate and on either side of

    the urethra are known as the _____ glands or as _____

    glands.

23. Name the three sections of the male urethra.

a. _____   b. _____

c. _____

24. State a function of the male urethra. _____

25. The male urethra is approximately _____ cm long.

Word Parts

1. In the spaces provided, write the definitions of these prefixes, roots, combining forms, and suffixes. Do not refer to the listings of medical words. Leave blank those words you cannot define.

2. After completing as many as you can, refer to the medical word listings to check your work. For each word missed or left blank, write the word and its definition several times on the margins of these pages or on a separate sheet of paper.

3. To maximize the learning process, it is to your advantage to do the following exercises as directed. To refer to the word building section before completing these exercises invalidates the learning process.

PREFIXES

Give the definitions of the following prefixes:

1. a- _____   2. an- _____

3. circum- _____   4. epi- _____

5. hydro- _____   6. hypo- _____

7. oligo- _____   8. par- _____

9. in- _____   10. eu- _____

11. heter- _____   12. homo- _____

13. tri- _____

ROOTS AND COMBINING FORMS

Give the definitions of the following roots and combining forms:

1. balan _____

2. cis _____

3. crypt _____

4. artific/i _____

5. didym _____

6. enchyma _____

7. orch _____

8. orchid _____

9. orchid/o _____

10. pen _____

11. phim _____

12. prostat _____

13. castr _____

14. spadias _____

15. sperm _____

16. seminat _____

17. spermat/o _____

18. sperm/i _____

19. testicul _____

20. varic/o _____

21. vas _____

22. vesicul _____

23. zo/o _____

24. zoon _____

25. ejaculat _____

26. gon/o _____

27. gynec/o _____

28. mast _____

29. sexu _____

30. mit _____

31. som _____

SUFFIXES

Give the definitions of the following suffixes:

1. -al _____

2. -ar _____

3. -blast _____

4. -cele _____

5. -cide _____

6. -ectomy _____

7. -genesis _____

8. -ia _____

9. -ion _____

10. -ism _____

11. -itis _____

12. -ate _____

13. -osis _____

14. -genic(s) _____

15. -rrhea _____

16. -tomy _____

17. -y _____

Identifying Medical Terms

In the spaces provided, write the medical terms for the following meanings:

1. _____ Inflammation of the glans penis

2. _____ Surgical excision of the epididymis

3. _____ Surgical excision of a testicle

4. _____ The foreskin over the glans penis

5. _____ A male who has been castrated

6. _____ A wart-like growth of the skin

7. _____ The sperm germ cell

8. _____ The male sex cell

9. _____ An agent that kills sperm

10. _____ Pertaining to a testicle

Spelling

In the spaces provided, write the correct spelling of these misspelled words:

1. crptorchism _____

2. hyospadias _____

3. orchdotomy _____

4. ugenics _____

5. tisomy _____

Matching

Select the appropriate lettered meaning for each word listed below.

_____ 1. circumcision

_____ 2. coitus

_____ 3. condom

_____ 4. gamete

_____ 5. genital warts

_____ 6. gonorrhea

_____ 7. infertility

_____ 8. prepuce

_____ 9. syphilis

_____ 10. trichomoniasis

a. Caused by the bacterium *Treponema pallidum*

b. A mature reproductive cell of the male or female

c. Sexual intercourse between a man and a woman

d. Caused by a parasitic protozoa

e. The surgical process of removing the foreskin of the penis

f. A thin, flexible protective sheath worn over the penis during copulation to help prevent impregnation or venereal disease

g. Caused by the human papilloma virus

h. The inability to produce a viable offspring

i. Causes purulent urethral discharge in the male and purulent vaginal discharge in the female

j. Caused by the bacterium *Chlamydia trachomatis*

k. The foreskin over the glans penis in the male

Abbreviations

Place the correct word, phrase, or abbreviation in the space provided.

1. benign prostatic hyperplasia _____

2. GC _____

3. human papillomavirus _____

4. HSV-2 _____

5. STDs _____

6. *Treponema pallidum* agglutination _____

7. TUR _____

8. UG _____

9. venereal disease _____

10. prostate-specific antigen _____

Diagnostic and Laboratory Tests

Select the best answer to each multiple choice question. Circle the letter of your choice.

1. A test performed on blood serum to detect syphilis.
   a. paternity
   b. semen
   c. FTA-ABS
   d. HSV-2

2. A test to determine whether a certain man could be the father of a specific child.
   a. paternity
   b. semen
   c. FTA-ABS
   d. HSV-2

3. An increased level indicates prostate disease or possibly prostate cancer.
   a. fluorescent treponemal antibody
   b. prostate-specific antigen
   c. semen
   d. testosterone toxicology

4. Used to determine infertility in men.
   a. paternity
   b. prostate-specific antigen
   c. semen
   d. testosterone toxicology

5. An increased level may indicate benign prostatic hyperplasia.
   a. fluorescent treponemal antibody
   b. prostate-specific antigen
   c. testosterone toxicology
   d. venereal disease research

CASE STUDY

BENIGN PROSTATIC HYPERPLASIA

Read the following case study and then answer the questions that follow.

A 58-year-old male was seen by a physician, and the following is a synopsis of the visit.

Present History: The patient states that he is having difficulty with urination. He is having a need to urinate often, especially at night, urgency, and a decrease in size and force of the urinary stream.

Signs and Symptoms: Frequency, urgency, and decrease in size and force of the urinary stream.

Diagnosis: Benign prostatic hyperplasia

Treatment: Proscar (finasteride) was ordered by the physician to help relieve the symptoms of benign prostatic hyperplasia. It lowers the levels of dihydrotestosterone (DHT), which is a major factor in enlargement of the prostate. Lowering of DHT leads to shrinkage of the enlarged prostate gland in most men. It may take 6 months or more to determine if it is working for an individual. The patient was scheduled for a follow-up visit in 6 months and informed that side effects of Proscar may include impotence and less desire for sex, and that this medication can alter the prostate-specific antigen test (PSA) that is used to screen for prostate cancer.

CASE STUDY QUESTIONS

1. Signs and symptoms of benign prostatic hyperplasia include frequency, _____, and decrease in size and force of the urinary stream.

2. Treatment included _____ (finasteride).

3. Side effects of this medication may include _____ and less desire for sex.

4. This medication can alter the _____-specific antigen test that is used to screen for prostate cancer.

 MedMedia Wrap-Up
www.prenhall.com/rice

Additional interactive resources and activities for this chapter can be found on the Companion Website. For animations, videos, audio glossary, and review, access the accompanying CD-ROM in this book.

Audio Glossary
Medical Terminology Exercises & Activities
Pathology Spotlight
Terminology Translator
Animations
Videos

Objectives
Medical Terminology Exercises & Activities
Audio Glossary
Drug Updates
Medical Terminology in the News

ONCOLOGY 17

OBJECTIVES

On completion of this chapter, you will be able to:

- Describe cancer.
- Describe the three main classifications of cancer.
- Describe cell differentiation.
- Describe the invasive process.
- Identify the staging system that evaluates the spread of a tumor.
- Describe various methods that may be used in diagnosing cancer.
- Describe the various forms of treatment for cancer.
- List several recommended cancer preventive methods.
- Analyze, build, spell, and pronounce medical words.
- Describe each of the conditions presented in the Pathology Spotlights.
- Complete the Pathology Checkpoint.
- Identify and define selected abbreviations.
- Successfully complete the study and review section.

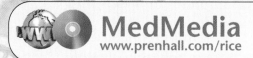

MedMedia
www.prenhall.com/rice

Additional interactive resources and activities for this chapter can be found on the Companion Website. For Terminology Translator, animations, videos, audio glossary, and review, access the accompanying CD-ROM in this book.

An Overview of Cancer

Cancer was first identified around 400 BC during the time of Hippocrates and is a Latin term meaning **a crab**. Early reports on cancer compared the disease to a crab because of its tendency to stretch out and spread like the crab's four pairs of legs. Today, cancer refers to any malignant tumor (neoplasm, oncoma). More than 200 different types of cancer have been identified; however, the majority of tumors can be classified into three main groups: **carcinomas**, which account for about 80 percent of cancers; **sarcomas**, which are the next largest group; and **mixed cancers**, which have characteristics of both carcinomas and sarcomas (see Classification of Cancer).

The incidence of cancer is now five times greater than it was 100 years ago. Cancer will strike one of every three Americans, according to recent statistics from the American Cancer Society. However, there is hope for those afflicted. Cancer has become one of the most curable of the major diseases in the United States, and those tumors that cannot be cured can be controlled through treatment, thereby giving the patient an extended life span. With early detection followed by immediate treatment, the cure rate for cancer is now one in every two. Highly advanced surgical techniques are being used to remove cancerous tissue, and it is usually possible to excise all the cancer cells when the malignancy is discovered in its earliest stages. *Chemotherapy* and *radiation therapy* are the other two principal means of treatment for patients with cancer. These treatments employ agents to kill cancerous cells that remain after surgery or in malignancies deemed inoperable. Other forms of treatment are under investigation as scientists continue their research into the causes of cancer. Although the exact cause or causes remain unknown, research has shown that some cancers can be prevented, especially those associated with environmental factors. Oncologists searching for the causes of cancer have identified numerous factors that play a role in the development of cancer. See Figure 17–1. These factors are generally grouped under three main classifications: environmental, hereditary, and biological. Viruses have long been suspected of playing a role in the development of cancer; however, the human T-cell leukemia-lymphoma virus (HTLV) is the first known to cause cancer in humans. It has been found to be present in the cells of individuals with certain types of leukemia and lymphoma. Fortunately, not everyone affected by HTLV develops cancer. Scientists are studying the complex biological relation among viruses, genes, and the development of cancer with the hope of uncovering information leading to the prevention, control, and possible cure of cancer. The American Cancer Society has published the following list of safeguards against cancer, which encourages individuals to take specific steps to safeguard their health and aids in the early detection of cancer.

Site	Action
Breast	Monthly self-examination
Uterus	Pap test once a year
Lung	Don't smoke cigarettes
Skin	Avoid excess sun
Colon-rectum	Procto annually, especially after 40
Mouth	Exams regularly
Whole body	Annual health checkup

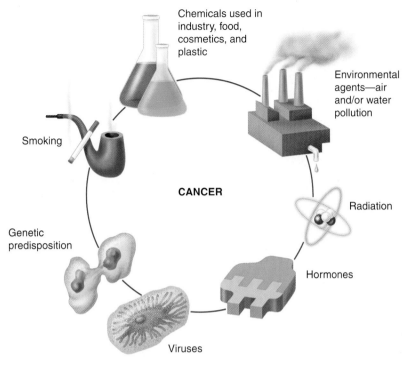

FIGURE 17–1

Possible causes of cancer. (Source: Pearson Education/PH College.)

CLASSIFICATION OF CANCER

The more than 200 types of cancer have been grouped into three main classifications: **carcinomas**, **sarcomas**, and **mixed cancers**.

Carcinomas

As mentioned earlier, **carcinomas** make up the great majority of all cancers and are malignant tumors of epithelial tissues. They are named according to the type of epithelial cell in which the malignancy occurs or the primary site of the tumor. For example, a cancer of squamous epithelium is a **squamous carcinoma**. See Figures 17–2 and 17–3. Likewise a cancer originating in the bronchus of the respiratory tract is a **bronchogenic carcinoma**. Epithelial tissue lines body surfaces including those of glands and organs; therefore, carcinomas make up the majority of the glandular cancers and are generally found in the breast, stomach, uterus, tongue, and skin.

Sarcomas

Sarcomas are a less prevalent type of cancer that develops from embryonic cells of connective tissue such as muscle, fat, bone, and blood vessels. They are named by adding the suffix -oma (tumor) with the root sarc (flesh) to the word part that identifies the tissue of origin. A cancer of the bone, for examples, is an **osteosarcoma**: osteo (CF), bone; sarc (R), flesh; and -oma (S), tumor.

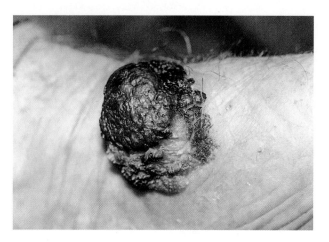

FIGURE 17–2

Squamous cell carcinoma. (Courtesy of Jason L. Smith, MD.)

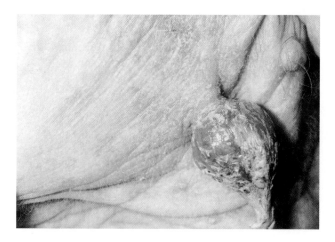

FIGURE 17–3

Squamous cell carcinoma. (Courtesy of Jason L. Smith, MD.)

Mixed Cancers

Mixed cancers originate in cells capable of differentiating into epithelial or connective tissue or when malignancies occur concurrently in adjacent tissue types. For example, stomach cancer may be a mixed cancer when carcinoma originates in the epithelial lining of the stomach wall and a **sarcoma** arises in the adjacent muscular layer underlying the epithelium.

Other Types

Other types of cancer may be classified as **leukemias, lymphomas,** or **melanomas.** Leukemias are cancers of the blood-forming tissues. Lymphomas are cancers of lymphoid tissue, and melanomas are cancers of black moles.

CELL DIFFERENTIATION

Normal cells reproduce themselves through an orderly process that assures growth, tissue repair, and cell reproduction or **mitosis.** Normal cells have a distinct appearance and a specialized function. In normal cell development, immature cells undergo normal changes as they mature and assume their specialized functions. This process is called **differentiation,** Knowledge of cell differentiation allows a pathologist or histologist, looking at a sample of tissue through a microscope, to identify the body area from which the tissue was removed. In cancer, there is an abnormal process wherein a cell or group of cells undergoes changes and no longer carries on normal cell functions. This failure of immature cells to develop specialized functions is called dedifferentiation. It is believed that this process involves a disturbance in the DNA of the affected cells. **Malignant cells** usually multiply rapidly, forming a mass of abnormal cells that enlarges, ulcerates, and sheds malignant cells to surrounding tissues. This process destroys the normal cells, with malignant cells taking their places. Microscopic analysis of a malignant cell reveals a loss of differentiation, anaplasia, nuclei of various sizes that are hyperchromatic, and cells in the process of rapid and disorderly division. Based on microscopic analysis, malignant tumors are further classified as grades I, II, III, or IV.

The following describes each of the four grades of tumors in this system:

Grade I. The most differentiated and the least malignant tumors. Only a few cells are undergoing mitosis; however, some abnormality does exist.

Grade II. Moderately undifferentiated. More cells are undergoing mitosis, and the pattern is fairly irregular.

Grade III. Many cells are undifferentiated, and tissue origin may be difficult to recognize. Many cells are undergoing mitosis.

Grade IV. The least differentiated and a high degree of malignancy.

This system of grading tumors is used to report the prognosis of the disease and also to determine whether the tumor is likely to respond to radiation therapy.

THE INVASIVE PROCESS

Two ways in which malignant cells spread to body parts are by **invasive growth** (*by active migration or direct extension*) and **metastasis**.

Invasive Growth

Invasive growth is the spreading process of a malignant tumor into adjacent normal tissue. Young malignant cells divide at the periphery of the tumor and spread by active migration or direct extension. In **active migration**, the malignant cells break away from the neoplasm, invade surrounding tissue, divide, form secondary neoplasms, and then reunite with the primary tumor as growth continues. In **direct extension**, multiplication of malignant cells is rapid, and there is subsequent spreading into surrounding tissues via the interstitial spaces accompanied by engulfment and destruction of normal cells. As a tumor's mass enlarges, its weight is supported by connective fibers that attach to surrounding structures. Adjacent veins and lymph vessels are invaded by these fibers and become pathways for the spread of malignant cells.

Metastasis

Metastasis is the process whereby cancer cells are spread from a primary site to distant secondary sites elsewhere in the body. This process usually occurs when malignant cells invade the bloodstream or lymph system and are transported to a secondary site where they become lodged and form a neoplasm. Malignant cells carried in the bloodstream may lodge in highly vascular organs such as the lungs or liver, and the development of a secondary neoplasm depends on the viability and the reception of the organ.

STAGING

Further reporting of the development and spread of cancer cells may be made through the use of a system that evaluates the spread of the tumor. The staging system uses the letters **T** (tumor), **N** (node), and **M** (metastasis) to indicate spread and uses numerical subscripts to indicate degree of tumor involvement. For example, $T_2N_1M_0$ indicates a primary tumor at stage 2, abnormality of regional lymph nodes at stage 1, and no evidence of distant metastasis.

CHARACTERISTICS OF NEOPLASMS

Neoplasms or tumors, as they are commonly called, may be **benign** or **malignant**. The following characteristics will distinguish the differences between benign and malignant neoplasms:

Benign Tumors	*Malignant Tumors*
1. Grow slowly	1. Grow rapidly
2. Encapsulated	2. Not encapsulated
3. Cells resemble the normal cells from which they arose	3. Cells undergo permanent change, abnormal rapid proliferation
4. Grow by expansion and cause pressure on surrounding tissue	4. Invasive growth and metastasis
5. Remain localized	5. Spread via the bloodstream
6. Do not recur when surgically removed	6. May recur when surgically removed if invasive growth has occurred
7. Tissue destruction is minimal	7. Tissue destruction is extensive if invasive growth has occurred
8. No cachexia	8. Cancer cachexia (extreme weakness, fatigue, wasting, and malnutrition)
9. Usually not a threat to life	9. Threat to life unless detected early and properly treated

As malignant cells proliferate and begin the invasive process, the patient is unaware of the development of the cancer. In its early stages, cancer is said to be silent; however, cytologic changes are occurring that could be detected if a tissue sample were taken and analyzed by a pathologist. With the proliferation of malignant cells and the continuation of the invasive process, tissues, organs, and surrounding structures become compressed, and ischemia may occur, causing necrosis, inflammation, ulceration, and bleeding. This bleeding is usually **occult** (*hidden*) and is not noted by the patient. The enlarging tumor eventually causes sufficient pressure on surrounding tissues and organs to create a feeling of numbness, tingling, and pain. Because the tumor itself does not have nerve endings, pain is not an early symptom of its development. Because of the silent development of cancer, the patient does not usually become aware of its symptoms until its systemic effects are evident. These systemic effects depend on the site and type of cancer but usually result in an imbalance in the patient's physiology, leading to subtle but noticeable changes that may warn of the disease.

The American Cancer Society lists seven warning signals of cancer. The first letters of each warning signal combine to spell the word CAUTION, and persons who develop any of the following symptoms should bring it to the attention of a physician immediately:

- **C**hange in bowel or bladder habits
- **A** sore that does not heal
- **U**nusual bleeding or discharge
- **T**hickening or lump in breast or elsewhere

- Indigestion or difficulty in swallowing
- Obvious change in a wart or mole
- Nagging cough or hoarseness

DIAGNOSIS

A variety of *diagnostic tools* and *procedures* is used to detect the possible presence of cancer. Principal among these are examination, visualization by endoscopy, laboratory analysis, biopsy, and diagnostic radiology.

Examination

An *annual physical examination* may be the best means of protecting one's state of health. The American Cancer Society publishes a cancer detection examination that recommends certain tests be included in an annual physical examination in addition to the medical history and usual tests.* These tests are listed below:

Skin. Entire skin

Head and neck. Eyes; nose; mouth, under all dentures; vocal cords with mirror, if hoarseness

Chest. Listen to heart and lungs; x-ray record of chest when indicated

Breast. Palpation of breasts and under arms for any abnormalities; biopsy of lump in breast when indicated; instruct and encourage breast self-examination; ages 40 to 49 get a mammogram every 1 to 2 years, after age 49 every year

Abdomen. Palpation for any abnormalities

Pelvis. Pelvic examination, including a Pap test for all women

Colon and rectum. Digital examination of rectum; proctosigmoidoscopic examination; x-ray record of colon or intestinal tract when indicated

Prostate. Digital examination of prostate; palpation of male testes; palpation of groin for enlarged lymph nodes; age 50 and over should have a prostate-specific antigen (PSA) blood test each year

Blood. For leukemia or anemia

Urinalysis. For indication of bladder or kidney cancer

Visualization by Endoscopy

Endoscopy provides the physician with a direct view of certain portions of the body. The following is a list of endoscopic procedures used to assess specific locations within the body:

Sigmoidoscopy. The process of using a sigmoidoscope to examine the lower 10 inches of the large intestines

Laryngoscopy. The process of using a laryngoscope to examine the interior of the larynx

Bronchoscopy. The process of using a bronchoscope to examine the bronchi

*This information was taken from American Cancer Society Professional Education publications.

Gastroscopy. The process of using a gastroscope to examine the interior of the stomach

Cystoscopy. The process of using a cystoscope to examine the bladder

Colposcopy. The process of using a colposcope to examine the cervix and vagina

Proctoscopy. The process of using a proctoscope to examine the anus and rectum

Colonoscopy. The process of using a colonoscope to examine the colon

Laparoscopy. The process of using a laparoscope to examine the abdomen

Laboratory Analysis

Laboratory analysis plays a key role in detecting specific types of cancer. The following are some of the laboratory tests used to diagnose cancer:

Pap smear/test. A cytologic screening test developed by Dr. George Papanicolaou and used to detect the presence of abnormal or cancerous cells from the cervix and vagina

Fecal occult blood test. A test used to detect occult (hidden) blood. This test may be used to check for cancer of the colon

Sputum cytology test. Microscopic examination of sputum to detect abnormal or cancerous cells of the bronchi and lungs

Blood serum test. Analysis of blood serum provides useful information about certain proteins synthesized by cancer

Abbot Lab's AFP-EIA test. An immunoassay test that uses alpha-fetoprotein to mark tumor cells when testing for cancer of the testicles

Bone marrow study. A test used to detect abnormal bone marrow cells, which may indicate leukemia

Urine assay tests. Tests providing useful information about catecholamines, which may indicate pheochromocytoma of the adrenal medulla

Gravlee jet washer. A device developed by Dr. Clark Gravlee to check for endometrial abnormalities as surface cells of the uterine cavity are studied under a microscope

Biopsy

The surgical removal of a small piece of tissue for microscopic examination is known as **biopsy.** It is the method of providing the proof of cancer in the diagnosis of the disease. The following different types of biopsy may be used for tissue removal:

Excisional biopsy. Surgical removal of a piece of tissue from the suspected body site

Incisional biopsy. A surgical incision to remove a section or wedge of tissue from the suspected body site

Needle biopsy. Puncture of a tumor for the removal of a core of tissue through the lumen of a needle

Cone biopsy. Removal of a cone of tissue from the uterine cervix

Sternal biopsy. Removal of a piece of bone marrow from the sternum

Endoscopic biopsy. Removal of a piece of tissue through an endoscope

Punch biopsy. Removal of a plug of tissue (epidermis, dermis, and subcutaneous tissue) from the skin

Diagnostic Radiology

Encompassing a wide range of tests and procedures, **diagnostic radiology** can reveal tumors that may not have been detected by other diagnostic procedures (see Chapter 18, Radiology and Nuclear Medicine).

TREATMENT

The treatment of cancer may be any one or a combination of the following methods: **surgery, chemotherapy, radiation therapy,** or **immunotherapy.** The treatment of choice will depend on the type of cancer, its location, its invasive process, and the state of health of the patient. The ultimate outcome of treatment is the killing of every cancer cell. Therefore the need to treat tumors at an early stage is critical. For example: a 1-cm breast tumor may contain 1,000,000,000 cancer cells before it is detected. A drug killing 99 percent of these cells would be considered an excellent drug, but 10,000,000 cancer cells would still remain in the body. The relationship between cell kill and chemotherapy is shown in Figure 17–4.

Surgery

Surgery may be the treatment of choice when the tumor is small and localized and the surrounding tissue is accessible for removal. The aim of surgery is the removal of all cancerous tissue plus some of the surrounding normal tissue. Surgery may also be used to alleviate some of the complications of cancer, such as the obstruction of an area caused by the enlargement of a tumor.

Chemotherapy

Chemotherapy may be the treatment of choice when the cancer is disseminated and cannot be surgically removed. It is also used when a tumor fails to respond to radiation therapy. Antineoplastic anticancer drugs do injury to individual cells, interfere with their vital functions, and kill or destroy malignant cells. See Figure 17–5. In rendering cancerous cells harmless, certain normal cells may also be destroyed. The normal cells with the greatest sensitivity to destruction are the hematopoietic cells, epithelial cells, and the hair follicles. The plan of treatment for patients undergoing chemotherapy is individualized. The aim of chemotherapy is to put the patient in remission so that life may continue without **exacerbation** of symptoms. The following are classifications of chemotherapeutic drugs used in the treatment of cancer.

Alkylating Agents

Alkylating agents are chemical compounds that cause chromosome breakage and prevent the formation of new DNA, thereby interfering with cell division. These agents are used in the treatment of leukemia, lymphoma, or disseminated malignancies. They affect all rapidly proliferating cells and often cause toxicity to the hematopoietic system. Bone marrow depression/suppression, anemia, leukopenia, thrombocytopenia, and pancytopenia may occur. Most alkylating agents disrupt cells within the gastrointestinal tract, thereby producing nausea and vomiting.

Examples: Myleran (busulfan), Leukeran (chlorambucil), Platinol (cisplatin), Cytoxan (cyclophosphamide), DTIC-Dome (decarbazine), Ifex (ifosfamide), Mustargen

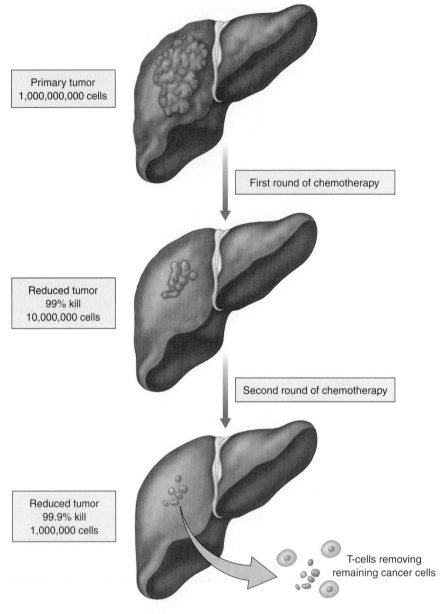

FIGURE 17–4

Cell kill and chemotherapy. (Source: Pearson Education/PH College.)

(mechlorethamine HCl), Alkeran (melphalan), Matulane (procarbazine), Temodar (temozolomide), and Tioplex (thiotepa).

ANTIMETABOLITES

Antimetabolites are substances that interfere with the metabolic process of the cell, thus preventing cell reproduction. They are used in the treatment of leukemia, disseminated solid tumors, and choriocarcinoma. They act only on dividing cells and are most effective in treating rapidly proliferating malignant cells. These agents often cause toxicity to the hematopoietic system. Bone marrow depression/suppression, anemia, leukopenia, thrombocytopenia, and pancytopenia may occur. They also cause nausea and vomiting.

Examples: Cytosar (cytarabine), 5-FU (fluorouracil), Hydrea (hydroxyurea), Purinethol (mercaptopurine), Rheumatrex (methotrexate), and Xeloda (capecitabine).

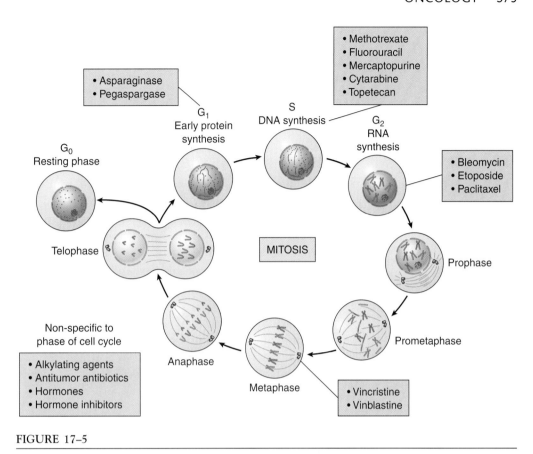

FIGURE 17–5

Antineoplastic agents and the cell cycle. (Source: Pearson Education/PH College.)

NITROSOUREAS

Nitrosoureas inhibit enzymes that are needed for DNA repair. These agents are able to travel to the brain, so they are used to treat brain tumors, as well as non-Hodgkin's lymphomas, multiple myeloma, and malignant melanoma.

Examples: BiCNU (carmustine), and CeeNU (lomustine).

ANTITUMOR ANTIBIOTICS

Certain **antibiotics** have an antineoplastic effect. These antibiotics are derived from species of microorganisms and are not to be confused with antibiotics used in the treatment of infections. Their action is not known, but it appears they act by interfering with one or more stages of RNA and/or DNA synthesis. They interfere with the malignant cell's ability to grow and reproduce. They are used in the treatment of leukemia, Wilm's tumor, choriocarcinoma, and cancer of the testes.

Examples: Blenoxane (bleomycin sulfate), Cosmegen (dactinomycin), Cerubidine (daunorubicin), DaunoXome (daunorubicin citrate liposomal), Doxil (doxorubicin HCl liposomal), Adriamycin (doxorubicin HCl), Ellence (epirubicin HCl), Mutamycin (mitomycin), Mithracin (plicamycin), and Valstar (valrubicin).

MITOTIC INHIBITORS

Mitotic inhibitors are plant alkaloids and natural products that can inhibit mitosis or inhibit enzymes that prevent protein synthesis, which is needed for cell reproduction. They are phase cycle specific and work during the mitosis (M) phase. They are used in the treatment of advanced breast cancer, carcinomas of the bladder, cervix, lung, and ovaries, melanoma, and non-Hodgkin's lymphoma. Adverse reactions that may occur are allergic reactions, skin rashes, edema, abnormally low neutrophil counts, abnormally low platelet counts, anemia, and peripheral nervous system disorders.

Examples: Taxotere (docetaxel), VePesid (etoposide), Taxol (paclitaxel), Velban (vinblastine), Oncovin (vincristine), and Navelbine (vinorelbine).

HORMONES

Hormones are used to treat endocrine-related tumors (carcinomas of the breast, prostate, endometrium, ovary, kidney, and thyroid) and nonendocrine malignant neoplasms (leukemia, lymphomas). They have been used in antineoplastic therapy because they are capable of suppressing the growth of certain tissues of the body without exerting cytotoxic action.

Corticosteroids (prednisone and prednisolone) are used in conjunction with antineoplastic agents in the treatment of acute lymphoblastic leukemia and malignant lymphoma. They produce a wide variety of adverse reactions after extended use, such as Cushingoid features, edema, hypertension, heart failure, potassium loss, paper-thin skin, euphoria, and poor wound healing.

Other hormones that may be used in antineoplastic therapy are *Premarin (conjugated estrogens), Teslac (testolactone), Depo-Provera (medroxyprogesterone acetate), and Megace (megestrol acetate).*

OTHER ANTINEOPLASTIC AGENTS

There are many other antineoplastic agents that are used in the treatment of various types of cancer.

Examples: Elspar (asparaginase), Proleukin and IL-2 (aldesleukin), Hexalen (altretamine), Roferon-A (interferon alfa-2a recombinant), Intron (interferon alfa-2b recombinant), Alferon N (interferon alfa-n3, human), Ergamisol (levamisole), Ontak (denileukin diftitox), Neupogen (filgrastim), Leukine (sargramostim), Herceptin (trastuzumab), and Nolvadex (tamoxifen citrate).

COMBINATION CHEMOTHERAPY

The combination of certain antineoplastic agents has proven to be effective in treating acute leukemia; Hodgkin's disease; non-Hodgkin's lymphoma; carcinoma of the breast, testis, and ovary; childhood neuroblastoma; Wilm's tumor; and osteogenic sarcoma. The physician who prescribes combination chemotherapy weighs the anticipated benefits against the possible additive toxic effects of the drugs.

Examples: TPE-Taxol (paclitaxel), Platinol (cisplatin), and VePesid (etoposide).

Immunotherapy

Immunotherapy is the treatment of disease by stimulation of the body's immune system. It may be used as an adjuvant to other types of treatment. There are three types of immunotherapy: **active specific**, **passive**, and **adoptive**.

ACTIVE IMMUNOTHERAPY

Active specific immunotherapy is the use of various agents to produce a specific host–immune response. The patient's own tumor cells, tumor antigens, oncogenic viruses, and bacterial products are a few of the agents that are being used to create an immune response of a specific nature.

PASSIVE IMMUNOTHERAPY

Passive immunotherapy is the use of serum or other products from an immunocompetent individual that are given to an immunodeficient individual to produce an immune response.

ADOPTIVE IMMUNOTHERAPY

Adoptive immunotherapy is the process of transferring a form of specific immune response from a donor to a recipient.

Other Forms of Treatment

INTRAOPERATIVE RADIATION THERAPY

This is the delivery of **tumoricidal** doses of radiation directly onto a tumor bed while the surgical wound is still open. The surgeon and radiotherapist decide on the target area, and then the radiotherapist positions the sterile treatment cone in the incision. The treatment is usually for 15 to 30 minutes, and the incision is closed after the treatment is completed.

PHOTODYNAMIC THERAPY

This is the use of a **red laser** to kill cancerous cells. **Hematoporphyrin derivative (Hpd)**, a light-sensitizing agent, is intravenously injected, and 3 days after the injection the physician uses the red laser. Normal cells eliminate Hpd and are not harmed during the treatment. Cancerous cells retain Hpd, and the red light kills them.

WHOLE BODY HYPERTHERMIA

This is the process of elevating the patient's body temperature to 108°F (42.2°C) to enhance the effect of radiation or chemotherapy. Cancer cells are sensitive to heat, so after radiation therapy, **hyperthermia** is employed to inhibit the cancer cells from repairing themselves. It is used before chemotherapy to increase the vulnerability of the cancer cells to the drug being used in the treatment process.

PREVENTION OF CANCER

Stop Smoking or Don't Ever Start

Smoking is the most preventable cause of death in man. In the United States, tobacco use is responsible for more than one in six deaths. Cigarette smoking is responsible for 90 percent of lung cancer among men and 79 percent among women. Smoking accounts for about 30 percent of all cancer deaths. Those who smoke two or more packs of cigarettes a day have lung cancer mortality rates 15 to 25 times greater than nonsmokers. According to the World Health Organization, approximately 2.5 million people each year worldwide die as a result of smoking.

Stop Using Smokeless Tobacco or Don't Ever Start

There has been a resurgence in the use of all forms of smokeless tobacco. The greatest cause of concern centers on the increased use of "dipping snuff." In this practice, tobacco that has been processed into a coarse, moist powder is placed between the cheek and gum, and nicotine, along with a number of carcinogens, is absorbed through the oral mucosa. Use of chewing tobacco or snuff increases the risk of cancer of the mouth, larynx (voice box), pharynx (throat), and esophagus (food tube).

Avoid Direct Sunlight and/or Use Protective Sunscreen

Epidemiologic evidence shows that sun exposure is a major factor in the development of melanoma and that incidence increases for those living near the equator. Almost all of the more than 700,000 cases of basal and squamous cell skin cancer diagnosed each year in the United States are sun related (ultraviolet radiation).

Avoid Ionizing Radiation and/or Limit Exposure

Excessive exposure to ionizing radiation can increase cancer risk. Excessive radon exposure in homes, schools, and one's workplace may increase the risk of lung cancer, especially in cigarette smokers.

"Eat-Right" Nutrition and Diet

More and more evidence shows that **proper nutrition** and **diet** can help prevent disease. One may reduce his or her cancer risk by:

- Maintaining desirable weight. Individuals 40 percent or more overweight increase their risk of colon, breast, prostate, gallbladder, ovary, and uterus cancer.
- Eat a variety of foods.
- Eat a variety of vegetables and fruits each day. The National Cancer Institute (NCI) suggest eating at least 5 servings of fruits and vegetables each day: "5 a Day for Better Health." Studies have shown that daily consumption of vegetables and fruits may decrease the risk of lung, prostate, esophagus, colorectal, and stomach cancers.
- Eat more foods that are high in fiber, such as whole grains, breads, vegetables, and fruits. High-fiber diets may reduce the risk of colon cancer.
- Cut down on total fat intake. It is recommended that only 30 percent or less of one's daily intake be from fat. A high-fat diet may contribute to breast, colon, and prostate cancer.
- If you drink, limit the consumption of alcohol to a minimum. The heavy use of alcohol, especially when accompanied by cigarette smoking or smokeless tobacco use, increases the risk of cancers of the mouth, larynx, pharynx, esophagus, colon, and liver.
- Limit the consumption of salt-cured, smoked, and nitrite-cured foods. In areas of the world where salt-cured and smoked foods are eaten frequently, there is higher incidence of cancer of the esophagus and stomach.

Avoid Occupational Hazards

Exposure to several different **industrial agents** (nickel, chromate, asbestos, vinyl chloride, etc.) increases risk of various cancers. Risk of lung cancer from **asbestos** is greatly increased when combined with cigarette smoking.

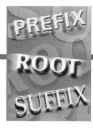

BUILDING YOUR MEDICAL VOCABULARY

This section provides the foundation for learning medical terminology. Medical words can be made up of four different types of word parts:

- Prefixes (P)
- Roots (R)
- Combining forms (CF)
- Suffixes (S)

By connecting various word parts in an organized sequence, thousands of words can be built and learned. In this text the word list is alphabetized so one can see the variety of meanings created when common prefixes and suffixes are repeatedly applied to certain word roots and/or combining forms. Words shown in pink are additional words related to the content of this chapter that are not built from word parts. These words are included to enhance your vocabulary. Note: An asterisk icon (✱) indicates words that are covered in the Pathology Spotlights section in this chapter.

MEDICAL WORD	WORD PARTS (WHEN APPLICABLE)			DEFINITION
	Part	Type	Meaning	
adenocarcinoma (ăd″ ĕ-nō-kăr″ sĭn-ō′ mă)	aden/o carcin -oma	CF R S	gland cancer tumor	A cancerous tumor of a gland
adjuvant therapy (ăd′ jū-vănt thĕr′ ă-pē)				Treatment that is given following the primary treatment. It is used to enhance the effectiveness of the primary treatment. In breast cancer, adjuvant therapy may include chemotherapy, radiation therapy, or hormone therapy.
anaplasia (ăn″ ă-plā′ zĭ-ă)	ana -plasia	P S	up formation	A characteristic of most cancerous cells in which there is a loss of differentiation
astrocytoma (ăs″ trō-sī-tō′ mă)	astro cyt -oma	P R S	star-shaped cell tumor	A tumor composed of star-shaped neuroglial cells
Burkitt's lymphoma (bŭrk′ ĭtz lĭm-fō′ mă)				A malignant tumor, most commonly found in Africa, that affects children. The characteristic symptom is a massive, swollen jaw.
carcinogen (kăr″ sĭn′ ō-jĕn)	carcin/o -gen	CF S	cancer formation	Any agent or substance that incites or produces cancer

MEDICAL WORD	WORD PARTS (WHEN APPLICABLE)			DEFINITION
	Part	Type	Meaning	
carcinoid (kăr′ sĭ-nōĭd)	carcin -oid	R S	cancer resemble	A tumor derived from the argentaffin cells in the intestinal tract, bile duct, pancreas, bronchus, or ovary.
carcinoma (kăr″ sĭ-nō′ mă)	carcin -oma	R S	cancer tumor	A cancerous tumor. See Figure 17–6.
chondrosarcoma (kŏn″ drō-săr-kō′ mă)	chondr/o sarc -oma	CF R S	cartilage flesh tumor	A cancerous tumor derived from cartilage cells
choriocarcinoma (kō″ rĭ-ō-kăr″ sĭ-nō′ mă)	chori/o carcin -oma	CF R S	chorion cancer tumor	A cancerous tumor of the uterus or at the site of an ectopic pregnancy
dedifferentiation (dē-dĭf″ ĕr-ĕn′ shē-ā′ shŭn)				The process whereby normal cells lose their specialization (differentiation) and become malignant
deoxyribonucleic acid (dē-ŏk″ sĭ-rī″ bō-nū-klē′ ĭk ăs′ ĭd)				A complex protein of high molecular weight that is found in the nucleus of every cell. DNA controls all the cell's activities and contains the genetic material necessary for the organism's heredity.
differentiation (dĭf″ ĕr-ĕn″ shē-ā″ shŭn)				The process whereby normal cells have a distinct appearance and specialized function
ductal carcinoma in situ (dŭk-tăl kăr′ sĭ-nō′ mă ĭn sī′ too)	duct -al carcin -oma in situ	R S R S P R	to lead pertaining to cancer tumor in place	Abnormal cells that involve only the lining of a duct. The cells have not spread outside the duct to other tissues in the breast. Also called DCIS or intraductal carcinoma. ✳ See Pathology Spotlight: Breast Cancer.
encapsulated (ĕn-kăp″ sū-lā′ tĕd)	en capsul -ate(d)	P R S	in a little box use, action	Enclosed within a sheath or capsule
Ewing's sarcoma (ū′ ingz săr-kō′ mă)				A primary bone cancer occurring in the pelvic area or in one of the long bones
exacerbation (ĕks-ăs″ ĕr-bā′ shŭn)				The process of increasing the severity of symptoms; a time when the symptoms of a disease are most prevalent

MEDICAL WORD	WORD PARTS (WHEN APPLICABLE)			DEFINITION
	Part	Type	Meaning	
fibrosarcoma (fĭ″ brō-săr-kō′ mă)	fibr/o sarc -oma	CF R S	fiber flesh tumor	A cancerous tumor arising from collagen-producing fibroblasts
fungating (fŭn′ gāt-ĭng)	fungat -ing	R S	mushroom, fungus quality of	The process of growing rapidly, like a fungus
glioblastoma (glī′ ō-blăs-tō′ mă)	gli/o -blast -oma	CF S S	glue immature cell tumor	A cancerous tumor of the brain, usually of the cerebral hemispheres
glioma (gli-ō′ mă)	gli -oma	R S	glue tumor	A cancerous tumor of the brain
hemangiosarcoma (hē-măn″ jĭ-ō- săr-kō′ mă)	hem angi/o sarc -oma	R CF R S	blood vessel flesh tumor	A cancerous tumor originating from blood vessels
Hodgkin's disease (hŏj′ kĭns dĭ-zēz″)				A form of lymphoma that occurs in young adults. See Figure 17–12. ✱ See Pathology Spotlight: Hodgkin's Disease.
human T-cell leukemia-lymphoma virus (HTLV) (hū′ măn tē′ sĕl lū-kē′ mĭ-ă lĭm-fō′ mă vī′ rŭs)				The first virus known to cause cancer in humans
hyperplasia (hī″ pĕr-plā′ zĭ-ă)	hyper -plasia	P S	excessive formation	Excessive formation and growth of normal cells
immuno-suppression (ĭm″ ū-nō-sŭ-prĕsh′ ŭn)	immun/o suppress -ion	CF R S	safe, immunity suppress process	The process of preventing formation of the immune response
immunotherapy (ĭm″ mū-nō-thĕr′ ă pē)	immun/o -therapy	CF S	safe, immunity treatment	Treatment of disease by active, passive, or adoptive immunity
infiltrative (ĭn′ fĭl-trā″ tĭve)	in filtrat -ive	P R S	into to strain through nature of	Pertaining to the process of extending or growing into normal tissue; invasive
in situ (ĭn sī′ too)				To stay within a site; refers to tumor cells that remain at a site and have not invaded adjacent tissue
interstitial (ĭn″ tĕr-stĭsh′ ăl)				Pertaining to between spaces

MEDICAL WORD	WORD PARTS (WHEN APPLICABLE)			DEFINITION
	Part	Type	Meaning	
invasive (ĭn-vā′ sĭv)				The spreading process of a malignant tumor into normal tissue
Kaposi's sarcoma (kăp′ ō-sēz săr-kō′ mă)				A malignant neoplasm that causes violaceous vascular lesions and general lymphadenopathy
leiomyosarcoma (lī″ ō-mī″ ō-săr-kō′ mă)	lei/o my/o sarc -oma	CF CF R S	smooth muscle flesh tumor	A cancerous tumor of smooth muscle tissue
lesion (lē′ zhŭn)				A wound; an injury, altered tissue, or a single infected patch of skin
leukemia (lū-kē′ mĭ-ă)	leuk -emia	R S	white blood condition	A disease of the blood characterized by overproduction of leukocytes; *cancer of the blood-forming tissues.* ✶ See Pathology Spotlight: Leukemia.
leukoplakia (lū″ kō-plā′ kĭ-ă)	leuk/o -plakia	CF S	white plate	White, thickened patches formed on the mucous membranes of the cheeks, gums, or tongue. These patches tend to become cancerous
liposarcoma (lĭp″ ō-săr-kō′ mă)	lip/o sarc -oma	CF R S	fat flesh tumor	A cancerous tumor of fat cells
lobular carcinoma in situ (lŏb′ ū-lăr kăr′ sĭ-nō′ mă ĭn sī′ too)	lobul -ar carcin -oma in situ	R S R S P R	small lobe pertaining to cancer tumor in place	Abnormal cells found in the lobules of the breast. This condition seldom becomes invasive cancer. However, having lobular carcinoma in situ increases one's risk of developing cancer in either breast. Also called LCIS.
lymphangiosarcoma (lĭm-făn″ jē-ō-săr-kō′ mă)	lymph angi/o sarc -oma	R CF R S	lymph vessel flesh tumor	A cancerous tumor of lymphatic vessels
lymphoma (lĭm-fō′ mă)	lymph -oma	R S	lymph tumor	A cancerous tumor of the lymph nodes
lymphosarcoma (lĭm″ fō-săr-kō′ mă)	lymph/o sarc -oma	CF R S	lymph flesh tumor	A cancerous disease of lymphatic tissue
malignant (mă-lĭg′ nănt)	malign -ant	R S	bad kind forming	Pertaining to a bad wandering; refers to the spreading process of cancer from one area of the body to another

MEDICAL WORD	WORD PARTS (WHEN APPLICABLE)			DEFINITION
	Part	**Type**	**Meaning**	
medulloblastoma (mĕ-dŭl″ ō-blăs-tō′ mă)	medull/o -blast -oma	CF S S	marrow immature cell tumor	A cancerous tumor of the brain, the fourth ventricle, and the cerebellum
melanoma (mĕl″ ă-nō′ mă)	melan -oma	R S	black tumor	A cancerous black mole or tumor. See Figure 17–7.
meningioma (mĕn-ĭn″ jĭ-ō′ mă)	mening/i -oma	CF S	membrane tumor	A cancerous tumor arising in the arachnoidal tissue of the brain
metastasis (mĕ-tăs′ tă-sis)	meta -stasis	P S	beyond control	The spreading process of cancer from a primary site to a secondary site
mucositis (mū″ kō-sī′ tĭs)	mucos -itis	R S	mucus inflammation	Inflammation of the oral mucosa caused by exposure to high-energy beams delivered by radiation therapy
mutagen (mū′ tă-jĕn)	muta -gen	R S	to change formation, produce	Any agent that causes a change in the genetic structure of an organism
mutation (mū-tā′ shŭn)	mutat -ion	R S	to change process	The process whereby the genetic structure is changed
mycotoxin (mī″ kō-tŏk′ sĭn)	myc/o tox -in	CF R S	fungus poison pertaining to	Pertaining to a fungus growing in food or animal feed that, if ingested, may cause cancer
myeloma (mī″ ĕ-lō′ mă)	myel -oma	R S	marrow tumor	A tumor arising in the hemopoietic portion of the bone marrow
myosarcoma (mī″ ō-săr-kō′ mă)	my/o sarc -oma	CF R S	muscle flesh tumor	A cancerous tumor of muscle tissue
neoplasm (nē′ ō-plăzm)	neo -plasm	P S	new a thing formed	A new thing formed, such as an abnormal growth or tumor
nephroblastoma (nĕf″ rō-blăs-tō′ mă)	nephr/o -blast -oma	CF S S	kidney immature cell tumor	A cancerous tumor of the kidney; *also called Wilm's tumor*
neuroblastoma (nū″ rō-blăs-tō′ mă)	neur/o -blast -oma	CF S S	nerve immature cell tumor	A cancerous tumor composed chiefly of neuroblasts; usually found in infants or young children
oligodendroglioma (ŏl″ ĭ-gō-dĕn″ drō-glī-ō′ mă)	oligo dendr/o gli -oma	P CF R S	little tree glue tumor	A cancerous tumor composed chiefly of neuroglial cells and located in the cerebrum
oncogenes (ŏng″ kō-jēn z′)	onc/o -genes	CF S	tumor produce	Cancer-causing genes

MEDICAL WORD	WORD PARTS (WHEN APPLICABLE)			DEFINITION
	Part	Type	Meaning	
oncogenic (ŏng″ kō-jĕn′ ĭk)	onc/o -genic	CF S	tumor formation, produce	The formation of tumors, especially cancerous tumors
osteogenic sarcoma (ŏs″ tē-ō-jĕn′ ĭk săr-kō′ mă)	oste/o -genic sarc -oma	CF S R S	bone formation, produce flesh tumor	A cancerous tumor composed of osseous tissue
Paget's disease (păj′ ĕts dĭ-zēz′)				An inflammatory bone disease that may precede the development of bone cancer. See Figure 17–8.
palliative (păl′ ĭ-ā-tĭv)	palliat -ive	R S	cloaked nature of	Pertaining to a form of treatment that will relieve or alleviate symptoms without curing
precancerous (prē-kăn′ sĕr-ŭs)	pre cancer -ous	P R S	before crab pertaining to	Pertaining to the state of a growth or condition before the onset of cancer
primary site (prī′ mă-rē sīt)				The original, initial, or principal site
proliferation (prō-lĭf″ ĕr-ā′ shŭn)	prolif (f)erat -ion	R R S	fruitful to bear process	The process of rapid production; to grow by multiplying
remission (rē- mĭsh′ ŭn)	remiss -ion	R S	remit process	The process of lessening the severity of symptoms. A time when symptoms of a disease are at rest
reticulosarcoma (rĕ-tĭk″ ū-lō-săr-kō′ mă)	reticul/o sarc -oma	CF R S	net flesh tumor	A cancerous tumor of the lymphatic system
retinoblastoma (rĕt″ ĭ-nō-blăs-tō′ mă)	retin/o -blast -oma	CF S S	retina immature cell tumor	A cancerous tumor of the retina
rhabdomyo- sarcoma (răb″ dō-mī″ ō-săr-kō′ mă)	rhabd/o my/o sarc -oma	CF CF R S	rod muscle flesh tumor	A cancerous tumor arising in striated muscle tissue
ribonucleic acid (RNA) (rī″ bō-nū′ klē′ ĭk ăs′ ĭd)				A nucleic acid found in all living cells that is responsible for protein synthesis. The three types are mRNA—messenger RNA; tRNA—transfer RNA; and rRNA—ribosomal RNA.

MEDICAL WORD	WORD PARTS (WHEN APPLICABLE)			DEFINITION
	Part	**Type**	**Meaning**	
sarcoma (săr-kō′ mă)	sarc -oma	R S	flesh tumor	A cancerous tumor arising from connective tissue
scirrhus (skĭr′ ŭs)				A hard, cancerous tumor composed of connective tissue
secondary site (sĕk′ ăn-dĕr″ ē sīt)				The second site usually derived from the primary site
seminoma (sĕm″ ĭ-nō′ mă)	semin -oma	R S	seed tumor	A cancerous tumor of the testis
sentinel node biopsy (sĕn′ tĭ-nĕl nōd bī′ ŏp-sē)				Allows the physician to pinpoint the first lymph node into which a tumor drains (*the sentinel node*), and remove only the nodes most likely to contain cancer cells. To locate the sentinel node, the physician injects a radioactive tracer in the area around the tumor. The tracer travels the same path to the lymph nodes that cancer cells would take, making it possible for the surgeon to determine the one or two nodes most likely to test positive. The surgeon will then remove the nodes most likely to be cancerous.
tamponade (cardiac) (tam′ pŏn-ād [kăr′ dē-ăk])				A pathologic condition of the heart in which there is accumulation of excess fluid in the pericardium. It may be caused by advanced cancer of the lung or a tumor that has metastasized to the pericardium.
teratoma (tĕr″ ă-tō′ mă)	terat -oma	R S	monster tumor	A cancerous tumor of the ovary or testis; may contain embryonic tissues of hair, teeth, bone, or muscle
thymoma (thī-mō′ mă)	thym -oma	R S	thymus tumor	A tumor of the thymus gland
trismus (trĭz′ mŭs)	trism -us	R S	grating pertaining to	Pertaining to the inability to open the mouth fully; occurs in patients with oral cancer who undergo a combination of surgery and radiation therapy
tumor (tū′ mor)				An abnormal growth, swelling, or enlargement

MEDICAL WORD	WORD PARTS (WHEN APPLICABLE)			DEFINITION
	Part	**Type**	**Meaning**	
viral (vī′ răl)	vir -al	R S	virus (poison) pertaining to	Pertaining to a virus, which means poison in Latin. A virus is a minute organism that may be responsible for 50% of all diseases.
Wilms' tumor (vĭlmz tū′ mor)				A cancerous tumor of the kidney occurring mainly in children
xerostomia (zē″ rō-stō′ mē-ă)	xer/o stom -ia	CF R S	dry mouth condition	A condition of dryness of the mouth; an oral change caused by radiation therapy or chemotherapy

Terminology Translator

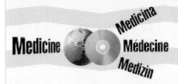

This feature, found on the accompanying CD-ROM, provides an innovative tool to translate medical words into Spanish, French, and German.

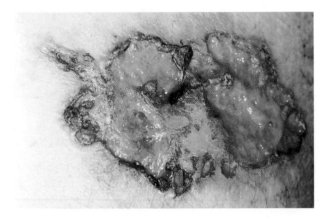

FIGURE 17–6

Basal cell carcinoma. (Courtesy of Jason L. Smith, MD.)

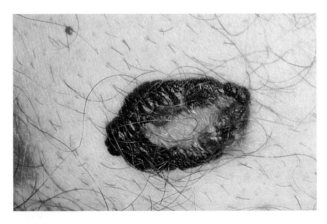

FIGURE 17–7

Melanoma. (Courtesy of Jason L. Smith, MD.)

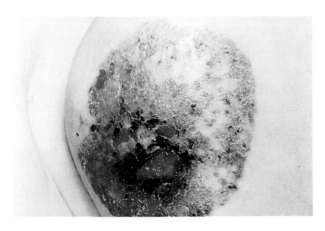

FIGURE 17–8

Paget's disease of the breast. (Courtesy of Jason L. Smith, MD.)

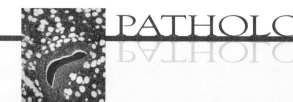

PATHOLOGY SPOTLIGHTS

Breast Cancer

This year approximately 211,300 women and approximately 1,300 men will be diagnosed with breast cancer. It kills about 39,800 women a year, and is the leading cause of death in women between the ages of 32 and 52.

In cancer, there is an abnormal process wherein a cell or group of cells undergoes changes and no longer carries on normal cell functions. This failure of immature cells to develop specialized functions is called dedifferentiation. It is believed that this process involves a disturbance in the DNA of the affected cells. Malignant cells usually multiply rapidly, forming a mass of abnormal cells that enlarges, ulcerates, and sheds malignant cells to surrounding tissues. This process destroys the normal cells, with malignant cells taking their place, and often results in the formation of a tumor.

If cancer is not detected and treated early, it will continue to grow, invade, and destroy adjacent tissue, and spread into surrounding lymph nodes. See Figure 17–9. It can be carried by the lymph and/or blood to other areas of the body and once this process, known as metastasis, has occurred, the cancer is usually advanced and/or disseminated and the 5-year survival rate is low. See Figure 17–10. Early detection of breast cancer is extremely important. The 5-year survival rate for women with localized and properly treated breast cancer is 92 percent.

Approximately 50 percent of malignant tumors of the breast appear in the upper, outer quadrant and extend into the armpit. Eighteen percent of breast cancers occur in the nipple area, 11 percent in the lower outer quadrant, and 6 percent in the inner quadrant.

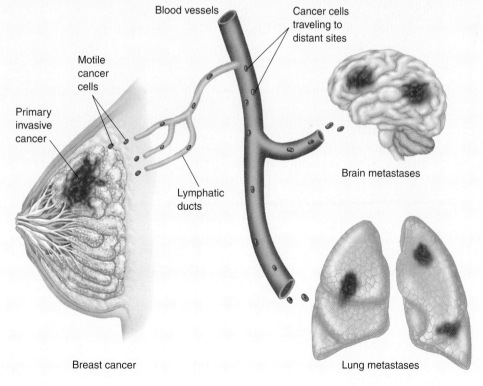

FIGURE 17–9

Invasion and metastasis by cancer cells. (Source: Pearson Education/PH College.)

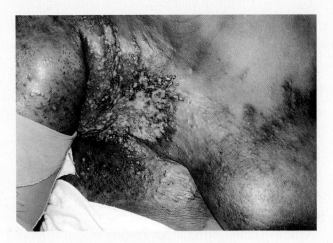

FIGURE 17–10

Metastatic breast cancer. (Courtesy of Jason L. Smith, MD.)

Signs and symptoms of breast cancer are generally insidious and may include:

- Unusual secretions from the nipple
- Changes in the nipple's appearance
- Nontender, movable lump
- Well-localized discomfort that may be described as burning, stinging, or aching sensation
- Dimpling or peau d'orange (orange-peel appearance) may be present over the area of cancer of the breast
- Asymmetry and an elevation of the affected breast
- Nipple retraction
- Pain in the later stages

Stages of breast cancer, according to the American Cancer Society, indicate the size of a tumor and how far the cancer has spread within the breast, to nearby tissues, and to other organs. Specific treatment is most often determined by the following stages of the disease:

Carcinoma in situ. Cancer is confined to the lobules (milk-producing glands) or ducts (passages connecting milk-producing glands to the nipple) and has not invaded nearby breast tissue.

Stage I. Tumor is smaller than or equal to 2 centimeters in diameter and underarm (axillary) lymph nodes test negative for cancer.

Stage II. Tumor is between 2 and 5 centimeters in diameter with or without positive lymph nodes, or tumor is greater than 5 centimeters without positive lymph nodes.

Stage III. This stage is divided into substages known as IIIA and IIIB:
- **IIIA.** Tumor is larger than 5 centimeters with positive movable lymph nodes, or tumor is any size with lymph nodes that adhere to one another or surrounding tissue.
- **IIIB.** Tumor of any size has spread to the skin, chest wall, or internal mammary lymph nodes (located beneath the breast and inside the chest).

Stage IV. Tumor, regardless of size, has metastasized (spread) to distant sites such as bones, lungs, or lymph nodes not near the breast.

Recurrent breast cancer. The disease has returned in spite of initial treatment.

Two genes have been identified as "breast cancer genes." BRCA-1 and BRCA-2 are genes that, when changed, place a woman at greater risk of developing breast cancer compared to women who do not have either mutation. One single genetic mishap is not enough for a cell to become cancerous. It takes several changes. Women who have inherited mutations within the BRCA-1 and BRCA-2 genes are at higher risk for breast cancer than those who don't have them. However, it still takes further events for cancer to occur in these women. There are internal factors, such as estrogen, and external factors that can contribute to this chain of events.

Women who have defective BRCA-1 or BRCA-2 genes have a higher rate of breast cancer. Now it appears that only 5 percent to 9 percent of all breast cancers occur because of the defective genes. Unfortunately, 80 percent to 90 percent of women who have the genes will get breast cancer.

However, 90 percent to 95 percent of all breast cancers occur in women over age 50 who do not have the genes. Testing negative for BRCA-1 or BRCA-2 does not mean that a person will not get breast cancer.

More than 90 percent of all breast lumps are discovered by women themselves. The majority of these lumps are benign (noncancerous) but of those that are not, early detection and treatment are essential.

Refer to the following BREAST acronym for easy-to-remember guidelines:

- **B**eing informed could save your life.
- **R**isk factors in order of importance:
  1. Family history—increased risk when breast cancer occurs before menopause in mother, sister, or daughter, especially if cancer occurs in both breasts
  2. Over age 50 and nullipara
  3. Having a first baby after age 30
  4. History of chronic breast disease, especially epithelial hyperplasia
  5. Exposure to ionizing radiation of more than 50 rad during adolescence
  6. Obesity
  7. Early menarche, late menopause
- **E**xamine your breast every month (BSE, Breast Self-Examination—see Figure 17–11).
- **A**ppearance
- **S**ize, shape, symmetry
- **T**enderness, thickening, texture changes

Hodgkin's Disease

Hodgkin's disease, sometimes called *Hodgkin's lymphoma*, is a cancer that starts in lymphatic tissue. Hodgkin's disease is a *malignant lymphoma* (cancer of lymphatic tissue). There are two kinds of lymphomas: *Hodgkin's disease* (named after Dr. Thomas Hodgkin, who first recognized it in 1832) and *non-Hodgkin's lymphomas*.

Because lymphatic tissue is present in many parts of the body, Hodgkin's disease can start almost anywhere, but most often starts in lymph nodes in the upper part of the body. The most common sites are in the chest, neck, or under the arms. Hodgkin's disease enlarges the lymphatic tissue, which can then cause pressure on important structures. It can spread through the lymphatic vessels to other lymph nodes. This is the major way it spreads. Most Hodgkin's disease spreads to nearby lymph node sites in the body, not distant ones. It rarely gets into the blood vessels, but when it does, it can spread to almost any other site in the body, including the liver and lungs. See Figure 17–12 for a picture of cutaneous Hodgkin's, in which it has spread to the patient's skin.

Lymph nodes enlarge for many reasons. Although Hodgkin's disease is one cause, enlarged lymph nodes are more commonly a result of the body fighting an infection.

The cancer cells in Hodgkin's disease are called *Reed-Sternberg cells*, after the two doctors who first described them in detail. Under a microscope they look different from

WHY DO THE BREAST SELF-EXAM?

There are many good reasons for doing a breast self-exam each month. One reason is that it is easy to do and the more you do it, the better you will get at it. When you get to know how your breasts normally feel, you will quickly be able to feel any change, and early detection is the key to successful treatment and cure.

REMEMBER: A breast self-exam could save your breast – and save your life. Most breast lumps are found by women themselves, but in fact, most lumps in the breast are not cancer. Be safe, be sure.

WHEN TO DO BREAST SELF-EXAM

The best time to do breast self-exam is right after your period, when breasts are not tender or swollen. If you do not have regular periods or sometimes skip a month, do it on the same day every month.

NOW, HOW TO DO BREAST SELF-EXAM

1. Lie down and put a pillow under your right shoulder. Place your right arm behind your head.

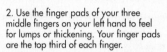

2. Use the finger pads of your three middle fingers on your left hand to feel for lumps or thickening. Your finger pads are the top third of each finger.

3. Press firmly enough to know how your breast feels. If you're not sure how hard to press, ask your health care provider. Or try to copy the way your health care provider uses the finger pads during a breast exam. Learn what your breast feels like most of the time. A firm ridge in the lower curve of each breast is normal.

4. Move around the breast in a set way. You can choose either the circle (A), the up and down line (B), or the wedge (C). Do it the same way every time. It will help you to make sure that you've gone over the entire breast area, and to remember how your breast feels.

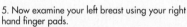

5. Now examine your left breast using your right hand finger pads.

6. If you find any changes, see your doctor right away.

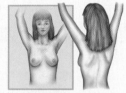

FOR ADDED SAFETY:

You should also check your breasts while standing in front of a mirror right after you do your breast self-exam each month. See if there are any changes in the way your breasts look: dimpling of the skin, changes in the nipple, or redness or swelling.

You might also want to do a breast self-exam while you're in the shower. Your soapy hands will glide over the wet skin, making it easy to check how your breasts feel.

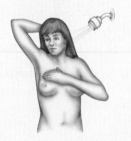

FIGURE 17–11

Breast self-examination.

cells of non-Hodgkin's lymphomas and other cancers. Most scientists now believe that Reed-Sternberg cells are a type of malignant *B lymphocyte*. Normal B lymphocytes are the cells that make antibodies that help fight infections.

Before 1970 few people with diagnosed Hodgkin's disease recovered. Today, more than 80 percent of people who receive initial treatment experience a complete remission. Advances in diagnosis, staging and treatment of Hodgkin's disease have helped to make this once uniformly fatal disease highly treatable with potential for full recovery.

Within 15 years following treatment, many of the people who die do so because of complications of the treatment, such as secondary cancers and heart failure, rather than of the dis-

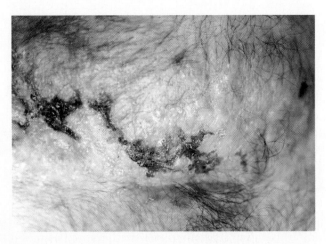

FIGURE 17–12

Cutaneous Hodgkin's disease. (Courtesy of Jason L. Smith, MD.)

ease itself. The challenge for researchers is to decrease the long-term complications of treatment without compromising the effectiveness of the therapy.

Leukemia

Leukemia is cancer that usually affects the white blood cells. White blood cells develop from stem cells in the bone marrow. Leukemia results when something goes wrong with the process of maturation from stem cell to white blood cell and a cancerous change occurs. The change often involves a rearrangement of pieces of chromosomes. Because the chromosomal rearrangements disturb the normal control of cell division, the affected cells multiply without restraint, becoming cancerous. They ultimately occupy the bone marrow, replacing the cells that produce normal blood cells. These leukemic (cancer) cells may also invade other organs, including the liver, spleen, lymph nodes, kidneys, and brain.

There are four major types of leukemia, named for how quickly they progress and which kind of white blood cell they affect. Acute leukemias progress rapidly; chronic leukemias progress slowly. Lymphocytic leukemias affect lymphocytes; myeloid (myelocytic) leukemias affect myelocytes. Myelocytes develop into granulocytes, another term for neutrophils.

Acute lymphocytic (lymphoblastic) **leukemia** is a life-threatening disease in which the cells that normally develop into lymphocytes become cancerous and rapidly replace normal cells in the bone marrow. It is the most common cancer in children, accounting for 25 percent of all cancers in children under age 15. It most often affects children between the ages of 3 and 5, but can also affect adolescents and, less commonly, adults.

Acute myeloid (myelocytic, myelogenous, myeloblastic, myelomonocytic) **leukemia** is a life-threatening disease in which myelocytes (the cells that normally develop into granulocytes) become cancerous and rapidly replace normal cells in the bone marrow. This type of leukemia affects people of all ages, but mostly adults. Exposure to large doses of radiation and use of some cancer chemotherapy drugs increase the likelihood of developing acute myeloid leukemia.

Chronic lymphocytic leukemia is characterized by a large number of cancerous mature lymphocytes (a type of white blood cell) and enlarged lymph nodes. More than three-fourths of the people who have this type of leukemia are over age 60; it affects men two to three times more often than women. This type of leukemia is rare in Japan and China and remains uncommon in Japanese people who have moved to the United States—a clue that genetics plays some role in its development.

Chronic myelocytic (myeloid, myelogenous, granulocytic) **leukemia** is a disease in which a cell in the bone marrow becomes cancerous and produces a large number of abnormal granulocytes (a type of white blood cell). This disease may affect people of any age and of either sex but is uncommon in children under 10 years old.

Testicular Cancer

Cancer of the testicles is the most common cancer in men aged 15 to 34. It accounts for only about 1 percent of all cancers in men, according to the National Cancer Institute. In a given year about 7,000 American men get the disease, with an estimated 325 deaths. Compared to prostate cancer, estimated to kill 40,400 of its 244,000 victims in a given year, testicular cancer is relatively rare. For unknown reasons, the disease is about four times more common in white men than in black men. The cause of testicular tumors is unknown.

Most testicular tumors are discovered by patients themselves, either by accident or while performing a self-examination on each testicle. See Figure 17–13. The usual presentation is of an enlarged, painless lump. The lump typically is pea-sized, but sometimes it might be as big as a marble or even an egg. Occasionally there may be pain. Besides lumps, if a man notices any other abnormality—an enlarged testicle, a feeling of heaviness or sudden collection of fluid in the scrotum, or a dull ache in the lower abdomen or groin—he should seek medical attention immediately. The origin and nature of scrotal masses must be determined as soon as possible because most testicular masses are malignant. Prognosis depends on the histology and extent of the tumor. Survival rates are approximately 95 percent at 5 years for seminomas and nonseminomas localized to the testis or low-volume metastases in the retroperitoneal area. The 5-year survival rate for extensive retroperitoneal metastases or pulmonary or other visceral metastases

Testicular Self-Examination

- Examine testicles while taking a warm shower or bath, or just after if using a mirror to compare size.

- The scrotum, testicles, and hands should be soapy to allow easy manipulation of the tissue.

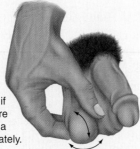

- Gently roll each testicle between the thumb and fingers of each hand. If one testicle is substantially larger than the other, or if any hard lumps are detected, consult a physician immediately.

- Normal scrotal contents may be confusing. Just above and behind the testicle is the epididymis. It feels soft and tender overall, although parts of it may be rather firm. This is normal. The spermatic cord, a small, round, moveable tube, extends up from the epididymis. It feels firm and smooth. Of greatest concern is any hard lump felt directly on the testicle, even if it is painless.

- Choose a day out of each month on which to examine yourself. Most men choose an easy day to remember, such as the first or last day of the month.

FIGURE 17–13

Procedure for testicular self-examination. (Source: Pearson Education/PH College.)

is poorer and varies with site, volume, and histology of the metastases. It is most important that testicular cancer be diagnosed early.

Testicular cancer is diagnosed by physical examination, ultrasonography, radioimmunoassay, abdominal and pelvic CT scans, and pathological examination of a tissue sample. The tissue sample is obtained by removing the entire affected testicle (inguinal orchiectomy). It is believed that a surgeon should not cut through the scrotum to remove a part of the testicle, because if cancer is present, a cut through the outer layer of the testicle may cause the disease to spread. Besides enabling diagnosis, testicle removal also can prevent further growth of the primary tumor.

Nearly all testicular tumors stem from germ cells, the special sperm-forming cells within the testicles. These tumors fall into one of two types, seminomas or nonseminomas. Other forms of testicular cancer, such as sarcomas or lymphomas, are extremely rare.

Seminomas account for about 40 percent of all testicular cancer and are made up of immature germ cells. Usually, seminomas are slow growing and tend to stay localized in the testicle for long periods.

Nonseminomas are a group of cancers that sometimes occur in combination, including choriocarcinoma, embryonal carcinoma, and yolk sac tumors. Nonseminomas arise from more mature, specialized germ cells and tend to be more aggressive than seminomas. According to the American Cancer Society, 60 to 70 percent of patients with nonseminomas have cancer that has spread to the lymph nodes.

Physicians measure the extent of the disease by conducting tests that allow the doctor to categorize, or "stage," the disease. These staging tests include blood analyses, imaging techniques, and sometimes additional surgery. Staging allows the doctor to plan the most appropriate treatment for each patient. Stages of testicular cancer are as follows:

Stage 1. Cancer confined to the testicle.

Stage 2. Disease spread to retroperitoneal lymph nodes, located in the rear of the body below the diaphragm.

Stage 3. Cancer spread beyond the lymph nodes to remote sites in the body, such as the lungs and/or liver.

Recurrent. Recurrent disease means that the cancer has come back after it has been treated. It may come back in the same place or in another part of the body.

No one treatment works for all testicular cancers. Seminomas and nonseminomas differ in their tendency to spread, their patterns of spread, and response to radiation therapy. Thus, they often require different treatment strategies, which doctors choose based on the type of tumor and the stage of disease.

Because they are slow growing and tend to stay localized, seminomas generally are diagnosed in stage 1 or 2. Treatment might be a combination of testicle removal, radiation, or chemotherapy. Stage 3 seminomas are usually treated with a combination of chemotherapy drugs.

Though most nonseminomas are not diagnosed at an early stage, cases confined to the testicle may need no further treatment other than testicle removal. These men must have careful follow-up for at least two years because about 10 percent of stage 1 patients have recurrences, which then are treated with chemotherapy. Stage 2 nonseminoma patients who have had testicle and lymph node removal may also need no further therapy. Some doctors recommend a short course of a combination of chemotherapy drugs for stage 2 patients to reduce the risk of recurrence. Most stage 3 nonseminomas can be cured with drug combinations.

The Food and Drug Administration (FDA) has approved several drugs to treat testicular cancer, including Ifex (ifosfamide), Vepesid (etoposide), Velban (vinblastine sulfate), Blenoxane (bleomycin sulfate), and Platinol (cisplatin).

✔ PATHOLOGY CHECKPOINT

Following is a concise list of the pathology-related terms that you've seen in the chapter. Review this checklist to make sure that you are familiar with the meaning of each term before moving on to the next section.

Conditions and Symptoms

- ❏ adenocarcinoma
- ❏ anaplasia
- ❏ astrocytoma
- ❏ Burkitt's lymphoma
- ❏ carcinoma
- ❏ chondrosarcoma
- ❏ choriocarcinoma
- ❏ ductal carcinoma in situ
- ❏ Ewing's sarcoma
- ❏ fibrosarcoma
- ❏ glioblastoma
- ❏ glioma
- ❏ hemangiosarcoma
- ❏ Hodgkin's disease
- ❏ hyperplasia
- ❏ Kaposi's sarcoma
- ❏ Leiomyosarcoma
- ❏ leukemia
- ❏ leukoplakia
- ❏ liposarcoma
- ❏ lobular carcinoma in situ
- ❏ lymphangiosarcoma
- ❏ lymphoma
- ❏ lymphosarcoma
- ❏ medulloblastoma
- ❏ melanoma
- ❏ meningioma

- ❏ mucositis
- ❏ myeloma
- ❏ myosarcoma
- ❏ neoplasm
- ❏ nephroblastoma
- ❏ neuroblastoma
- ❏ oligodendroglioma
- ❏ osteogenic sarcoma
- ❏ Paget's disease
- ❏ reticulosarcoma
- ❏ retinoblastoma
- ❏ rhabdomyosarcoma
- ❏ sarcoma
- ❏ scirrhus
- ❏ seminoma
- ❏ tamponade (cardiac)
- ❏ teratoma
- ❏ thymoma
- ❏ trismus
- ❏ tumor
- ❏ Wilm's tumor
- ❏ xerostomia

Diagnosis and Treatment

- ❏ adjuvant therapy
- ❏ carcinogen
- ❏ dedifferentiation
- ❏ differentiation

- ❏ encapsulated
- ❏ exacerbation
- ❏ fungating
- ❏ human T cell leukemia-lymphoma virus
- ❏ immunosuppression
- ❏ immunotherapy
- ❏ infiltrative
- ❏ in situ
- ❏ interstitial
- ❏ invasive
- ❏ lesion
- ❏ malignant
- ❏ metastasis
- ❏ mutagen
- ❏ mutation
- ❏ mycotoxin
- ❏ oncogenes
- ❏ oncogenic
- ❏ palliative
- ❏ precancerous
- ❏ primary site
- ❏ proliferation
- ❏ remission
- ❏ secondary site
- ❏ sentinel node biopsy
- ❏ virus

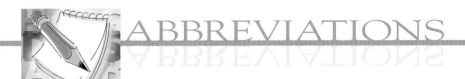

ABBREVIATION	MEANING	ABBREVIATION	MEANING
Adeno-CA	adenocarcinoma	IL-2	interleukin-2
AFP	alpha-fetoprotein	LAK	lymphokine-activated killer (cells)
Bx	biopsy		
CA	cancer	LCIS	lobular carcinoma in situ
chem	chemotherapy	mets	metastases
DCIS	ductal carcinoma in situ	RNA	ribonucleic acid
DNA	deoxyribonucleic acid	St	stage (of disease)
HD	Hodgkin's disease	TNF	tumor necrosis factor
Hpd	hematoporphyrin derivative	TNM	tumor, node, metastasis
HTLV	human T-cell leukemia-lymphoma virus		

STUDY AND REVIEW

An Overview of Oncology

Write your answers to the following questions. Do not refer to the text.

1. Name the three main classifications of cancer.

   a. _____   b. _____   c. _____

2. Define cell differentiation. _____

   _____

3. Define dedifferentiation. _____

   _____

4. Name three ways that malignant cells spread to body parts.

   a. _____   b. _____   c. _____

5. List the seven warning signals for cancer.

   a. _____   b. _____

   c. _____   d. _____

   e. _____   f. _____

   g. _____

6. Name four methods that may be used in the treatment of cancer.

   a. _____   b. _____

   c. _____   d. _____

Word Parts

1. In the spaces provided, write the definitions of these prefixes, roots, combining forms, and suffixes. Do not refer to the listings of medical words. Leave blank those words you cannot define.

2. After completing as many as you can, refer to the medical word listings to check your work. For each word missed or left blank, write the word and its definition several times on the margins of these pages or on a separate sheet of paper.

3. To maximize the learning process, it is to your advantage to do the following exercises as directed. To refer to the word building section before completing these exercises invalidates the learning process.

PREFIXES

Give the definitions of the following prefixes:

1. ana- _____

2. astro- _____

3. hyper- _____

4. neo- _____

5. oligo- _____

6. pre- _____

7. en- _____

8. in- _____

9. meta- _____

ROOTS AND COMBINING FORMS

Give the definitions of the following roots and combining forms:

1. aden/o _____

2. angi/o _____

3. cancer _____

4. carcin _____

5. carcin/o _____

6. chondr/o _____

7. chori/o _____

8. cyt _____

9. dendr/o _____

10. fibr/o _____

11. gli _____

12. gli/o _____

13. hem _____

14. immun/o _____

15. lei/o _____

16. leuk _____

17. leuk/o _____

18. lip/o _____

19. lymph _____

20. lymph/o _____

21. medull/o _____

22. melan _____

23. mening/i _____

24. mucos _____

25. myc/o _____

26. myel _____

27. my/o _____

28. capsul _____

29. nephr/o _____

30. neur/o _____

31. onc/o _____

32. oste/o _____

33. reticul/o _____

34. retin/o _____

35. rhabd/o _____

36. sarc _____

37. duct _____

38. semin _____

39. stom _____   40. terat _____

41. thym _____   42. tox _____

43. trism _____   44. xer/o _____

45. lobul _____   46. situ _____

47. fungat _____   48. suppress _____

49. filtrat _____   50. malign _____

51. muta _____   52. mutat _____

53. palliat _____   54. prolif _____

55. f (erat) _____   56. remiss _____

57. vir _____

SUFFIXES

Give the definitions of the following suffixes:

1. -blast _____   2. -emia _____

3. -gen _____   4. -genes _____

5. -genic _____   6. -ia _____

7. -in _____   8. -itis _____

9. -oma _____   10. -ous _____

11. -plakia _____   12. -plasia _____

13. -plasm _____   14. -ate (d) _____

15. -therapy _____   16. -us _____

17. -al _____   18. -ar _____

19. -ing _____   20. -ion _____

21. -ive _____   22. -ant _____

23. -stasis _____   24. -oid _____

Identifying Medical Terms

In the spaces provided, write the medical terms for the following meanings:

1. _____ Any agent or substance that incites or produces cancer

2. _____ A cancerous tumor derived from cartilage cells

3. _____ A cancerous tumor of the brain

4. _____ A hard, cancerous tumor composed of connective tissue

5. _____ Cancer of the blood-forming tissues

6. _____ A cancerous tumor of lymphoid tissue

7. _____ A cancerous black mole or tumor

8. _____ A cancerous tumor of muscle tissue

9. _____ A cancerous tumor composed of osseous tissue

10. _____ A cancerous tumor arising from connective tissue

Spelling

In the spaces provided, write the correct spelling of these misspelled words.

1. anplasia _____

2. fibrsarcoma _____

3. lymphsarcoma _____

4. myloma _____

5. oncgenic _____

6. semioma _____

Matching

Select the appropriate lettered meaning for each word listed below.

_____ 1. Hodgkin's disease

_____ 2. exacerbation

_____ 3. differentiation

_____ 4. in situ

_____ 5. interleukin-2

_____ 6. photodynamic therapy

_____ 7. recombinant interferon

_____ 8. tumor necrosis factor

_____ 9. Kaposi's sarcoma

_____ 10. malignant

a. The spreading process of cancer from one area of the body to another

b. A lymphokine produced by macrophages

c. A genetically engineered immune-boosting drug that stimulates the patient's immune system

d. The process whereby normal cells have a distinct appearance and specialized function

e. A form of lymphoma that occurs in young adults

f. The use of a red laser to kill cancerous cells

g. To stay within a site

h. A malignant neoplasm that causes violaceous vascular lesions and general lymphadenopathy

i. The process of increasing the severity of symptoms

j. A genetically engineered immune system activator

k. Any agent that causes a change in the genetic structure of an organism

Abbreviations

Place the correct word, phrase, or abbreviation in the space provided.

1. adenocarcinoma _____

2. biopsy _____

3. CA _____

4. chem _____

5. deoxyribonucleic acid _____

6. IL-2 _____

7. lymphokine-activated killer _____

8. mets _____

9. TNF _____

10. tumor, node, metastases _____

MedMedia
Wrap-Up
www.prenhall.com/rice

Additional interactive resources and activities for this chapter can be found on the Companion Website. For animations, videos, audio glossary, and review, access the accompanying CD-ROM in this book.

Audio Glossary
Medical Terminology Exercises & Activities
Pathology Spotlight
Terminology Translator
Animations
Videos

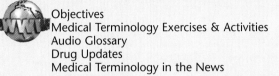

Objectives
Medical Terminology Exercises & Activities
Audio Glossary
Drug Updates
Medical Terminology in the News

RADIOLOGY AND NUCLEAR MEDICINE 18

OBJECTIVES

On completion of this chapter, you will be able to:

- Define radiology.
- Describe dangers and safety precautions associated with x-rays.
- Describe the positions used in radiography.
- Describe diagnostic radiology.
- Describe interventional radiology.
- Describe nuclear medicine.
- Define radiation therapy.
- Describe important factors that must be considered when determining the use of radiotherapy for the cancer patient.
- Define the techniques of radiotherapy: external and internal.
- List 13 side effects of radiation.
- Analyze, build, spell, and pronounce medical words.
- Describe each of the conditions presented in the Radiology & Nuclear Medicine Spotlights.
- Complete the Medical Vocabulary Checkpoint.
- Identify and define selected abbreviations.
- Successfully complete the study and review section.

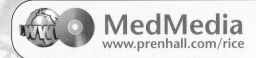

MedMedia
www.prenhall.com/rice

Additional interactive resources and activities for this chapter can be found on the Companion Website. For Terminology Translator, animations, videos, audio glossary, and review, access the accompanying CD-ROM in this book.

An Overview of Radiology and Nuclear Medicine

RADIOLOGY

Radiology is the study of x-rays, radioactive substances, radioactive isotopes, and ionizing radiation. Sometimes called **roentgenology**, this medical specialty was developed after the discovery of an unknown ray in 1895 by Wilhelm Konrad Roentgen, a German physicist, who called his discovery an x-ray. An x-ray is produced by the collision of a stream of electrons against a target (usually an anode of one of the heavy metals) contained within a vacuum tube. This collision produces electromagnetic rays of short wavelengths and high energy. The physician who specializes in radiology, roentgen diagnosis, and roentgen therapy is called a **radiologist**. A **roentgenologist** is a physician who has specialized only in the use of x-rays for diagnosis and the treatment of disease.

Characteristics of X-Rays

1. X-rays are an invisible form of radiant energy with short wavelengths traveling at 186,000 miles per second. They are able to penetrate different substances to varying degrees.

2. X-rays cause **ionization** of the substances through which they pass. Ionization is a process resulting in the gain or loss of one or more electrons in neutral atoms. The gain of an electron creates a negative electrical charge, whereas the loss of an electron results in a positively charged particle. These negatively or positively charged particles are called ions.

3. X-rays cause fluorescence of certain substances, thus allowing for the process known as **fluoroscopy** (Fig. 18–1). With this technique, internal structures show up as dark images on a glowing screen as x-rays pass through the area being examined. Fluoroscopy also allows the physician an opportunity to visualize internal structures that are in motion. It is also possible to make permanent records of the fluoroscopic examination for future study.

4. X-rays travel in a straight line, thus allowing the x-ray beam to be directed at a specific site during radiotherapy or to produce high-quality shadow images on film (radiographs).

5. X-rays are able to penetrate substances of different densities. In the body, x-rays pass through air in the lungs, fluids such as blood and lymph, and fat around muscles. Such substances are said to be **radiolucent**. Substances that obstruct the passage of radiant energy, in other words absorb radiant energy, such as calcium in bones, lead, or barium, are **radiopaque**. Control of the voltage and amperage applied to the x-ray tube, plus the duration of the exposure, allow images of body structures of varying densities. A contrast medium can be introduced into the body to enhance certain x-ray images. This characteristic allows x-rays to be used as a diagnostic tool.

6. X-rays can destroy body cells. Radiation can be used in the treatment of malignant tumors. In these cases, the x-ray voltage is administered by a radiotherapist using radiotherapy machines such as a linear accelerator or the betatron. Care must be exercised in the administration of radiotherapy, as x-rays can destroy healthy as well as abnormal tissue.

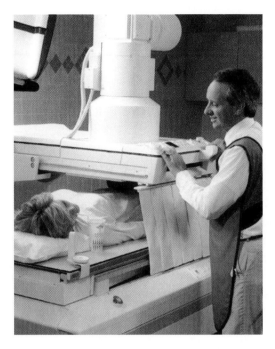

FIGURE 18–1

Advantx™ radiography/fluoroscopy system. (Courtesy of GE Medical Systems.)

Dangers and Safety Precautions

Because **x-rays** are invisible and produce no sound or smell, those working around and with them need to take certain precautions to avoid unnecessary exposure. Listed are some of the dangers known to be associated with x-rays and the safety precautions designed to prevent unnecessary exposure.

PROLONGED EXPOSURE

Prolonged and continued exposure to x-rays can cause damage to the gonads and/or depress the hematopoietic system, which can cause leukopenia and/or leukemia. Personnel involved with radiation therapy should spend the minimal amount of time necessary when caring for patients receiving internal radiation therapy. The farther away one is from the source of radiation, the less the degree of exposure.

SECONDARY RADIATION

X-rays can scatter or be diverted from their normal straight paths when they strike radiopaque objects. This scatter or secondary radiation tends to add unwanted density to the image; therefore, a device known as a **grid** is positioned between the x-ray machine and the patient to absorb scatter before it reaches the x-ray film. The **Potter-Bucky diaphragm**, commonly known as the Bucky, is the most frequently used grid. It consists of alternating strips of lead and radiolucent material. The lead strips are arranged parallel to the stream of x-rays and are kept in motion by a mechanism to prevent them from becoming superimposed on the exposed film.

SAFETY PRECAUTIONS

Not all scatter or secondary radiation is absorbed by a grid; therefore, those working in areas adjacent to x-ray equipment risk unintentional exposure from this source unless proper safety precautions are observed. Generally, these safety precautions include the five described below.

Film Badge.   A **film badge** is a device, usually pinned to the clothing, that is sensitive to ionizing radiation and monitors exposure to beta and gamma rays. A periodic analysis of the film badge reveals the amount of radiation the individual has received.

Lead Barrier.   Persons who operate x-ray machines do so from behind barriers equipped with a lead-treated window for viewing the patient.

Lead-lined Room.   X-ray equipment should be housed in an area featuring lead-lined walls, floors, and doors to prevent the escape of radiation from the room.

Protective Clothing.   Lead-lined gloves and aprons are worn by people who hold or position patients for x-ray examination, especially if they hold a patient, such as a child, while an x-ray is being taken.

Gonad Shield.   The reproductive organs are radiosensitive and must be protected by a lead shield while x-rays are being taken. X-rays can cause damage to the genetic material within the reproductive organs, which could lead to birth defects or cancer.

Positions Used in Radiography

ANTEROPOSTERIOR (AP) POSITION

In the **anteroposterior position**, the patient is placed with the anterior (front) part of the body facing the x-ray tube and the posterior (back) of the body facing the film. X-rays will pass through the body from the front to the back in reaching the film.

POSTEROANTERIOR (PA) POSITION

In the **posteroanterior position**, the patient is placed with the posterior (back) portion of the body facing the x-ray tube and the anterior (front) of the body facing the film. The x-rays will pass through the body from the back to the front to reach the film.

LATERAL POSITION

In the **lateral position**, the x-ray beam passes from one side of the patient's body to the opposite side to reach the film. Placing the patient's right side next to the film and passing x-rays through the body from left to right is known as the right lateral position. Placing the patient's left side next to the film and passing x-rays through the body from right to left is known as the left lateral position.

SUPINE POSITION

In the **supine position**, the patient rests on the back, face upward, allowing the x-rays to pass through the body from the front to the back.

PRONE POSITION

In the **prone position**, the patient is placed lying face down with the head turned to one side. The x-rays will pass from the back to the front side of the body.

OBLIQUE POSITION

In the **oblique position**, the patient is placed so that the body or body part to be imaged is at an angle to the x-ray beam.

Diagnostic Imaging

Diagnostic imaging involves the use of x-rays, ultrasound, radiopharmaceuticals, radiopaque media, and computers to provide the radiologist with images of internal body organs and processes. These images are used in identifying and locating tumors, fractures, hematomas, disease processes, and other abnormalities within the body. In recent years, advances in the field of electronics have produced a variety of computer-assisted x-ray machines to enhance the images obtained by the radiologist. These sophisticated machines now make possible noninvasive procedures for the visualization of organs and processes that were previously not accessible or that required exploratory surgical procedures for examination. Of the computer-assisted radiology equipment now in general use, the computed tomography (CT) scanner and the magnetic resonance imaging (MRI) machine offer the greatest range of diagnostic potential. A brief description of each of these diagnostic tools is given below.

COMPUTED TOMOGRAPHY

When first introduced, **computed tomography** was hailed as the most significant advance in diagnostic medicine since the discovery of x-rays. It combines an advanced x-ray scanning system with a powerful minicomputer and vastly improved imaging quality while making it possible to view parts of the body and abnormalities not previously open to radiography. The CT scanner combines tomography, the process of imaging structures by focusing on a specific body plane and blurring all details from other planes, with a microprocessor that provides high-speed analysis of the tissue variances scanned (Fig. 18–2).

MAGNETIC RESONANCE IMAGING (MRI)

MRI is a technique that offers greater safety, as it does not use x-rays, while providing images and data on body structures such as the heart, large blood vessels, brain, and soft tissue. The MRI is a device that emits FM radiowaves of a certain frequency that are directed at a specific body area that is contained within a magnetic field. After the radiowaves are turned off, hydrogen nuclei in the patient emit weak radiowaves or microwaves that are analyzed by a computer and transformed into cross-sectional pictures.

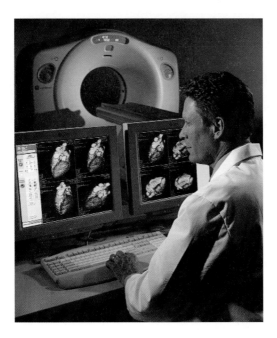

FIGURE 18–2

LightSpeed[16TM] computed tomography system. (Courtesy of GE Medical Systems.)

ULTRASOUND

Ultrasound literally means "beyond sound." It is sound whose frequency is beyond the range of human hearing. Ultrasound is widely used in diagnostic imaging for evaluation of a patient's internal organs. Its energy is transmitted into the patient and, because various internal organs and structures reflect and scatter sound differently, returning echoes can be used to form an image of a particular structure. These ultrasonic echoes are then recorded as a composite picture of the internal organ and/or structure.

Ultrasonography is the process of using ultrasound to produce a record of ultrasonic echoes as they strike tissues of different densities. The record produced by this process is called a **sonogram** or **echogram**. An adaptation of ultrasound technology is **Doppler echocardiography**. It is a noninvasive technique for determining the blood flow velocity in different locations in the heart. This same technique can be used in determining the uterine artery blood flow velocity during pregnancy, as well as to determine the fetal heart rate.

OTHER IMAGING TECHNIQUES

Other diagnostic imaging techniques being used include **thermography**, in which detailed images of body parts are developed from data showing the degree of heat and cold present in areas being studied, and **scintigraphy**, which involves the production of two-dimensional images of tissue areas from the scintillations emitted by a radiopharmaceutical, internally administered, that concentrates in a targeted site.

Interventional Radiology

Interventional radiology is a branch of medicine where certain diseases are treated non-operatively. An interventional radiologist (IR) uses radiologic imaging to guide catheters, balloons, stents, filters, and other tiny instruments through the body's vascular system and/or other systems. An **interventional radiologist** is a physician

SOME INTERVENTIONAL PROCEDURES

Angiography	An x-ray exam of the arteries; a catheter is used to enter the artery and a contrast agent (radiopaque substance) is injected to make the artery visible on x-ray
Balloon Angioplasty	Opens blocked or narrowed blood vessels
Chemoembolization	Delivery of cancer-fighting agents directly to the tumor site
Embolization	Delivery of clotting agents directly to an area that is bleeding or to block blood flow to a problem area, such as a fibroid tumor
Fallopian Tube Catheterization	Opens blocked fallopian tubes, a cause of infertility in women
Needle Biopsy	Diagnostic test for breast or other cancers that is an alternative to surgical biopsy
Stent-graft	A procedure that reinforces a ruptured or ballooning section of an artery with a fabric-wrapped stent, a small cage-like tube to patch the vessel
Thrombolysis	Dissolves blood clots
Transjugular Intrahepatic Portosystemic Shunt (TIPS)	Improves blood flow for patients with severe liver dysfunction
Varicocele Occlusion	A treatment for varicose veins in the testicles, a cause of infertility in men
Vena Cava Filters	Prevent blood clots from reaching the heart

who has had special training in imaging and who specializes in treating diseases percutaneously.

The procedures and/or surgeries are performed in an interventional suite, generally on an outpatient basis. General anesthesia is usually not necessary, and conscious sedation and/or local anesthesia is more commonly used. These procedures are cost effective and are increasingly replacing traditional surgery.

NUCLEAR MEDICINE

Nuclear medicine uses atomic particles that emit electromagnetic radiation on disintegration. The radiant energy thus released is used for diagnostic, investigative, and therapeutic purposes. It may be administered externally from radiation machines such as the betratron and the linear accelerator or internally from small radionuclides implanted within the body near the site to be irradiated.

Radiation Therapy

The treatment of disease by the use of ionizing radiation may be called **radiotherapy**, **x-ray therapy**, **cobalt treatment**, or simply **radiation therapy**. In all cases, the aim of this treatment is to deliver a precise, calculated dose of radiation to diseased tissue, such as a tumor, while causing the least possible damage to surrounding normal tissue. **Radiation** can be defined as the process whereby energy is beamed from its source through space and matter to a selected target area. Substances that emit radiation are said to be radioactive. In radiation therapy, the radioactive substances used emit three types of rays: **alpha, beta, and gamma**.

ALPHA RAYS

Alpha rays are the least penetrating of the three types and can be absorbed by a thin sheet of material. They consist of *positively* charged helium particles released by atomic disintegration of radioactive material.

BETA RAYS

Beta rays are able to penetrate body tissues for a few millimeters and consist of *negatively* charged electrons released when atoms of radioactive substances undergo disintegration.

GAMMA RAYS

Gamma rays are electromagnetic waves emitted by atoms of radioactive elements as they undergo disintegration. They are similar to x-rays but originate from the element's nucleus, whereas x-rays derive from the element's orbit. Gamma rays are without mass or electrical charge and have great penetrating power. They can pass through most substances, including the body, but are absorbed by lead.

Radiotherapy and Cancer

Malignant cells are more sensitive to radiation than are normal cells. They seem less able to repair themselves; therefore, *radiation* is frequently used in the treatment of patients with cancer, as either a *curative* or a *palliative* mode of therapy. Certain types of cancer cells can be destroyed by radiation therapy, thus preventing the unrestrained growth of such tumors. In other cancers, radiation has only a palliative effect, preventing cell growth, reducing pain, pressure, and bleeding, but not providing complete tumor destruction. Important factors that must be considered when determining the use of radiotherapy for the cancer patient include the following:

- The tumor must be surrounded by normal tissue that can tolerate the radiation and then repair itself.
- The tumor must not be widely spread. If the tumor has metastasized, radiation may be used as a palliative form of treatment.
- The tumor must be moderately sensitive to radiation (a radiosensitive tumor).

Radiotherapy is often the treatment of choice for cancers of the skin, uterus, cervix, or larynx or those located within the oral cavity. With other types of cancer, radiotherapy is frequently used in combination with other forms of treatment, including surgery and chemotherapy (Figs. 18–3 and 18–4).

Techniques of Radiotherapy

There are two methods for the administration of radiation: **external radiation therapy** (ERT) and **internal radiation therapy** (IRT). The following is an overview of these two methods.

EXTERNAL RADIATION THERAPY (ERT)

With the **ERT** *method*, the patient receives calculated doses of radiation from a machine located at some distance from the site of the tumor. The patient is carefully prepared for treatment by a radiation therapist, sometimes assisted by the **dosimetrist** or a radiation physicist. The precise size and location of the tumor are determined, and the **port**, or point of entry for the radiation, is marked using a dye or tattoo. In formulating the

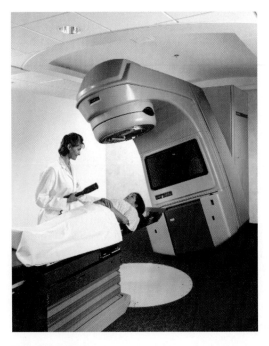

FIGURE 18–3

Clinac® 21 EX high-performance accelerator, integrated cancer therapy system. (Courtesy of Varian Medical Systems of Palo Alto, CA. © 2003, Varian Medical Systems. All rights reserved.)

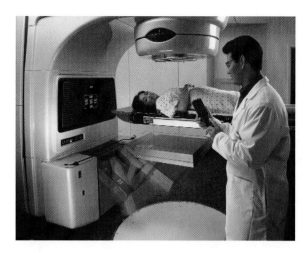

FIGURE 18–4

Clinac® 23 EX linear accelerator. Used for the delivery of computer-driven intensity-modulated radiation therapy (IMRT), as well as conventional therapy in the treatment of cancer. (Courtesy of Varian Medical Systems of Palo Alto, CA. © 1999, Varian Medical Systems. All rights reserved.)

treatment plan, a computer is used to calculate the radiation dosage that will be needed to effect maximal destruction of malignant cells and minimal damage to surrounding normal tissue. Special lead blockers or shields may be constructed by a radiation physicist to protect surrounding normal tissue from the harmful effects of radiation.

INTERNAL RADIATION THERAPY (IRT)

The **IRT** *method* of treatment can have two forms of administration known as **sealed** and **unsealed radiation therapy**. Sealed radiation therapy involves the implantation of sealed containers of radioactive material near the tumor site within the body. Unsealed radiation therapy involves the introduction of a liquid containing a radioactive substance into the patient through the mouth, via the bloodstream, or by instillation into a body cavity.

Sealed Radiation Therapy.   Radioactive material such as *radium, cesium-137, cobalt-60,* and *iridium-192* is sealed in small gold containers called seeds or within molds, plaques, needles, or other devices designed to hold the radioactive substance near the malignancy. In some cases, the radiation source may be implanted within the diseased tissue. In other cases, special devices or applicators have been designed to hold the implant in position for the desired period of treatment.

Unsealed Radiation Therapy.   *Radioactive iodine-131, radioactive phosphorus-32,* and *radioactive gold-198* are some of the substances used in the unsealed form of internal radiation therapy. *Phosphorus-32* may be intravenously administered for use in the treatment of leukemia or lymphoma. *Gold-198* and/or *phosphorus-32* may be placed in colloidal suspension and instilled in a body cavity for the palliative treatment of certain malignancies. *Iodine-131* may be orally administered, usually in conjunction with a thyroidectomy.

Side Effects of Radiation

Because radiotherapy unavoidably affects normal tissue while destroying malignant cells, patients usually experience some unpleasant **side effects.** The degree of severity associated with the side effects will depend on the individual, the cancer, its location, and the amount of radiation. The following is a listing of some side effects that may occur as a result of radiation therapy:

1. Anorexia
2. Nausea
3. Vomiting
4. Diarrhea
5. Malaise
6. Mild erythema
7. Edema
8. Ulcers
9. Alopecia
10. Taste blindness
11. Stomatitis
12. Mucositis
13. Xerostomia

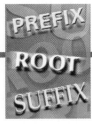

BUILDING YOUR MEDICAL VOCABULARY

This section provides the foundation for learning medical terminology. Medical words can be made up of four different types of word parts:

- Prefixes (P)
- Roots (R)
- Combining forms (CF)
- Suffixes (S)

By connecting various word parts in an organized sequence, thousands of words can be built and learned. In this text the word list is alphabetized so one can see the variety of meanings created when common prefixes and suffixes are repeatedly applied to certain word roots and/or combining forms. Words shown in pink are additional words related to the content of this chapter that are not built from word parts. These words are included to enhance your vocabulary. Note: an asterisk icon (✳) indicates words that are covered in Radiology & Nuclear Medicine Spotlights section in this chapter.

MEDICAL WORD	WORD PARTS (WHEN APPLICABLE)			DEFINITION
	Part	Type	Meaning	
alpha ray (ăl′ fərā)				A ray of positively charged particles of helium moving at a high speed. It is the least penetrating ray and is stopped by skin or a single sheet of paper.
ampere (ăm′ pēr)				The unit of strength of electricity
angiocardiogram (ăn″ jĭ-ō-kăr′ dĭ-ō-grăm)	angi/o	CF	vessel	An x-ray record of the heart and great vessels that is made visible through the use of a radiopaque contrast medium
	cardi/o	CF	heart	
	-gram	S	record	

MEDICAL WORD	WORD PARTS (WHEN APPLICABLE)			DEFINITION
	Part	Type	Meaning	
angiogram (ăn′ jĭ-ō-grăm)	angi/o -gram	CF S	vessel record	An x-ray record of the blood vessels made visible through the use of an injected radiopaque contrast medium
angiography (ăn″ jĭ-ŏg′ ră-fē)	angi/o -graphy	CF S	vessel recording	The process of making an x-ray record of blood vessels
aplastic anemia (ă-plăs′ tĭk ăn-nē′ mĭ-ă)				A type of anemia in which there is aplasia or destruction of the bone marrow; may be caused by chemotherapeutic agents, x-rays, or other sources of ionizing radiation
arteriography (ăr″ tē-rĭ-ŏg′ ră-fē)	arteri/o -graphy	CF S	artery recording	The process of making an x-ray record of the arteries
arthrography (ăr-thrŏg′ ră-fē)	arthr/o -graphy	CF S	joint recording	The process of making an x-ray record of a joint
barium sulfate (bā′ rĭ-ŭm sŭl′ fāt)				A radiopaque barium compound used as a contrast medium in x-ray examination of the digestive tract
beam (bēm)				A ray of light; in radiology and nuclear medicine, a beam is radiant energy emitted by a group of atomic particles traveling a parallel course
beta ray (bā′ tă rā)				A ray of negatively charged electrons moving at a high speed. It penetrates only a few millimeters of body tissue.
betatron (bā′ tă-trŏn)				A megavoltage machine used in administering external radiation therapy
brachytherapy (brăk″ ĭ thĕr′ ă-pē)	brachy -therapy	P S	short treatment	Radiation therapy in which the radioactive substance is inserted into a body cavity or organ. The source of radiation is located a short distance from the body area being treated.
bronchogram (brŏng′ kō-grăm)	bronch/o -gram	CF S	bronchi record	An x-ray record of the bronchial tree that is made visible through the use of a radiopaque contrast medium
cassette (kă-sĕt′)				A light-proof case or holder for x-ray film
cathode (kăth′ ōd)				The negative pole of an electrical current

MEDICAL WORD	WORD PARTS (WHEN APPLICABLE)			DEFINITION
	Part	Type	Meaning	
cholangiogram (kō-lăn′ jĭ-ō-grăm)	chol angi/o -gram	R CF S	gall, bile vessel record	An x-ray record of the bile ducts that is made visible through the use of a radiopaque contrast medium
cholecystogram (kō″ lē-sĭs′ tō-grăm)	chole cyst/o -gram	R CF S	gall bladder record	An x-ray record of the gallbladder that is made visible through the use of a radiopaque contrast medium
cinematoradio-graphy (sĭn″ ĭ-măt″ ō-rā″ dĭ-ŏg′ ră-fē)	cinemat/o radi/o -graphy	CF CF S	motion ray recording	The process of making an x-ray record of an organ in motion
cineradiography (sĭn″ ē-rā″ dē-ŏg′ ră-fē)	cine radi/o -graphy	R CF S	motion ray recording	The process of making a motion picture record of successive x-ray images appearing on a fluoroscopic screen
cobalt-60 (kō′ balt)				A radionuclide that serves as the radioactive substance in teletherapy machines. It is also used for implantation (interstitial) in the treatment of some malignancies.
contrast medium (kōn′ trăst mēd′ ĭ-ūm)				A radiopaque substance used in certain x-ray procedures to permit visualization of organs or structures
curie (Ci) (kūr′ ē)				A unit of radioactivity
cyclotron (sī′ klō-trŏn)				A megavoltage machine used in administering external radiation therapy
decontamination (dē″ kŏn-tăm″ ĭ-nā′ shŭn)				The process of freeing an object, area, or person of some contaminating substance (*bacteria, poisonous gas, or radioactive substances*)
digital subtraction angiography (dĭj′ ĭ-tăl sŭb-trăk′ shŭn ăn″ jĭ-ŏg′ ră-fē)	digit -al sub tract -ion angi/o -graphy	R S P R S CF S	finger or toe pertaining to below to draw process vessel recording	A method by which the computer performs instantaneous subtraction of the x-ray images, giving high-quality x-ray images of blood vessels with less x-ray dye
dose (dōs)				The amount of medication or radiation that is to be administered

MEDICAL WORD	WORD PARTS (WHEN APPLICABLE)			DEFINITION
	Part	Type	Meaning	
echoencepha-lography (ĕk″ ō-ĕn-sĕf″ ă-lŏg′ ră-fē)	ech/o encephal/o -graphy	CF CF S	echo brain recording	The process of using ultrasound to determine the presence of a centrally located mass in the brain
echography (ĕk-ŏg′ ră-fē)	ech/o -graphy	CF S	echo recording	The process of using ultrasound as a diagnostic tool. A record is made of the echo produced when sound waves are reflected back through tissues of different density.
external radiation (ĕk-stur′ năl rā-dĭ-ā′ shŭn)				The process of administering radiation to the patient via a radiation machine that is located outside the body
film (film)				A thin, cellulose-coated, light-sensitive sheet or slip of material used in taking pictures
film badge (film badj)				A device that is sensitive to ionizing radiation. It is worn by one who is around x-rays to monitor the degree of exposure to beta and gamma rays.
fluorescence (floo″ ō-rĕs′ ĕnts)				The property of certain substances to emit light as a result of exposure to and absorption of radiant energy
fluoroscopy (floo-räs′ kə-pē)	fluor/o -scopy	CF S	fluorescence to view	The process of examining internal structures by viewing the shadows cast on a fluorescent screen after the x-ray has passed through the body
fractionation (frăk″ shŭn-ā′ shŭn)				The process of delivering a fraction or portion of a dose of radiation over time to minimize untoward radiation effects on normal tissue
gamma ray (găm′ ăh rā)				An electromagnetic wave without mass or electrical charge. It is the most penetrating ray and can pass through the whole body. It can be stopped by lead.
Geiger counter (gī′ gĕr kown′ tĕr)				An instrument used to detect, measure, and record ionizing radiation; also called a Geiger-Müler counter
half-life (haf′ līf)				The time required for half of the radioactivity of a substance to be reduced by radioactive decay

MEDICAL WORD	WORD PARTS (WHEN APPLICABLE)			DEFINITION
	Part	Type	Meaning	
hysterosalpin-gogram (hĭs″ tĕr-ō-săl-pĭn′ gō-grăm)	hyster/o salping/o -gram	CF CF S	uterus fallopian tube record	An x-ray record of the uterus and fallopian tubes that is made visible through the use of a radiopaque contrast medium
implant (ĭm-plănt′)				To place within a body cavity or organ; also means to transfer, to graft, or to insert
intracavitary (ĭn″ tră-kăv′ ĭt-ă-rē)	intra cavit -ary	P R S	within cavity pertaining to	Pertaining to within a cavity
intravenous pyelogram (ĭn″ tră-vē′ nŭs pī′ ĕ-lō-grăm)	intra ven -ous pyel/o -gram	P R S CF S	within vein pertaining to renal pelvis record	An x-ray record of the kidney and renal pelvis that is made visible through the use of an injected radiopaque contrast medium
in vitro (ĭn vē′ trō)				Within a glass
ion (ī-ŏn)				An atomic particle consisting of an atom or a group of atoms that carry an electrical charge, either negative or positive
ionization (ī″ ŏn-ĭ-zā′ shŭn)	ionizat -ion	R S	ion (going) process	The process of breaking up molecules into their component parts
ionizing radiation (ī′ ŏn-ī-zĭng rā″ dĭ-ā′ shŭn)				A powerful invisible energy capable of producing ions
ionometer (ĭŏn′ ō-mē-tĕr)	ion/o -meter	CF S	ion instrument to measure	An instrument used to measure the amount of radiation used by x-rays or radioactive substances
ionotherapy (ī″ ŏn-ō-thĕr′ ă-pē)	ion/o -therapy	CF S	ion treatment	Treatment by introducing ions into the body
iontoradiometer (ī-ŏn″ tō-rā″ dĭ-ŏm′ ĭ-tĕr)	iont/o radi/o -meter	CF CF S	ion ray instrument to measure	An instrument used to measure the amount and intensity of x-rays
irradiation (i-rā″ dē-ā′ shŭn)	ir (in) radiat -ion	P R S	into to emit rays process	A process of using x-rays, radium rays, ultraviolet rays, gamma rays, or infrared rays in the diagnosis or therapeutic treatment of a patient

MEDICAL WORD	WORD PARTS (WHEN APPLICABLE)			DEFINITION
	Part	Type	Meaning	
isotope (ī′ sō-tōp)				One of a series of nuclides that are chemically identical yet differ in atomic weight and electrical charge. Radioactive isotopes are composed of unstable atoms, and most are artificially produced. Example: cobalt-60 is a radioactive isotope artificially produced from naturally occurring cobalt-59.
kilovolt (kĭl′ ō-vōlt)	kil/o volt	CF R	one thousand volt	1,000 V
kilowatt (kĭl′ ō-wătt)	kil/o watt	CF R	one thousand watt	1,000 W
lead (lĕd)				A metallic chemical element
linear accelerator (lĭn′ ē-ar ăk-sĕl′ ĕr-ā″ tŏr)				A megavoltage machine used in administering external radiation therapy. See Figures 18–3 and 18–4.
lymphangiogram (lĭm-făn″ jē-ō-grăm)	lymph angi/o -gram	R CF S	lymph vessel record	An x-ray record of the lymph vessels that is made visible through the use of radiopaque contrast medium
lymphangiography (lĭm-făn″ jē-ŏg′ ră-fē)	lymph angi/o -graphy	R CF S	lymph vessel recording	The process of making an x-ray record of the lymph vessels
magnetic resonance imaging (MRI) (măg-nĕt′ ĭk rĕz′ ŏ-năns)				A technique that uses radiowaves and a magnet. A device emits FM radiowaves of a certain frequency that are directed at a specific body area contained within an external magnetic field. After the radiowaves are turned off, hydrogen nuclei in the patient emit weak radiowaves or microwaves that are analyzed by a computer and transformed into cross-sectional pictures. ✱ See Radiology & Nuclear Medicine Spotlight: Magnetic Resonance Imaging (MRI).
mammography (măm-ŏg′ ră-fē)	mamm/o -graphy	CF S	breast recording	The process of obtaining pictures of the breast through the use of x-rays. ✱ See Radiology & Nuclear Medicine Spotlight: Mammography.
megavoltage (mĕg′ ă-vōl″ tĭj)				Pertains to 1,000,000 V

MEDICAL WORD	WORD PARTS (WHEN APPLICABLE)			DEFINITION
	Part	Type	Meaning	
milliampere (mĭl″ ĭ-ăm′ pēr)	milli ampere	P R	one-thousandth ampere	0.001 A
millicurie (mĭl″ ĭ-kū′ rē)	milli curie	P R	one-thousandth curie	0.001 Ci
myelogram (mī′ ĕ-lō-grăm)	myel/o -gram	CF S	spinal cord record	An x-ray record of the spinal cord that is made visible through the use of a radiopaque contrast medium
orthovoltage (or″ thō-vōl′ tĭj)	orth/o volt -age	CF R S	straight volt related to	Pertains to a voltage range of 140 to 400 kV. In radiation therapy, it is used in administering low-energy radiation for palliative treatment of cancer.
oscilloscope (ŏ-sĭl′ ō-skōp)	oscill/o -scope	CF S	to swing instrument	An instrument used to record an electrical wave visually on a fluorescent screen of a cathode-ray tube
photofluorogram (fō″ tō-floo′ ĕr-ō-grăm)	phot/o fluor/o -gram	CF CF S	light fluorescence record	An x-ray record of images seen during fluoroscopic examination
physicist (fīz′ ĭ-sĭst)	physic -ist	R S	nature one who specializes	One who specializes in the science of physics
port (pôrt)				In radiation therapy, refers to the skin area of entry for the radiation
rad (răd)				Refers to the amount of radiation absorbed. The letters stand for **r**adiation **a**bsorbed **d**ose.
radiation (rā-dĭ-ā′ shŭn)	radiat -ion	R S	radiant process	The process whereby radiant energy is propagated through space or matter
radioactive (rā″ dĭ-ō-ăk′ tĭv)	radi/o act -ive	CF R S	ray acting nature of	Characterized by emitting radiant energy
radiodermatitis (rā″ dĭ-ō-dur′ mă-tī′ tĭs)	radi/o dermat -itis	CF R S	ray skin inflammation	Inflammation of the skin caused by exposure to x-rays or radioactive substances
radiograph (rā′ dĭ-ō-grăf)	radi/o -graph	CF S	ray record	A picture produced on a sensitized film or plate by rays; *an x-ray record*

MEDICAL WORD	WORD PARTS (WHEN APPLICABLE)			DEFINITION
	Part	**Type**	**Meaning**	
radiographer (rā″ dĭ-ŏg′ ră-fĕr)	radi/o -graph -er	CF S S	ray record one who	One who is skilled in making x-ray records
radiography (rā″ dĭ-ŏg′ ră-fē)	radi/o -graphy	CF S	ray recording	The process of making an x-ray record
radiologist (rā″ dĭ-ŏl′ ō-jĭst)	radi/o log -ist	CF R S	ray study of one who specializes	One who specializes in radiology
radiology (rā″ dĭ-ŏl′ ō-jē)	radi/o -logy	CF S	ray study of	The study of x-rays, radioactive substances, radioactive isotopes, and ionizing radiation
radiolucent (rā″ dĭ-ō-lū′ sĕnt)	radi/o lucent	CF R	ray to shine	Property of permitting the passage of radiant energy
radionuclide (rā″ dĭ-ō-nū′ klĭd)	radi/o nucl -ide	CF R S	ray nucleus having a particular quality	A radioactive species of an atomic nucleus identified by its atomic number, mass, and energy state
radiopaque (rā″ dĭ-ō-pāk′)	radi/o paque	CF R	ray dark	Property of obstructing the passage of radiant energy
radioscopy (rā″ dĭ-ŏs′ kō-pē)	radi/o -scopy	CF S	ray to view, examine	The process of viewing and examining the inner structures of the body through the process of x-rays
radiotherapy (rā″ dĭ-ō-thĕr′ ă-pē)	radi/o -therapy	CF S	ray treatment	The treatment of disease by the use of x-rays, radium, and other radioactive substances
radium (rā′ dĭ-ŭm)				A radioactive isotope used in the treatment of certain malignant diseases
roentgen (R) (rĕnt′ gĕn)				The international unit for describing exposure dose of x-ray or γ-radiation
roentgenology (rĕnt″ gĕn-ŏl′ ō-jē)	roent gen/o -logy	R CF S	roentgen kind study of	The study of roentgen rays for diagnostic and therapeutic purposes
scan (skăn)				A process of using a moving device or a sweeping beam of radiation to produce images of organs or structures of the body. ✱ See Figure 18–5, in Radiology & Nuclear Medicine Spotlight: Bone Scan.

MEDICAL WORD	WORD PARTS (WHEN APPLICABLE)			DEFINITION
	Part	Type	Meaning	
shield (shĕld)				A protective structure used to prevent or reduce the passage of particles or radiation
sialography (sī″ ă-lŏg′ ră-fē)	sial/o -graphy	CF S	salivary recording	The process of making an x-ray record of the salivary ducts and glands
sonogram (sōn′ ō-grăm)	son/o -gram	CF S	sound record	A record produced by ultrasonography
tagging (tag′ ing)				The process of tracing a radioactive isotope that has become involved in metabolic or chemical actions
teletherapy (tĕl″ ĕ-thĕr′ ă-pē)	tele -therapy	R S	distant treatment	Radiation therapy in which the radioactive substance is at a distance from the body area being treated
thermography (thĕr-mŏg′ ră-fē)	therm/o -graphy	CF S	heat recording	The process of recording heat patterns of the body's surface; useful in the detection of cancer of the breast
tomography (tō-mŏg′ ră-fē)	tom/o -graphy	CF S	to cut recording	The process of cutting across and producing images of single tissue planes
ultrasonic (ŭl″ tră-sŏn′ ĭk)	ultra son -ic	P R S	beyond sound pertaining to	Pertaining to sounds beyond 20,000 cycles/sec
ultrasonography (ŭl″ tră-sŏn-ŏg′ ră-fē)	ultra son/o -graphy	P CF S	beyond sound recording	The process of using ultrasound to produce a record of ultrasonic echoes as they strike tissues of different densities. ✱ See Figures 18–11 and 18–12 in Radiology & Nuclear Medicine Spotlight: Ultrasound.
venography (vē-nŏg′ ră-fē)	ven/o -graphy	CF S	vein recording	The process of making an x-ray record of veins
volt (V) (vōlt)				The electromotive force or unit of pressure for the flow of electricity
watt (W) (wătt)				The unit of electrical power. One watt is equal to a current of 1 A under 1 V of pressure.
x-ray (x′ rā)				An electromagnetic wave of high energy produced by the collision of a beam of electrons with a target in a vacuum tube (x-ray tube)

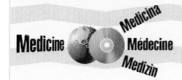

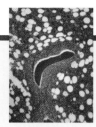

RADIOLOGY & NUCLEAR MEDICINE SPOTLIGHTS

Bone Scan

A **bone scan** is a test used to find cancer, infection, or injuries in the bone. It may also be used to check a person's response to treatment for certain bone conditions. See Figure 18–5.

A healthcare provider may recommend this test to:

- Detect whether cancer has spread to the bone
- Find an infection in the bone
- Detect a tumor in the bone
- Follow a person's response to treatment for conditions like Paget's Disease, a condition that destroys bone
- Find a fracture or injury to the bone

A bone scan takes about an hour, not including pre-scan waiting time. A radioactive substance is injected into a vein in the arm of the person having a bone scan. Usually, the test begins after a wait of 2 to 3 hours. In the case of a 3-phase study, though, the test begins right away and then resumes after a wait of 2 hours.

Before the test, the person will undress completely and put on an exam gown. All jewelry and metal objects—including pierced body jewelry—must be removed so they will not interfere with the exam. A woman will be asked if she is pregnant. When the test starts, the person having a bone scan lies flat on his or her back on a table. A special camera is positioned so the entire body can be scanned. Rays from the radioactive substance are detected by the camera, which sends pictures to a computer.

In a normal study, the table will not move during each scan. Depending on the health issue in question, though, more focused views may be needed and the scanner may move 10 to 15 centimeters (4 to 6 inches) per minute while pictures are being taken.

In the 3-phase study, the first scans are done every 5 seconds for 60 seconds. A blood pool image, a special image to follow the radioactive substance while it travels through the blood vessels, is done next. Then the person needs to wait for 2 hours before scans are resumed. After the bone scan is done, the person will be asked to wait to get dressed until the technologist is sure the pictures are adequate.

This test can:

- Show specific areas of irregular bone metabolism, which may suggest certain diseases based on the pattern of abnormality
- Detect abnormal blood flow to a particular bony region
- Help evaluate metabolic diseases that affect bone, such as certain thyroid conditions
- Detect the spread of cancer to the bones and evaluate results of cancer treatment
- Diagnose bone changes from a condition called reflex sympathetic dystrophy, a disorder of nerves that may cause pain, usually in the hands or feet

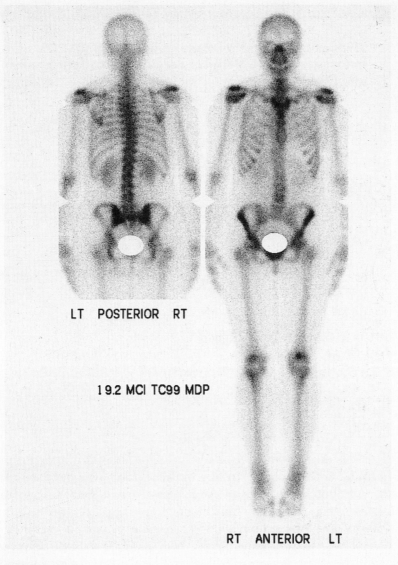

LT   POSTERIOR   RT

I 9.2 MCI TC99 MDP

RT   ANTERIOR   LT

FIGURE 18–5

Nuclear medicine bone scan. (Courtesy of Teresa Resch.)

Computed Tomography (CT) Scan

Computed tomography (CT) is a computer-aided x-ray technique. X-rays consist of electromagnetic waves of energy that penetrate the body to varying extents depending upon the density of the structures being viewed. The result provides black and white images of interior portions of the body. A CT scan produces detailed cross-sectional views of the body, similar to slices of bread.

The technology behind CT scans has advanced rapidly in recent years. Older machinery used to take minutes to obtain enough information for a single "slice." Now, the same image can be produced in seconds. Newer scanners called spiral or helical scanners are so fast that they can scan the entire chest during one held breath. These devices can also produce three-dimensional scans.

CT scans are performed to evaluate:

- Abnormalities that showed up on other other types of x-rays
- Injuries (see Figures 18–6 and 18–7)
- Tumors related to cancer. CT scans can indicate the progress of some cancers if the cancers spread or metastasize, and the effectiveness of treatment.

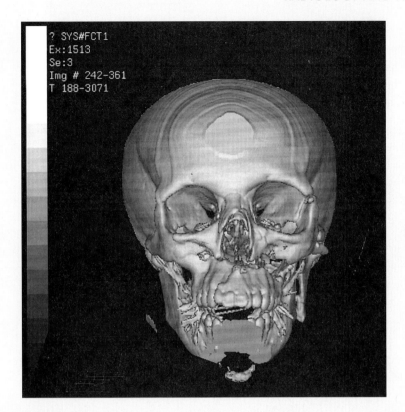

FIGURE 18–6

3D CT scan, multiple facial fractures. (Courtesy of Teresa Resch.)

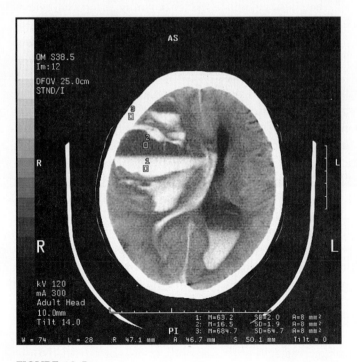

FIGURE 18–7

CT scan of head showing massive bleed with midline shift. (Courtesy of Teresa Resch.)

- Bony abnormalities
- Brain abnormalities
- Abdominal symptoms. Use of CT scans in these cases can often prevent exploratory surgery.
- Suspicious chest abnormalities

A person having the test will be asked to refrain from eating or drinking for 4 hours before the scan. All jewelry and metal objects that may interfere with the exam need to be removed beforehand, as well. Women will be asked if they are pregnant. A person having a CT scan will need to undress and put on an exam gown.

Next, the person will lie on a narrow table. The table will slide through a machine that looks like a doughnut. This is called the gantry. While in the gantry, an x-ray tube travels around the individual, creating computer-generated x-ray images. Some types of exams require the patient to receive an intravenous injection of iodinated contrast, which is a dye that makes some tissues show up better. Scans of the intestines sometimes call for the person to drink diluted iodinated contrast solution prior to the exam. After the exam, the technologist will view the pictures. If they are adequate, the person is free to leave.

Magnetic Resonance Imaging (MRI)

Magnetic resonance imaging (MRI) is a noninvasive imaging technique. The MRI machine is used to view organs, bone and other internal body structures. The imaged body part is exposed to radio waves while in a magnetic field. The picture is produced by energy emitted from hydrogen atoms in the human body. The patient is not exposed to radiation during this test.

MRI can be used for a variety of purposes. An MRI of the brain, known as a cranial MRI, may be ordered by a healthcare provider to evaluate a person's tumor, seizure disorder, or headache symptoms. See Figure 18–8. An MRI of the spine may be requested to examine a disc problem in a person's spine. If an individual has sustained injury to the shoulder or knee, an MRI is frequently used to study these large joints. Disease of the heart, chest, abdomen, and pelvis are also commonly evaluated with MRI.

Before the test, the physician will assess for any drug or food allergies (especially shellfish, or foods with added iodine such as table salt), or if the person has experienced claustrophobia, or anxiety in enclosed spaces. If this is a problem, mild sedating medication may be given. A woman will be asked if she is pregnant.

The person will be asked to remove all metal objects such as belts, jewelry, and any pieces of removable dental work. Internal metal objects that cannot be removed may distort the final images. The person should inform the MRI technologist about any previous surgery which required placement of metal, such as a hip pinning. Since the magnetic field can damage watches and credit cards, these objects are not taken into the MRI scanner.

Typically, the person having the test does not need to restrict food or fluids before an MRI scan. Certain tests, such as an MRI-guided biopsy, will require certain food and fluid restrictions. The person should consult the healthcare provider for instructions prior to the MRI.

As the test begins, the person lies on a flat platform. The platform then slides into a doughnut-shaped magnet where the scanning takes place. To prevent image distortion on the final images, the person must lie very still for the duration of the test. Commonly, a special substance called a contrast agent is administered prior to or during the test. The contrast agent is used to enhance internal structures and improve image quality. Typically, this material is injected into a vein in the arm.

The scanning process is painless. However, the part of the body being imaged may feel a bit warm. This sensation is harmless and normal. Loud banging and knocking noises are heard by the person during many stages of the exam. Earplugs are provided for people who find the noises disturbing.

A radiologist analyzes the MRI images. Frequently, the MRI will help to better evaluate a disease or disorder affecting organs and blood vessels. MRI is particularly useful in evaluating

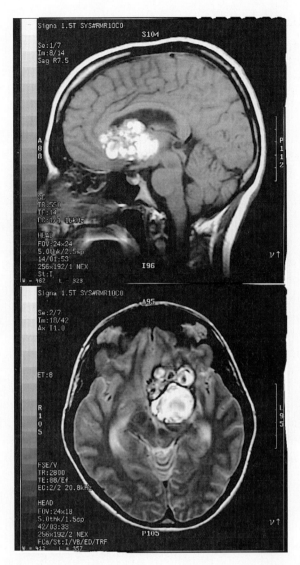

FIGURE 18–8

MRI head showing large hemorrhagic lesion. (Courtesy of Teresa Resch.)

the size and location of tumors, as well as bleeding at various clotting stages. The healthcare provider and the radiologist will use this information to help guide the next course of action for the individual's condition.

Mammogram

Mammogram is a type of x-ray for the breasts. See Figure 18–9. There are two types of mammograms: screening and diagnostic. A screening mammogram usually involves two x-rays of each breast. A diagnostic mammogram involves more x-rays.

A screening mammogram is generally used to detect breast cancer or other changes in the breast tissue in women who do not have symptoms. A diagnostic mammogram may be ordered when a screening mammogram shows something abnormal in the breast. It may also be ordered if the woman has symptoms, such as the following:

- A discharge from the nipple other than breast milk
- A lump or swelling in the breast or underarm area
- Nipple pain

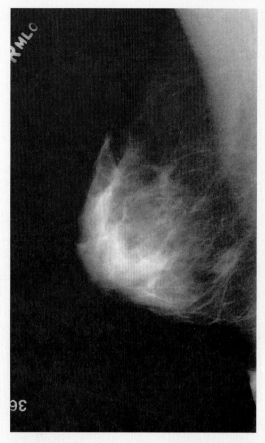

FIGURE 18–9

Normal mammogram. (Courtesy of Teresa Resch.)

- Redness or scaliness of the nipple or breast skin
- Retraction, or turning inward, of the nipple
- Skin irritation or dimpling

A mammographer is an individual who is responsible for taking the x-ray and a radiologist is an individual who is responsible for making an accurate assessment of the film. It is recommended that the mammographer and radiologist be specifically trained in mammography and breast evaluation and be certified by the American College of Radiology. To ensure quality performance, the x-ray machine, processor, screens, and cassettes must be state-of-the-art equipment and should be properly evaluated on a regular basis.

The American Cancer Society and the National Cancer Institute endorse the following breast cancer screening guidelines:

- Practice monthly breast self-examination (BSE).
- Between the ages of 40 and 49, have your breasts examined by a health professional every year and get a mammogram every 1 or 2 years.
- After age 49, have a mammogram (along with a manual breast examination) every year.

Breast cancer screening with mammograms has reduced deaths from breast cancer in women 40 to 69 years of age. A mammogram can detect changes in the breast, such as cancer, often before a lump can be felt. It can also show calcifications, or mineral deposits, cysts, or fluid-filled masses, leaking breast implants, and noncancerous tumors or growths. See Figure 18–10.

For a screening mammography, the woman undresses to the waist and puts on a gown that opens from the front. The technologist places one breast on an x-ray film cassette, which resembles a metal shelf. The woman rests her breast on the film cassette. Usually the woman

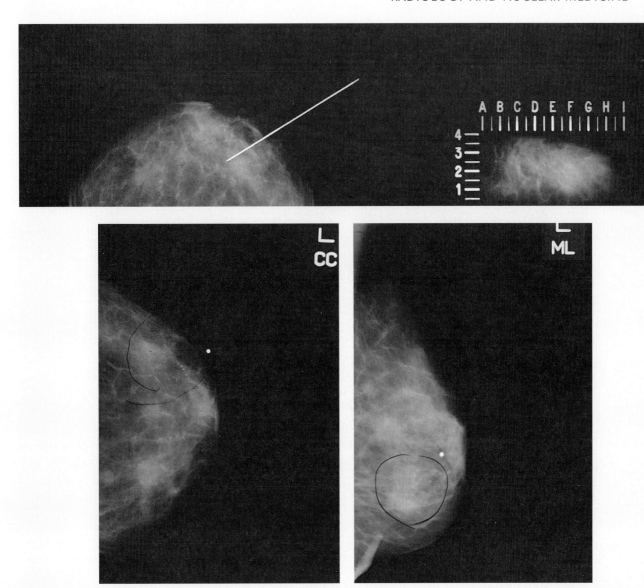

FIGURE 18–10

Mammogram showing cancer with microcalcifications. (Courtesy of Teresa Resch.)

stands during this procedure. A plastic paddle briefly squeezes the breast from above to flatten it out. This allows a clearer x-ray to be taken. Two views are usually taken of each breast for a screening mammogram. A diagnostic mammogram requires more views and more detail than the screening exam. With modern mammography equipment used specifically for breast x-rays, very low levels of radiation are used.

New techniques are being studied in a search for better diagnosis of breast abnormalities. Examples of these new techniques include the following:

- Digital mammography, which records images in computer code instead of on x-ray film
- MRI imaging, which uses a large magnet and radio frequencies to produce pictures of the breast tissue
- Positron emission tomography, or PET, which uses radioactive materials to create computer images
- Radionuclides, which uses contrast agents
- Ultrasound, which uses ultrasound waves instead of x-rays

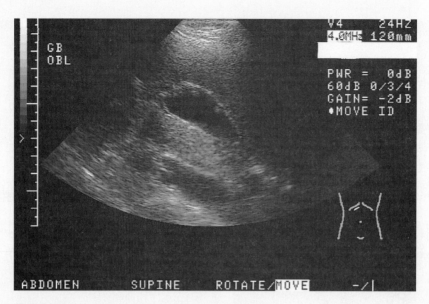

FIGURE 18–11

Ultrasound, abdomen supine. (Courtesy of Teresa Resch.)

It is recommended that a mammogram be scheduled one week after a woman's last period. Women should not wear powder, deodorant, lotion, or perfume under the arms or on the breasts. Wearing a two-piece outfit is suggested. Prior to the exam, all jewelry and metal objects should be removed.

Approximately 1,300 men a year are diagnosed with breast cancer. When a male is scheduled for a mammogram, he may be embarrassed, as he may feel that breast cancer is a female disease, and not a man's. The male breast generally does not contain as much adipose tissue as the female; therefore, it may be difficult to place the man's breast onto the film holder and obtain the proper amount of compression.

Ultrasound

Also referred to as a sonogram, **ultrasound** involves the use of high-frequency sound waves to create images of organs and systems within the body. See Figures 18–11 and 18–12.

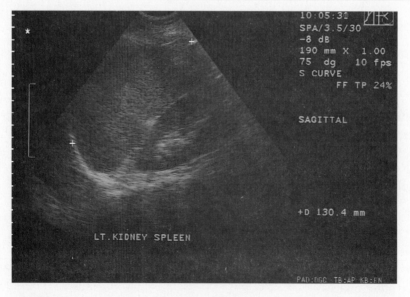

FIGURE 18–12

Ultrasound, left kidney and spleen. (Courtesy of Teresa Resch.)

An ultrasound machine creates images that allow various organs in the body to be examined. The machine sends out high-frequency sound waves, which reflect off body structures. A computer receives these reflected waves and uses them to create a picture. Unlike with an x-ray, there is no ionizing radiation exposure with this test.

The test is done in the ultrasound or radiology department. The patient lies down for the procedure. A clear, water-based conducting gel is applied to the skin over the area being examined to help with the transmission of the sound waves. A handheld probe called a transducer is then moved over the area being examined. The patient may be asked to change position so that other areas can be examined.

Preparation for the procedure will depend on the body region being examined. There is generally little discomfort with ultrasound procedures. The conducting gel may feel slightly cold and wet.

Results are considered normal if the organs and structures in the region being examined are normal in appearance. The significance of abnormal results will depend on the body region being examined and the nature of the problem.

✓ MEDICAL VOCABULARY CHECKPOINT

Following is a list of the medical vocabulary that you've seen in the chapter. Review this checklist to make sure that you are familiar with the meaning of each term.

Medical Vocabulary

- ❏ alpha ray
- ❏ aplastic anemia
- ❏ ampere
- ❏ angiocardiogram
- ❏ angiogram
- ❏ angiography
- ❏ arteriography
- ❏ arthrography
- ❏ barium sulfate
- ❏ beam
- ❏ beta ray
- ❏ betatron
- ❏ brachytherapy
- ❏ bronchogram
- ❏ carcinoid
- ❏ cassette
- ❏ cathode
- ❏ cholangiogram
- ❏ cholecystogram

- ❏ cinematoradiography
- ❏ cineradiography
- ❏ cobalt-60
- ❏ contrast medium
- ❏ curie
- ❏ cyclotron
- ❏ decontamination
- ❏ digital subtraction angiography
- ❏ dose
- ❏ echoencephalography
- ❏ echography
- ❏ external radiation
- ❏ film
- ❏ film badge
- ❏ fluorescence
- ❏ fluoroscopy
- ❏ fractionation
- ❏ gamma ray
- ❏ Geiger counter

- ❏ half-life
- ❏ hysterosalpingogram
- ❏ implant
- ❏ intracavitary
- ❏ intravenous pyelogram
- ❏ in vitro
- ❏ ion
- ❏ ionization
- ❏ ionizing radiation
- ❏ ionometer
- ❏ ionotherapy
- ❏ iontoradiometer
- ❏ irradiation
- ❏ isotope
- ❏ kilovolt
- ❏ kilowatt
- ❏ lead
- ❏ linear accelerator
- ❏ lymphangiogram
- ❏ lymphangiography

- ❏ magnetic resonance imaging
- ❏ mammography
- ❏ megavoltage
- ❏ milliampere
- ❏ millicurie
- ❏ myelogram
- ❏ orthovoltage
- ❏ oscilloscope
- ❏ photofluorogram
- ❏ physicist
- ❏ port
- ❏ rad
- ❏ radiation
- ❏ radioactive

- ❏ radiodermatitis
- ❏ radiograph
- ❏ radiographer
- ❏ radiography
- ❏ radiologist
- ❏ radiology
- ❏ radiolucent
- ❏ radionuclide
- ❏ radiopaque
- ❏ radioscopy
- ❏ radiotherapy
- ❏ radium
- ❏ roentgen
- ❏ roentgenology

- ❏ scan
- ❏ shield
- ❏ sialography
- ❏ sonogram
- ❏ tagging
- ❏ teletherapy
- ❏ thermography
- ❏ tomography
- ❏ ultrasonic
- ❏ ultrasonography
- ❏ venography
- ❏ volt
- ❏ watt
- ❏ x-ray

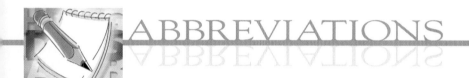

ABBREVIATIONS

ABBREVIATION	MEANING
AP	anteroposterior
Ba	barium
BE	barium enema
Ci	curie
CT	computed tomography
ERT	external radiation therapy
IR	interventional radiologist
IRT	internal radiation therapy
kV	kilovolt
kW	kilowatt
lat	lateral
mA	milliampere

ABBREVIATION	MEANING
mAs	milliampere second
mCi	millicurie
MRI	magnetic resonance imaging
PA	posteroanterior
PET	positron emission tomography
Ra	radium
rad	radiation absorbed dose
SBFT	small-bowel follow-through
TIPS	transjugular intrahepatic portosystemic shunt
US	ultrasound

STUDY AND REVIEW

An Overview of Radiology and Nuclear Medicine

Write your answers to the following questions. Do not refer to the text.

1. Define radiology. _____

   _____

2. Name three characteristics of x-rays.

   a. _____   b. _____

   c. _____

3. Name two dangers of x-rays.

   a. _____   b. _____

4. List five safety precautions designed to prevent unnecessary exposure to x-rays.

   a. _____   b. _____

   c. _____   d. _____

   e. _____

5. Name four diagnostic tools used in diagnostic radiology.

   a. _____   b. _____

   c. _____   d. _____

6. Define radiation therapy. _____

   _____

Word Parts

1. In the spaces provided, write the definition of these prefixes, roots, combining forms, and suffixes. Do not refer to the listings of medical words. Leave blank those words you cannot define.

2. After completing as many as you can, refer to the medical word listings to check your work. For each word missed or left blank, write the word and its definition several times on the margins of these pages or on a separate sheet of paper.

3. To maximize the learning process, it is to your advantage to do the following exercises as directed. To refer to the word building section before completing these exercises invalidates the learning process.

PREFIXES

Give the definitions of the following prefixes:

1. brachy- _____

2. sub- _____

3. intra- _____

4. milli- _____

5. ultra- _____

6. ir- (in-) _____

ROOTS AND COMBINING FORMS

Give the definitions of the following roots and combining forms:

1. act _____

2. ampere _____

3. angi/o _____

4. digit _____

5. arteri/o _____

6. arthr/o _____

7. bronch/o _____

8. cardi/o _____

9. cavit _____

10. chol _____

11. chole _____

12. cine _____

13. cinemat/o _____

14. tract _____

15. curie _____

16. cyst/o _____

17. dermat _____

18. ionizat _____

19. ech/o _____

20. orth/o _____

21. encephal/o _____

22. fluor/o _____

23. gen/o _____

24. volt _____

25. hyster/o _____

26. ion/o _____

27. iont/o _____

28. kil/o _____

29. nucl _____

30. log _____

31. lucent _____

32. lymph _____

33. mamm/o _____

34. myel/o _____

35. oscill/o _____

36. paque _____

37. phot/o _____

38. physic _____

39. pyel/o _____

40. radiat _____

41. radi/o _____

42. roent _____

43. salping/o _____

44. sial/o _____

45. son _____

46. son/o _____

47. tele _____

48. therm/o _____

49. tom/o _____

50. ven _____

51. ven/o _____

52. volt _____

53. watt _____

SUFFIXES

Give the definitions of the following suffixes:

1. -ary _____

2. -er _____

3. -genic _____

4. -al _____

5. -gram _____

6. -graph _____

7. -graphy _____

8. -ic _____

9. -ion _____

10. -ist _____

11. -itis _____

12. -ive _____

13. -logy _____

14. -meter _____

15. -age _____

16. -ous _____

17. -scope _____

18. -scopy _____

19. -therapy _____

20. -ide _____

Identifying Medical Terms

In the spaces provided, write the medical terms for the following meanings:

1. _____ The process of making an x-ray record of blood vessels

2. _____ The process of making an x-ray record of a joint

3. _____ An x-ray record of the gallbladder that is made visible through the use of a radiopaque contrast medium

4. _____ Pertaining to within a cavity

5. _____ Treatment by introducing ions into the body

6. _____ 1000 V

7. _____ 1000 W

8. _____ The process of obtaining pictures of the breast through the use of x-rays

9. _____ 0.001 Ci

10. _____ One who specializes in the science of physics

11. _____ The process whereby radiant energy is propagated through space or matter

12. _____ Caused or produced by radioactivity

13. _____ One who is skilled in making x-ray records

14. _____ Property of permitting the passage of radiant energy

15. _____ Property of obstructing the passage of radiant energy

16. _____ A record produced by ultrasonography

Spelling

In the spaces provided, write the correct spelling of these misspelled words:

1. hystersalpingram _____

2. echgraphy _____

3. lymphangography _____

4. myleogram _____

5. tovl _____

6. radiactive _____

7. radigraphy _____

8. silography _____

9. tomgraphy _____

10. vengraphy _____

Matching

Select the appropriate lettered meaning for each word listed below.

_____ 1. ampere

_____ 2. cathode

_____ 3. beam

_____ 4. cassette

_____ 5. rad

_____ 6. lead

_____ 7. radium

_____ 8. scan

_____ 9. shield

_____ 10. tagging

a. A protective structure used to prevent or reduce the passage of particles or radiation

b. A radioactive isotope used in the treatment of certain malignant diseases

c. A ray of light

d. Unit of strength of electricity

e. Negative pole of an electrical current

f. Loss of energy

g. A light-proof case or holder for x-ray film

h. The process of tracing a radioactive isotope that has become involved in metabolic or chemical reactions

i. A process of using a moving device or a sweeping beam of radiation to produce images of organs or structures of the body

j. Amount of radiation absorbed

k. A metallic chemical element

Abbreviations

Place the correct word, phrase, or abbreviation in the space provided.

1. anteroposterior _____

2. barium _____

3. computed tomography _____

4. kV _____

5. lat _____

6. Ra _____

7. magnetic resonance imaging _____

8. PA _____

9. curie _____

10. PET _____

MedMedia
Wrap-Up
www.prenhall.com/rice

Additional interactive resources and activities for this chapter can be found on the Companion Website. For animations, videos, audio glossary, and review, access the accompanying CD-ROM in this book.

Audio Glossary
Medical Terminology Exercises & Activities
Radiology & Nuclear Medicine Spotlight
Terminology Translator
Animations
Videos

Objectives
Medical Terminology Exercises & Activities
Audio Glossary
Drug Updates
Medical Terminology in the News

ANSWER KEY

■ CHAPTER 1

WORD PARTS

Prefixes

1. without
2. away from
3. against
4. self
5. bad
6. a hundred
7. through
8. different
9. bad
10. small
11. one thousandth
12. many, much
13. new
14. beside
15. before
16. together
17. three
18. apart
19. upon
20. out
21. in, into

Roots and Combining Forms

1. stuck to
2. armpit
3. center
4. chemical
5. a shaping
6. formation, produce
7. a thousand
8. large

9. death
10. law
11. rule
12. tumor
13. organ
14. fever
15. heat, fire
16. ray
17. to examine
18. putrefaction
19. hot, heat
20. place
21. cough
22. infection
23. people
24. cause
25. to cut
26. bad kind
27. greatest
28. least
29. palm
30. guarding

Suffixes

1. related to
2. pertaining to
3. pertaining to
4. surgical puncture
5. a key
6. a course
7. shape
8. to flee
9. formation, produce
10. knowledge
11. a step

12. a weight
13. recording
14. condition
15. pertaining to
16. process
17. condition of
18. nature of, quality of
19. liter
20. study of
21. instrument to measure
22. condition of
23. pertaining to
24. disease
25. to carry
26. instrument
27. decay
28. treatment
29. pertaining to
30. condition

IDENTIFYING MEDICAL TERMS

1. adhesion
2. asepsis
3. axillary
4. chemotherapy
5. heterogeneous
6. malformation
7. microscope
8. multiform
9. neopathy
10. oncology

SPELLING

1. antiseptic
2. autonomy

3. centimeter
4. diaphoresis
5. milligram
6. necrosis
7. paracentesis
8. radiology

MATCHING

1.	f	6.	k
2.	d	7.	b
3.	j	8.	i
4.	g	9.	c
5.	a	10.	e

ABBREVIATIONS

1. abnormal
2. axillary
3. Bx
4. cardiovascular disease
5. diagnosis-related groups
6. ENT
7. FP
8. g
9. gynecology
10. pediatrics

■ CHAPTER 2

ANATOMY AND PHYSIOLOGY

1. body . . . cells . . . sustain
2. cell membrane
3. protoplasm . . . cytoplasm . . . karyoplasm
4. karyoplasm
5. cell reproduction. . . . control over activity within the cell's cytoplasm
6. a. protection
   b. absorption
   c. secretion
   d. excretion
7. connective
8. a. striated (voluntary)
   b. cardiac
   c. smooth (involuntary)
9. excitability . . . conductivity

10. A tissue serving a common purpose
11. A group of organs functioning together for a common purpose
12. a. integumentary
    b. skeletal
    c. muscular
    d. digestive
    e. cardiovascular
    f. blood and lymphatic
    g. respiratory
    h. urinary
    i. endocrine
    j. nervous
    k. reproductive
13. a. above, in an upward direction
    b. in front of, before
    c. toward the back
    d. toward the head
    e. nearest the middle
    f. to the side
    g. nearest the point of attachment
    h. away from the point of attachment
    i. the front side
    j. the back side
14. midsagittal plane
15. transverse or horizontal
16. coronal or frontal
17. a. thoracic
    b. abdominal
    c. pelvic
18. a. cranial
    b. spinal

WORD PARTS

Prefixes

1. both
2. up
3. two
4. color
5. down, away from
6. apart
7. outside

8. within
9. similar, same
10. middle
11. through
12. first
13. one

Roots and Combining Forms

1. fat
2. man
3. life
4. tail
5. cell
6. cell
7. to pour
8. formation, produce
9. tissue
10. water
11. cell's nucleus
12. side
13. disease
14. nature
15. to drink
16. body
17. place
18. a turning
19. body organs
20. toward the front
21. head
22. away from the point of origin
23. backward
24. to strain through
25. horizon
26. below
27. groin
28. within
29. side
30. toward the middle
31. organ
32. to show
33. behind, toward the back
34. near the point of origin
35. near the surface
36. upper
37. a composite whole
38. near the belly side

Suffixes

1. pertaining to
2. use, action
3. formation, produce
4. pertaining to
5. process
6. study of
7. form, shape
8. resemble
9. like
10. condition of
11. pertaining to
12. a thing formed, plasma
13. body
14. control, stopping
15. incision
16. a doer
17. pertaining to
18. type

IDENTIFYING MEDICAL TERMS

1. android
2. bilateral
3. cytology
4. ectomorph
5. karyogenesis
6. somatotrophic
7. unilateral

SPELLING

1. adipose
2. caudal
3. cytology
4. diffusion
5. histology
6. mesomorph
7. perfusion
8. proximal
9. somatotrophic
10. unilateral

MATCHING

1. c   6. i
2. d   7. g
3. e   8. h
4. f   9. j
5. a   10. b

ABBREVIATIONS

1. abd
2. anatomy and physiology
3. central nervous system
4. CV
5. GI
6. lateral
7. respiratory
8. endoplasmic reticulum
9. anteroposterior
10. posteroanterior

■ CHAPTER 3

ANATOMY AND PHYSIOLOGY

1. The skin
2. a. hair
   b. nails
   c. sebaceous glands
   d. sweat glands
3. a. protection
   b. regulation
   c. sensory reception
   d. secretion
4. epidermis . . . dermis
5. a. stratum corneum
   b. stratum lucidum
   c. stratum granulosum
   d. stratum germinativum
6. Keratin
7. Melanin
8. dermis
9. a. papillary layer
   b. reticular layer
10. lunula

WORD PARTS

Prefixes

1. without, lack of
2. self
3. out
4. down
5. out
6. excessive
7. under
8. within
9. around
10. below

Roots and Combining Forms

1. extremity
2. ray
3. gland
4. white
5. cancer
6. heat
7. juice
8. corium
9. skin
10. skin
11. skin
12. skin
13. skin
14. skin
15. fox mange
16. red
17. sweat
18. jaundice
19. tumor
20. horn
21. white
22. study of
23. black
24. black
25. fungus
26. nail
27. little cell
28. nail
29. thick
30. a louse
31. cord
32. wrinkle
33. hard
34. oil
35. old
36. hot, heat
37. to pull
38. hair
39. nail
40. yellow
41. dry
42. to lie

43. little bag
44. a covering
45. yellow
46. plate
47. millet (tiny)
48. itching
49. end, distant
50. vessel

Suffixes

1. pertaining to
2. pain
3. pertaining to
4. pertaining to
5. skin
6. pertaining to
7. sensation
8. pencil, grafting knife
9. condition
10. pertaining to
11. process
12. condition of
13. one who specializes
14. inflammation
15. study of
16. dilatation
17. resemble
18. tumor
19. condition of
20. pertaining to
21. surgical repair
22. flow, discharge
23. instrument to cut

IDENTIFYING MEDICAL TERMS

1. actinic dermatitis
2. cutaneous
3. dermatitis
4. dermatology
5. pruritus
6. hyperhidrosis
7. hypodermic
8. icteric
9. onychitis
10. pachyderma
11. thermanesthesia
12. xanthoderma

SPELLING

1. causalgia
2. dermomycosis
3. ecchymosis
4. excoriation
5. hyperhidrosis
6. melanoma
7. onychomycosis
8. rhytidoplasty
9. scleroderma
10. seborrhea

MATCHING

1. d
2. f
3. e
4. h
5. j
6. i
7. b
8. g
9. a
10. c

ABBREVIATIONS

1. FUO
2. TTS
3. hypodermic
4. I & D
5. SG
6. intradermal
7. T
8. UV
9. foreign body
10. psoralen-ultraviolet light

DIAGNOSTIC AND LABORATORY TESTS

1. c
2. d
3. a
4. b
5. a

■ CHAPTER 4

ANATOMY AND PHYSIOLOGY

1. 206
2. a. axial
   b. appendicular
3. a. flat . . . ribs, scapula, parts of the pelvic girdle, bones of the skull
   b. long . . . tibia, femur, humerus, radius
   c. short . . . carpal, tarsal
   d. irregular . . . vertebrae, ossicles of the ear
   e. sesamoid . . . patella

   *Optional answer to question 3:

   f. sutural or wormian . . . between the flat bones of the skull
4. a. shape, support
   b. protection
   c. storage
   d. formation of blood cells
   e. attachment of skeletal muscles
   f. movement, through articulation
5. a. the ends of a developing bone
   b. the shaft of a long bone
   c. the membrane that forms the covering of bones, except at their articular surfaces
   d. the dense, hard layer of bone tissue
   e. a narrow space or cavity throughout the length of the diaphysis
   f. a tough connective tissue membrane lining the medullary canal and containing the bone marrow
   g. the reticular tissue that makes up most of the volume of bone
6. Numbers of the matching answers:
   a. 6
   b. 11
   c. 4
   d. 13
   e. 8
   f. 10
   g. 9
   h. 14
   i. 1
   j. 12

k. 2

l. 3

m. 7

n. 5

7. a. synarthrosis

b. amphiarthrosis

c. diarthrosis

8. Abduction

9. the process of moving a body part toward the midline

10. Circumduction

11. the process of bending a body part backward

12. Eversion

13. the process of straightening a flexed limb

14. Flexion

15. the process of turning inward

16. Pronation

17. the process of moving a body part forward

18. Retraction

19. the process of moving a body part around a central axis

20. Supination

WORD PARTS

Prefixes

1. without
2. apart
3. water
4. between
5. beyond
6. around
7. many, much
8. under, beneath
9. together
10. back

ROOTS AND COMBING FORMS

1. vinegar cup
2. gristle
3. extremity, point
4. extremity
5. stiffening, crooked
6. joint
7. joint
8. a pouch

9. heel bone
10. to place
11. cancer
12. wrist
13. wrist
14. cartilage
15. cartilage
16. little key
17. fastened
18. tail bone
19. tail bone
20. glue
21. to lead
22. to bind together
23. rib
24. rib
25. crescent
26. light
27. skull
28. skull
29. finger or toe
30. finger or toe
31. femur
32. carrying
33. fibula
34. ray
35. humerus
36. ilium
37. ilium
38. ischium
39. a hump
40. lamina (thin plate)
41. bending
42. loin
43. loin
44. lower jawbone
45. jawbone
46. jaw
47. marrow
48. marrow
49. discharge
50. elbow
51. bone
52. kneecap
53. to draw
54. foot

55. closely knit row
56. a passage
57. spine
58. radius
59. sacrum
60. flesh
61. shoulder blade
62. curvature
63. curvature
64. spine
65. vertebra
66. sternum
67. sternum
68. tendon
69. tibia
70. elbow
71. elbow
72. vertebra
73. vertebra
74. sword

Suffixes

1. pertaining to
2. pertaining to
3. pain
4. pertaining to
5. pertaining to
6. immature cell, germ cell
7. surgical puncture
8. related to
9. process
10. pain
11. excision
12. swelling
13. formation, produce
14. formation, produce
15. mark, record
16. to write
17. pertaining to
18. inflammation
19. nature of
20. instrument
21. softening
22. pertaining to
23. resemble
24. tumor
25. shoulder

26. condition of
27. lack of
28. growth
29. formation
30. surgical repair
31. formation
32. instrument to cut
33. incision

IDENTIFYING MEDICAL TERMS

1. acroarthritis
2. ankylosis
3. arthritis
4. calcaneal
5. chondral
6. coccygodynia
7. costal
8. craniectomy
9. dactylic
10. hydrarthrosis
11. intercostal
12. ischialgia
13. lumbar
14. myeloma
15. osteoarthritis
16. osteomyelitis or myelitis
17. osteopenia
18. pedal
19. xiphoid

SPELLING

1. acromion
2. arthroscope
3. bursitis
4. chrondroblast
5. connective
6. cranioplasty
7. dislocation
8. ischial
9. myelitis
10. osteochondritis
11. phosphorus
12. patellar
13. phalangeal
14. rachigraph
15. scoliosis
16. spondylitis

17. symphysis
18. tenonitis
19. ulnocarpal
20. vertebral

MATCHING

1. i   6. h
2. j   7. g
3. e   8. a
4. c   9. d
5. b   10. f

ABBREVIATIONS

1. CDH
2. DJD
3. long leg cast
4. osteoarthritis
5. PEMFs
6. rheumatoid arthritis
7. SPECT
8. thoracic vertebra, first
9. temporomandibular joint
10. Tx

DIAGNOSTIC AND LABORATORY TESTS

1. c
2. d
3. c
4. b
5. b

■ CHAPTER 5

ANATOMY AND PHYSIOLOGY

1. a. skeletal
   b. smooth
   c. cardiac
2. 42
3. a. nutrition
   b. oxygen
4. a. origin
   b. insertion
5. voluntary or striated
6. aponeurosis
7. a. body
   b. origin
   c. insertion

8. a. A muscle that counteracts the action of another muscle.
   b. A muscle that is primary in a given movement.
   c. A muscle that acts with another muscle to produce movement.
9. involuntary, visceral, or unstriated
10. a. digestive tract
    b. respiratory tract
    c. urinary tract
    d. eye
    e. skin
11. Cardiac
12. a. movement
    b. maintain posture
    c. produce heat

WORD PARTS

Prefixes

1. lack of
2. away from
3. toward
4. against
5. separation
6. two
7. slow
8. with
9. through
10. difficult
11. into
12. within
13. water
14. four
15. with, together
16. three

Roots and Combining Forms

1. agony
2. arm
3. clavicle
4. to cut through
5. neck
6. finger or toe
7. to lead
8. work

9. a band
10. skin
11. discharge
12. fiber
13. fiber
14. equal
15. a rind
16. lifter
17. an addition
18. breast
19. hot, heat
20. to measure
21. muscle
22. muscle
23. muscle
24. muscle
25. nerve
26. nerve
27. disease
28. to loosen
29. rod
30. to turn
31. a turning
32. flesh
33. hardening
34. to gain
35. convulsive
36. sternum
37. tendon
38. tone, tension
39. twisted
40. to draw
41. will
42. joint fluid
43. twisted

Suffixes

1. pain
2. pertaining to
3. pertaining to
4. weakness
5. immature cell, germ cell
6. head
7. binding
8. pain
9. chemical
10. treatment

11. to write, record
12. condition
13. pertaining to
14. process
15. agent
16. inflammation
17. condition
18. motion
19. motion
20. study of
21. process
22. softening
23. resemble
24. tumor
25. a doer
26. condition of
27. weakness
28. disease
29. a fence
30. surgical repair
31. stroke, paralysis
32. suture
33. pertaining to
34. tension, spasm
35. order
36. instrument to cut
37. incision
38. nourishment, development
39. condition of
40. condition of

IDENTIFYING MEDICAL TERMS

1. atonic
2. bradykinesia
3. dactylospasm
4. dystrophy
5. intramuscular
6. levator
7. myasthenia
8. myology
9. myoparesis
10. myoplasty
11. myosarcoma
12. myotomy
13. polyplegia
14. tenodesis

15. synergetic
16. triceps

SPELLING

1. fascia
2. myokinesis
3. dermatomyositis
4. rhabdomyoma
5. sarcolemma
6. sternocleidomastoid
7. dystrophin
8. torticollis

MATCHING

1. d   6. a
2. i   7. h
3. g   8. c
4. e   9. b
5. j   10. f

ABBREVIATIONS

1. above elbow
2. aspartate aminotransferase
3. Ca
4. EMG
5. full range of motion
6. musculoskeletal
7. ROM
8. sh
9. total body weight
10. triceps jerk

DIAGNOSTIC AND LABORATORY TESTS

1. b   4. c
2. d   5. a
3. b

■ **CHAPTER 6**

ANATOMY AND PHYSIOLOGY

1. a. mouth
   b. pharynx
   c. esophagus
   d. stomach
   e. small intestine
   f. large intestine
2. a. salivary glands
   b. liver

c. gallbladder

d. pancreas

3. a. digestion

b. absorption

c. elimination

4. A small mass of masticated food ready to be swallowed

5. A series of wave-like muscular contractions that are involuntary

6. Hydrochloric acid and gastric juices

7. duodenum

8. chyme

9. circulatory system

10. cecum, colon, rectum, and the anal canal

11. liver

12. Stores and concentrates bile

13. Produces digestive enzymes

14. a. It plays an important role in metabolism.

b. It manufactures bile.

c. It stores iron, vitamins B_{12}, A, D, E, and K

15. small intestine

16. parotid, sublingual, submandibular

17. a. insulin

b. glucagon

WORD PARTS

Prefixes

1. lack of

2. up

3. down

4. difficult

5. above

6. excessive, above

7. deficient, below

8. bad

9. through

10. around

11. after

12. through

13. below

Roots and Combining Forms

1. to suck in

2. gland

3. starch

4. orange-yellow

5. appendix

6. appendix

7. gall, bile

8. to cast, throw

9. cheek

10. abdomen, belly

11. lip

12. gall, bile

13. common bile duct

14. colon

15. colon

16. colon

17. colon

18. bladder

19. tooth

20. to press together

21. diverticula

22. duodenum

23. intestine

24. to remove dregs

25. esophagus

26. to carry

27. stomach

28. stomach

29. gums

30. tongue

31. sweet, sugar

32. blood

33. liver

34. liver

35. hernia

36. ileum

37. ileum

38. lip

39. flank, abdomen

40. to loosen

41. tongue

42. fat

43. study of

44. middle

45. pancreas

46. to digest

47. pharynx

48. meal

49. to vomit

50. rectum, anus

51. pylorus, gate keeper

52. rectum

53. saliva

54. sigmoid

55. spleen

56. mouth

57. poison

58. a breaking out

59. worm

60. breath

61. vein liable to bleed

62. nourishment

63. to chew

64. to disable; paralysis

65. hair

66. nest

67. to roll

68. tooth

Suffixes

1. pertaining to

2. pertaining to

3. pain

4. pertaining to

5. enzyme

6. hernia

7. resemble

8. condition of

9. excision

10. vomiting

11. shape

12. formation, produce

13. pertaining to

14. pertaining to

15. process

16. condition of

17. one who specializes

18. inflammation

19. nature of, quality of

20. study of

21. destruction, to separate

22. enlargement, large

23. tumor
24. appetite
25. condition of
26. flow
27. to digest
28. pertaining to
29. to eat
30. instrument
31. to view, examine
32. contraction
33. new opening
34. incision
35. pertaining to

IDENTIFYING MEDICAL TERMS

1. amylase
2. anabolism
3. anorexia
4. appendectomy
5. appendicitis
6. biliary
7. celiac
8. colorrhaphy
9. dysphagia
10. hepatitis
11. herniotomy
12. postprandial
13. proctalgia
14. splenomegaly
15. sigmoidoscope

SPELLING

1. biliary
2. colonoscopy
3. enteroclysis
4. gastroenterology
5. hepatotoxin
6. laxative
7. peristalsis
8. sialadenitis
9. vagotomy
10. vermiform

MATCHING

1. e
2. f
3. d
4. b
5. i
6. h
7. j
8. a
9. g
10. c

ABBREVIATIONS

1. ac
2. bowel movement
3. bowel sounds
4. cib
5. GB
6. HAV
7. nasogastric
8. nothing by mouth
9. pc
10. TPN

DIAGNOSTIC AND LABORATORY TESTS

1. a
2. c
3. d
4. c
5. c

■ CHAPTER 7

ANATOMY AND PHYSIOLOGY

1. a. heart
   b. arteries
   c. veins
   d. capillaries
2. a. endocardium
   b. myocardium
   c. pericardium
3. 300
4. atria . . . interatrial
5. ventricles . . . interventricular
6. a. superior and inferior vena cavae
   b. right atrium
   c. tricuspid valve
   d. right ventricle
   e. pulmonary semilunar valve
   f. left and right pulmonary arteries
   g. lungs
   h. left and right pulmonary veins
   i. left atrium
   j. bicuspid or mitral valve
   k. left ventricle
   l. aortic valve
   m. aorta
   n. capillaries
7. autonomic nervous system
8. sinoatrial node
9. Purkinje system
10. a. radial . . . on the radial side of the wrist
    b. brachial . . . in the antecubital space of the elbow
    c. carotid . . . in the neck
11. a. the pressure exerted by the blood on the walls of the vessels
    b. the difference between the systolic and diastolic readings
12. man's fist . . . 60 to 100
13. 100 and 140 . . . 60 and 90
14. transport blood from the right and left ventricles of the heart to all body parts
15. transport blood from peripheral tissues to the heart

WORD PARTS

Prefixes

1. lack of
2. two
3. slow
4. together
5. within
6. within
7. outside
8. excessive, above
9. deficient, below
10. around
11. difficult
12. half
13. fast
14. three

Roots and Combining Forms

1. vessel
2. to choke, quinsy
3. vessel
4. opening
5. aorta
6. artery

7. artery
8. artery
9. fatty substance, porridge
10. fatty substance, porridge
11. atrium
12. atrium
13. heart
14. heart
15. heart
16. dark blue
17. listen to
18. to widen
19. electricity
20. a throwing in
21. sweet, sugar
22. blood
23. to hold back
24. bile
25. study of
26. moon
27. thin
28. mitral valve
29. muscle
30. circular
31. sour, sharp, acid
32. vein
33. vein
34. sound
35. lung
36. rhythm
37. hardening
38. a curve
39. pulse
40. narrowing
41. chest
42. to draw, to bind
43. to limp
44. pressure
45. clot of blood
46. to expand
47. small vessel
48. vessel
49. echo
50. vein
51. body
52. ventricle

53. fibrils (small fibers)
54. blood
55. power
56. infarct (necrosis of an area)
57. fat
58. first
59. to shut up
60. oxygen
61. throbbing
62. a partition
63. contraction
64. end
65. clot of blood
66. solid (fat)

Suffixes

1. pertaining to
2. pertaining to
3. pertaining to
4. immature cell, germ cell
5. surgical puncture
6. small
7. point
8. measurement
9. dilatation
10. excision
11. blood condition
12. relating to
13. formation, produce
14. chemical
15. to write
16. recording
17. condition
18. pertaining to
19. having a particular quality
20. process
21. condition of
22. one who specializes
23. inflammation
24. nature of, quality of
25. study of
26. softening
27. enlargement, large
28. instrument to measure
29. tumor
30. one who
31. condition of
32. disease

33. surgical repair
34. to pierce
35. instrument
36. contraction, spasm
37. incision
38. tissue
39. pertaining to

IDENTIFYING MEDICAL TERMS

1. angioma
2. angioblast
3. angioplasty
4. angiostenosis
5. arteriotomy
6. arteritis
7. bicuspid
8. cardiologist
9. cardiomegaly
10. cardiopulmonary
11. constriction
12. embolism
13. phlebitis
14. tachycardia
15. vasodilator

SPELLING

1. anastomosis
2. atherosclerosis
3. atrioventricular
4. endocarditis
5. extracorporeal
6. ischemia
7. myocardial
8. oxygen
9. phlebitis
10. palpitation

MATCHING

1. d	6. c
2. e	7. a
3. f	8. i
4. g	9. j
5. b	10. h

ABBREVIATIONS

1. AMI
2. A-V, AV
3. blood pressure
4. coronary artery disease

5. CC
6. electrocardiogram
7. high-density lipoprotein
8. H & L
9. myocardial infarction
10. tissue plasminogen activator

DIAGNOSTIC AND LABORATORY TESTS
1. c
2. a
3. b
4. c
5. b

■ CHAPTER 8

ANATOMY AND PHYSIOLOGY
1. a. erythrocytes
   b. thrombocytes
   c. leukocytes
2. transport oxygen and carbon dioxide
3. 5
4. 80 to 120 days
5. body's main defense against the invasion of pathogens
6. 8000
7. a. neutrophils
   b. eosinophils
   c. basophils
   d. lymphocytes
   e. monocytes
8. play an important role in the clotting process
9. 200,000 to 500,000
10. a. A
    b. B
    c. AB
    d. O
11. a. It transports proteins and fluids
    b. It protects the body against pathogens
    c. It serves as a pathway for the absorption of fats
12. a. spleen
    b. tonsils
    c. thymus

WORD PARTS

Prefixes
1. lack of
2. against
3. self
4. up
5. beyond
6. excessive
7. deficient
8. one
9. all
10. many
11. before
12. across

Roots and Combining Forms
1. gland
2. gland
3. clumping
4. other
5. vessel
6. unequal
7. base
8. lime, calcium
9. color
10. to pour
11. clots, to clot
12. flesh, creatine
13. cell
14. cell
15. cell
16. rose-colored
17. red
18. globe
19. little grain, granular
20. blood
21. blood
22. blood
23. white
24. white
25. fat
26. study of
27. lymph
28. lymph
29. large
30. neither
31. kernel, nucleus
32. eat, engulf
33. a thing formed, plasma
34. net
35. putrefying
36. whey, serum
37. iron
38. fiber
39. spleen
40. sea
41. clot
42. clot
43. thymus
44. fiber
45. tonsil
46. formation
47. immunity
48. vessel
49. whey
50. a developing
51. vessel
52. small vessel

Suffixes
1. capable
2. forming
3. immature cell, germ cell
4. body
5. swelling
6. to separate
7. cultivation
8. cell
9. excision
10. blood condition
11. work
12. formation, produce
13. protection
14. protein
15. tissue
16. pertaining to
17. chemical
18. process
19. one who specializes
20. inflammation
21. study of
22. destruction
23. enlargement
24. tumor

25. condition of
26. lack of
27. removal
28. attraction
29. attraction
30. formation
31. bursting forth
32. control, stopping
33. incision

IDENTIFYING MEDICAL TERMS

1. agglutination
2. allergy
3. antibody
4. anticoagulant
5. antigen
6. basocyte
7. coagulable
8. creatinemia
9. eosinophil
10. granulocyte
11. hematologist
12. hemoglobin
13. hyperglycemia
14. hyperlipemia
15. leukocyte
16. lymphostasis
17. mononucleosis
18. prothrombin
19. splenopexy
20. thrombocyte

SPELLING

1. allergy
2. creatinemia
3. extravasation
4. erythrocytosis
5. thromboplastin
6. hematocrit
7. hemorrhage
8. leukemia
9. lymphadenotomy
10. anaphylaxis

MATCHING

1. h   4. g
2. d   5. f
3. e   6. c

7. b   9. j
8. a   10. i

ABBREVIATIONS

1. AIDS
2. BSI
3. chronic myelogenous leukemia
4. Hb, Hgb
5. hematocrit
6. HIV
7. *Pneumocystis carinii* pneumonia
8. prothrombin time
9. red blood cell (count)
10. RIA

DIAGNOSTIC AND LABORATORY TESTS

1. d
2. c
3. c
4. b
5. a

■ CHAPTER 9

ANATOMY AND PHYSIOLOGY

1. a. nose
   b. pharynx
   c. larynx
   d. trachea
   e. bronchi
   f. lungs
2. To furnish oxygen for use by individual cells and to take away their gaseous waste product, carbon dioxide
3. The process whereby the lungs are ventilated and oxygen and carbon dioxide are exchanged between the air in the lungs and the blood within capillaries of the alveoli
4. The process whereby oxygen and carbon dixodide are exchanged between the bloodstream and the cells of the body

5. a. Serves as an air passageway
   b. Warms and moistens inhaled air
   c. Its cilia and mucous membrane trap dust, pollen, bacteria, and foreign matter
   d. It contains olfactory receptors that sort out odors
   e. It aids in phonation and the quality of voice
6. a. nasopharynx
   b. oropharynx
   c. laryngopharynx
7. a. Serves as a passageway for air
   b. Serves as a passageway for food
   c. Aids in phonation by changing its shape
8. Acts as a lid to prevent aspiration of food into the trachea
9. A narrow slit at the opening between the true vocal folds
10. The production of vocal sounds
11. Serves as a passageway for air
12. right bronchus . . . left bronchus
13. Provide a passageway for air to and from the lungs
14. Cone-shaped, spongy organs of respiration lying on either side of the heart
15. A serous membrane composed of several layers
16. diaphragm
17. mediastinum
18. 3 . . . 2
19. alveoli
20. To bring air into intimate contact with blood so that oxygen and carbon dioxide can be exchanged in the alveoli
21. temperature, pulse, respiration, and blood pressure
22. a. The amount of air in a single inspiration or expiration

b. The amount of air remaining in the lungs after maximal expiration

c. The volume of air that can be exhaled after a maximal inspiration

23. medulla oblongata . . . pons
24. 30 to 80
25. 15 to 20

WORD PARTS

Prefixes

1. lack of
2. upon
3. through
4. difficult
5. within
6. good
7. out
8. below, deficient
9. excessive
10. in
11. fast

Roots and Combining Forms

1. to draw in
2. small, hollow air sac
3. coal
4. imperfect
5. bronchi
6. bronchi
7. bronchiole
8. bronchi
9. dust
10. dark blue
11. breathe
12. blood
13. larynx
14. larynx
15. larynx
16. lobe
17. sac
18. fiber
19. nose
20. straight
21. middle
22. a little swelling
23. palate
24. breast
25. pharynx
26. pharynx
27. nipple
28. partition
29. speech
30. pleura
31. pleura
32. pleura
33. lung, air
34. lung
35. lung
36. lung
37. pus
38. nose
39. a curve, hollow
40. breath
41. breathing
42. chest
43. to air
44. almond, tonsil
45. trachea
46. trachea
47. snore
48. flesh

Suffixes

1. pertaining to
2. pain
3. hernia
4. surgical puncture
5. pain
6. dilation
7. excision
8. pertaining to
9. condition
10. process
11. inflammation
12. instrument to measure
13. condition of
14. tumor
15. dripping
16. surgical repair
17. a doer
18. breathing
19. to spit
20. flow, discharge
21. instrument
22. new opening
23. incision
24. pertaining to

IDENTIFYING MEDICAL TERMS

1. alveolus
2. bronchiectasis
3. bronchitis
4. dysphonia
5. eupnea
6. hemoptysis
7. inhalation
8. laryngitis
9. pneumothorax
10. rhinoplasty
11. rhinorrhea
12. sinusitis

SPELLING

1. bronchoscope
2. diaphragmatocele
3. expectoration
4. laryngeal
5. orthopnea
6. pleuritis
7. pulmonectomy
8. rhoncus
9. tachypnea
10. tracheal

MATCHING

1. h		6. b	
2. i		7. d	
3. k		8. a	
4. f		9. e	
5. c		10. g	

ABBREVIATIONS

1. AFB
2. cystic fibrosis
3. CXR
4. COLD
5. endotracheal
6. postnasal drip, paroxysmal nocturnal dyspnea
7. R
8. sudden infant death syndrome

9. SOB

10. tuberculosis

DIAGNOSTIC AND LABORATORY TESTS

1. b
2. c
3. c
4. d
5. a

■ CHAPTER 10

ANATOMY AND PHYSIOLOGY

1. a. kidneys
   b. ureters
   c. bladder
   d. urethra
2. Extraction of certain wastes from the bloodstream, conversion of these materials to urine, and transport of the urine from the kidney, via the ureters, to the bladder for elimination
3. a. true capsule
   b. perirenal fat
   c. renal fascia
4. A notch
5. Sac-like collecting portion of the kidney
6. arteries, veins, convoluted tubules, and glomerular capsules
7. inner
8. The structural and functional unit of the kidney
9. renal corpuscle . . . tubule
10. glomerulus . . . Bowman's capsule
11. To remove the waste products of metabolism from the blood plasma
12. filtration . . . reabsorption
13. 95. . . . 5
14. 1000 to 1500
15. Narrow, muscular tubes that transport urine from the kidneys to the bladder

16. Muscular, membranous sac that serves as a reservoir for urine
17. Small, triangular area near the base of the bladder
18. Convey urine and semen
19. Convey urine
20. urinary meatus
21. Physical, chemical, and microscopic examination of urine
22. a. yellow to amber
    b. clear
    c. 5.0 to 7.0
    d. 1.003 to 1.030
    e. aromatic
    f. 1000 to 1500 mL/day
23. a. renal
    b. transitional
    c. squamous
24. diabetes mellitus
25. renal disease, acute glomerulonephritis, pyelonephritis

WORD PARTS

Prefixes

1. without
2. against
3. through
4. through
5. difficult, painful
6. within
7. water
8. outside of
9. not
10. scanty
11. through
12. beyond
13. excessive

Roots and Combining Forms

1. sifted out
2. protein
3. bacteria
4. bile
5. calcium
6. colon
7. to hold
8. bladder

9. body
10. bladder
11. skin
12. glomerulus, little ball
13. glomerulus, little ball
14. sweet, sugar
15. blood
16. ketone
17. stone
18. study of
19. blood
20. passage
21. to urinate
22. kidney
23. kidney
24. night
25. peritoneum
26. perineum
27. sound
28. to draw, to bind
29. pus
30. renal pelvis
31. kidney
32. hardening
33. trigone
34. urine
35. urinate
36. urine
37. ureter
38. urethra
39. urethra
40. urine
41. urine
42. urine
43. urine

Suffixes

1. pertaining to
2. pain
3. pertaining to
4. hernia
5. pain
6. like, resemble
7. pertaining to
8. excision
9. blood condition
10. a mark, record

11. pertaining to
12. chemical
13. process
14. one who specializes
15. inflammation
16. stone
17. study of
18. destruction, to separate
19. crushing
20. process
21. instrument to measure
22. tumor
23. condition of
24. disease
25. surgical repair
26. instrument
27. condition
28. new opening
29. incision
30. urine

IDENTIFYING MEDICAL TERMS

1. antidiuretic
2. cystectomy
3. cystitis
4. dysuria
5. glomerulitis
6. hypercalciuria
7. micturition
8. nephrolith
9. periurethral
10. pyuria
11. ureteropathy
12. urethralgia
13. urologist

SPELLING

1. excretory
2. enuresis
3. glycosuria
4. hematuria
5. incontinence
6. nephrocystitis
7. nocturia
8. ureteroplasty
9. urinalysis
10. urobilin

MATCHING

1. d	6. g
2. e	7. j
3. b	8. c
4. f	9. h
5. a	10. i

ABBREVIATIONS

1. ADH
2. blood urea nitrogen
3. CRF
4. cystoscopic examination
5. genitourinary
6. hemodialysis
7. IVP
8. peritoneal dialysis
9. hydrogen ion concentration
10. UA

DIAGNOSTIC AND LABORATORY TESTS

1. c
2. c
3. b
4. c
5. b

■ CHAPTER 11

ANATOMY AND PHYSIOLOGY

1. a. pituitary
   b. pineal
   c. thyroid
   d. parathyroid
   e. islets of Langerhans
   f. adrenals
   g. ovaries
   h. testes
2. a. thymus
   b. placenta during pregnancy
   c. gastrointestinal mucosa
3. It involves the production and regulation of chemical substances (hormones) that play an essential role in maintaining homeostasis.
4. A chemical transmitter that is released in small amounts and transported via the bloodstream to a targeted organ or other cells.
5. It synthesizes and secretes releasing hormones, releasing factors, release-inhibiting hormones, and release inhibiting factors.
6. Because of its regulatory effects on the other endocrine glands
7. a. growth hormone (GH)
   b. adrenocorticotropin (ACTH)
   c. thyroid-stimulating hormone (TSH)
   d. follicle-stimulating hormone (FSH)
   e. luteinizing hormone (LH)
   f. prolactin (PRL)
   g. melanocyte-stimulating hormone (MSH)
8. a. antidiuretic hormone (ADH)
   b. oxytocin
9. melatonin . . . serotonin
10. It plays a vital role in metabolism and regulates the body's metabolic processes.
11. a. thyroxine (T_4)
    b. triiodothyronine (T_3)
    c. calcitonin
12. serum calcium . . . phosphorus
13. blood sugar
14. glucocorticoids, mineralocorticoids, and the androgens
15. a. Regulates carbohydrate, protein, and fat metabolism
    b. Stimulates output of glucose from the liver
    c. Increases the blood sugar level
    d. Regulates other physiologic body processes

*Optional answers to question 15:

e. Promotes the transport of amino acids into extracellular tissue

f. Influences the effectiveness of catecholamines such as dopamine, epinephrine, and norepinephrine

g. Has an anti-inflammatory effect

h. Helps the body cope during times of stress

16. a. use of carbohydrates

   b. absorption of glucose

   c. gluconeogenesis

   d. potassium and sodium metabolism

17. Aldosterone

18. A substance or hormone that promotes the development of male characteristics

19. a. dopamine

   b. epinephrine

   c. norepinephrine

20. a. It elevates the systolic blood pressure.

   b. It increases the heart rate and cardiac output.

   c. It increases glycogenolysis, thereby hastening release of glucose from the liver. This action elevates the blood sugar level and provides the body with a spurt of energy.

*Optional answers to question 20:

   d. It dilates the bronchial tubes.

   e. It dilates the pupils.

21. estrogen . . . progesterone

22. testosterone

23. a. thymosin

   b. thymopoietin

24. a. gastrin

   b. secretin

   c. pancreozymincholecyst-okinin

   d. enterogastrone

WORD PARTS

Prefixes

1. toward
2. through
3. within
4. good, normal
5. out, away from
6. out, away from
7. excessive
8. deficient, under
9. all
10. beside
11. before
12. upon
13. water

Roots and Combining Forms

1. acid
2. extremity
3. gland
4. gland
5. cortex
6. flesh
7. cretin
8. man
9. to secrete
10. to secrete
11. small
12. milk
13. old age
14. giant
15. little acorn
16. sweet, sugar
17. seed
18. hairy
19. insulin
20. cortex
21. insulin
22. potassium
23. drowsiness
24. study of
25. mucus
26. eye
27. pine cone
28. kidney
29. phlegm
30. kidney
31. kidney
32. mad desire
33. thymus
34. to bear
35. thyroid, shield
36. thyroid, shield
37. poison
38. nourishment
39. masculine
40. body
41. testicle
42. solid
43. thyroid, shield
44. vessel
45. to press

Suffixes

1. pertaining to
2. formation, produce
3. pertaining to
4. to go
5. excision
6. swelling
7. blood condition
8. formation, produce
9. condition
10. pertaining to
11. condition of
12. one who specializes
13. inflammation
14. study of
15. hormone
16. enlargement, large
17. resemble
18. tumor
19. condition of
20. disease
21. pertaining to
22. growth
23. chemical
24. flow, discharge
25. pertaining to

IDENTIFYING MEDICAL TERMS

1. adenosis
2. cretinism
3. diabetes
4. endocrinology
5. euthyroid
6. exocrine
7. gigantism

8. glucocorticoid
9. hyperkalemia
10. hypogonadism
11. lethargic
12. thymitis

SPELLING

1. catecholamines
2. cretinism
3. exophthalmic
4. hypothyroidism
5. myxedema
6. pineal
7. pituitary
8. thyroid
9. oxytocin
10. virilism

MATCHING

1. e
2. f
3. b
4. g
5. h
6. i
7. c
8. j
9. d
10. a

ABBREVIATIONS

1. BMR
2. DM
3. fasting blood sugar
4. glucose tolerance tests
5. PBI
6. parathormone
7. radioimmunoassay
8. STH
9. thyroid function studies
10. vasopressin

DIAGNOSTIC AND LABORATORY TESTS

1. a
2. c
3. c
4. b
5. c

■ **CHAPTER 12**

ANATOMY AND PHYSIOLOGY

1. a. central
   b. peripheral

2. neurons
3. a. cause contractions in muscles
   b. cause secretions from glands and organs
   c. inhibit the actions of glands and organs
4. An axon is a long process reaching from the cell body to the area to be activated.
5. A dendrite resembles the branches of a tree and has short, unsheathed processes that transmit impulses to the cell body.
6. Sensory nerves transmit impulses to the central nervous system.
7. interneurons
8. a. a single elongated process
   b. a bundle of nerve fibers
   c. groups of nerve fibers
9. brain . . . spinal cord
10. a. receives impulses
    b. processes information
    c. responds with appropriate action
11. a. dura mater
    b. arachnoid
    c. pia mater
12. a. cerebrum
    b. diencephalon
    c. midbrain
    d. cerebellum
    e. pons
    f. medulla oblongata
    g. reticular formation
13. frontal lobe
14. somesthetic area
15. auditory . . . language
16. vision
17. a. is relay center for all sensory impulses
    b. relays motor impulses from the cerebellum to the cortex
18. a. is a regulator
    b. produces neurosecretions

c. produces hormones
19. coordination of voluntary movement
20. a. regulates and controls breathing
    b. regulates and controls swallowing
    c. regulates and controls coughing
    d. regulates and controls sneezing
    e. regulates and controls vomiting
21. a. conducts sensory impulses
    b. conducts motor impulses
    c. is a reflex center
22. 120 . . . 150
23. a. olfactory
    b. optic
    c. oculomotor
    d. trochlear
    e. trigeminal
    f. abducens
    g. facial
    h. acoustic
    i. glossopharyngeal
    j. vagus
    k. accessory
    l. hypoglossal
24. a. cervical
    b. brachial
    c. lumbar
    d. sacral
25. a. controls sweating
    b. controls the secretions of glands
    c. controls arterial blood pressure
    d. controls smooth muscle tissue
26. a. sympathetic
    b. parasympathetic

WORD PARTS

Prefixes

1. lack of
2. lack of
3. star-shaped

4. slow
5. down
6. difficult
7. upon
8. half
9. water
10. excessive
11. within
12. small
13. little
14. beside
15. beside
16. many
17. fire
18. four
19. below
20. together

Roots and Combining Forms

1. extremity
2. to walk
3. marketplace
4. dura, hard
5. imperfect
6. center
7. head
8. side
9. little brain
10. little brain
11. cerebrum
12. color
13. self
14. shaken violently
15. skull
16. skull
17. cell
18. tree
19. a disk
20. dura, hard
21. I, self
22. electricity
23. brain
24. brain
25. feeling
26. numbness
27. knot
28. glue

29. seizure
30. sleep
31. globus pallidus
32. thin plate
33. lobe
34. study of
35. membrane
36. membrane
37. membrane
38. mind
39. memory
40. spinal cord
41. spinal cord
42. muscle
43. nerve
44. nerve
45. nerve
46. papilla
47. dusky
48. gray
49. mind
50. mind
51. hardening
52. a thorn
53. vertebra
54. body
55. sleep
56. sympathy
57. vagus, wandering
58. little belly

Suffixes

1. pertaining to
2. pain
3. pain
4. pertaining to
5. weakness
6. germ cell
7. hernia
8. cell
9. binding
10. excision
11. swelling
12. feeling
13. glue
14. mark, record
15. to write

16. recording
17. condition
18. pertaining to
19. process
20. condition
21. one who specializes
22. inflammation
23. motion
24. motion
25. seizure
26. a sheath, husk
27. diction
28. study of
29. strike
30. softening
31. madness
32. nourishment, development
33. measurement
34. to view, examine
35. mind
36. tumor
37. condition of
38. weakness
39. disease
40. to eat
41. speak
42. fear
43. action
44. strength
45. order
46. incision
47. pertaining to
48. condition

IDENTIFYING MEDICAL TERMS

1. amnesia
2. analgesia
3. aphagia
4. ataxia
5. cephalalgia
6. cerebellar
7. craniectomy
8. dyslexia
9. encephalitis
10. epidural
11. hemiparesis

12. meningitis
13. neuralgia
14. neuritis
15. neurocyte
16. neurology
17. neuroma
18. neurosis
19. polyneuritis
20. psychology
21. vagotomy
22. ventriculometry

SPELLING

1. anesthesia
2. atelomyelia
3. cerebrospinal
4. craniotomy
5. epilepsy
6. meningioma
7. meningomyelocele
8. neuropathy
9. poliomyelitis
10. ventriculometry

MATCHING

1. g	6. h
2. d	7. j
3. c	8. f
4. b	9. a
5. e	10. i

ABBREVIATIONS

1. AD
2. ALS
3. central nervous system
4. cerebral palsy
5. CT
6. HDS
7. intracranial pressure
8. lumbar puncture
9. multiple sclerosis
10. PET

DIAGNOSTIC AND LABORATORY TESTS

1. a	4. d
2. b	5. c
3. c	

■ CHAPTER 13

ANATOMY AND PHYSIOLOGY

1. hearing . . . equilibrium
2. a. external
   b. middle
   c. inner
3. a. auricle
   b. external acoustic meatus
   c. tympanic membrane
4. auricle
5. a. lubrication
   b. protection
6. a. malleus
   b. incus
   c. stapes
7. to transmit sound vibrations
8. a. transmitting sound vibrations
   b. equalizing air pressure
   c. control of loud sounds
9. cochlea, vestibule, and the semicircular canals
10. a. cochlear duct
    b. semicircular ducts
    c. utricle and saccule
11. organ of Corti
12. vestibule
13. eighth cranial nerve
14. the position of the ear
15. a. endolymph
    b. perilymph

WORD PARTS

Prefixes

1. within
2. within
3. around
4. twice
5. one

Roots and Combining Forms

1. hearing
2. to hear
3. to hear
4. hearing
5. the ear
6. gall, bile
7. land snail
8. electricity
9. maze
10. maze
11. larynx
12. study of
13. breast
14. fungus
15. drum membrane
16. drum membrane
17. nerve
18. ear
19. ear
20. pharynx
21. voice
22. old
23. pus
24. nose
25. hardening
26. stirrup
27. fat
28. a jingling
29. drum
30. ear
31. equal
32. balance
33. window
34. middle
35. drum

Suffixes

1. pertaining to
2. pain
3. hearing
4. pain
5. excision
6. a mark, record
7. recording
8. pertaining to
9. one who specializes
10. inflammation
11. stone
12. study of
13. serum, clear fluid

14. instrument to measure
15. measurement
16. form
17. tumor
18. condition of
19. surgical repair
20. flow
21. instrument
22. instrument to cut
23. incision
24. pertaining to
25. pertaining to
26. small
27. tissue
28. process
29. condition of

IDENTIFYING MEDICAL TERMS

1. audiologist
2. audiometry
3. auditory
4. endaural
5. labyrinthitis
6. myringoplasty
7. myringotome
8. otodynia
9. otolaryngology
10. otopharyngeal
11. otoscope
12. perilymph
13. stapedectomy
14. tympanectomy
15. tinnitus

SPELLING

1. acoustic
2. audiology
3. cholesteatoma
4. electrocochleography
5. labyrinthitis
6. myringoplasty
7. otomycosis
8. otosclerosis
9. tympanic
10. tympanitis

MATCHING

1. h   6. b
2. e   7. j
3. i   8. c
4. a   9. d
5. g   10. f

ABBREVIATIONS

1. AC
2. AD
3. left ear
4. AU
5. ear, nose, throat
6. eyes, ears, nose, throat
7. HD
8. oto
9. serous otitis media
10. UCHD

DIAGNOSTIC AND LABORATORY TESTS

1. a
2. b
3. c
4. d
5. b

■ CHAPTER 14

ANATOMY AND PHYSIOLOGY

1. orbit, muscles, eyelids, conjunctiva, and the lacrimal apparatus
2. fatty tissue
3. optic nerve . . . ophthalmic artery
4. a. support
   b. rotary movement
5. intense light, foreign particles, . . . impact
6. A mucous membrane that acts as a protective covering for the exposed surface of the eyeball
7. Structures that produce, store, and remove the tears that cleanse and lubricate the eye
8. eyeball, its structures, and the nerve fibers

9. vision
10. optic disk
11. The process of sharpening the focus of light on the retina
12. Answers to the matching question:
    1. c
    2. e
    3. b
    4. a
    5. f
    6. d
    7. h
    8. i
    9. j
    10. g

WORD PARTS

Prefixes

1. lack of, without
2. two
3. double
4. out
5. in
6. inward
7. beyond
8. within
9. three
10. out
11. half
12. lack of
13. behind

Roots and Combining Forms

1. dull
2. to join together
3. unequal
4. eyelid
5. eyelid
6. choroid
7. cold
8. pupil
9. cornea
10. ciliary body
11. ciliary body
12. to remove the kernel of
13. tear

14. less, smaller
15. electricity
16. focus
17. angle
18. iris
19. iris
20. cornea
21. cornea
22. tear
23. study of
24. measure
25. to shut
26. muscle
27. blind
28. eye
29. eye
30. eye
31. eye
32. eye
33. lens
34. lentil, lens
35. light
36. old
37. pupil
38. retina
39. retina
40. sclera
41. point
42. tone
43. turn
44. uvea
45. foreign material
46. dry
47. dilation, widen
48. to nod
49. straight
50. disintegrate
51. to clot
52. radiating out from a center
53. lens
54. fiber
55. a squinting
56. hair

Suffixes

1. pertaining to
2. pertaining to

3. pertaining to
4. germ cell
5. condition
6. excision
7. mark, record
8. recording
9. condition
10. pertaining to
11. process
12. condition of
13. one who specializes
14. inflammation
15. study of
16. destruction, to separate
17. formation
18. instrument to measure
19. tumor
20. eye, vision
21. condition of
22. disease
23. fear
24. surgical repair
25. stroke, paralysis
26. prolapse, drooping
27. instrument
28. pertaining to
29. incision
30. tissue

IDENTIFYING MEDICAL TERMS

1. amblyopia
2. bifocal
3. blepharoptosis
4. corneal
5. dacryoma
6. diplopia
7. emmetropia
8. intraocular
9. keratitis
10. keratoplasty
11. lacrimal
12. ocular
13. photophobia

SPELLING

1. astigmatism
2. cycloplegia

3. iridectomy
4. ophthalmologist
5. phacosclerosis
6. pupillary
7. retinoblastoma
8. scleritis
9. tonometer
10. uveal

MATCHING

1. e	6. d
2. f	7. g
3. j	8. b
4. h	9. a
5. c	10. i

ABBREVIATIONS

1. DVA
2. emmetropia
3. hypermetropia (hyperopia)
4. IOL
5. L & A
6. myopia
7. right eye
8. OS
9. OU
10. exotropia

DIAGNOSTIC AND LABORATORY TESTS

1. c
2. b
3. c
4. d
5. d

■ CHAPTER 15

ANATOMY AND PHYSIOLOGY

1. a. ovaries
   b. fallopian tubes
   c. uterus
   d. vagina
   e. vulva
   f. breasts
2. To perpetuate the species through sexual or germ cell reproduction

3. a. body
   b. isthmus
   c. cervix
4. The bulging surface of the body of the uterus extending from the internal os of the cervix upward above the fallopian tubes
5. a. broad ligaments
   b. round ligaments
   c. uterosacral ligaments
   d. ligaments that attach to the bladder
6. a. peritoneum
   b. endometrium
   c. myometrium
7. a. menstruation
   b. functions as a place for the protection and nourishment of the fetus during pregnancy
   c. uterine wall contracts rhythmically and powerfully to expel the fetus from the uterus
8. a. The process of bending forward of the uterus at its body and neck
   b. The process of bending the body of the uterus backward at an angle, with the cervix usually unchanged from its normal position
   c. The process of turning the fundus forward toward the pubis, with the cervix tilted up toward the sacrum
   d. The process of turning the uterus backward, with the cervix pointing forward toward the symphysis pubis
9. uterine tubes or oviducts
10. a. serosa
    b. muscular
    c. mucosa
11. Finger-like processes that work to propel the discharged ovum into the fallopian tube
12. fertilization

13. a. Serves as a duct for the conveyance of the ovum from the ovary to the uterus
    b. Serve as ducts for the conveyance of spermatozoa from the uterus toward each ovary
14. Almond-shaped organs attached to the uterus by the ovarian ligament
15. a. primary
    b. growing
    c. graafian
16. pituitary gland (anterior lobe)
17. a. production of ova
    b. production of hormones
18. musculomembranous . . . vestibule
19. a. female organ of copulation
    b. passageway for discharge of menstruation
    c. passageway for birth of the fetus
20. a. mons pubis
    b. labia major
    c. labia minora
    d. vestibule
    e. clitoris
21. perineum
22. A surgical procedure to prevent tearing of the perineum and to facilitate delivery of the fetus
23. mammary glands
24. areola . . . nipple
25. a. prolactin
    b. insulin
    c. glucocorticoids
26. A thin yellowish secretion containing mainly serum and white blood cells; the "first milk"
27. a. menstruation
    b. proliferation
    c. luteal or secretory
    d. premenstrual or ischemic

28. A condition that affects certain women and may cause distressful symptoms such as nausea, constipation, diarrhea, anorexia, headache, appetite cravings, backache, muscular aches, edema, insomnia, clumsiness, malaise, irritability, indecisiveness, mental confusion, and depression

WORD PARTS
Prefixes
1. lack of
2. out
3. before
4. together
5. against
6. difficult, painful
7. within
8. within
9. many
10. new
11. none
12. scanty
13. beside
14. around
15. after
16. before
17. first
18. false
19. backward
20. three

ROOTS AND COMBINING FORMS
1. to miscarry
2. lamb
3. Bartholin's glands
4. receive
5. cervix
6. a coming together
7. vagina
8. cul-de-sac
9. bladder
10. vulva
11. a bed
12. fibrous tissue
13. belonging to birth

14. female
15. life
16. hymen
17. womb, uterus
18. womb, uterus
19. study of
20. breast
21. breast
22. month
23. month
24. month
25. womb, uterus
26. uterus
27. muscle
28. birth
29. birth
30. ovum, egg
31. ovary
32. ovary
33. to bear
34. labor
35. cessation
36. pelvis
37. germ cell
38. to shine
39. rectum
40. tube
41. tube
42. displaced
43. formation, produce
44. uterus
45. vagina
46. sexual intercourse
47. turning
48. lump
49. beginning
50. in labor
51. pregnant
52. external genitals
53. second
54. sound
55. substituted

Suffixes

1. pertaining to
2. use

3. hernia
4. surgical puncture
5. pregnancy
6. excision
7. formation, produce
8. record
9. condition
10. pertaining to
11. process
12. one who specializes
13. inflammation
14. study of
15. measurement
16. tumor
17. condition of
18. surgical repair
19. to burst forth
20. sac
21. flow
22. instrument
23. pertaining to
24. incision
25. resemble
26. pertaining to

IDENTIFYING MEDICAL TERMS

1. abortion
2. antepartum
3. cervicitis
4. dysmenorrhea
5. fibroma
6. gynecology
7. hymenectomy
8. mammoplasty
9. menorrhea
10. neonatal
11. oogenesis
12. postpartum

SPELLING

1. amniocentesis
2. bartholinitis
3. dystocia
4. episiotomy
5. hysterotomy
6. menorrhagia
7. oophoritis

8. salpingitis
9. vaginitis
10. venereal

MATCHING

1. f
2. j
3. d
4. c
5. e

6. a
7. g
8. h
9. b
10. i

ABBREVIATIONS

1. abortion
2. AFP
3. abdominal hysterectomy
4. CS; C-section
5. diethylstilbestrol
6. EDC
7. pregnancy one
8. gynecology
9. IUD
10. PID

DIAGNOSTIC AND LABORATORY TESTS

1. b
2. c
3. a
4. c
5. d

■ CHAPTER 16

ANATOMY AND PHYSIOLOGY

1. a. testes
   b. various ducts
   c. urethra
   d. bulbourethral gland
   e. prostate gland
   f. seminal vesicles
2. a. sacrotum
   b. penis
3. To provide the sperm cells necessary to fertilize the ovum, thereby perpetuating the species
4. A pouch-like structure located behind the penis

5. corpora cavernosa penis and the corpus spongiosum
6. 15 to 20
7. glans penis
8. The loose skin folds that cover the penis
9. A lubricating fluid
10. a. It is the male organ of copulation
    b. It is the site of the orifice for the elimination of urine and semen from the body.
11. They are two ovoid-shaped organs located in the scrotum. Each testis is about 4 cm long and 2.5 cm wide.
12. Seminiferous tubules
13. a. It is responsible for the development of secondary male characteristics during puberty.
    b. It is essential for normal growth and development of the male accessory sex organs.
    c. It plays a vital role in the erection process of the penis.
    d. It affects the growth of hair on the face.
    e. It affects muscular development and vocal timbre.
14. rete testis
15. A coiled tube lying on the posterior aspect of the testis
16. a. It is a storage site for sperm.
    b. It is a duct for the passage of sperm.
17. ductus deferens or the vas deferens
18. a. ductus deferens
    b. arteries
    c. veins
    d. lymphatic vessels
    e. nerves
19. Production of a slightly alkaline fluid
20. It is about 4 cm wide and weighs about 20 g. It is composed of glandular, connective, and muscular tissues and lies behind the urinary bladder.
21. Enlargement of the prostate that sometimes occurs in older men
22. bulbourethral . . . Cowper's
23. a. prostatic
    b. membranous
    c. penile
24. It transmits urine and semen out of the body.
25. 20

WORD PARTS

Prefixes

1. lack of
2. lack of
3. around
4. upon
5. water
6. under
7. scanty
8. beside
9. into
10. good
11. different
12. similiar, same
13. three

Roots and Combining Forms

1. glans
2. to cut
3. hidden
4. not natural
5. testis
6. to pour
7. testicle
8. testicle
9. testicle
10. penis
11. a muzzle
12. prostate
13. to prune
14. a rent (opening)
15. seed
16. seed
17. seed, sperm
18. sperm
19. testicle
20. twisted vein
21. vessel
22. vesicle
23. animal
24. life
25. to throw out
26. genitals
27. female
28. breast
29. sex
30. thread
31. body

Suffixes

1. pertaining to
2. pertaining to
3. immature cell, germ cell
4. hernia
5. to kill
6. excision
7. formation, produce
8. condition
9. process
10. condition of
11. inflammation
12. use
13. condition of
14. formation, produce
15. flow
16. incision
17. pertaining to

IDENTIFYING MEDICAL TERMS

1. balanitis
2. epididymectomy
3. orchidectomy
4. prepuce
5. eunuch
6. condyloma
7. spermatoblast
8. spermatozoon
9. spermicide
10. testicular

SPELLING

1. cryptorchism
2. hypospadias
3. orchidotomy
4. eugenics
5. trisomy

MATCHING

1. e	6. i
2. c	7. h
3. f	8. k
4. b	9. a
5. g	10. d

ABBREVIATIONS

1. BPH
2. gonorrhea
3. HPV
4. herpes simplex virus-2
5. sexually transmitted diseases
6. TPA
7. transurethral resection
8. urogenital
9. VD
10. PSA

DIAGNOSTIC AND LABORATORY TESTS

1. c
2. a
3. b
4. c
5. c

■ CHAPTER 17

AN OVERVIEW OF CANCER

1. a. carcinomas
   b. sarcomas
   c. mixed cancers
2. The process whereby normal cells have a distinct appearance and specialized function
3. The process whereby normal cells lose their specialization and become malignant
4. a. active migration

b. direct extension
c. metastasis
5. a. Change in bowel or bladder habits
   b. A sore that does not heal
   c. Unusual bleeding or discharge
   d. Thickening or lump in breast or elsewhere
   e. Indigestion or difficulty in swallowing
   f. Obvious change in a wart or mole
   g. Nagging cough or hoarseness
6. a. surgery
   b. chemotherapy
   c. radiation therapy
   d. immunotherapy

WORD PARTS

Prefixes

1. up
2. star-shaped
3. excessive
4. new
5. little
6. before
7. in
8. in
9. beyond

ROOTS AND COMBINING FORMS

1. gland
2. vessel
3. crab
4. cancer
5. cancer
6. cartilage
7. chorion
8. cell
9. tree
10. fiber
11. glue
12. glue
13. blood
14. safe
15. smooth

16. white
17. white
18. fat
19. lymph
20. lymph
21. marrow
22. black
23. membrane
24. mucus
25. fungus
26. marrow
27. muscle
28. a little box
29. kidney
30. nerve
31. tumor
32. bone
33. net
34. retina
35. rod
36. flesh
37. to lead
38. seed
39. mouth
40. monster
41. thymus
42. poison
43. grating
44. dry
45. small lobe
46. place
47. mushroom, fungus
48. suppress
49. to strain through
50. bad kind
51. to change
52. to change
53. cloaked
54. fruitful
55. to bear
56. remit
57. virus (poison)

Suffixes

1. immature cell
2. blood condition
3. formation

4. produce

5. formation, produce

6. condition

7. pertaining to

8. inflammation

9. tumor

10. pertaining to

11. plate

12. formation

13. a thing formed

14. use, action

15. treatment

16. pertaining to

17. pertaining to

18. pertaining to

19. quality of

20. process

21. nature of

22. forming

23. control

24. resemble

IDENTIFYING MEDICAL TERMS

1. carcinogen

2. chondrosarcoma

3. glioma

4. scirrhus

5. leukemia

6. lymphoma

7. melanoma

8. myosarcoma

9. osteogenic sarcoma

10. sarcoma

SPELLING

1. anaplasia

2. fibrosarcoma

3. lymphosarcoma

4. myeloma

5. oncogenic

6. seminoma

MATCHING

1. e   6. f

2. i   7. j

3. d   8. b

4. g   9. h

5. c   10. a

ABBREVIATIONS

1. Adeno-CA

2. Bx

3. cancer

4. chemotherapy

5. DNA

6. interleukin-2

7. LAK

8. metastases

9. tumor necrosis factor

10. TNM

■ CHAPTER 18

AN OVERVIEW OF RADIOLOGY AND NUCLEAR MEDICINE

1. The study of x-rays, radioactive substances, radioactive isotopes, and ionizing radiation

2. a. invisible

   b. cause ionization

   c. cause fluorescence

   *Alternate characteristics to those listed:

   d. travel in a straight line

   e. able to penetrate substances

   f. destroy cells

3. a. Can depress the hematopoietic system, cause leukopenia, leukemia

   b. Can damage the gonads

4. a. wearing a film badge

   b. lead screens

   c. lead-lined room

   d. protective clothing

   e. gonad shield

5. a. computed tomography

   b. magnetic resonance imaging

   c. thermography

   d. scintigraphy

6. Treatment of disease by the use of ionizing radiation

WORD PARTS

Prefixes

1. short

2. below

2. within

4. one-thousandth

5. beyond

6. into

ROOTS AND COMBINING FORMS

1. acting

2. ampere

3. vessel

4. finger or toe

5. artery

6. joint

7. bronchi

8. heart

9. cavity

10. gall, bile

11. gall

12. motion

13. motion

14. to draw

15. curie

16. bladder

17. skin

18. ion (going)

19. echo

20. straight

21. brain

22. fluorescence

23. kind

24. volt

25. uterus

26. ion

27. ion

28. one thousand

29. nucleus

30. study of

31. to shine

32. lymph

33. breast

34. spinal cord

35. to swing

36. dark

37. light

38. nature

39. renal pelvis

40. radiant

41. ray

42. roentgen
43. fallopian tube
44. salivary
45. sound
46. sound
47. distant
48. heat
49. to cut
50. vein
51. vein
52. volt
53. watt

SUFFIXES

1. pertaining to
2. one who
3. formation, produce
4. pertaining to
5. record
6. record
7. recording
8. pertaining to
9. process
10. one who specializes
11. inflammation
12. nature of
13. study of
14. instrument to measure
15. related to
16. pertaining to
17. instrument
18. to view, examine
19. treatment
20. having a particular quality

IDENTIFYING MEDICAL TERMS

1. angiography
2. arthrography
3. cholecystogram
4. intracavitary
5. ionotherapy
6. kilovolt
7. kilowatt
8. mammography
9. millicurie
10. physicist
11. radiation
12. radioactive
13. radiographer
14. radiolucent
15. radiopaque
16. sonogram

SPELLING

1. hysterosalpingogram
2. echography

3. lymphangiography
4. myelogram
5. volt
6. radioactive
7. radiography
8. sialography
9. tomography
10. venography

MATCHING

1. d   6. k
2. e   7. b
3. c   8. i
4. g   9. a
5. j   10. h

ABBREVIATIONS

1. AP
2. Ba
3. CT
4. kilovolt
5. lateral
6. radium
7. MRI
8. posteroanterior
9. Ci
10. positron emission tomography

CASE STUDY ANSWERS

■ CHAPTER 3

1. pruritus
2. vesicle
3. contact dermatitis
4. antipruritic
5. corticosteroid
6. a. stay away from poison ivy
   b. when working outside, wear clothing that covers arms and legs
   c. after working in the yard, immediately take a bath or shower to remove any possible contamination of skin with poison ivy
7. erythroderma
8. edema

■ CHAPTER 4

1. humpback
2. one 5mg tablet orally, taken daily
3. Vitamin A
4. Vitamin C
5. Calcium

■ CHAPTER 5

1. waddling
2. electromyography
3. a. minimize deformities
   b. preserve mobility

■ CHAPTER 6

1. pyrosis
2. gastrointestinal
3. acidity
4. Mylanta
5. 300

■ CHAPTER 7

1. dyspnea
2. electrocardiogram
3. nitroglycerin
4. seek medical attention without delay

■ CHAPTER 8

1. diarrhea
2. immune
3. AZT and/or zidovudine
4. Pre-existing conditions can make them less tolerant of drugs.

■ CHAPTER 9

1. anorexia
2. *Mycobacterium tuberculosis*
3. isoniazid
4. purified protein derivative

■ CHAPTER 10

1. sensation
2. urinalysis

3. sulfonamide
4. Because of the short length of the female urethra
5. *Escherichia coli (E. coli)*
6. To avoid contaminating the urinary meatus with colon bacteria

■ CHAPTER 11

1. polydipsia
2. glucose
3. diet
4. polydipsia
5. polyuria
6. polyphagia

■ CHAPTER 12

1. memory
2. electroencephalogram
3. assistance
4. Because brain cells die and the connections between cells are lost
5. To prevent the breakdown of acetylcholine in the brain and to keep the levels of this chemical messenger high, even while the cells that produce the messenger continue to become damaged or die
6. To help family members and health care professionals recognize warning signs of Alzheimer's Disease, so that

people with dementia and their families receive information, care, and support as early as possible

■ CHAPTER 13
1. tinnitus
2. otoscopy
3. analgesic; pain
4. antibiotic; infection
5. earache; pain in the ear

■ CHAPTER 14
1. photophobia
2. complete
3. ultrasonic
4. It is aspirated.
5. unusual intolerance of light; fear of light

■ CHAPTER 15
1. dyspareunia
2. gynecologic

3. diet, dietary supplements
4. phytoestrogens
5. stabilizing

■ CHAPTER 16
1. urgency
2. Proscar
3. impotence
4. prostate

GLOSSARY OF WORD PARTS

PREFIXES

a	no, not, without, lack of, apart
ab	away from
ad	toward, near
ambi	both
an	no, not, without, lack of
ana	up
ant	against
ante	before
anti	against
apo	separation
astro	star-shaped
auto	self
bi	two, double
bin	twice
brachy	short
brady	slow
cac	bad
cata	down
centi	a hundred
chromo	color
circum	around
con	with, together
contra	against
de	down, away from
deca	ten
di (a)	through, between
dia	through, between

dif	apart, free from, separate
dipl	double
di (s)	two, apart
dis	apart
dys	bad, difficult, painful
ec	out, outside, outer
ecto	out, outside, outer
em	in
en	within
end	within, inner
endo	within, inner
ep	upon, over, above
epi	upon, over, above
eso	inward
eu	good, normal
ex	out, away from
exo	out, away from
extra	outside, beyond
hemi	half
heter	different
hetero	different
homo	similar, same
homeo	similar, same, likeness, constant
hydr	water
hydro	water
hyp	below, deficient

hyper	above, beyond, excessive
hypo	below, under, deficient
in	in, into, not
infra	below
infer	below
inter	between
intra	within
ir (in)	into
macro	large
mal	bad
mega	large, great
meso	middle
meta	beyond, over, between, change
micro	small
milli	one-thousandth
mon (o)	one
mono	one
multi	many, much
neo	new
nulli	none
olig	little, scanty
oligo	little, scanty
pan	all
par	around, beside
para	beside, alongside, abnormal

per	through	pyro	fire	sym	together
peri	around	quadri	four	syn	together, with
poly	many, much,	quint	five	tachy	fast
	excessive	re	back	tetra	four
post	after, behind	retro	backward	trans	across
pre	before	semi	half	tri	three
primi	first	sub	below, under,	ultra	beyond
pro	before		beneath	uni	one
proto	first	supra	above, beyond		
pseudo	false	super	above, beyond		

WORD ROOTS/COMBINING FORMS

abdomin	abdomen	andr	man	atri/o	atrium
abort	to miscarry	andr/o	man	aud/i	to hear
absorpt	to suck in	ang	vessel	audi/o	to hear
acanth	a thorn	ang/i	vessel	auditor	hearing
acetabul	vinegar cup	angin	to choke, quinsy	aur	ear
acid	acid	angi/o	vessel	aur/i	ear
acoust	hearing	anis/o	unequal	auscultat	listen to
acr	extremity, point	ankyl	stiffening, crooked	aut	self
acr/o	extremity, point	an/o	anus	axill	armpit
act	acting	anter/i	toward the front	bacter/i	bacteria
actin	ray	anthrac	coal	balan	glans penis
aden	gland	aort	aorta	bartholin	Bartholin's glands
aden/o	gland	aort/o	aorta	bas/o	base
adhes	stuck to	append	appendix	bil	bile, gall
adip	fat	arachn	spider	bil/i	bile, gall
agglutinat	clumping	arche	beginning	bi/o	life
agon	agony	arter	artery	blast/o	germ cell
agor/a	market place	arter/i	artery	blephar	eyelid
albin	white	arteri/o	artery	blephar/o	eyelid
albumin	protein	arthr	joint	bol	to cast, throw
alimentat	nourishment	arthr/o	joint	brach/i	arm
all	other	artific/i	not natural	bronch	bronchi
alveol	small, hollow air sac	aspirat	to draw in	bronch/i	bronchi
ambyl	dull	atel	imperfect	bronchiol	bronchiole
ambul	to walk	atel/o	imperfect	bronch/o	bronchi
amni/o	lamb	ather	fatty substance,	bucc	cheek
ampere	ampere		porridge	burs	a pouch
amputat	to cut though	ather/o	fatty substance,	calc	lime, calcium
amyl	starch		porridge	calc/i	calcium
anastom	opening	atri	atrium	calcan/e	heel bone

cancer	crab	circulat	circular	crur	leg
capn	smoke	cirrh	orange-yellow	cry/o	cold
capsul	a little box	cirrh/o	orange-yellow	crypt	hidden
carcin	cancer	cis	to cut	cubit	elbow, to lie
carcin/o	cancer	claudicat	to limp	culd/o	cul-de-sac
card	heart	clavicul	little key	curie	curie
card/i	heart	cleid/o	clavicle	cutane	skin
cardi/o	heart	coagul	to clot	cyan	dark blue
carp	wrist	coagulat	to clot	cycl	ciliary body
carp/o	wrist	coccyg/e	tailbone	cycl/o	ciliary body
cartil	gristle	coccyg/o	tail bone	cyst	bladder, sac
castr	to prune	cochle/o	land snail	cyst/o	bladder, sac
caud	tail	coit	a coming together	cyt	cell
caus	heat	col	colon	cyth	cell
cavit	cavity	coll/a	glue	cyt/o	cell
celi	abdomen, belly	collis	neck	dacry	tear
cellul	little cell	col/o	colon	dactyl	finger or toe
centr	center	colon	colon	dactyl/o	finger or toe
centr/i	center	colon/o	colon	defecat	to remove dregs
cephal	head	colp/o	vagina	dem	people
cept	receive	concuss	shaken violently	dendr/o	tree
cerebell	little brain	condyle	knuckle	dent	tooth
cerebell/o	little brain	con/i	dust	dent/i	tooth
cerebr/o	cerebrum	conjunctiv	to join together	derm	skin
cervic	cervix, neck	connect	to bind together	derm/a	skin
cheil	lip	constipat	to press together	dermat	skin
chem/o	chemical	continence	to hold	dermat/o	skin
chlor/o	green	cor	pupil	derm/o	skin
chol	gall, bile	coriat	corium	dextr/o	to the right
chole	gall, bile	corne	cornea	diast	to expand
chol/e	gall, bile	corpor	body	didym	testis
choledoch/o	common bile duct	corpor/e	body	digit	finger or toe
chondr	cartilage	cortic	cortex	dilat	to widen
chondr/o	cartilage	cortis	cortex	disk	a disk
chord	cord	cost	rib	dist	away from the point
chori/o	chorion	cost/o	rib		of origin
choroid	choroid	cox	hip	diverticul	diverticula
choroid/o	choroid	cran/i	skull	dors	backward
chromat	color	crani/o	skull	dors/i	backward
chrom/o	color	creat	flesh	duct	to lead
chym	juice	creatin	flesh, creatine	duoden	duodenum
cine	motion	crine	to secrete	dur	dura, hard
cinemat/o	motion	crin/o	to secrete	dur/o	dura, hard

dwarf	small	flex	to bend	halat	breathe
dynam	power	fluor/o	fluorescence	hallux	great (big) toe
ech/o	echo	foc	focus	hem	blood
ectop	displaced	follicul	little bag	hemat	blood
eg/o	I, self	format	a shaping	hemat/o	blood
ejaculat	to throw out	fungat	mushroom, fungus	hem/o	blood
electr/o	electricity	fus	to pour	hemorrh	vein liable to bleed
eme	to vomit	galact/o	milk	hepat	liver
embol	to cast, to throw	ganglion	knot	hepat/o	liver
emulsificat	disintergrate	gastr	stomach	herni/o	hernia
encephal	brain	gastr/o	stomach	hidr	sweat
encephal/o	brain	gen	formation, produce	hirsut	hairy
enchyma	to pour	gene	formation, produce	hist/o	tissue
enter	intestine	genet	formation, produce	hol/o	whole
enucleat	to remove the kernel of	genital	belonging to birth	horizont	horizon
		gen/o	kind	humer	humerus
eosin/o	rose-colored	ger	old age	hydr	water
episi/o	vulva, pudenda	gest	to carry	hymen	hymen
equ/i	equal	gester	to bear	hypn	sleep
erget	work	gigant	giant	hyster	womb, uterus
erg/o	work	gingiv	gums	hyster/o	womb, uterus
eructat	a breaking out	glandul	little acorn	icter	jaundice
erysi	red	gli	glue	ile	ileum
erythr/o	red	gli/o	glue	ile/o	ileum
esophag/e	esophagus	glob	globe	ili	ilium
esophag/o	esophagus	globin	globule	ili/o	ilium
esthesi/o	feeling	globul	globe	illus	foot
estr/o	mad desire	glomerul	glomerulus, little ball	immun/o	safe, immunity
eti/o	cause			infarct	infarct (necrosis of an area)
eunia	a bed	glomerul/o	glomerulus, little ball		
excret	sifted out			infect	infection
f(erat)	to bear	gloss/o	tongue	infer/i	below
fasc	a band (fascia)	gluc/o	sweet, sugar	inguin	groin
fasci/o	a band (fascia)	glyc	sweet, sugar	insul	insulin
femor	femur	glyc/o	glucose, sweet, sugar	insulin/o	insulin
fenestrat	window	glycos	sweet, sugar	integument	covering
fibr	fibrous tissue, fiber	gonad	seed	intern	within
fibrillat	fibrils (small fibers)	goni/o	angle	ionizat	ion (going)
fibrin/o	fiber	gon/o	genitals	ion/o	ion
fibr/o	fiber	granul/o	little grain, granular	iont/o	ion
fibul	fibula	gravida	pregnant	irid	iris
filtrat	to strain through	gryp	curve	irid/o	iris
fixat	fastened	gynec/o	female	isch	to hold back

ischi	ischium	log	study	micturit	to urinate
is/o	equal	log/o	word	miliar	millet (tiny)
jaund	yellow	lopec	fox mange	minim	least
kal	potassium	lord	bending	mi/o	less, smaller
kary/o	cell's nucleus	lucent	to shine	mit	thread
kel	tumor	lumb	loin	mitr	mitral valve
kerat	cornea	lumb/o	loin	mnes	memory
kerat/o	horn, cornea	lump	lump	mucos	mucus
keton	ketone	lun	moon	mucus	mucus
kil/o	a thousand	lymph	lymph, clear fluid	muscul	muscle
kinet	motion	lymph/o	lymph, clear fluid	muscul/o	muscle
kyph	a hump	malign	bad kind	muta	to change
labi	lip	mamm/o	breast	mutat	to change
labyrinth	maze	mandibul	lower jawbone	my	muscle
labyrinth/o	maze	man/o	thin	myc	fungus
lacrim	tear	mast	breast	myc/o	fungus
lamin	lamina, thin plate	masticat	to chew	mydriat	dilation, widen
lamp (s)	to shine	mast/o	breast	myel	bone marrow, spinal cord
lapar/o	flank, abdomen	maxill	jawbone		
laryng	larynx	maxilla	jaw	myel/o	marrow
laryng/e	larynx	maxim	greatest	my/o	muscle
laryng/o	larynx	meat	passage	my/os	muscle
later	side	meat/o	passage	myring	drum membrane
laxat	to loosen	med	middle	myring/o	drum membrane
lei/o	smooth	medi	toward the middle	myx	mucus
lemma	rind, sheath, husk	medull	marrow	narc/o	numbness
lent	lens	medull/o	marrow	nas/o	nose
lept	seizure	melan	black	nat	birth
letharg	drowsiness	melan/o	black	nat/o	birth
leuk	white	men	month	necr	death
leuk/o	white	mening	membrane (meninges)	necr/o	death
levat	lifter			nephr	kidney
libr/i	balance	mening/i	membrane	nephr/o	kidney
lingu	tongue	mening/o	membrane	neur	nerve
lip	fat	menise	crescent	neur/i	nerve
lipid	fat	men/o	month	neur/o	nerve
lip/o	fat	ment	mind	neutr/o	neither
lith	stone	mes	middle	nid	nest
lith/o	stone	mes/o	middle	noct	night
lob	lobe	mester	month	nom	law
lob/o	lobe	metr	to measure, womb, uterus	norm	rule
lobul	small lobe			nucl	nucleus
locat	to place	metr/i	womb, uterus	nucle	kernel, nucleus

nyctal	blind	para	to bear	physi/o	nature
nystagm	to nod	paralyt	to disable, paralysis	pil/o	hair
occlus	to shut up	partum	labor	pine	pine cone
ocul	eye	parturit	in labor	pineal	pineal body
odont	tooth	patell	kneecap, patella	pin/o	to drink
olecran	elbow	path	disease	pituitar	phlegm
onc/o	tumor	path/o	disease	plak	plate
onych	nail	pause	cessation	plasma	a thing formed, plasma
onych/o	nail	pector	chest		
o/o	ovum, egg	pectorat	breast	plast	a developing
oophor	ovary	ped	foot, child	pleur	pleura
ophthalm	eye	ped/i	foot, child	pleura	pleura
ophthalm/o	eye	pedicul	a louse	pleur/o	pleura
opt	eye	pelv/i	pelvis	plicat	to fold
opt/o	eye	pen	penis	pneum/o	lung, air
or	mouth	penile	penis	pneumon	lung
orch	testicle	pept	to digest	poiet	formation
orchid	testicle	perine	perineum	poli/o	gray
orchid/o	testicle	periton/e	peritoneum	pollex	thumb
organ	organ	phac	lens	por	a passage
orth	straight	phac/o	lens	porphyr	purple
orth/o	straight	phag	to eat, engulf	poster/i	behind, toward the back
oscill	to swing	phag/o	to eat, engulf		
oscill/o	to swing	phak	lentil, lens	prand/i	meal
oste	bone	phalang/e	closely knit row	presby	old
oste/o	bone	pharyng/o	pharynx	press	to press
ot	ear	pharyng	pharynx	proct	anus, rectum
ot/o	ear	phas	speech	proct/o	anus, rectum
ovar	ovary	phen/o	to show	prolif	fruitful
ovul	ovary	phe/o	dusky	prophylact	guarding
ovulat	ovary	phim	a muzzle	prostat	prostate
ox	oxygen	phleb	vein	prosth/e	an addition
ox/i	oxygen	phleb/o	vein	prot/e	first
oxy	sour, sharp, acid	phon	voice	proxim	near the point of origin
pachy	thick	phone	voice		
pancreat	pancreas	phon/o	sound	prurit	itching
paque	dark	phor	carrying	psych	mind
palat/o	palate	phos	light	psych/o	mind
palliat	cloaked	phot/o	light	pudend	external genitals
pallid/o	globus, pallidus	phragm	partition	pulm/o	lung
palm	palm	phragmat/o	partition	pulmon	lung
palpitat	throbbing	phras	speech	pulmonar	lung
papill	papilla	physic	nature	pupill	pupil

purpur	purple	scapul	shoulder blade	spondyl/o	vertebra
py	pus	scler	hardening	staped	stirrup
pyel	renal pelvis	scler/o	hardening, sclera	steat	fat
pyel/o	renal pelvis	scoli	curvature	sten	narrowing
pylor	pylorus, gate keeper	scoli/o	curvature	ster	solid
py/o	pus	scop	to examine	stern	sternum
pyret	fever	seb/o	oil	stern/o	sternum
pyr/o	heat, fire	secund	second	sterol	solid (fat)
rach	spine	semin	seed	steth	chest
rachi	spine	seminat	seed	steth/o	chest
radi	radius	senile	old	stigmat	point
rad/i	radiating out from a center	senil	old	stom	mouth
		sept	putrefaction	stomat	mouth
radiat	radiant	septic	putrefying	strabism	a squinting
radic/o	spinal nerve root	ser (a)	whey	strict	to draw, to bind
radicul	spinal nerve root	ser/o	whey, serum	superfic/i	near the surface
radi/o	ray	sert	to gain	super/i	upper
rect/o	rectum	sexu	sex	suppress	suppress
relaxat	to loosen	sial	saliva	surrog	substituted
remiss	remit	sial/o	salivary	sympath	sympathy
ren	kidney	sider/o	iron	synov	joint fluid
ren/o	kidney	sigmoid	sigmoid	syst	contraction
respirat	breathing	sigmoid/o	sigmoid	system	a composite whole
reticul/o	net	sin/o	a curve	systol	contraction
retin	retina	sinus	a hollow curve	tel	end, distant
retin/o	retina	situ	place	tele	distant
rhabd/o	rod	som	body	tempor	temples
rheumat	discharge	somat	body	tend/o	tendon
rheumat/o	discharge	somat/o	body	tendin	tendon
rhin/o	nose	somn	sleep	ten/o	tendon
rhonch	snore	son	sound	tenon	tendon
rhytid/o	wrinkle	son/o	sound	tenos	tendon
roent	roentgen	spadias	a rent, an opening	tens	tension
rotat	to turn	spastic	convulsive	tentori	tentorium, tent
rrhyth	rhythm	sperm	seed (sperm)	terat	monster
rrhythm	rhythm	spermi	seed (sperm)	testicul	testicle
rube/o	red	spermat	seed (sperm)	test/o	testicle
sacr	sacrum	spermat/o	seed (sperm)	thalass	sea
salping	tube, fallopian tube	sphygm/o	pulse	thel/i	nipple
salping/o	tube, fallopian tube	spin	spine, a thorn	therm	hot, heat
salpinx	tube, fallopian tube	spir/o	breath	therm/o	hot, heat
sarc	flesh	splen/o	spleen	thorac	chest
sarc/o	flesh	spondyl	vertebra	thorac/o	chest

thorax	chest	tubercul	a little swelling	venere	sexual intercourse
thromb	clot	tuss	cough	ven/i	vein
thromb/o	clot	tympan	ear drum	ven/o	vein
thym	thymus, mind, emotion	tympan/o	drum	ventilat	to air
		uln	ulna, elbow	ventr	near or on the belly
thyr	thyroid, shield	uln/o	ulna, elbow		side of the body
thyr/o	thyroid, shield	umbilic	navel	ventricul	ventricle
thyrox	thyroid, shield	ungu	nail	ventricul/o	little belly
tibi	tibia	ur	urine	vermi	worm
tinnit	a jingling	ure	urinate	vers	turning
toc	birth	urea	urea	vertebr	vertebra
tom/o	to cut	uret	urine	vertebr/o	vertebra
ton	tone, tension	ureter	ureter	vesic	bladder
ton/o	tone	ureter/o	ureter	vesicul	vesicle
tonsill	tonsil, almond	urethr	urethra	vir	virus (poison)
topic	place	urethr/o	urethra	viril	masculine
top/o	place	urin	urine	viscer	body organs
tors	twisted	urinat	urine	volt	volt
tort/i	twisted	urin/o	urine	volunt	will
tox	poison	ur/o	urine	volvul	to roll
toxic	poison	uter	uterus	vuls	to pull
trach/e	trachea	uter/o	uterus	watt	watt
trache/o	trachea	uve	uvea	xanth/o	yellow
tract	to draw	vagin	vagina	xen	foreign material
trephinat	a bore	vag/o	vagus, wandering	xer	dry
trich	hair	varic/o	twisted vein	xer/o	dry
trich/o	hair	vas	vessel	xiph	sword
trigon	trigone	vascul	small vessel	zo/o	animal
trism	grating	vas/o	vessel	zoon	life
trop	turning	vector	a carrier		
troph	a turning	ven	vein		

SUFFIXES

-able	capable	-ary	pertaining to	-cele	hernia, tumor, swelling
-ac	pertaining to	-ase	enzyme		
-ad	pertaining to	-asthenia	weakness	-centesis	surgical puncture
-age	related to	-ate	use, action	-ceps	head
-al	pertaining to	-ate (d)	use, action	-cide	to kill
-algesia	pain	-betes	to go	-clasia	a breaking
-algia	pain	-blast	immature cell, germ cell	-clave	a key
-ant	forming			-cle	small
-ar	pertaining to	-body	body	-clysis	injection

-cope	strike	-ic	pertaining to	-opsy	to view
-crit	to separate	-ide	having a particular	-or	one who, a doer
-culture	cultivation		quality	-ory	like, resemble
-cusis	hearing	-in	chemical, pertaining	-orexia	appetite
-cuspid	point		to	-ose	like
-cyesis	pregnancy	-ine	pertaining to	-osis	condition
-cyst	bladder	-ing	quality of	-ous	pertaining to
-cyte	cell	-ion	process	-paresis	weakness
-derma	skin	-ism	condition	-pathy	disease
-dermis	skin	-ist	one who specializes,	-penia	lack of, deficiency
-desis	binding		agent	-pepsia	to digest
-dipsia	thirst	-itis	inflammation	-pexy	surgical fixation
-drome	a course	-ity	condition	-phagia	to eat
-dynia	pain	-ive	nature of, quality of	-phasia	to speak
-ectasia	dilatation	-kinesia	motion	-pheresis	removal
-ectasis	dilatation,	-kinesis	motion	-phil	attraction
	distention	-lalia	to talk	-philia	attraction
-ectasy	dilation	-lemma	a sheath, rind	-phobia	fear
-ectomy	surgical excision	-lepsy	seizure	-phoresis	to carry
-edema	swelling	-lexia	diction	-phragm	a fence
-emesis	vomiting	-liter	liter	-phraxis	to obstruct
-emia	blood condition	-lith	stone	-phylaxis	protection
-er	relating to, one who	-logy	study of	-physis	growth
-ergy	work	-lymph	clear fluid	-plakia	plate
-esthesia	feeling	-lysis	destruction, to	-plasia	formation, produce
-form	shape		separate	-plasm	a thing formed,
-fuge	to flee	-malacia	softening		plasma
-gen	formation, produce	-mania	madness	-plasty	surgical repair
-genes	produce	-megaly	enlargement, large	-plegia	stroke, paralysis
-genesis	formation, produce	-meter	instrument to	-pnea	breathing
-genic	formation, produce		measure	-poiesis	formation
-glia	glue	-metry	measurement	-praxia	action
-globin	protein	-mnesia	memory	-ptosis	prolapse, drooping
-gnosis	knowledge	-morph	form, shape	-ptysis	to spit, spitting
-grade	a step	-noia	mind	-puncture	to pierce
-graft	pencil, grafting knife	-oid	resemble	-rrhage	to burst forth, burst-
-gram	a weight, mark,	-ole	opening		ing forth
	record	-oma	tumor	-rrhagia	to burst forth, burst-
-graph	to write, record	-omion	shoulder		ing forth
-graphy	recording	-on	pertaining to	-rrhaphy	suture
-hexia	condition	-one	hormone	-rrhea	flow, discharge
-ia	condition	-opia	eye, vision	-rrhexis	rupture
-iasis	condition	-opsia	eye, vision	-scope	instrument

-scopy	to view, examine	-systole	contraction	-trophy	nourishment, development
-sepsis	decay	-taxia	order		
-sis	condition	-therapy	treatment	-type	type
-some	body	-thermy	heat	-um	tissue
-spasm	tension, spasm, contraction	-tic	pertaining to	-ure	process
		-tome	instrument to cut	-uria	urine
-stalsis	contraction	-tomy	incision	-us	pertaining to
-stasis	control, stopping	-tone	tension	-y	condition, pertaining to, process
-staxis	dripping, trickling	-tripsy	crushing		
-sthenia	strength	-troph (y)	nourishment, development		
-stomy	new opening				

ABBREVIATIONS AND SYMBOLS

A

a	ampere; anode; anterior; aqua; area; artery
AB	abortion; abnormal
Ab	antibody
ABC	aspiration biopsy cytology
ABGs	arterial blood gases
ABLB	alternate binaural loudness balance
ABO	blood group
ABR	auditory brainstem response
ac	before meals (ante cibum); acute
AC	air conduction; anticoagulant
Acc	accommodation
ACG	angiocardiography
Ach	acetylcholine
ACL	anterior cruciate ligament
ACR	American College of Rheumatology
ACS	American Cancer Society
ACTH	adrenocorticotropic hormone
AD	right ear (auris dexter); Alzheimer's Disease; advance directive
ADA	American Diabetes Association
ad lib	as desired; freely
adeno-CA	adenocarcinoma
ADH	antidiuretic hormone (vasopressin)
ADHD	attention-deficit hyperactivity disorder
ADP	adenosine diphosphate
AE	above the elbow
AF	atrial fibrillation
AFB	acid-fast bacillus (TB organism)
AFP	alpha-fetoprotein
A/G	albumin/globulin ratio
Ag	antigen
AGN	acute glomerulonephritis
AH	abdominal hysterectomy
AHF	antihemophilic factor VIII
AHG	antihemophillic globulin factor VIII
AI	artificial insemination; aortic insufficiency
AIDS	acquired immunodeficiency syndrome
AIH	artificial insemination homologous
AK	above knee
AKA	above-knee amputation
alk phos	alkaline phosphatase
ALD	aldolase
ALL	acute lymphocytic leukemia
ALS	amyotrophic lateral sclerosis
ALT	argon laser trabeculoplasty; alanine aminotransferase
AMA	American Medical Association
AMD	age-related macular degeneration
AMI	acute myocardial infarction
AML	acute myelogenous leukemia
ANS	autonomic nervous system
A&P	auscultation and percussion; anatomy and physiology
AP	anteroposterior
APTT	activated partial thromboplastin time
ARD	acute respiratory disease
ARDS	acute respiratory distress syndrome
ARF	acute renal failure
ARMD	age-related macular degeneration
AS	aortic stenosis; left ear (auris sinistra)
As, Ast, astigm	astigmatism
Ascus	atypical squamous cells of undetermined significance
ASD	atrial septal defect
ASH	asymmetrical septal hypertrophy
ASHD	arteriosclerotic heart disease
AST	aspartate aminotransferase
ATN	acute tubular necrosis
ATP	adenosine triphosphate
AU	both ears (auris unitas)

AV	atrioventricular; arteriovenous
AVMs	arteriovenous malformations
AVR	aortic valve replacement

B

Ba	barium
BAC	blood alcohol concentration
BaE	barium enema
baso	basophil
BBB	bundle branch block
BBT	basal body temperature
BC	bone conduction
BE	below elbow; barium enema
BG, bG	blood glucose; blood sugar
bid	twice a day
BIN, bin	twice a night
BK	below knee
BKA	below-knee amputation
BM	bowel movement
BMD	bone mineral density (test)
BMR	basal metabolic rate
BNO	bladder neck obstruction
BP	blood pressure
BPH	benign prostatic hyperplasia (hypertrophy)
BRP	bathroom privileges
BS	bowel sounds
BSE	breast self-examination
BSI	body systems isolation
BSP	bromsulphalein
BT	bleeding time
BUN	blood urea nitrogen
Bx	biopsy

C

$\bar{c}$	with (cum)
C1, C2, etc.	first cervical vertebra; second cervical vertebra
C&S	culture and sensitivity
CA	cancer; carcinoembryonic antigen
Ca	calcium
CABG	coronary artery bypass graft
CAD	coronary artery disease
CAM	complementary and alternative medicines
cap	capsule
CAPD	continuous ambulatory peritoneal dialysis
cath	catheterization; catheter
CBC	complete blood count
CBS	chronic brain syndrome

cc	cubic centimeter
CC	cardiac catheterization; chief complaint; clean catch
CCU	coronary care unit
CDC	Centers for Disease Control and Prevention
CDH	congenital dislocation of the hip
CEA	carcinoembryonic antigen
CF	cystic fibrosis
CGN	chronic glomerulonephritis
CHD	coronary heart disease
chem	chemotherapy
CHF	congestive heart failure
CHO	carbohydrate
chol	cholesterol
Ci	curie
Cib	food (cibus)
CIN	cervical intraepithelial neoplasia
CIS	carcinoma in situ
CK	creatine kinase
Cl	chlorine
CLL	chronic lymphocytic leukemia
cm	centimeter
CMG	cystometrogram
CML	chronic myelogenous leukemia
CMP	cardiomyopathy
CNS	central nervous system
c/o	complains of
CO	cardiac output
CO_2	carbon dioxide
COLD	chronic obstructive lung disease
COPD	chronic obstructive pulmonary disease
CP	cerebral palsy
CPD	cephalopelvic disproportion
CPK	creatine phosphokinase
CPM	continuous passive motion
CPR	cardiopulmonary resuscitation
CPS	cycles per second
CR	computerized radiography
CRF	chronic renal failure; corticotropin-releasing factor
CS, C-section	cesarean section
CSF	cerebrospinal fluid
CT	computed tomography
CTS	carpal tunnel syndrome
CUC	chronic ulcerative colitis
CV	cardiovascular
CVA	cerebrovascular accident (stroke)
CVD	cardiovascular disease
CVP	central venous pressure
CVS	chorionic villus sampling
CWP	childbirth without pain

CXR	chest x-ray film; chest radiograph
cysto	cystoscopic examination

D

/d	per day
D	diopter (lens strength)
db, dB	decibel
DBS	deep brain stimulation
D&C	dilatation (dilatation) and curettage
D&E	dilation and evacuation
dc	discontinue
DC	discharge
DCIS	ductal carcinoma in situ
DDS	Doctor of Dental Surgery; dorsal cord stimulation
decub	decubitus
derm	dermatology
DES	diethylstilbestrol
DHT	dihydrotestosterone
DI	diabetes insipidus; diagnostic imaging
diff	differential count (white blood cells)
dil	dilute; diluted
DJD	degenerative joint disease
DM	diabetes mellitus
DNA	deoxyribonucleic acid
DNR	do not resuscitate
DO	doctor of osteopathy
DOA	dead on arrival
DOB	date of birth
DRE	digital rectal examination
DRGs	diagnostic related groups
DSA	digital subtraction angiography
DTaP	diphtheria, tetanus and pertussis (vaccine)
DTRs	deep tendon reflexes
DUB	dysfunctional uterine bleeding
DVA	distance visual acuity
DVT	deep vein thrombosis
Dx	diagnosis

E

EBV	Epstein-Barr virus
ECC	extracorporeal circulation
ECCE	extracapsular cataract extraction
ECF	extracellular fluid; extended care facility
ECG, EKG	electrocardiogram
ECHO	echocardiogram
E. coli	*Escherichia coli*
ECSL	extracorporeal shockwave lithotriptor
ECT	electroconvulsive therapy

ED	erectile dysfunction
EDC	estimated date of confinement
EEG	electroencephalogram; electroencephalograph
EENT	eye, ear, nose and throat
EGD	esophagogastroduodenoscopy
ELISA	enzyme-linked immunosorbent assay
EM	emmetropia
EMG	electromyography
ENG	electronystagmography
ENT	ear, nose and throat
EOM	extraocular movement, extraocular muscles
eos, eosin	eosinophil
ERCP	endoscopic retrograde cholangiopancreatography
ERT	estrogen replacement therapy; external radiation therapy
ERV	expiratory reserve volume
ESL, ESWL	extracorporeal shock-wave lithotripsy
ESR, SR, sed rate	erythrocyte sedimentation rate; sedimentation rate
ESRD	end-stage renal disease
EST	electroshock therapy
ESWL	extracorporeal shockwave lithotripsy
ET	esotropia; endotracheal
ETF	eustachian tube function

F

F	Fahrenheit
FACP	Fellow, American College of Physicians
FACS	Fellow, American College of Surgeons
FBS	fasting blood sugar
FDA	Food and Drug Administration
FEF	forced expiratory flow
FEKG	fetal electrocardiogram
FEV	forced expiratory volume
FH	family history
FHR	fetal heart rate
FHS	fetal heart sound
FHT	fetal heart tone
FMS	fibromyalgia syndrome
FROM	full range of motion
FS	frozen section
FSH	follicle-stimulating hormone
FTA-ABS	fluorescent treponemal antibody absorption
FTND	fulltern normal delivery

FUO	fever of undetermined origin		HNP	herniated nucleus pulposus (herniated disk)
FVC	forced vital capacity		H_2O	water
Fx	fracture		Hpd	hematoporphyrin derivative
			H. pylori	*Heliocobacter pylori*
G			HPV	human papillomavirus
g	gram		HRT	hormone replacement therapy
GB	gallbladder		hs	at bedtime
GC	gonorrhea		HSG	hysterosalpingography
GCSF	granulocyte colony-stimulating factor		HSV-2	herpes simplex virus-2
GERD	gastroesophageal reflux disease		Ht	height
GGT	gamma-glutamyl transferase		HT	hypermetropia (hyperopia)
GH	growth hormone		HTLV	human T-cell leukemia-lymphoma virus
GI	gastrointestinal			
GIFT	gamete intrafallopian transfer		Hx	history
GnRF	gonadotropin-releasing factor		hypo	hypodermic
GOT	glutamic oxaloacetic transaminase			
Gpi	globus pallidus		**I**	
GPT	glutamic pyruvic transaminase			
gr	grain		IAS	interatrial septum
grav I	pregnancy one		IBS	irritable bowel syndrome
GTT	glucose tolerance test		IC	interstitial cystitis
gtt	drops (guttae)		ICCE	intracapsular cataract cryoextraction
GU	genitourinary		ICF	intracellular fluid
GYN	gynecology		ICP	intracranial pressure
			ICSH	interstitial cell-stimulating hormone
			ICU	intensive care unit
			ID	intradermal
H			I&D	incision and drainage
h	hour		IDDM	insulin-dependent diabetes mellitus
H	hypodermic; hydrogen		Ig	immunoglobulin
H&L	heart & lungs		IH	infectious hepatitis
HAA	hepatitis-associated antigen		IHSS	idiopathic hypertropic subaortic stenosis
HAV	hepatitis A virus			
HBIG	hepatitis B immune globulin		IL-2	interleukin-2
HBOT	hyperbaric oxygen therapy		IM	intramuscular
HBP	high blood pressure		inj	injection
HBV	hepatitis B virus		I&O	intake and output
HCG	human chorionic gonadotropin		IOL	intraocular lens
HCl	hydrochloric acid		IOP	intraocular pressure
HCO_3	bicarbonate		IPD	intermittent peritoneal dialysis
HCT, Hct	hematocrit		IPPB	intermittent positive-pressure breathing
HD	hip disarticulation; hearing distance; Hodgkin's disease			
			IQ	intelligence quotient
HDL	high-density lipoprotein		IR	interventional radiologist
HDN	hemolytic disease of the newborn		IRDS	infant respiratory distress syndrome
HDS	herniated disk syndrome		IRT	internal radiation therapy
HEENT	head, eyes, ears, nose and throat		IRV	inspiratory reserve volume
HF	heart failure		IS	intercostal space
Hg	mercury		ITP	idiopathic thrombocytopenia purpura
HGB, Hgb, Hb	hemoglobin			
HIV	human immunodeficiency virus		IU	international unit
HLA	human leukocyte antigen		IUD	intrauterine device
HMD	hyaline membrane disease			

IUGR	intrauterine growth rate; intrauterine growth retardation
IV	intravenous
IVC	inferior vena cava; intravenous cholangiography; intraventricular catheter
IVF	in vitro fertilization
IVP	intravenous pyelogram
IVS	interventricular septum
IVU	intravenous urogram

J

J	joule
JNC	Joint National Committee

K

K	potassium
KD	knee disarticulation
kg	kilogram
KS	Kaposi's sarcoma
KUB	kidney, ureter and bladder
kV	kilovolt

L

L, l	liter
L1, L2, etc.	first lumbar vertebra, second lumbar vertebra, etc.
LA	left atrium
L&A	light and accommodation
lab	laboratory
LAC	long arm cast
LAK	lymphokine-activated killer (cells)
LAT, lat	lateral
lb	pound
LB	large bowel
LBBB	left bundle branch block
LCIS	lobular carcinoma in situ
LD	lactate dehydrogenase
LDH	lactic dehydrogenase
LDL	low-density lipoprotein
LE	lupus erythematosus; lower extremity; left eye
LEDs	light-emitting diodes
LES	lower esophageal sphincter
LH	luteinizing hormone
LH-RH	luteinizing hormone-releasing hormone
liq	liquid; fluid
LLC	long leg cast
LLQ	left lower quadrant

LMP	last menstrual period
LOM	limitation or loss of motion
LP	lumbar puncture
LPE	laser peripheral iridotomy
LPF	low-power field
LRQ	lower right quadrant
L, lt	left
LTH	lactogenic hormone
LUQ	left upper quadrant
LV	left ventricle
lymphs	lymphocytes

M

M	molar; thousand; muscle
m	male; meter; minim
mA	milliampere
mAs	milliampere second
MBC	maximal breathing capacity
MCH	mean corpuscular hemoglobin
MCHC	mean corpuscular hemoglobin concentration
mCi	millicurie
MCV	mean corpuscular volume
MD	medical doctor; muscular dystrophy
mEq	milliequivalent
mets	metastases
MG	myasthenia gravis
mg	milligram (0.001 gram)
MH	marital history
MI	myocardial infarction; mitral insufficiency
MIF	melanocyte-stimulating hormone release-inhibiting factor
mix astig	mixed astigmatism
mL, ml	milliliter (0.001 liter)
mm	millimeter (0.001 meter; 0.039 inch)
mMol	millimole
MMR	measles, mumps, and rubella (vaccine)
mol wt	molecular weight
mono	monocyte
MR	mental retardation
MRI	magnetic resonance imaging
MS	mitral stenosis; multiple sclerosis; musculoskeletal
MSH	melanocyte-stimulating hormone
mV	millivolt
MV	minute volume
MVP	mitral valve prolapse
MVV	maximal voluntary ventilation
MY	myopia

N

n	nerve
Na	sodium
NANBH	non-A, non-B hepatitis virus
NB	newborn
nCi	nanocurie
NCV	nerve conduction velocity
NIDDM	non-insulin-dependent diabetes mellitus
NG	nasogastric (tube)
NH_4	ammonia
NHLBI	National Heart, Lung and Blood Institute
NIH	National Institute of Health
NMR	nuclear magnetic resonance
NPH	nonprotein nitrogen
NPO, npo	nothing by mouth (nil per os)
NPT	nocturnal penile tumescence
NPUAP	National Pressure Ulcer Advisory Panel
NSAIDs	nonsteroidal anti-inflammatory drugs
N&V	nausea & vomiting
NVA	near visual acuity

O

O	pint
O_2	oxygen
OA	osteoarthritis
OB	obstetrics
OB-GYN	obstetrics and gynecology
OC	oral contraceptive
OCD	obsessive-compulsive disorder
OCPs	oral contraceptive pills
od	once a day
OD	right eye (oculus dexter); overdose
OHS	open heart surgery
OM	otitis media
O&P	ova and parasites
OR	operating room
ORTH, ortho	orthopedics; orthopaedics
os	mouth opening; bone
OS	left eye (oculus sinister)
OTC	over the counter
oto	otology
OU	both eyes (oculi unitas); each eye (oculus uterque)
OV	office visit
oz	ounce

P

P	pulse; phosphorus
PA	posteroanterior; pernicious anemia
PAC	premature arterial contraction
Pap	Papanicolaou (smear)
PAT	paroxysmal atrial tachycardia
Path	pathology
PBI	protein bound iodine
pc	after meals (post cibum)
PCL	posterior cruciate ligament
PCP	*Pneumocystis carinii* pneumonia
PCV	packed cell volume
PD	peritoneal dialysis
PDR	*Physicians' Desk Reference*
PE	physical examination; pulmonary embolism
PEEP	positive end-expiratory pressure
PEG	percutaneous endoscopic gastrostomy
PERRLA	pupils equal, regular, react to light and accommodation
PET	positron emission tomography
PE tube	polyethylene tube
PFT	pulmonary function test
pH	hydrogen ion concentration, degree of acidity
PH	past history
PID	pelvic inflammatory disease
PIF	prolactin release-inhibiting factor
PKU	phenylketonuria
PM, pm	afternoon, evening
PMH	past medical history
PMI	point of maximal impulse
PMN	polymorphonuclear neutrophil
PMP	previous menstrual period
PMR	physical medicine and rehabilitation
PMS	premenstrual syndrome
PND	paroxysmal nocturnal dyspnea; postnasal drip
PNS	peripheral nervous system
PO, po	orally, by mouth (per os)
poly	polymorphonuclear
PP	postprandial (after meals)
PPD	purified protein derivative (TB test)
PPI	proton pump inhibitors
pr	per rectum
PRF	prolactin-releasing factor
prn	as necessary, as required, when necessary
PSA	prostate-specific antigen
PT	physical therapy; prothrombin time
pt	patient; pint

PTC	percutaneous transhepatic cholangiography
PTCA	percutaneous transluminal coronary angioplasty
PTH	parathormone
PTS	permanent threshold shift
PTT	partial thromboplastin time
PUD	peptic ulcer disease
PUL	percutaneous ultrasonic lithotropsy
PVC	premature ventricular contraction
PVD	peripheral vascular disease

Q

q	every
qam,qm	every morning
qd	every day (quaque die)
qh	every hour
q2h	every 2 hours
qid	four times a day
qns	quantity not sufficient
qpm, qn	every night
qs	quantity sufficient
qt	quart

R

R	respiration
R, rt	right
Ra	radium
RA	right atrium; rheumatoid arthritis
rad	radiation absorbed dose
RAI	radioactive iodine
RAIU	radioactive iodine uptake
RBC	red blood cell; red blood cell (count)
RD	respiratory disease
RDA	recommended dietary or daily allowance
RDS	respiratory distress syndrome
RE	right eye
REM	rapid eye movement
Rh	Rhesus (factor)
RIA	radioimmunoassay
RLQ	right lower quadrant
RNA	ribonucleic acid
R/O	rule out
ROM	range of motion; read only memory
RP	retrograde pyelogram
RPM	revolutions per minute
RQ	respiratory quotient

RT	radiation therapy
RUQ	right upper quadrant
RV	right ventricle
Rx	take thou; prescribe; treatment; therapy

S

$\bar{s}$	without
SA,S-A	sinoatrial (node)
SAC	short arm cast
SAD	seasonal affective disorder
SAH	subarachnoid hemorrhage
SALT	serum alanine aminotransferase
SARS	severe acute respiratory syndrome
SAST	serum aspartate aminotransferase
SBFT	small-bowel follow-through
SC, sc, subq	subcutaneous
SCD	sudden cardiac death
SD	shoulder disarticulation; standard deviation
seg, poly	polymorphonuclear neutrophil
segs	segmented (mature RBCs)
SG	skin graft
SGOT	serum glutamic oxaloacetic transaminase
SGPT	serum glutamic pyruvic transaminase
sh	shoulder
SH	serum hepatitis
SIDS	sudden infant death syndrome
SK	streptokinase
SLE	systemic lupus erythematosus
SMBG	self-monitoring of blood glucose
SOB	shortness of breath
SOM	serous otitis media
sono	sonogram, sonography
SOP	standard operating procedure
sp gr, SG	specific gravity
SPP	suprapubic prostatectomy
SR	sedimentation rate
ss	one half
St	stage (of disease)
ST	esotropia
staph	staphylococcus
stat	immediately
STDs	sexually transmitted diseases
STH	somatotropin hormone
strep	streptococcus
STS	serologic test for syphilis
STSG	split thickness skin graft
subcu, subq	subcutaneous

SVC	superior vena cava
SVD	spontaneous vaginal delivery
Sx	signs, symptoms
syr	syrup

T

T	temperature
T1, T2, etc.	thoracic vertebrae first, thoracic vertebrae second, etc.
T_3	triiodothyronine
T_3RU	triiodothyronine resin uptake
T_4	thyroxine
T&A	tonsillectomy and adenoidectomy
tab	tablet
TAH	total abdominal hysterectomy
TB	tuberculosis
TBW	total body weight
TENS	transcutaneous electrical nerve stimulation
TFS	thyroid function studies
THA	total hip arthroplasty
THR	total hip replacement
TIAs	transient ischemic attacks
tid	three times a day
TIMS	topical immunomodulators
TIPS	transjugular intrahepatic portosystemic shunt
TJ	triceps jerk
TKA	total knee arthroplasty
TKR	total knee replacement
TLC	tender loving care; total lung capacity
TMJ	temporomandibular joint
TNF	tumor necrosis factor
TNM	tumor, node, metastasis
TNS	transcutaneous nerve stimulation
top	topically
TPA	*Treponema pallidum* agglutination (test)
TPA, tPA	tissue plasminogen activator
TPN	total parenteral nutrition
TPR	temperature, pulse, respiration
tr, tinct	tincture
TSE	testicular self-exam
TSH	thyroid stimulating hormone
TSS	toxic shock syndrome
TTH	thyrotropic hormone
TTS	temporary threshold shift
TUIP	transurethral incision of the prostate
TUMP	transurethral microwave thermotherapy
TUNA	transurethral needle ablation
TUR, TURP	transurethral resection of the prostate
TV	tidal volume
Tx	traction; treatment; transplant

U

U	units
UA	urinalysis
UC	uterine contractions
UCHD	usual childhood diseases
UG	urogenital
UGI	upper gastrointestinal
U&L, U/L	upper and lower
ULQ	upper left quadrant
ung	ointment
URI	upper respiratory infection
URQ	upper right quadrant
US	ultrasound
USP	United States Pharmacopeia
UTI	urinary tract infection
UV	ultraviolet

V

v	vein
VA	visual acuity
VC	vital capacity
VCD	vacuum constriction device
VCG	vectorcardiogram
VCU, VCUG	voiding cystourethrogram
VD	venereal disease
VDRL	Venereal Disease Research Laboratory (syphilis test)
VF	visual field
VHD	ventricular heart disease
VLDL	very low density lipoprotein
vol	volume
vol %	volume percent
VMA	vanillylmandelic acid
VP	vasopressin
VSD	ventricular septal defect
VT	ventricular tachycardia

W

WBC	white blood cell; white blood (cell) count
WDWN	well developed, well nourished
WNL	within normal limits
wt	weight
w/v	weight by volume

X

x	multiplied by
XM	cross match for blood (type and cross match)
XP	xeroderma pigmentosum
XR	x-ray
XT	exotropia
XX	female sex chromosomes
XY	male sex chromosomes

Y

YAG	yttrium-aluminum-garnet (laser)
YOB	year of birth
yr	year

Z

z	atomic number

Charting Abbreviations and Symbols

āā	of each
ac	before meals (ante cibum)
AD	right ear (auris dextra)
ADL	activities of daily living
ad lib	as desired
adm	admission
AE	above elbow
AJ	ankle jerk
AK	above knee
alt dieb	every other day
alt hor	every other hour
alt noc	every other night
AM, am	before noon (ante meridiem); morning
AMA	against medical advice
AMB	ambulate; ambulatory
ant	anterior
AP	anteroposterior
A-P	anterior-posterior
approx	approximately
AQ, aq	water
ASAP	as soon as possible
AS or LE	left ear (auris sinistra)
AV	atrioventricular
BE	below elbow
bid	twice a day
bin	twice a night
BK	below knee
BM	bowel movement
BMR	basal metabolic rate
BRP	bathroom privileges

C	Centigrade, Celsius or calorie (kilocalorie)
caps	capsules
CBR	complete bed rest
CC	chief complaint; clean catch (urine)
CCU	cardiac (coronary) care unit
c/o	complains of
cont	continue
dc	discontinue
DC	discharge from hospital
DNA	does not apply
DNR	do not resuscitate
DNS	did not show
Dr	doctor
D/W	dextrose in water
Dx	diagnosis
EOM	extraocular movement
ER	emergency room
Ex	examination
F	Fahrenheit
FHS	fetal heart sounds
FHT	fetal heart tones
GB	gallbladder
GI	gastrointestinal
GU	genitourinary
h, hr	hour
hpf	high power field
hs	hour of sleep; bedtime (hora somni)
hypo	hypodermic injection
ICU	intensive care unit
IM	intramuscular
I&O	intake and output
IU	international unit
IV	intravenous
L	left
L&A	light and accommodation
LAT	lateral
L&W	living and well
LLQ	left lower quadrant
LMP	last menstrual period
LOA	left occipitoanterior
LPF	low power field (10x)
LUQ	left upper quadrant
MTD	right ear drum (membrana tympani dexter)
MTS	left ear drum (membrana tympani sinister)
neg	negative
NG	nasogastric
NPO	nothing by mouth
NS	normal saline
OD	right eye (oculus dexter)
OP	outpatient

OR	operating room	tabs	tablets
OS or OL	left eye (oculus sinister, oculus laevus)	TC&DB	turn, cough, deep breathe
		tid	three times a day
OU	each eye (oculus uterque)	tinct	tincture
P	pulse	TPN	total parenteral nutrition
PA	posteroanterior	trans	transverse
pc	after meals (post cibum)	ULQ	upper left quadrant
PI	present illness	ung	ointment
po	by mouth (per os)	URQ	upper right quadrant
PO	postoperative	VS	vital signs
PM, pm	afternoon or evening (post meridiem)	WBC	white blood cell; white blood (cell) count
prn	as necessary, as required, when necessary	WM, BM	white male, black male
q	every (quaque)	WF, BF	white female, black female
qd	every day (quaque die)	×	times, power
qh	every hour (quaque hora)	−	negative
q2h	every 2 hours	+	positive
q4h	every 4 hours	F	female
qid	four times a day (quarter in die)	M	male
qm	every morning (quaque mane)	+/−	positive or negative
qn	every night (quaque nocte)	*	birth
R	right; respiration	†	death
RBC	red blood cell; red blood (cell) count	%	percent
		#	number; pound
Rh	Rhesus blood factor (Rh + or Rh −)	&	and
RLQ	right lower quadrant	<	less than
R/O	rule out	=	equal
ROM	range of motion	>	greater than
RUQ	right upper quadrant	?	question
SC, sc, subq	subcutaneous	@	at
SOB	shortness of breath	^	increase
SOS	if necessary (si opus sit)	™	trade mark
stat	immediately	©	copyright
Sx	signs, symptoms	®	registered
T, temp	temperature	¶	paragraph

LABORATORY REFERENCE VALUES

ABBREVIATIONS USED IN REPORTING LABORATORY VALUES

cm^3	cubic centimeter
cu μ	cubic microns
dL	deciliter
fL	femtoliter
g	gram
g/dL	grams per deciliter
IU	International Unit
kg	kilogram
L	liter
mol (M)	mole
mEq	milliequivalent
mg	milligram
mg/dL	milligram per deciliter
mm	millimeter
mmol	millimole
mm^3	cubic millimeter
mm Hg	millimeter of mercury
ng	nanogram
ng/dL	nanogram per deciliter
ng/mL	nanogram per milliliter
pg	picogram
U	unit
U/L	units per liter
uIU/mL	units International Unit per milliliter
μg (mcg)	microgram

HEMATOLOGY TESTS

	Normal Ranges
Erythrocytes–Red blood cells (RBC)	
Females	4.2–5.4 million/mm^3
Males	4.6–6.2 million/mm^3
Children	4.5–5.1 million/mm^3

Hemoglobin (HGB, Hgb)	
Females	12.0–14.0 g/dL
Males	14.0–16.0 g/dL
Hematocrit (HCT)	37.0–54 %
Females	37–47 %
Males	40–54 %
Leukocytes–White blood cells (WBC)	4500–11,000/mm^3
Differential	
Neutrophils	54–62 %
Lymphocytes	20–40 %
Monocytes	2–10 %
Eosinophils	1–2 %
Basophils	0–1 %
Thrombocytes–Platelets	200,000–400,000/mm^3
Mean corpuscular volume (MCV)	80–97 fL
Mean corpuscular hemoglobin (MCH)	27.0–31.2 pg
Mean corpuscular hemoglobin concentration (MCHC)	31.8–37.4 g/dL

COAGULATION TESTS

Bleeding time	2.75–8.0 min
Coagulation time	5–15 min
Prothrombin time (PT)	12–14 sec

CHEMISTRIES

	Normal Ranges
Sodium (Na)	136–145 mEq/L
Potassium (K)	3.5–5.0 mEq/L
Calcium (Ca)	9.0–11.0 mg/dL
Chloride (Cl)	100–108 mmol/L
CO_2	21–32 mmol/L
Phosphate (PO_4)	3.0–4.5 mg/dL
Glucose (fasting)	70–115 mg/dL
Blood urea nitrogen (BUN)	8–20 mg/dL
Creatinine	0.9–1.5 mg/dL
Creatine phosphokinase (CPK)	
Females	30–135 U/L
Males	55–170 U/L
Anion gap	10–17 mEq/L
Alkaline phosphatase (ALP)	20–90U/L
Alanine aminotransferase (ALT, SGPT)	5–30 U/L
Albumin	3.5–5.5 g/dL
Globulin	1.4–4.8 g/dL
A/G ratio	0.7–2.0 g/dL
Aspartate aminotransferase (AST, SGOT)	10–30 U/L
Bilirubin	0.3–1.1 mg/dL
Cholesterol	<200 mg/dL
High density lipoprotein (HDL)	>60 mg/dL
Low density lipoprotein (LDL)	<100 mg/dL
Triglycerides	<150 mg/dL
Uric acid	
Females	1.5–7.0 mg/dL
Males	2.5–8.0 mg/dL
Lactate dehydrogenase (LDH)	100–190 U/L
Thyroxine (T_4)	4.4–9.9 µg/dL
Free T_4	0.8–1.8 ng/dL
Thyroid stimulating hormone (TSH)	0.5–6.0 uIU/mL
Prostate specific antigen (PSA) Male	0.0–4.0 ng/mL
Testosterone	241–827 ng/dL

URINALYSIS

	Normal Ranges
Color	Yellow to amber
Turbidity (Appearance)	Clear
Specific gravity	1.003–1.030
Reaction (pH)	5.0–7.0
Odor	Faintly aromatic
Protein	Negative
Glucose	Negative
Ketones	Negative
Bilirubin	Negative
Blood	Negative
Urobilinogen	0.1–1.0
Nitrite	Negative
Leukocytes	Negative

INDEX

SINGLE PC LICENSE AGREEMENT AND LIMITED WARRANTY

READ THIS LICENSE CAREFULLY BEFORE OPENING THIS PACKAGE. BY OPENING THIS PACKAGE, YOU ARE AGREEING TO THE TERMS AND CONDITIONS OF THIS LICENSE. IF YOU DO NOT AGREE, DO NOT OPEN THE PACKAGE. PROMPTLY RETURN THE UNOPENED PACKAGE AND ALL ACCOMPANYING ITEMS TO THE PLACE YOU OBTAINED THEM. *THESE TERMS APPLY TO ALL LICENSED SOFTWARE ON THE DISK EXCEPT THAT THE TERMS FOR USE OF ANY SHAREWARE OR FREEWARE ON THE DISKETTES ARE AS SET FORTH IN THE ELECTRONIC LICENSE LOCATED ON THE DISK:*

1. GRANT OF LICENSE and OWNERSHIP: The enclosed computer programs and data ("Software") are licensed, not sold, to you by Pearson Education, Inc. ("We" or the "Company") and in consideration of your purchase or adoption of the accompanying Company textbooks and/or other materials, and your agreement to these terms. We reserve any rights not granted to you. You own only the disk(s) but we and/or our licensors own the Software itself. This license allows you to use and display your copy of the Software on a single computer (i.e., with a single CPU) at a single location for <u>academic</u> use only, so long as you comply with the terms of this Agreement. You may make one copy for back up, or transfer your copy to another CPU, provided that the Software is usable on only one computer

2. RESTRICTIONS: You may <u>not</u> transfer or distribute the Software or documentation to anyone else. Except for backup, you may <u>not</u> copy the documentation or the Software. You may <u>not</u> network the Software or otherwise use it on more than one computer or computer terminal at the same time. You may <u>not</u> reverse engineer, disassemble, decompile, modify, adapt, translate, or create derivative works based on the Software or the Documentation. You may be held legally responsible for any copying or copyright infringement which is caused by your failure to abide by the terms of these restrictions.

3. TERMINATION: This license is effective until terminated. This license will terminate automatically without notice from the Company if you fail to comply with any provisions or limitations of this license. Upon termination, you shall destroy the Documentation and all copies of the Software. All provisions of this Agreement as to limitation and disclaimer of warranties, limitation of liability, remedies or damages, and our ownership rights shall survive termination.

4. LIMITED WARRANTY AND DISCLAIMER OF WARRANTY: Company warrants that for a period of 60 days from the date you purchase this SOFTWARE (or purchase or adopt the accompanying textbook), the Software, when properly installed and used in accordance with the Documentation, will operate in substantial conformity with the description of the Software set forth in the Documentation, and that for a period of 30 days the disk(s) on which the Software is delivered shall be free from defects in materials and workmanship under normal use. The Company does not warrant that the Software will meet your requirements or that the operation of the Software will be uninterrupted or error-free. Your only remedy and the Company's only obligation under these limited warranties is, at the Company's option, return of the disk for a refund of any amounts paid for it by you or replacement of the disk. THIS LIMITED WARRANTY IS THE ONLY WARRANTY PROVIDED BY THE COMPANY AND ITS LICENSORS, AND THE COMPANY AND ITS LICENSORS DISCLAIM ALL OTHER WARRANTIES, EXPRESS OR IMPLIED, INCLUDING WITHOUT LIMITATION, THE IMPLIED WARRANTIES OF MERCHANTABILITY AND FITNESS FOR A PARTICULAR PURPOSE. THE COMPANY DOES NOT WARRANT, GUARANTEE OR MAKE ANY REPRESENTATION REGARDING THE ACCURACY, RELIABILITY, CURRENTNESS, USE, OR RESULTS OF USE, OF THE SOFTWARE.

5. LIMITATION OF REMEDIES AND DAMAGES: IN NO EVENT, SHALL THE COMPANY OR ITS EMPLOYEES, AGENTS, LICENSORS, OR CONTRACTORS BE LIABLE FOR ANY INCIDENTAL, INDIRECT, SPECIAL, OR CONSEQUENTIAL DAMAGES ARISING OUT OF OR IN CONNECTION WITH THIS LICENSE OR THE SOFTWARE, INCLUDING FOR LOSS OF USE, LOSS OF DATA, LOSS OF INCOME OR PROFIT, OR OTHER LOSSES, SUSTAINED AS A RESULT OF INJURY TO ANY PERSON, OR LOSS OF OR DAMAGE TO PROPERTY, OR CLAIMS OF THIRD PARTIES, EVEN IF THE COMPANY OR AN AUTHORIZED REPRESENTATIVE OF THE COMPANY HAS BEEN ADVISED OF THE POSSIBILITY OF SUCH DAMAGES. IN NO EVENT SHALL THE LIABILITY OF THE COMPANY FOR DAMAGES WITH RESPECT TO THE SOFTWARE EXCEED THE AMOUNTS ACTUALLY PAID BY YOU, IF ANY, FOR THE SOFTWARE OR THE ACCOMPANYING TEXTBOOK. BECAUSE SOME JURISDICTIONS DO NOT ALLOW THE LIMITATION OF LIABILITY IN CERTAIN CIRCUMSTANCES, THE ABOVE LIMITATIONS MAY NOT ALWAYS APPLY TO YOU.

6. GENERAL: THIS AGREEMENT SHALL BE CONSTRUED IN ACCORDANCE WITH THE LAWS OF THE UNITED STATES OF AMERICA AND THE STATE OF NEW YORK, APPLICABLE TO CONTRACTS MADE IN NEW YORK, AND SHALL BENEFIT THE COMPANY, ITS AFFILIATES AND ASSIGNEES. HIS AGREEMENT IS THE COMPLETE AND EXCLUSIVE STATEMENT OF THE AGREEMENT BETWEEN YOU AND THE COMPANY AND SUPERSEDES ALL PROPOSALS OR PRIOR AGREEMENTS, ORAL, OR WRITTEN, AND ANY OTHER COMMUNICATIONS BETWEEN YOU AND THE COMPANY OR ANY REPRESENTATIVE OF THE COMPANY RELATING TO THE SUBJECT MATTER OF THIS AGREEMENT. If you are a U.S. Government user, this Software is licensed with "restricted rights" as set forth in subparagraphs (a)-(d) of the Commercial Computer-Restricted Rights clause at FAR 52.227-19 or in subparagraphs (c)(1)(ii) of the Rights in Technical Data and Computer Software clause at DFARS 252.227-7013, and similar clauses, as applicable.

Should you have any questions concerning this agreement or if you wish to contact the Company for any reason, please contact in writing: Prentice-Hall, New Media Department, One Lake Street, Upper Saddle River, NJ 07458.